HEMATOLOGY
FOR MEDICAL
TECHNOLOGISTS

HEMATOLOGY FOR MEDICAL TECHNOLOGISTS

BY

CHARLES E. SEIVERD

Research Associate, The Horizon Laboratories, Phoenix, Arizona;
Formerly Chief Technologist, Doctor's Clinical Laboratory,
Glendale, Arizona

Fourth Edition

188 Illustrations, 4 in Color

21 Color Plates

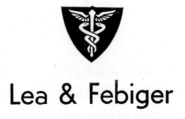

Lea & Febiger

Philadelphia

First Edition, 1952
Second Edition, 1958
Reprinted, 1958
Reprinted, 1960
Reprinted, 1961
Reprinted, 1962
Third Edition, 1964
Reprinted, 1964
Reprinted, 1966
Reprinted, 1968
Reprinted, 1969
Reprinted, 1970
Fourth Edition, 1972
Reprinted, 1973
Reprinted, 1975
Reprinted, 1977
Reprinted, 1979

ISBN 0–8121–03785

Library of Congress Catalog Card Number: 78–170739

Published in Great Britain by Henry Kimpton Publishers, London

Printed in the United States of America

DEDICATION

As I walked down the street of life, these men stood at the corners and showed me the way:

Dr. C. A. Seiverd
Rev. W. W. Wood
Dr. Maurice Powers
Prof. Harry A. Charipper
Dr. H. Ivan Brown

May this volume serve as a small token of appreciation for their counsel and guidance.

Preface to the Fourth Edition

THE purpose of this book is twofold.

One, to present those aspects of hematology which are significant to the medical technologist.

Two, to prepare the student for the hematology section of a National Registry or State Board Examination.

The text is directly concerned with obtaining blood from the patient, performing 47 blood tests, and recognizing the blood picture in 28 blood diseases.

This edition meets the academic and practical requirements of the various National Registry Examinations and the various State Board Examinations.

In preparing this edition, I have continued to comply with the requests of medical technologists and students.

At the request of medical technologists, the blood tests have been brought up to date, the section on blood diseases has been greatly expanded, and the irrelevant material has been discarded.

The discarded material consists mostly of tests that have outgrown the hematology department and are now being performed in the serology, parasitology, or blood bank department.

At the request of students, the Appendix now contains 500 review questions for National Registry and State Board Examinations.

Each review question is accompanied by a reference. The reference is the exact page in the text where the particular question was discussed and answered. Thus, an area of academic weakness may be quickly detected and readily reviewed.

The review questions are also accompanied by a set of answers which may be used as a quick reference in oral quizzes.

By presenting the review questions and text material under one cover, the student is given an opportunity to take a peek at the review questions before studying the text material.

The concept of peeking at review questions before studying the text material has recently become a cornerstone of the latest "discovery" in modern education.

The backbone of the book continues to be a functional presentation of the subject matter.

This practical approach to teaching and learning may be "taking the student by the hand" as a worthy reviewer stated.

But the practical approach is effective. It by-passes the irrelevant material, stimulates the process of learning, and simplifies the task of teaching. In short, it works.

Furthermore, the practical approach has proven successful in a new and nebulous profession where the only true test is the trial by market. In short, it sells.

The practical approach to teaching and learning may even become a future "discovery" in the field of education.

During the conception and growth of this text, I received a great deal of assistance and wish to make the following acknowledgments.

In the preparation of this edition, I received suggestions from several hundred students and technologists; I also received suggestions and assistance from many physicians.

I am grateful to every one and feel especially obligated to Mrs. Doris Haver, Dr. David P. Stiff, Mr. Bernie Conroy, Dr. Alexander S. Wiener, Mr. John Hannan, Mr. Robert Pribbenow, Mrs. Sharon Gilliland, Dr. Thomas Chayka, and Dr. Paul Gill.

And, looking back to previous editions, I am grateful to many people—especially the simon-pures.

I feel especially obligated to Mr. James Corbett, Mr. George Herold, Mr. John Myers Myers, Prof. Fred Crawford, Mrs. Gertrude Denning, Mr. Julian DeVries, Mr. Robert Pribbenow, Prof. Harry A. Charipper, and Mr. John Hannan.

In conclusion, I would appreciate suggestions for the improvement of the text.

CHARLES E. SEIVERD

The Horizon Laboratories
P. O. Box 1703
Phoenix, Arizona 85001

Contents

x   Contents

List of Colors

PART 1

Introduction

What is hematology? Why is it important? Whom does it concern?

Hematology is pronounced hem″ah-tol′o-je. The word comes from the Greek: *hemat* meaning blood, and *ology* meaning study. Thus, hematology is the study of blood.

Our study of blood is concerned with the blood tests that are performed in the hematology section of a medical laboratory.

These tests may tell of many things. They may speak of health. They may indicate disease. In guarded terms, they mention death. They reveal a patient's progress. They point to the road of recovery. They even select the blood that saves a life.

These vital secrets are entrusted to the men and women of a new profession—medical technology.

This profession accepts a sacred trust. It serves a noble cause. And it plays a leading role in the drama of life, death, and disease.

Our study will begin with the following chapters:

> Chapter 1 Characteristics of Blood
> Chapter 2 Collection of Blood
> Chapter 3 Preparation of Blood

The student review questions for the above chapters are numbered 1–24 and begin on page 726 of the Appendix.

Chapter 1

Characteristics of Blood

WHAT is blood? Where does it come from? What does it do?
This chapter considers the composition, formation, and function of blood.

COMPOSITION OF BLOOD

The average man has about 5 quarts of blood. This may be separated into 3 quarts of plasma and 2 quarts of cells. The plasma is a liquid and the cells are solids.

The plasma is made up of water, foods, wastes, hormones, antibodies, and enzymes.

The cells are classified as white cells, red cells, and platelets. In size, the cells vary as follows:

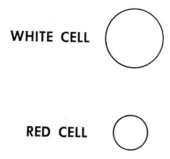

WHITE CELL

RED CELL

PLATELET

In quantity, however, the red cells greatly predominate. For every 500 red cells there are approximately 30 platelets and only 1 white cell.

The composition of the blood is illustrated in Figure 1.

FORMATION OF BLOOD

The plasma is derived from the intestine and organs of the body. From the intestine comes water and foods. And from the organs of the body come wastes, hormones, antibodies, and enzymes.

The red cells, platelets, and most of the white cells are formed in the marrow of our bones. The most common sources of supply are the ribs, breastbone, and backbone.

How are the blood cells formed?

In an effort to answer this question, two theories have been evolved:

The first theory states that a single mother cell produces all blood cells. This theory is known as the monophyletic (mon″o-fi-let′ik) theory.

The second theory states that several mother cells are involved, each

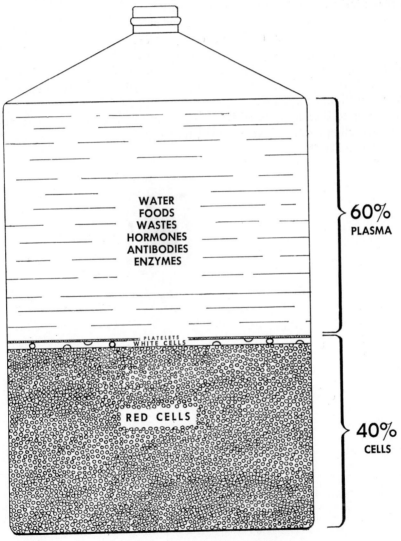

WATER
FOODS
WASTES
HORMONES
ANTIBODIES
ENZYMES

60%
PLASMA

PLATELETS
WHITE CELLS

RED CELLS

40%
CELLS

FIG. 1.—Composition of blood.

mother cell producing its own "tribe" of cells. This theory is known as the polyphyletic (pol″e-fi-let′ik) theory.

FUNCTION OF BLOOD

The blood may be thought of as the body's most versatile servant. It conveys the raw materials of protoplasm to countless millions of cells operating as factories to manufacture life itself. The cells empty their waste products into its everflowing stream, and this obliging servant carries them to the kidneys and other organs of elimination.

The blood transfers hormones from their organs of production to their organs of consumption. It aids in regulating the water content, temperature, and alkalinity of the tissues. In time of danger, it serves as a mechanized army, transporting white cells and antibodies to battle infection and disease. Quite often, it furnishes factors of coagulation to mend an abrasion, laceration, or incision.

In order to discharge these duties, this faithful servant works day and night, traveling endless miles over the highways of an intricate system of arteries, capillaries, and veins.

Chapter 2

Collection of Blood

THIS chapter considers the collection of blood. The discussion covers the following:

Introduction
Reassuring the Patient
Obtaining Blood from a Finger
Introduction to the Venipuncture
Syringe Method of Making a Venipuncture
B-D Vacutainer Method of Making a Venipuncture
Obtaining Blood from an Infant

INTRODUCTION

All too often a patient leaves a laboratory with this thought: "That darn blood-hound, sticking me 3 times. And laughing and joking about it too."

Does this seem humorous?

Suppose this patient has just lost her baby? Suppose she has cancer and only a few months to live? Suppose she has leukemia, a disease terminating in death?

Would it still seem humorous?

Obviously, it would not. This is not a joking matter. It is a serious and delicate undertaking.

In the withdrawal of blood, you should strive for the skill of a surgeon and the sympathy of a saint.

Your skill may be developed. You must study. You must observe. You must practice.

Your sympathy may be acquired. You must realize that the patient is sick, that he deserves to be treated with kindness and consideration. You must use tact . . . patience . . . understanding.

You should carefully study the methods of obtaining blood which are given on the following pages. You should delay the actual withdrawal of blood, however, until you have mastered the technique of diluting the blood and making a blood smear. These procedures will be considered in chapters 4 through 7.

REASSURING THE PATIENT

Before drawing blood, you should reassure the patient and endeavor to relieve any apprehension which may be present.

If the patient is an adult, you may reassure him with a pleasant smile, an introductory remark, or simply the stock statement: "This won't hurt very much."

If the patient is a child, you should take extra precautions, for a thoughtless moment may cause the child to harbor a life-long fear of the puncture.

Some technologists gain the child's confidence by asking about his school or games. Other technologists tell a child that it won't hurt any more than being stuck with his mother's sewing needle. Still other technologists use a supply of candy and lollipops to relieve pain and apprehension.

You should never tell a child that it will not hurt. In most cases, this is false. It is best to tell him that it will hurt—but just for a second—and that you will tell him when it will hurt.

In drawing blood from an infant, you should reassure the parent, if present.

Your thoughtful gestures will take very little time; and they will be greatly appreciated by the patient.

OBTAINING BLOOD FROM A FINGER

Some tests may be performed with a few drops of blood. Other tests require several cubic centimeters of blood.

When a test calls for a few drops of blood, the blood is obtained from a finger or lobe of the ear.

The finger is preferred for several reasons. First, there is less chance of the blood dripping on the patient's clothing. Second, the patient can see the procedure. In most cases, this makes him less apprehensive.

The finger puncture consists of 8 steps:

Step 1: Assembling the equipment
Step 2: Preparing the finger
Step 3: Puncturing the finger
Step 4: Eliminating the first drop
Step 5: Producing a large rounded drop
Step 6: Withdrawing the blood
Step 7: Preventing further bleeding
Step 8: Labelling the specimens

These 8 steps will be considered in detail on the following pages.

You will find that most of the steps are broken down into a *discussion* and a *procedure*.

For the present, carefully read the entire material. When it is time for your first finger puncture, carefully review the entire material. Then follow the *procedure* in each step.

You may feel a little nervous for your first finger puncture. This is normal. You should realize, however, that your objective is to help people. And that drawing blood is the first step in the process.

STEP 1: ASSEMBLING THE EQUIPMENT

Discussion of Step 1

In most schools, you will begin your study by doing blood counts from a test tube of blood. By the time you make your first finger puncture, you will be prepared to do a complete blood count. Consequently, in the following procedure, we have assumed that you will be performing a complete blood count.

The equipment for the finger puncture and complete blood count is usually kept in a blood tray such as the one illustrated in Figure 2.

The blood tray should be kept neat and clean. As the solutions and supplies are used, they should be replaced. *The blood tray should always be checked for solutions and supplies before and after it is used.*

There is nothing more irritating to a technologist than to get an emergency call and find that the blood tray must first be replenished with solutions and supplies.

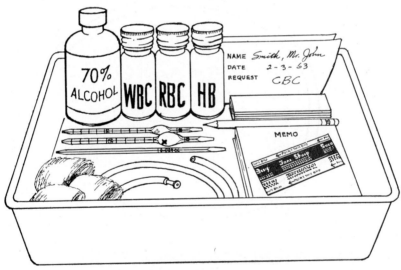

FIG. 2.—Blood tray containing equipment for the finger puncture and complete blood count.

2a

Procedure for Step 1

1. Assemble the equipment listed in Figure 4.

2. Place the above equipment within easy reach.

3. Remove the lids from the bottles so you will not waste time in diluting the blood.

4. If the rubber sucking tube has been used by someone else, dip the mouthpiece in the 70% alcohol.

5. Attach the rubber sucking tube to the white cell pipet as illustrated below (Fig. 3).

6. Lay the assembled white cell pipet and rubber sucking tube on the table ready for use.

7. Turn to step 2, preparing the finger.

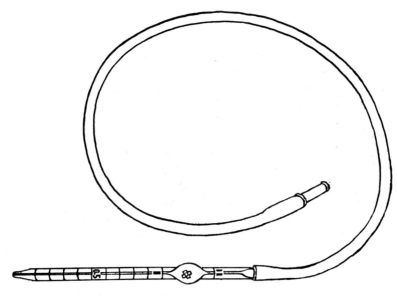

FIG. 3.—White cell pipet attached to rubber sucking tube.

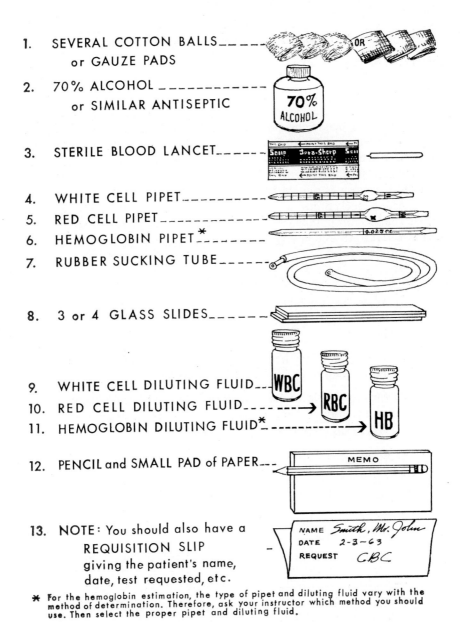

1. SEVERAL COTTON BALLS_ _ _ _ _
    or GAUZE PADS

2. 70% ALCOHOL _ _ _ _ _ _ _ _ _ _ _
    or SIMILAR ANTISEPTIC

3. STERILE BLOOD LANCET_ _ _ _ _ _

4. WHITE CELL PIPET_ _ _ _ _ _ _ _ _ _

5. RED CELL PIPET_ _ _ _ _ _ _ _ _ _ _

6. HEMOGLOBIN PIPET_ _ _ _ _ _ _ _*

7. RUBBER SUCKING TUBE_ _ _ _ _ _

8. 3 or 4 GLASS SLIDES_ _ _ _ _ _ _

9. WHITE CELL DILUTING FLUID_ _ _

10. RED CELL DILUTING FLUID_ _ _ _ _ _ _ _ →

11. HEMOGLOBIN DILUTING FLUID*_ _ _ _ _ _ _ _ _ _ _ _ →

12. PENCIL and SMALL PAD of PAPER_ _ _

13. NOTE: You should also have a
    REQUISITION SLIP
    giving the patient's name,
    date, test requested, etc.

    NAME *Smith, Mr. John*
    DATE   2-3-63
    REQUEST   *CBC*

* For the hemoglobin estimation, the type of pipet and diluting fluid vary with the method of determination. Therefore, ask your instructor which method you should use. Then select the proper pipet and diluting fluid.

FIG. 4.—Equipment for the finger puncture and complete blood count.

STEP 2:   PREPARING THE FINGER

Discussion of Step 2

The puncture is usually made on the middle finger of the right hand.

To increase the circulation, the fleshy portion of the middle finger is massaged. The massaging process must be *heavy* and *deep* so that the finger tip becomes red with blood. The ball or pad of the finger is then cleansed with a piece of cotton which has been moistened with 70% alcohol or some similar antiseptic. Finally, it is dried with a piece of *dry* cotton.

When the finger is punctured, the blood must form a rounded drop so that it can be sucked into a pipet. If the finger is wet, the blood will not form a rounded drop; it will run down the sides of the finger. Consequently, it is essential to thoroughly dry the finger.

Procedure for Step 2

1. With your left thumb and index finger, grasp the patient's middle finger about 3 inches above the tip of the finger (Fig. 5).

2. With your right hand, hold the sides of the patient's middle finger as illustrated in Figure 5.

3. Moving your left hand toward the tip of the patient's finger, apply a <u>heavy deep</u> massaging motion on the fleshy portion of the finger.

4. Repeat the above massaging process 5 or 6 times.

5. After you have massaged the finger, pick up a piece of cotton and moisten it with 70% alcohol.

6. With the moistened cotton, cleanse the ball or pad of the middle finger.

7. <u>With a piece of dry cotton, thoroughly dry the ball or pad of the middle finger.</u>

8. Reassure the patient with the usual: "This won't hurt very much."

9. Turn to step 3, puncturing the finger.

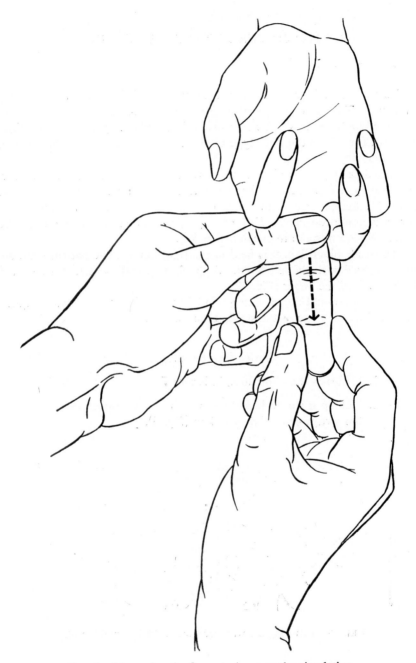

FIG. 5.—Massaging the finger to increase the circulation.

STEP 3:   PUNCTURING THE FINGER

Discussion of Step 3

A sterile blood lancet is used for the puncture.   It is usually thrown away after use.   This is done to prevent the spread of disease.

If the blood lancet is to be used again, it must be autoclaved or sterilized by heat, for this is the only type of sterilization that will kill the virus of infectious hepatitis.

Since a deep puncture is not any more painful than a superficial puncture, it is best to go deep enough the first time and thereby avoid puncturing the patient a second time.   Most blood lancets have a flange or guard which prevents going too deep.   Failure to go deep enough the first time is the most frequent mistake the beginner makes.

The sterile blood lancet is held in the right hand.   The patient's middle finger is held with the left hand.   A quick *deep* stab is then made on the ball or pad of the finger (Fig. 7).

The finger should be hit with a trip hammer effect, that is, with a quick drop and a quick rise of the sterile blood lancet.

Procedure for Step 3

1. Observe the illustration in Figure 7.

2. Pick up a sterile blood lancet.   If it is wrapped, remove the wrapper as shown below (Fig. 6).

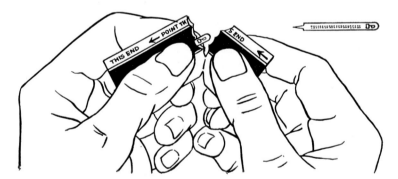

FIG. 6.—Removing the wrapper from a sterile blood lancet.

3. With your right hand, <u>firmly</u> grasp the sterile blood lancet (Fig. 7).

4. With your left hand, <u>firmly</u> grasp the patient's middle finger (Fig. 7).

5. With a quick drop and a quick rise of the sterile blood lancet, make a DEEP stab on the ball of the finger (Fig. 7).

6. Turn to step 4, eliminating the first drop.

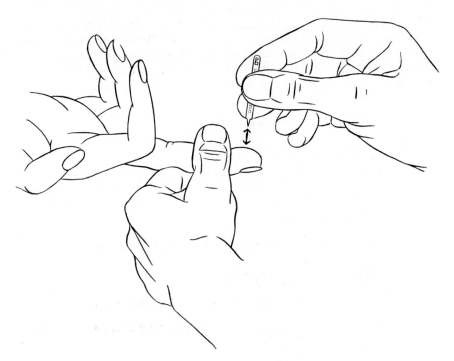

FIG. 7.—Puncturing the finger.

STEP 4:   ELIMINATING THE FIRST DROP

Discussion of Step 4

The first drop of blood may contain tissue juices; it may also be contaminated with extraneous materials which have been clinging to the surface of the skin.   When blood contains tissue juices and foreign particles, it is not a true representative sample of the patient's blood.   Therefore, the first drop of blood is wiped away.

After the first drop of blood has been wiped away, the area should be wiped dry with the piece of dry cotton.   This will enable the ensuing blood to form a rounded drop and not dribble over the side of the finger.

At this point in the procedure, many female students appear to be so nervous that they delay the procedure with giggles and conversation.

The student should realize that, once the puncture is made, *he should work with speed because the blood will clot in a matter of minutes.*

Procedure for Step 4

If the blood flows freely:

1. Take a piece of dry cotton and wipe away the first drop (Fig. 8).

2. Wipe the area dry.

3. Turn to step 5, producing a large rounded drop.

If the blood does not flow freely:

1. Massage toward the puncture to induce bleeding.

2. Take a piece of dry cotton and wipe away the first drop.

3. Wipe the area dry.

4. Turn to step 5, producing a large rounded drop.

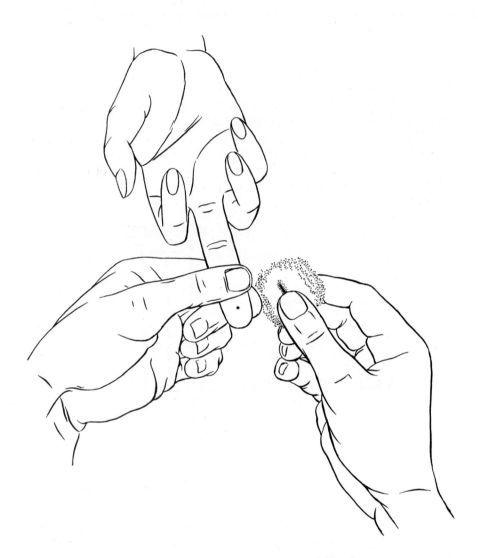

FIG. 8.—Eliminating the first drop of blood.

STEP 5:   PRODUCING A LARGE ROUNDED DROP

Discussion of Step 5

A large rounded drop of blood is produced as follows:

With your left hand, you *firmly and deeply* massage the fleshy portion of the patient's finger.   You repeat this DEEP massaging process several times. This forces blood toward the tip of the finger.

The last time you massage the finger, you clamp down *hard* at the line in the first joint of the patient's finger.   This dams off the blood.

Then, with your right hand, you *gently* squeeze the sides of the finger. This causes the blood to flow out of the puncture.

Thus,

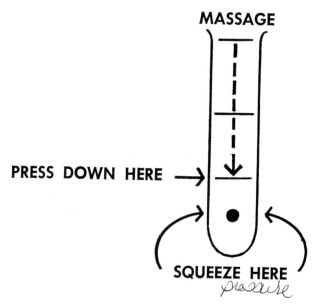

You should *not* squeeze too hard with your right hand.   If you do, it will cause the flow of tissue juices.   This tends to make the blood clot, thus defeating your purpose.

Whenever you squeeze with your right hand, always make sure that the blood is dammed off by *firm* pressure with your left hand.   If the blood is not dammed off, it will simply flow back toward the heart and not come out of the puncture.

Procedure for Step 5

1. With your right hand, hold the sides of the patient's middle finger as illustrated in Figure 9.

2. With your left thumb and index finger, grasp the patient's finger about 3 inches above the puncture.

3. Using your left thumb and index finger, DEEPLY massage the fleshy portion of the patient's finger. Repeat this massaging process several times.

4. The last time you massage the finger, clamp down <u>hard</u> at the line in the first joint of the patient's finger.

5. With your right hand, gently squeeze the sides of the patient's finger (Fig. 9).

6. A large rounded drop of blood should form at the site of the puncture.

7. Turn to step 6, withdrawing the blood.

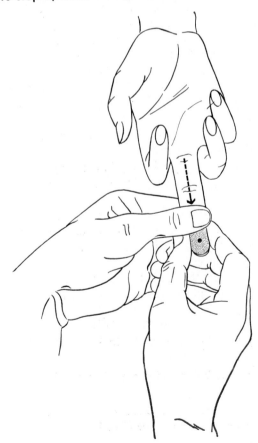

FIG. 9.—Producing a large rounded drop of blood.

STEP 6: WITHDRAWING THE BLOOD

Discussion of Step 6

You have already learned to make blood preparations from blood in a test tube. Now you will learn to make blood preparations from finger tip blood.

In this step, you will take blood from a finger puncture and make the following blood preparations:

1. Diluted blood for a white cell count
2. Diluted blood for a red cell count
3. Diluted blood for a hemoglobin determination
4. Blood smear for a differential white cell count and a stained red cell examination

The diluted blood for the first 3 tests is made by sucking the blood into a pipet. The technique of sucking finger tip blood into the pipet is illustrated in Figure 10.

In Figure 10, note the position of the technologist's fingers on the pipet. Holding the pipet in this manner enables him to see the markings on the pipet and thereby make the proper dilution.

In Figure 10, also note that the technologist is bracing a finger of his right hand on the side of the patient's finger. This enables him to move his hand with any slight movement of the patient's finger and thereby keep the tip of the pipet in the drop of blood. This technique is especially helpful in withdrawing blood from children, for they tend to move during the procedure.

In making your dilutions, it is essential that you hold the pipet and brace your finger as illustrated in Figure 10.

You hold the tip of the pipet loosely in the drop of blood. You do *not* press the tip of the pipet against the puncture because it will stop the flow of blood.

The blood smear is made by placing a drop of blood on a slide and smearing the blood over the slide. This, of course, you have done previously. The technique of getting a drop of finger tip blood on a slide is illustrated in Figure 11.

In Figure 11, note that the small drop of finger tip blood is being obtained by simply placing one end of the slide on the drop of blood.

Procedure for Step 6

1. Pick up the white cell pipet attached to the rubber sucking tube.
2. Put the mouthpiece of the rubber sucking tube in your mouth.
3. With your right hand, hold the pipet so you can see the markings on the pipet (Fig. 10).

4. With your left hand, grasp the patient's middle finger as illustrated below in Figure 10.

5. Put the tip of the pipet in the drop of blood, <u>resting your finger on the patient's finger as illustrated in Figure 10.</u>

6. Suck up blood to the 0.5 mark. Then suck up white cell diluting fluid to the 11.0 mark. Detach the rubber sucking tube from the white cell pipet. Place the pipet on the table.

7. Attach a red cell pipet to the rubber sucking tube.

8. To produce another rounded drop of blood for your red cell count, first dry the puncture with a piece of <u>dry</u> cotton. Then <u>deeply</u> massage the finger. Dam off the blood with your left hand. Gently squeeze with your right hand.

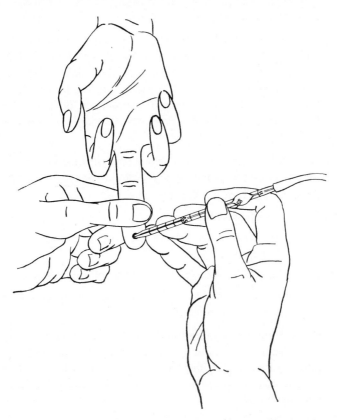

FIG. 10.—Sucking blood from a finger puncture into a white cell pipet.

9. When you have produced the rounded drop of blood, proceed as follows:

10. With your right hand, hold the pipet.

11. With your left hand, hold the patient's finger.

12. Put the tip of the pipet in the drop of blood, resting your finger on the patient's finger.

13. Suck up blood to the 0.5 mark.   Then suck up RBC diluting fluid to the 101 mark.

14. Detach the rubber sucking tube from the red cell pipet. Shake the pipet a few seconds.   Place the pipet on the table.

15. Note: The Haden-Hausser method of performing a hemoglobin determination uses the contents of the white cell pipet.   Consequently, if you are performing your hemoglobin determination by the Haden-Hausser method, you can skip the next step.

16. Attach the hemoglobin pipet to the rubber sucking tube. Then dry the puncture with a piece of dry cotton.   Now massage to produce another rounded drop of blood. Suck the required amount of blood into the pipet. Expel the blood into the required amount of diluting fluid. Rinse the pipet several times by sucking up and then expelling the solution.

17. To produce another rounded drop of blood: Dry the puncture with a piece of dry cotton.   Deeply massage. Dam off the blood.   Gently squeeze.

18. Pick up a glass slide.

19. Touch one end of the slide to the drop of blood as illustrated in Figure 11.

20. Place the slide containing the drop of blood on the table.

21. Pick up another slide.   Using this slide as a spreader, make your blood smear.

22. Note: If you are unable to make all your blood preparations from one finger puncture, simply make another finger puncture.   With practice, however, you should be able to obtain all the necessary blood preparations from one puncture.

23. Turn to step 7, preventing further bleeding.

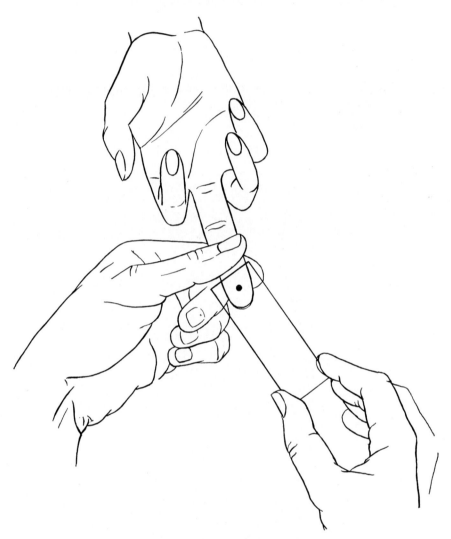

FIG. 11.—Technique of getting a drop of finger tip blood on a glass slide.

STEP 7:   PREVENTING FURTHER BLEEDING

Procedure for Step 7

1. Place the piece of cotton moistened with alcohol on the puncture.

2. Ask the patient to hold the cotton on the puncture until bleeding stops (Fig. 12).

3. Thank the patient.

4. Turn to step 8, labelling the specimens.

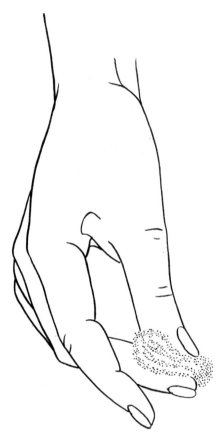

FIG. 12.—Preventing further bleeding.

STEP 8: LABELLING THE SPECIMENS

Procedure for Step 8

1. When handling pipets that contain diluted blood, keep the pipets in a <u>horizontal position.</u> Otherwise, the diluted blood may flow out of the pipet.

2. Now pick up one of the pipets and, keeping it in a <u>horizontal position,</u> push it into a piece of paper as illustrated below. (This keeps the tip of the pipet from touching anything. If the tip of the pipet touches something, the fluid may drain out.)

3. In a similar manner, push the other pipets into the same piece of paper (Fig. 13).

4. Write the patient's name on the piece of paper.

5. Allow the blood smear to dry (takes a few minutes).

6. Using an ordinary pen or pencil, write the patient's name on the <u>blood</u> as illustrated below.

7. Place the blood preparations in a convenient place until you are ready to perform the tests.

8. Clean up your table or workbench.

9. Check the blood tray for supplies and, if necessary, replenish it with cotton, alcohol, etc.

10. Put your equipment away.

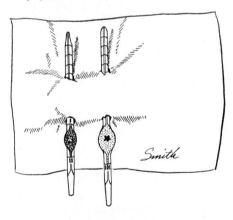

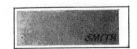

Fig. 13.—Labelling the blood specimens.

INTRODUCTION TO THE VENIPUNCTURE

Some tests require a few drops of blood; other tests require a few cubic centimeters of blood.

If a few drops of blood are required, the blood is obtained from a finger. If a few cubic centimeters of blood are required, the blood is obtained from a vein.

The following veins are used:

> veins of the forearm
>
> veins of the wrist
>
> veins of the hand
>
> veins of the ankle

The veins of the forearm are larger than the veins of the wrist, hand, or ankle. Consequently, the veins of the forearm are usually chosen.

The veins of the forearm, however, can not always be used. For example, they may be difficult to find, they may be sore from repeated venipunctures, or they may be bandaged. In such cases, the veins of the wrist, back of the hand, or ankle are used.

When blood is obtained from a vein, the procedure is called a venipuncture (ven′ĭ-punk″tūr).

The venipuncture may be made by either the syringe method or the Vacutainer method.

If the syringe method is used, a needle is attached to a syringe and inserted into a vein. Then the plunger of the syringe is pulled back. This creates a suction which draws blood into the syringe.

If the Vacutainer method is used, one end of a two-way needle is attached to the rubber stopper of a vacuum tube. The other end of the two-way needle is inserted into a vein. Then the needle is connected directly to the vacuum tube. The vacuum creates a suction which draws blood into the tube.

The syringe method of making a venipuncture should be thoroughly mastered before trying the Vacutainer method.

The procedures for the syringe method and Vacutainer method are given on the following pages.

A new and ingenious method of collecting blood from a vein has recently been developed.

The technologist simply inserts a needle into a vein and the blood is automatically collected into several test tubes.

This new method is called Techmate and complete information may be obtained by writing to Systematiks, 3524 N. Meridian Street, Indianapolis, Indiana 46208.

SYRINGE METHOD OF MAKING A VENIPUNCTURE

The syringe method of making a venipuncture consists of 13 steps:

Step 1. Assembling the Equipment

Step 2. Positioning and Identifying the Patient

Step 3. Preparing the Needle and Syringe

Step 4. Applying the Tourniquet

Step 5. Selecting the Vein

Step 6. Applying the Antiseptic

Step 7. Inserting the Needle

Step 8. Withdrawing the Blood

Step 9. Releasing the Tourniquet

Step 10. Withdrawing the Needle

Step 11. Transferring the Blood

Step 12. Cleaning the Needle and Syringe

Step 13. Checking the Patient's Wound

Each of the above steps will be broken down into a *discussion* and a *procedure*.

For the present, carefully read the entire material. When it is time for your first venipuncture, carefully review the entire material. Then follow the *procedure* in each step.

You may feel a little nervous for your first venipuncture. This is normal. Practically everyone feels nervous the first time.

After you have made your first venipuncture, you should re-read this entire material. The re-reading will strengthen your learning. It will also bring out any shortcomings in your technique.

3

STEP 1: ASSEMBLING THE EQUIPMENT

Discussion of Step 1

The equipment for the venipuncture is usually kept in a blood tray such as the one illustrated in Figure 14.

The equipment for the venipuncture is listed in Figure 15.

If the venipuncture is to be made on a patient in a hospital room or ward, you should always check the blood tray for the essential equipment before leaving the laboratory.

In addition to the above equipment, you should have a requisition slip giving the patient's name, date, doctor's name, tests requested, and room number (if in a hospital).

It is also advisable to have a bottle of smelling salts in case the patient faints.

Procedure for Step 1

1. Assemble the equipment listed in Figure 15.

2. Place the above equipment within easy reach.

3. Turn to step 2, positioning and identifying the patient.

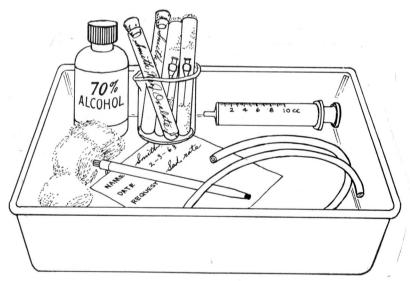

Fig. 14.—Blood tray containing equipment for the venipuncture.

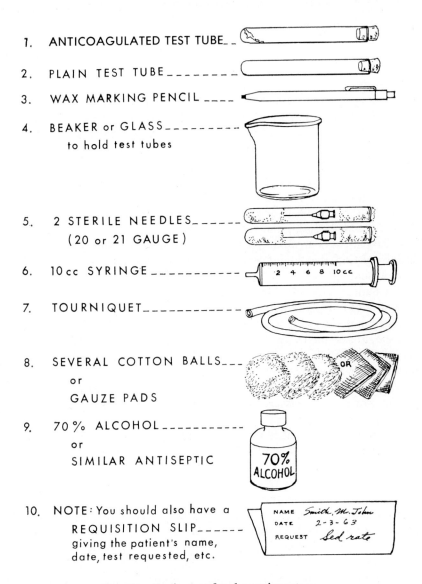

1. ANTICOAGULATED TEST TUBE _ _

2. PLAIN TEST TUBE _ _ _ _ _ _ _ _ _

3. WAX MARKING PENCIL _ _ _ _

4. BEAKER or GLASS _ _ _ _ _ _ _ _ _
     to hold test tubes

5. 2 STERILE NEEDLES _ _ _ _ _ _
     (20 or 21 GAUGE)

6. 10 cc SYRINGE _ _ _ _ _ _ _ _ _ _

7. TOURNIQUET _ _ _ _ _ _ _ _ _ _ _

8. SEVERAL COTTON BALLS _ _ _
     or
     GAUZE PADS

9. 70 % ALCOHOL _ _ _ _ _ _ _ _ _ _
     or
     SIMILAR ANTISEPTIC

10. NOTE: You should also have a
     REQUISITION SLIP _ _ _ _ _ _
     giving the patient's name,
     date, test requested, etc.

FIG. 15.—Equipment for the venipuncture.

STEP 2: POSITIONING AND IDENTIFYING THE PATIENT

Discussion of Step 2

In making a venipuncture, you should remain in a standing position. This gives you greater freedom and also a better command of the situation.

You should have the patient assume a comfortable position. The positioning of a bed patient and walking patient is discussed below.

If the patient is a bed patient, you should ask him to move to the edge of the bed. Then you should make any adjustments which will enable you to work with freedom of action. This may include moving a table, chair, or even the bed (Fig. 16).

You should place the blood tray where it is handy and yet not in danger of being upset by any unexpected movements of the patient. A blood tray placed on the lower portion of the bed spread, for example, may be upset if the patient kicks during the venipuncture.

If the patient is a walking patient, you should have him sit down. In a sitting position, the patient is not only more comfortable, but much safer in case of fainting.

If a patient feels faint, help him put his head between his knees. If a patient does faint, hold a bottle of smelling salts below his nose.

You should have the walking patient sit alongside a small table. Then you should ask him to put one of his arms on the table and hold it straight. As he does this, you should put a small pillow, roll of towels, or several books under his elbow to keep the arm extended (Fig. 17).

While the above adjustments are being made to the bed patient or walking patient, you should reassure him and endeavor to relieve any apprehension which may be present.

You should *always* have an order or requisition slip for the tests to be performed. And you should *always* check the name on the requisition slip with the patient's name.

For example, suppose the name on the requisition slip reads *Mrs. Jane Smith.* You should ask the patient: "Are you Mrs. Jane Smith?"

If the patient is delirious, unconscious, or unable to talk, you should check his identity with the nurse on duty.

After you have identified the patient, you should write the patient's name on the test tube (or tubes) which will receive the blood. This is extremely important! In blood transfusions, for example, a mislabelled test tube could result in the patient's death!

In addition to writing the patient's name on the test tube (or tubes) which will receive the blood, many laboratories further label each test tube with a *patient's number* which is pasted on the test tube.

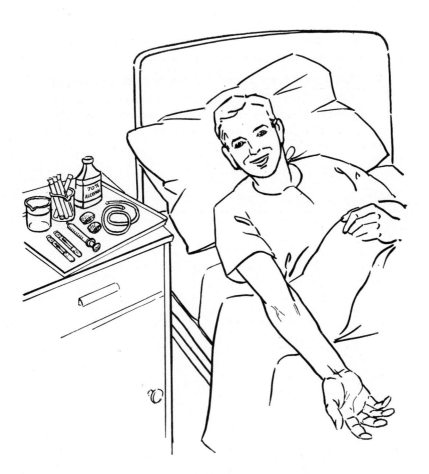

FIG. 16.—Positioning a bed patient for the venipuncture.

Procedure for Step 2

1. If the patient is in bed: Ask him to move to the edge of the bed. Place the blood tray where it is handy and yet not in danger of being upset by the patient. Make any adjustments which will enable you to work with freedom of action. Then go to point 3 below.

2. If the patient is not in bed: Ask him to sit down alongside a table. Then ask him to put one of his arms on the table and hold it straight. Now place a support (small pillow, roll of towels, several books) under the elbow to keep the arm extended (see Fig. 17).

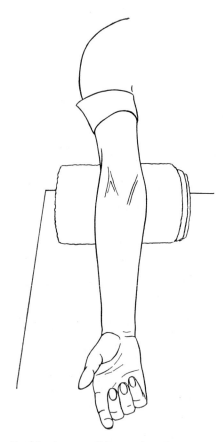

FIG. 17.—Positioning a walking patient for the venipuncture.

3. Reassure the patient and endeavor to relieve any apprehension which may be present.

4. Read the name on the requisition slip.

5. Ask the patient if he is the person whose name appears on the requisition slip.

6. Using the marking pencil, <u>write the patient's name on an anticoagulated test tube and also on a plain test tube. If your laboratory also requires a numerical identification of the patient, put the patient's number on the test tubes.</u>

7. Write the word anticoagulant (or oxalate) on the anticoagulated test tube.

8. Remove the stoppers from the test tubes.

9. Place the test tubes in a beaker or glass (Fig. 18).

10. Turn to step 3, preparing the needle and syringe.

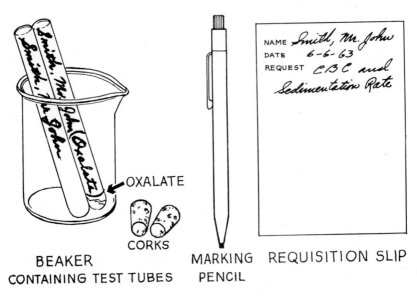

OXALATE

CORKS

BEAKER
CONTAINING TEST TUBES

MARKING
PENCIL

REQUISITION SLIP

NAME *Smith, Mr. John*
DATE *6-6-63*
REQUEST *CBC and Sedimentation Rate*

Fig. 18.—Test tubes labelled with the patient's name.

STEP 3:   PREPARING THE NEEDLE AND SYRINGE

Discussion of Step 3

Before use, all needles and syringes should be sterilized by one of the following methods:

1. Dry heating in an oven at 170° C. for 2 hours
2. Autoclaving at 15 pounds pressure for 20 minutes

To sterilize needles and syringes, many small laboratories use an ordinary household pressure cooker in place of an autoclave. The needles and syringes are brought to 15 pounds pressure and allowed to "cook" for 20 minutes. Then they are placed in a beaker and heated in an oven or over a Bunsen burner. This removes the moisture.

The needle and syringe should always be dry because moisture may rupture or hemolyze many of the red cells.

The needle should be sharp; a dull needle may hurt the patient. If a needle is dull or has burrs, it should be sharpened on an oil stone.

A needle consists of 3 parts: the bevel, shaft, and hub. The parts of a needle and the actual sizes of needles are illustrated in Fig. 19.

The gauge number gives the diameter of the needle. The smaller the gauge number, the greater the diameter. Either a 20 gauge needle or a 21 gauge needle is used for the veins of the forearm. A 25 gauge needle is used for the veins of the wrist, hand, or ankle (Fig. 19).

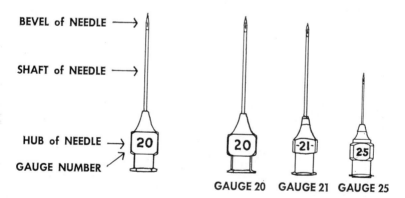

FIG. 19.—Actual size of needles used for the venipuncture.

The choice of a syringe is governed by the amount of blood required. A 10 cc. syringe is most frequently used. However, if a large amount of blood is required, a 20 cc. syringe is employed.

A syringe consists of a barrel and a plunger. The barrel and plunger must fit snugly and therefore they are "mated." The number on the barrel must correspond with the number on the plunger.

The plunger, barrel, and assembled syringe are illustrated in Figure 20.

The student should study the various parts of the needles and syringe which are illustrated in Figures 19 and 20, for this information will be necessary to follow the forthcoming procedure.

When the needle and syringe have been chosen, the needle is removed from its sterile test tube and *firmly* adjusted to the tip of the syringe—care being taken to keep the shaft of the needle sterile.

A check is then made to see that the needle is not clogged. This is done by moving the plunger up and down and attempting to force air through the needle. If the needle is clogged, the plunger will not move. In such cases, another needle should be selected.

The needle and syringe are then placed on a table in such a manner that the needle is kept sterile. This may be accomplished by slipping the point of the needle back into the test tube (from whence it was removed) or placing the syringe on the edge of the table so the needle extends over the edge.

Disposable needles and syringes are now being used by most laboratories. These, of course, are thrown away after use, thus saving the time and labor involved in sterilization. (A disposable needle and syringe cost about 15¢.)

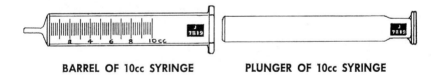

BARREL OF 10cc SYRINGE   PLUNGER OF 10cc SYRINGE

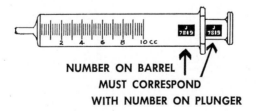

NUMBER ON BARREL
MUST CORRESPOND
WITH NUMBER ON PLUNGER

PLUNGER IN BARREL OF 10cc SYRINGE

Fig. 20.—Syringe used for the venipuncture.

Procedure for Step 3

1. Remove the cotton plug from the test tube containing the sterile needle.

2. Place the tip of the syringe in the test tube. Now invert the test tube so the needle slips onto the tip of the syringe (see below).

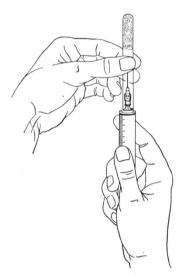

3. Remove the test tube (see below).

4. Place the test tube on the table.

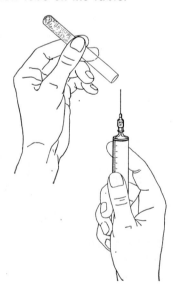

5. Fix the needle firmly on the tip of the syringe by holding the hub of the needle and twisting the syringe to the right (see below).

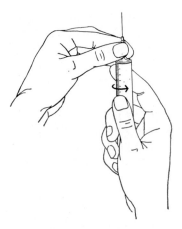

6. Check to see if the needle is clogged by moving the plunger up and down and attempting to force air through needle. If the needle is clogged, you will not be able to move the plunger. In such cases, get another needle.

7. Pick up the test tube which held the needle. Insert the needle in the test tube to keep it sterile. Place on table (see below).

8. Turn to step 4, applying the tourniquet.

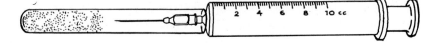

STEP 4: APPLYING THE TOURNIQUET

Discussion of Step 4

It is desirable to enlarge the veins of the forearm so that they may become more prominent. This is accomplished by allowing the blood to enter the arm by way of the arteries and blocking its return by way of the veins. A piece of rubber tubing known as a tourniquet serves the purpose.

The tourniquet is applied around the arm just above the bend in the elbow.

The tourniquet should not be too tight nor too loose. It should be just tight enough to stop the flow of blood. In other words, the tourniquet should be about as tight as an uncomfortable garter.

The patient should be instructed to clench his fist as this aids in building up the pressure.

If the student does not know how to tie a tourniquet, he will lose the confidence of the patient. Consequently, the student should practice tying a tourniquet before his first venipuncture.

Some students practice the procedure by tying the tourniquet around their left leg just above the knee.

The technique of tying a tourniquet requires 10 steps. These 10 steps are illustrated in Figure 21.

Procedure for Step 4

1. Tell the patient to clench his fist.

2. Apply the tourniquet above the bend in the elbow as illustrated in the 10 steps of Figure 21.

3. Then turn to step 5, selecting the vein.

Step 1: Put the tourniquet under the patient's arm just above the bend in the elbow. With each hand, grasp an end of the tourniquet and *pull up so tension is applied to the tourniquet. This tension must be maintained throughout the procedure (see below).*

Step 2: Keeping the tension on the tourniquet, hold both ends of the tourniquet with your *left* hand (see below).

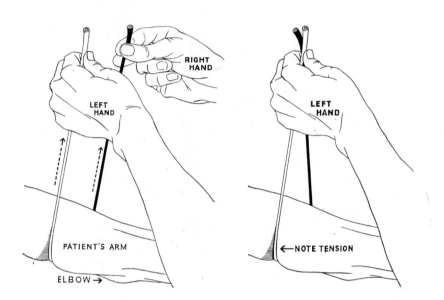

FIG. 21.—Tying a tourniquet.

Step 3: With your right hand, grasp the right side of the tourniquet where it touches the patient's arm. Now pull this right side up slightly and release it from your left hand (see below).

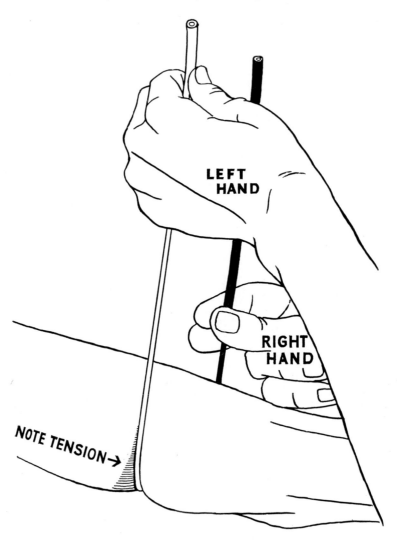

Fig. 21 (continued).—Tying a tourniquet.

Step 4: Now cross this right side over on _top_ of the left side as shown in the illustration below.

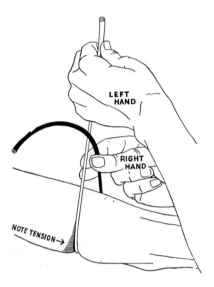

Step 5: Grasp both sides of the tourniquet with your right hand and pull up slightly to maintain the tension (see below).

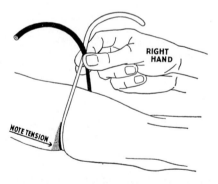

Fig. 21 (continued).—Tying a tourniquet.

Step 6: With your _left hand_, reach through the loop (see below).

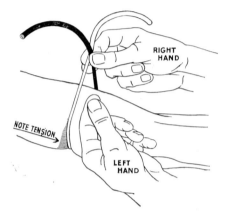

Step 7: And grasp the side which is colored black in the illustration below

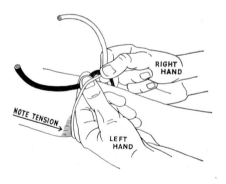

FIG. 21 (continued).—Tying a tourniquet.

Step 8: Pull this black side toward yourself until it reaches **the position** shown in the illustration below.

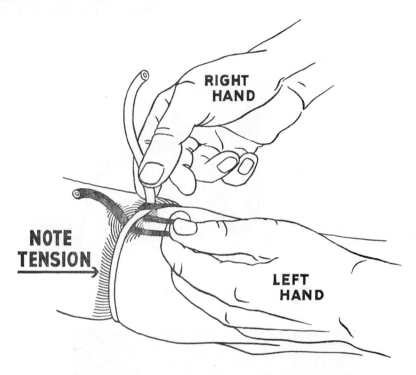

Step 9: *Gradually* release your hands.   And, if necessary, straighten or smooth out the loop.

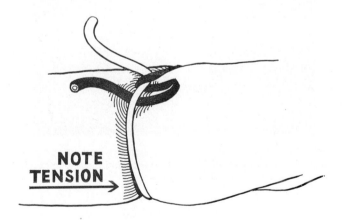

Fig. 21 (continued).—Tying a tourniquet.

Step 10: Check to see that your completed tourniquet has the tension illustrated below.

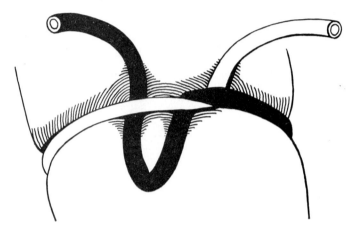

FIG. 21 (continued).—Tying a tourniquet.

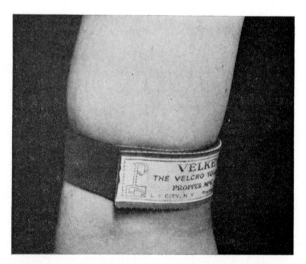

FIG. 22.—A Propper Velket Tourniquet applied to a patient's arm. This tourniquet is a band of gum rubber which may be easily and quickly applied. It may be purchased from your local medical supply house.

STEP 5: SELECTING THE VEIN

Discussion of Step 5

The large veins of the forearm are illustrated below in Figure 23.

The most prominent vein is usually chosen. If the veins are extremely large, however, one of the smaller veins is usually chosen.

In about 1 patient in 10, the veins can not be seen. They usually can be felt, however, by touching or palpating with the index finger. They will then reveal themselves as elastic tubes beneath the surface of the skin.

If the veins are difficult to find, the following technique may help to locate them: (1) opening and closing the fist, (2) massaging toward the heart, (3) slapping the area. The latter paralyzes the walls of the veins and makes them more prominent.

If a vein can not be located in one arm, the tourniquet should be released and applied to the other arm. The veins in this arm should then be inspected.

If a vein can not be seen or felt in either arm, the veins of the wrist or the veins in the back of the hand should be used. The veins of the wrist are illustrated in Figure 23 below.

When the veins of the wrist are used, the tourniquet should be applied just above the wrist. The patient should make a tight fist and bend his fist downward. This pulls the skin tightly over the veins and makes them stand out. Then the most prominent vein should be fixed with the thumb of your left hand and a 25 or 26 gauge needle should be used for the insertion.

It may sometimes be difficult to find the veins of fat people, colored persons, and children. In such cases, experience is the only teacher.

The student should never hesitate to ask for the help of a technologist or physician.

Sometimes a technologist may have an "off day" and be unable to locate a vein. When this occurs, he should call for the help of a fellow worker or physician.

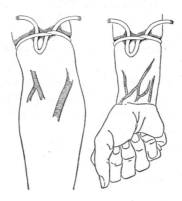

FIG. 23.—Veins of the forearm and wrist.

Procedure for Step 5

__If the veins are visible, proceed as follows:__

1. Select one of the larger veins (Fig. 24).

2. Place the index finger of your left hand on the vein.

3. Now press up and down on the vein several times and feel the path of the vein.

4. Turn to step 6, applying the antiseptic.

__If the veins are not visible, proceed as follows:__

1. Tell the patient to continuously open and close his fist.

2. Select a spot where you think a vein is located (Fig. 24).

3. Now, with the index finger of your left hand, apply a probing up and down pressure.

4. If you feel an elastic tube giving under the pressure of your finger, you have located a vein.

5. You should then press up and down on the vein several times and feel the path of the vein.

6. And then go to step 6, applying the antiseptic.

7. If you have difficulty in locating a vein, proceed as follows:
   a. Ask the patient to continue opening and closing his fist.
   b. Starting near the wrist, apply several HEAVY massaging motions toward the bend in the elbow.
   c. Then smartly slap the area below the bend in the elbow several times.
   d. Repeat the above massaging and slapping procedure several times.
   e. Now, with your index finger, probe the areas (Fig. 24) below the bend in the elbow and try to feel a vein.
   f. If you can feel a vein, continue probing and try to feel the path of the vein.
   g. Then proceed to step 6, applying the antiseptic.
   h. If you can not locate a vein, remove the tourniquet and try the other arm.

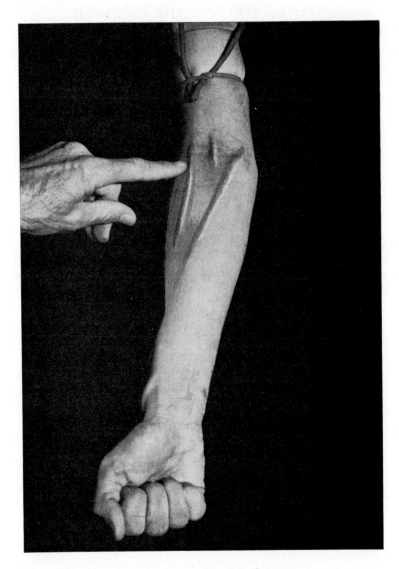

Fig. 24.—Actual photograph of the veins of the forearm.

1. Note the 3 prominent veins in this forearm. These veins, of course, will be easy to "hit".
2. The veins in some forearms, however, will be buried and therefore invisible.
3. To find a buried vein: (1) Note the *positions* of the above 3 veins. (2) Press down and probe these 3 positions with your index finger. (3) When you feel an elastic rubber-like tube, you have located a vein.

STEP 6:   APPLYING THE ANTISEPTIC

Discussion of Step 6

A cotton ball or gauze pad is moistened with 70% alcohol or some similar antiseptic.   This is rubbed on the selected vein.

You may feel a vein as often as you like.   After you feel it, however, you should rub the alcohol pad on it again.

Procedure for Step 6

1. Moisten a piece of cotton with 70% alcohol or some similar antiseptic.

2. Thoroughly rub the moistened cotton on the vein you have selected (Fig. 25).

3. If you wish to feel the vein again, do so; but after you feel it, rub the moistened cotton on it again.

4. Lay the piece of moistened cotton just to your left of the patient's arm because you will need it later on in the procedure (Fig. 25).

5. Turn to step 7, inserting the needle.

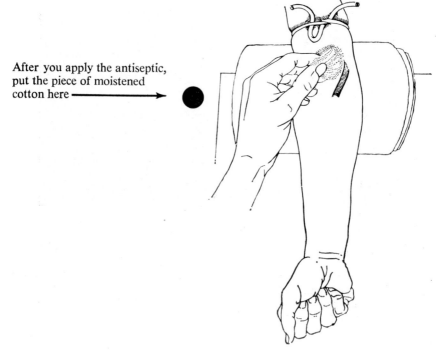

After you apply the antiseptic, put the piece of moistened cotton here ——————➤ ●

FIG. 25.—Applying the antiseptic for the venipuncture.

STEP 7: INSERTING THE NEEDLE

Discussion of Step 7

The right hand holds the syringe.

The bevel of the needle may face up or down. Some technologists prefer to have the bevel face up. They feel this helps "steer the needle." Other technologists prefer to have the bevel face down. They feel this removes the possibility of the bevel contacting the upper wall of the vein and thereby hindering the flow of blood (see Fig. 26 below).

Since the beginner must make a choice, we will suggest that he hold the bevel of the needle face down.

Air must never be pumped into a vein (a few cubic centimeters of air pumped into a vein of some patients could cause death!). To guard against pumping air into a vein, the plunger should be kept all the way down in the barrel of the syringe. It is held in this position with either the little finger or heel of the right hand (see Fig. 28, page 49).

The ball of the index finger is placed alongside the hub of the needle. This helps guide the passage of the needle (see Fig. 28, page 49).

A proposed point of entry into the vein should be selected.

If the visible area of the vein is extensive (several inches long), the proposed point of entry should be on the thickest portion of the vein.

If the visible area of the vein is small (less than an inch), the proposed point of entry should be *just below* the visible area. This is important! Entering the vein *below* the visible area prevents "over-riding" the vein, that is, going past the vein. (See Fig. 29, page 50.)

If the vein is not visible, the proposed point of entry should be *just below* the spot where you can feel the vein.

Because the veins are not held firmly by the flesh, they must be held in position.

Some technologists fix the vein by grasping the patient's arm just below the bend in the elbow and pulling the skin taut.

Other technologists fix the vein as follows: They place their left thumb about 1 inch below their proposed point of entry into the vein. Then they press down on the vein with their thumb and pull the skin toward themselves. This stretches the skin over the vein and holds it in position.

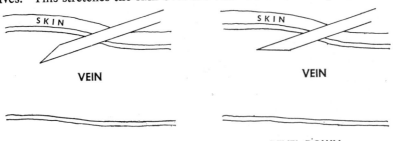

BEVEL UP   BEVEL DOWN

Fig. 26.—Vein being entered with bevel of needle facing up
and bevel of needle facing down.

The latter method of fixing the vein is probably the best. It is illustrated in Fig. 29, page 50.

The needle should be held *in line with the vein, that is, the needle should be pointing in exactly the same direction as the vein is running* (see Fig. 27 below).

The needle is held in line with the vein for two reasons: (1) It keeps the pressure on the vein in one direction—downward. Therefore, the vein can only move in one direction—downward. (2) It enables the vein to be entered from above rather than from the side. This gives the operator more "hitting area."

The syringe should be held so that it makes a 15 degree angle with the patient's arm. This is a 15 degree angle:

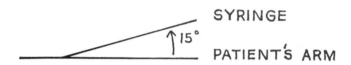

The proper angle of the syringe is important. If the angle is too small, the needle will slide along the top of the vein. If the angle is too great, the needle will go through the vein.

When the above techniques have been observed, the needle is placed on the vein and pushed firmly and deliberately forward. As the needle is pushed forward, the vein gives a little. Soon the needle penetrates the skin, then the wall of the vein. Finally, the needle enters the vein.

As the needle enters the vein, a little "give" may be felt. And sometimes the blood will spurt into the neck of the syringe.

Note: Some veins, especially men's, may be quite tough and it may be necessary to push quite hard. Failure to push the needle all the way into the vein is the most frequent mistake the beginner makes.

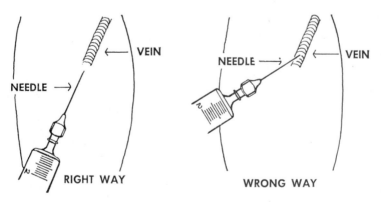

Fig. 27.—Proper method of pointing the needle prior to the venipuncture.

Procedure for Step 7

1. Pick up the syringe with your right hand. Remove the test tube covering the needle. Place the test tube on the table. Now hold the syringe so that the bevel of the needle is face down.

2. With the little finger or heel of your right hand, hold the plunger all the way down in the barrel of the syringe (see Fig. 28 below).

3. Now put your index finger alongside the hub of the needle (see Fig. 28 below).

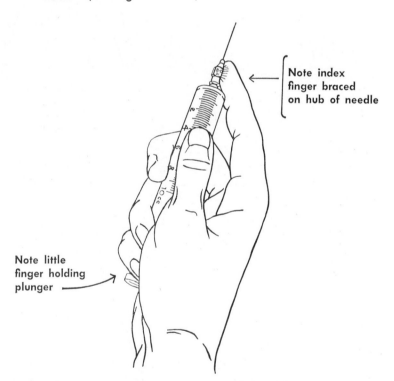

Note index
finger braced
on hub of needle

Note little
finger holding
plunger

FIG. 28.—Holding the plunger in the barrel of the syringe and putting the index finger alongside hub of needle.

4. Select a proposed point of entry (see Fig. 29 below).

5. Now put your left thumb about 1 inch below your proposed point of entry, press down firmly with your thumb, and pull the skin toward yourself (see Fig. 29 below).

6. Point the needle in <u>exactly</u> the same direction as the vein is running (see Fig. 29 below).

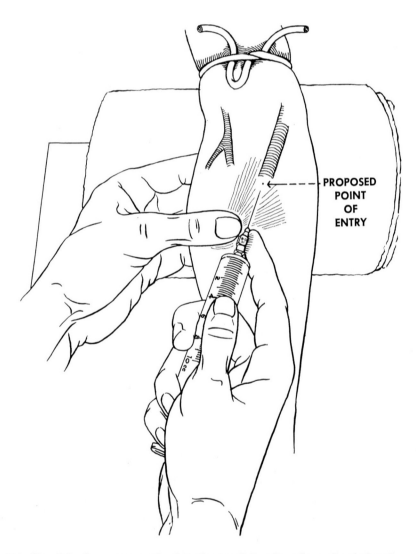

PROPOSED
POINT
OF
ENTRY

FIG. 29.—Selecting a proposed point of entry, fixing the vein, and pointing the needle in exactly the same direction as the vein is running.

7. Hold the syringe at a 15 degree angle with the patient's arm (see Fig. 30 below).

8. Without hesitation, push the needle firmly and deliberately into the vein.

9. When you have the needle in the vein, turn to step 8, withdrawing the blood.

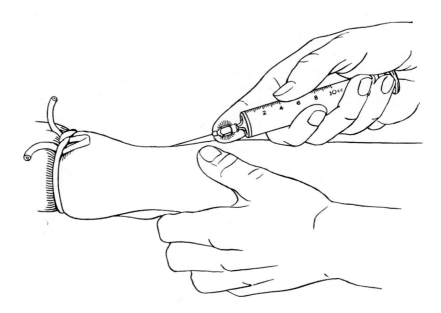

FIG. 30.—Holding the syringe at a 15 degree angle with the patient's arm and pushing the needle into the vein.

STEP 8:   WITHDRAWING THE BLOOD

Discussion of Step 8

When you perform your first venipuncture, you will be so occupied during the next 3 steps that you will not be able to refer to the book. Consequently, you should study the next 3 steps with extra diligence, trying to retain a picture of the *procedures* in your mind.

When the needle is in the vein, you put your *left* hand on the plunger and pull slowly back. If the plunger seems to stick, you should twist it slightly as you pull it back.

Now study the A, B, and C possibilities discussed below.

A. *If blood enters syringe:*

As the blood is withdrawn, *you should keep your index finger alongside the hub of the needle and brace it on the arm of the patient* (Fig. 31).

Bracing your index finger on the patient's arm serves a very useful purpose. It enables you to move your hand, syringe, and needle with any slight movement of the patient's arm. This helps keep the needle in the vein.

You will find the above technique especially helpful in withdrawing blood from children, for they often move their arm during a venipuncture.

As the blood is withdrawn, *you should keep your eye on the needle as much possible. This will help you keep the needle in the vein.*

You should not wiggle the needle around or put pressure on the needle, for this pushes the sharp edges of the needle against the walls of the vein and can be quite painful.

For your first few venipunctures, withdraw blood until the syringe is almost half full (about 6 cc.). Then you can use about half of this to make anticoagulated blood and the remainder to make serum. With anticoagulated blood and serum, you can perform most hematologic tests. Only a few drops of anticoagulated blood are needed to perform a complete blood count (CBC).

B. *If blood does not enter syringe:*

If blood fails to enter the syringe when you pull the plunger back, the needle is not in the vein. Using the index finger of your left hand, you should then feel to find the point of the needle.

When you locate the point of the needle, you should correct one of the 3 following mistakes:

(1) If it appears that the needle has not gone far enough, you should push the needle in further. Failure to push the needle in far enough is the most frequent mistake the beginner makes.

(2) If it appears that the needle has gone to the right or left of the vein, you should *partially* remove the needle, *fix the vein*, and make the proper insertion.

(3) If it appears that the needle has gone through the vein, you should proceed as follows: Slowly pull back the plunger and, *at the same time,* slowly withdraw the needle. By pulling back on the plunger, you create a suction in the syringe. This suction draws blood into the syringe when the point of the needle is drawn back into the vein. The needle, of course, should not be withdrawn entirely out of the arm.

If the above techniques fail and blood does not enter the syringe, you should release the tourniquet and completely withdraw the needle. Then you should make another venipuncture, using either the same arm or the other arm of the patient.

C. *If blood starts to enter syringe and then stops:*

Sometimes the blood will start to enter the syringe and then stop. This may be caused by any one of 3 different factors:

(1) The bevel of the needle may be pressing against the wall of the vein and preventing the flow of blood. If so, you should *very gently* wiggle the needle and, at the same time, pull back on the plunger.

(2) The needle may have slipped out of the vein. If so, you should *fix the vein* and carefully reinsert the needle.

(3) The needle may have gone through the vein. If so, you should slowly pull back the plunger and simultaneously withdraw the needle until the needle is again in the vein.

Question: How can you tell which of the above 3 factors are involved? Answer: The only answer is the "touch" which comes with experience.

If the above techniques fail to resume the flow of blood into the syringe, you should release the tourniquet, apply the piece of cotton moistened with alcohol, and carefully withdraw the needle. Then you should transfer any blood that you did get to the anticoagulated test tube.

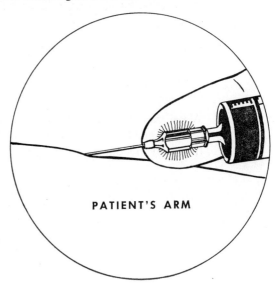

PATIENT'S ARM

Fig. 31.—Keeping index finger alongside hub of needle and bracing index finger on arm of patient.

Procedure for Step 8

1. With your <u>left</u> hand, slowly pull back the plunger of the syringe (Fig. 32).

   Note: If the plunger seems to stick, twist it slightly as you pull it out.

2. <u>If blood enters syringe:</u>

   Keep the index finger of your right hand alongside the hub of the needle and brace it on the arm of the patient. Keep your eye on the point of the needle as much as possible. Do not wiggle the needle or put pressure on the needle. Continue pulling on the plunger until the syringe is almost half full (about 6 cc.). Then turn to step 9, releasing the tourniquet.

3. <u>If blood does not enter syringe:</u>

   Feel with the index finger of your left hand to determine the position of the point of the needle.

   a. If it appears that you have not gone far enough, <u>fix the vein</u> and push the needle in farther.

   b. If it appears that you have gone to the right or left of the vein, draw the needle back slightly. Then re-direct the needle, <u>fix the vein,</u> and push the needle into the vein.

   c. If it appears that you have gone through the vein, proceed as follows: Slowly pull back the plunger and simultaneously withdraw the needle until the point of the needle is in the vein.

   When you do get in the vein, slowly pull back the plunger until the syringe is almost half full (about 6 cc.). Then turn to step 9, releasing the tourniquet.

Note: If you are unable to get in the vein, tell the patient to open his fist, <u>release the tourniquet, gently</u> apply the cotton moistened with alcohol to the puncture, and slowly withdraw the needle. Remove the needle from the syringe and attach another sterile needle. Apply the tourniquet. Then make a second attempt, using either the same vein or another vein.

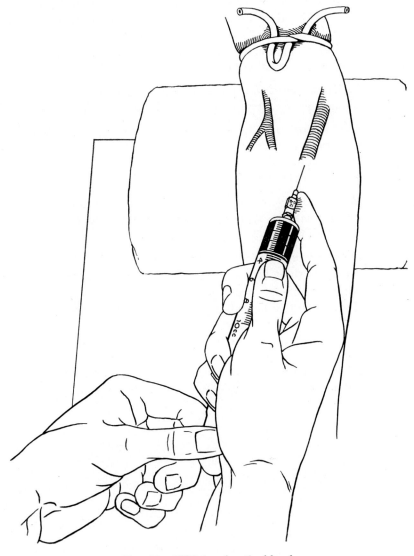

Fig. 32.—Withdrawing the blood.

4. If blood enters syringe and then stops:

   a. The bevel of the needle may be pressing against the wall of the vein. Therefore, very gently wiggle the needle and, at the same time, pull back on the plunger. If the blood does not resume its flow into the syringe, feel with the index finger of your left hand to determine the position of the point of the needle.

   b. If it appears that you have let the needle slip out of the vein, fix the vein and carefully reinsert the needle.

   c. If it appears that you have gone through the vein, proceed as follows: Slowly pull back the plunger and simultaneously withdraw the needle until the point of the needle is back in the vein.

   When you have corrected the fault, slowly pull back the plunger until the syringe is almost half full (about 6 cc.). Then turn to step 9, releasing the tourniquet.

   Note: If you are unable to get back in the vein, tell the patient to open his fist, release the tourniquet, apply the cotton moistened with alcohol to the puncture, and slowly withdraw the needle. Transfer any blood that you did get to the anticoagulated tube, pull the plunger about halfway out of the barrel, mix the blood and anticoagulant, and clean the needle and syringe. If you still need more blood, make another venipuncture, using another needle and syringe.

STEP 9:   RELEASING THE TOURNIQUET

Discussion of Step 9

Before the needle is withdrawn, the pressure must be released. Otherwise, the blood would continue to flow from the hole made by the needle. The pressure is released by having the patient open his clenched fist and by your pulling on either end of the tourniquet. Pulling on the tourniquet, of course, releases the tourniquet (Fig. 33).

Procedure for Step 9

1. When you have the syringe almost half full (about 6 cc.), tell the patient to open his fist.

2. With your left hand, pull on either end of the tourniquet. This, of course, will release the tourniquet.

3. Turn to step 10, withdrawing the needle.

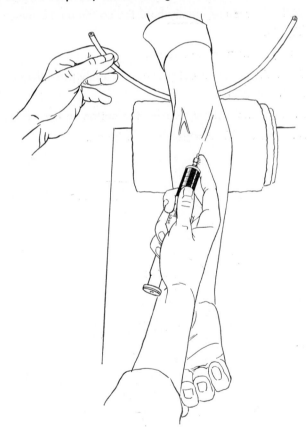

Fig. 33.—Releasing the tourniquet before withdrawing the needle.

5

STEP 10:   WITHDRAWING THE NEEDLE

Discussion of Step 10

When the tourniquet has been released, the next step is to withdraw the needle.   If the needle is jerked out of the arm, the sharp point of the needle may partially sever the vein.   Consequently, the needle should be withdrawn with a slow gentle motion.

As the needle is being withdrawn, the antiseptic pad should be *gently* applied to the puncture.   Heavy pressure at this point should be avoided because it may cause the sharp point of the needle to cut the vein.   However, when the needle is out of the arm, *firm pressure* should be applied to the antiseptic pad so that it will stop the flow of blood.

Procedure for Step 10

1. With your left hand, pick up the piece of cotton moistened with alcohol.

2. Without pressure, <u>gently</u> hold the cotton on the puncture (Fig. 34).

3. Slowly withdraw the needle.

4. When the needle is out of the arm, <u>firmly</u> press the cotton on the puncture.

5. Then ask the patient to press the cotton on the puncture.

6. Turn to step 11, transferring the blood.

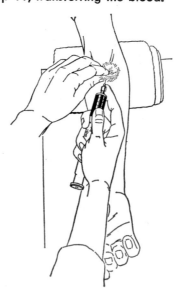

Fig. 34.—Withdrawing the needle after the venipuncture.

STEP 11: TRANSFERRING THE BLOOD

Discussion of Step 11

While the patient is applying pressure to the wound, you proceed with the following:

With the little finger of your right hand, you hold the plunger so it does not slip out of the barrel (see Fig. 35, page 60).

Then you remove the needle from the syringe and place it on the table.

If the needle is not removed, the sharp point of the needle and the speed of the blood hitting the test tube may rupture or hemolyze many red cells.

After the needle has been removed, you expel about half of the blood into the anticoagulated test tube and the remaining blood into the plain test tube. These test tubes should already be *labelled with the patient's name* (see Fig. 36, page 61).

When the blood has been expelled from the syringe, you pull the plunger of the syringe about half-way out of the barrel. (This prevents the drying blood from "freezing" the syringe.) Then you momentarily set the syringe aside.

Since anticoagulated blood is being made, the blood and anticoagulant *must be immediately mixed* to keep the blood from clotting. You mix the blood and anticoagulant by placing a stopper in the mouth of the test tube and *completely inverting the test tube 10 to 12 times.*

You do nothing to the blood in the plain test tube. This blood will clot in about 30 minutes and centrifuging will produce the serum.

In this step, you must work rather fast; otherwise, the anticoagulated blood may clot before you mix it.

Procedure for Step 11

1. With the little finger of your right hand, hold the plunger so it does not slip out of the barrel (Fig. 35).

2. With your left hand, remove the needle from the syringe.

3. Place the needle on the table.

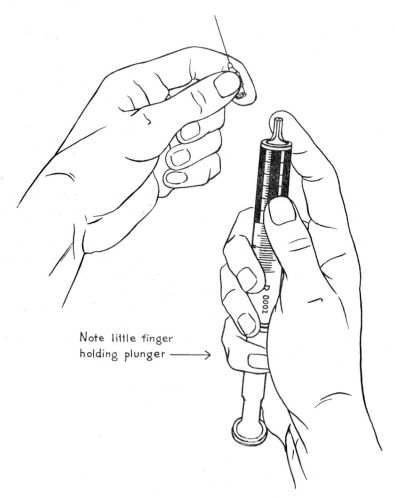

Note little finger holding plunger ⟶

Fig. 35.—Holding the plunger so it does not slip out of the barrel and removing the needle from the syringe.

4. Place the tip of the syringe in the anticoagulated test tube.

5. Then transfer the syringe to your left hand (Fig. 36).

6. Hold the syringe at an angle so the blood will hit against the side of the test tube (Fig. 36).

7. With your right hand, push the plunger and expel about half the blood into the anticoagulated test tube.

8. Now place the tip of the syringe in the plain test tube.

9. Expel the remaining blood into the plain test tube.

10. Pull the plunger of the syringe about half-way out of the barrel.

11. Then set the syringe on the table.

12. Immediately place a stopper in the mouth of the anticoagulated test tube and completely invert the test tube 10 to 12 times.   Do not shake!

13. Do nothing to the blood in the plain test tube.   This blood will clot (takes about 30 minutes).   Then centrifuging will produce the serum.

14. Turn to step 12, cleaning the needle and syringe.

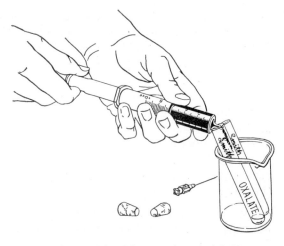

Fig. 36.—Transferring blood from syringe to labelled test tubes.

STEP 12:   CLEANING THE NEEDLE AND SYRINGE

Discussion of Step 12

After the blood and anticoagulant have been mixed, the needle and syringe are immediately washed with cold tap water and then with distilled water. If the cleaning process is not possible at the moment, the blood should be flushed out of the needle and the plunger should be separated from the barrel of the syringe.   This prevents the needle from becoming clogged and the syringe from becoming "frozen."

If the needle does become clogged, the dried blood may be removed with a 6 inch wire known as a stylet.   A stylet looks like this:

The stylet is simply pushed through the needle several times.

If a syringe becomes "frozen," it may be loosened by one of the following 4 methods:

Method 1: Soak for 1 or 2 hours in hot water (about 70° C. or 158° F.).

Method 2: Soak overnight in a 50–50 solution of rubbing alcohol and glycerin.

Method 3: Use a mechanical device known as a syringe opener.   Syringe openers (and directions for their use) may be obtained from Becton, Dickinson and Company, Rutherford, N.J.   The price is about $3.25.

Method 4:

1. Obtain a 500 cc. beaker or suitable container.   Add water until it is about ¾ full.   Heat to about 80° C. (176° F.).
2. Get a thick towel and fold it several times.
3. Obtain a rubber sucking tube which is normally used for diluting the blood in the white cell count.   This rubber sucking tube will be used to help get a good grip on the plunger.
4. Wrap the rubber sucking tube tightly around the end of the plunger.
5. With your right hand, hold the rubber sucking tube on the end of the plunger.
6. Now dip the syringe in the hot water for about 5 seconds (Fig. 37).

   Note: This causes the barrel to expand; the plunger does not expand because it does not receive sufficient heat in the 5 seconds time.

7. Remove the syringe from the water and quickly perform the following:

8. With your left hand, put the folded towel over the barrel and hold tight.
9. With your right hand, twist and pull the plunger.

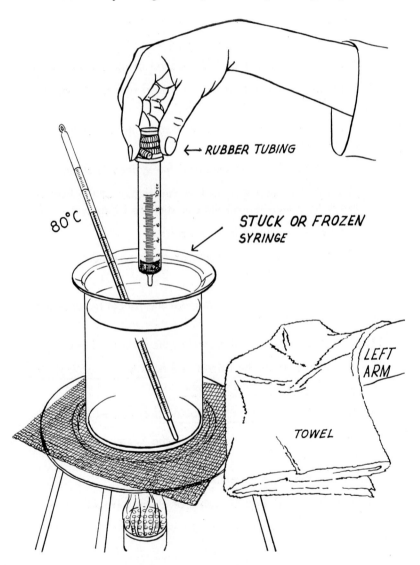

FIG. 37.—Loosening a frozen syringe.

Procedure for Step 12

1. Take the needle and syringe to the sink.

2. Place the needle on a table or clean surface.

3. Remove the plunger from the barrel of the syringe.

4. Let water from the faucet (tap water) run into the barrel until the barrel is about $\frac{3}{4}$ full.

5. Put the plunger in the barrel and force the water through the barrel.

6. Repeat the above process until the syringe is clean.

    Note: If some blood is stuck in the bottom of the barrel, get a long wooden applicator stick and loosen it.

7. Remove the plunger from the barrel.

8. Place the plunger on a table or clean surface.

9. Pick up the needle.

10. Hold the hub of the needle under the faucet to force out most of the blood.

11. Using tap water, fill the barrel of the syringe about $\frac{3}{4}$ full.

12. Put the needle on the barrel and <u>hold it there so it does not fall off and dull the point.</u>

13. <u>Holding the needle on the barrel,</u> proceed as follows:

14. Pick up the plunger and force the water through the needle (Fig. 38).

15. Remove the needle from the syringe.

16. Place the needle on the table or clean surface.

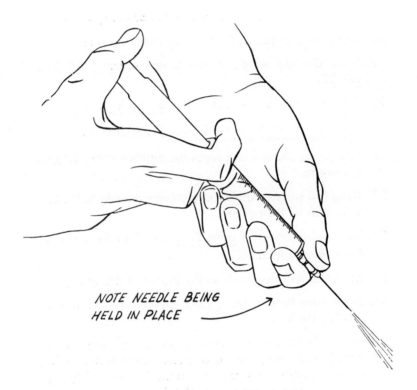

NOTE NEEDLE BEING
HELD IN PLACE

FIG. 38.—Cleaning the needle and syringe.

17. Remove the plunger from the barrel of the syringe.

18. Place the plunger on the table or clean surface.

19. Using distilled water, fill the barrel about ¾ full (see Fig. 39).

20. Put the needle on the barrel and hold it in place.

21. Holding the needle on the barrel, proceed as follows:

22. Pick up the plunger and force the distilled water through the needle.

23. Using tap water, wash off any blood adhering to the outside shaft of the needle.

24. Then put the needle, point first, back into the test tube from whence it came.

25. Separate the plunger from the barrel of the syringe.

26. Set the needle and syringe in a beaker until it is time to sterilize them.

27. Note: After the above cleaning process, the needle and syringe are ready for sterilization. Some technologists, however, prefer to further clean the needle and syringe with soap and water before sterilization.

28. Turn to step 13, checking the patient's wound.

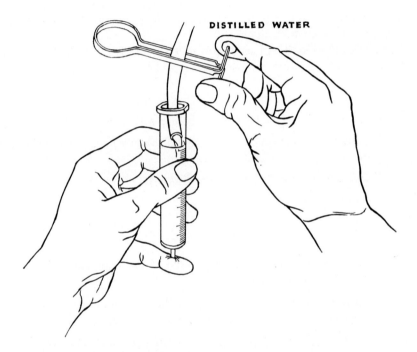

DISTILLED WATER

FIG. 39.—Filling the barrel of the syringe with distilled water.

STEP 13:   CHECKING THE PATIENT'S WOUND

Discussion of Step 13

After the patient has applied pressure for 3 to 5 minutes, the technologist should check the wound to make certain that bleeding has ceased.

When bleeding has ceased, the area should be cleansed with a fresh piece of cotton moistened with alcohol.

Sometimes the blood will seep into the flesh and leave a black and blue mark known as a hematoma.   A hematoma may be caused by:

(*a*) Failure to have the needle completely in the vein

(*b*) Failure to release the tourniquet before withdrawing the needle

(*c*) Jerking the needle out of the vein and thereby partially severing the vein

(*d*) Failure to apply pressure for a sufficient length of time

(*e*) Repeated punctures of the vein

Procedure for Step 13

1. After you have cleaned the needle and syringe, check the patient's wound (Fig. 40).

2. If bleeding has not ceased, have the patient continue the application of pressure until bleeding stops.

3. When bleeding has stopped, moisten a piece of cotton with alcohol and cleanse the area.

4. Thank the patient.

5. Note: If the patient is a child, put a "band-aid" on the wound and give the child a lollipop.

6. Clean up your table or workbench.

7. Check the blood tray for supplies and, if necessary, replenish it with cotton, needles, etc.

8. Put your equipment away.

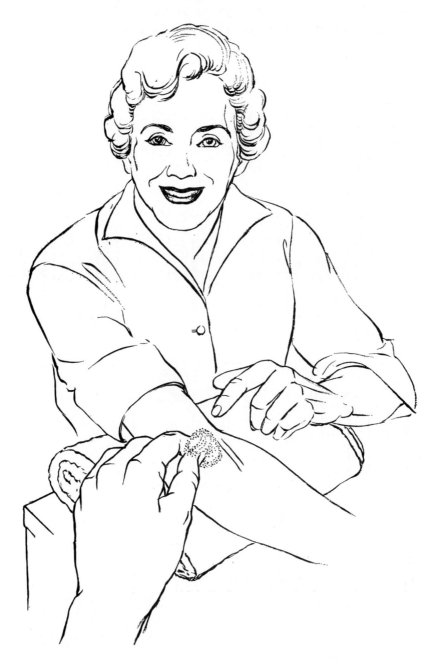

FIG. 40.—Checking the patient's wound after the venipuncture.

B-D VACUTAINER METHOD OF MAKING A VENIPUNCTURE

(Courtesy of Becton, Dickinson and Company)

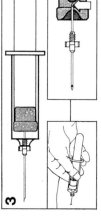

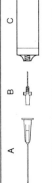

3

Push tube forward until top of stopper meets guide line. Let go. Tube stopper will retract below guide line—leave it in that position.

At this stage, the full point of the needle is embedded in the stopper (see cross section) thus avoiding blood leakage upon venipuncture and preventing premature loss of vacuum.

Alternate Method

If needle and adapter are used, follow these instructions in place of steps 1 and 2.

Description of parts:
A. Luer Hub Needle
B. VACUTAINER Adapter
C. Plastic Holder

Thread adapter into holder...tighten firmly!
Attach Luer Needle to Adapter slip as you would needle to a syringe. Place tube in holder with needle touching stopper, then proceed to step 3, above.

how to assemble

1

Description of parts:
A. Evacuated Glass Tube with Rubber Stopper
B. Plastic Holder with Guide Line
C. Double-Pointed Needle

2

Thread needle into holder ... tighten firmly!
Place tube in holder with needle touching stopper.

Fig. 41.—How to assemble B-D Vacutainer.

how to use

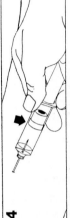

4

Where vein cannot be located — to conserve vacuum — remove tube from rear cannula (see arrow) before withdrawing needle from tissue.

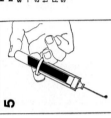

5

How to obtain blood drops for red and white cell counts, blood smears, etc. After tube is filled — grasp holder as illustrated and press firmly on bottom of tube. After each drop, release pressure and repeat for successive drops.

Additional Information

Incomplete Venipuncture, which may cause the tube to fill slowly or partially, may be corrected by deeper vein entry.
Transfixing of the vein may be corrected by pulling back slowly with needle until flow of blood indicates vein lumen re-entry.
Multiple Specimens (2, 3 or more) may be taken with one venipuncture and without loss of blood by releasing tourniquet while first tube is filling, and switching tubes while needle remains in vein.
Vein occlusion can be minimized by using VACUTAINER Adapter and smaller gauge needles (23, 24 or 25 gauge), thus slowing up flow of blood.
Proper degree of vacuum in each VACUTAINER Tube is doubly assured by the B-D Can Pack.

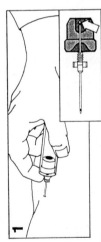

1

With rear point embedded in stopper, enter tissue — and immediately on tissue entry complete puncture of diaphragm.

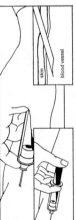

2

If in vein — blood flows immediately. Note: Technologist with small hands, proceed as you would with a hypodermic syringe. Holder provides finger grip and tube acts as plunger (see inset).

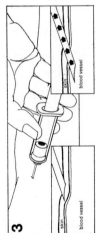

3

skin
blood vessel

If in tissue instead of vein — blood will not be drawn. Proceed until venipuncture is signaled by intake of blood into VACUTAINER Tube, as shown.

FIG. 42.—How to use B-D Vacutainer.

OBTAINING BLOOD FROM AN INFANT

If only a few drops are needed for examination, the blood is obtained by puncturing the infant's heel or big toe. This is done in a manner similar to obtaining blood from a finger.

If more than a few drops are required, the blood is obtained by either the capillary tube method or the venipuncture method. About 1 cc. of blood may be obtained by the capillary tube method. And about 10 cc. of blood may be obtained by the venipuncture method.

The procedures for the capillary tube method and the venipuncture method are given below.

PROCEDURE FOR THE CAPILLARY TUBE METHOD

1. Get the blood tray containing equipment for a finger puncture.

2. If anticoagulated blood is being prepared: Get about 12 anticoagulated capillary tubes. (These are thin tubes about 4 inches long. They are coated on the inside with some anticoagulant.)

3. If serum is being prepared: Get about 12 plain capillary tubes.

4. Moisten a piece of cotton with 70% alcohol.

5. With the moistened cotton, cleanse the infant's heel or big toe.

6. With a piece of dry cotton, dry the heel or big toe.

7. Using a sterile blood lancet, puncture the heel or big toe.

8. With a piece of dry cotton, wipe away the first drop of blood.

9. Massage the heel or big toe to produce a rounded drop of blood.

10. Take one of the capillary tubes (anticoagulated tube if you want anticoagulated blood; plain tube if you want serum).

11. Put one end of the tube in the drop of blood and tilt the other end of the tube downward so the blood will flow into the tube (Fig. 43).

12. When the capillary tube is full, place it in a horizontal position so the blood will not run out.

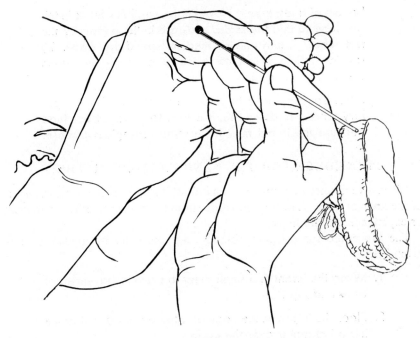

FIG. 43.—Capillary tube method of obtaining blood from an infant.

13. Using the above technique, fill about 10 capillary tubes.

14. Place a piece of cotton moistened with alcohol on the puncture and hold it there until bleeding ceases.

15. Ask the nurse or infant's mother to check the wound in about 10 minutes.

16. If anticoagulated blood is being prepared, let the contents of each tube drain into a small test tube.

    Note: Do not put your mouth directly on the capillary tube because the infant may have some contagious disease. You may have to get a rubber sucking tube (used to dilute the blood for the white cell count) and blow the blood out of each capillary tube.

17. If serum is being prepared, seal off one end of each capillary tube by either of the following methods: (a) Push one end of the tube in some soft clay or (b) hold one end in a flame until the glass melts. When you have one end of each tube sealed off, allow the blood to clot (takes about 30 minutes). Then stuff a little cotton in the

bottom of a test tube. Now put the capillary tubes in this test tube so that the *sealed ends* are in the *bottom* of the test tube. Centrifuge at medium speed for about 15 minutes. Then break off each tube where the serum begins and let drain into a small test tube.

Note: You may have to blow the serum out of the capillary tubes. In doing this, it is best to use a rubber tube because the infant may have some contagious disease.

PROCEDURE FOR THE VENIPUNCTURE METHOD

When a venipuncture is made on an infant, it is usually made on the veins of the scalp or neck. This venipuncture should be performed by a physician or experienced technologist.

The procedure for obtaining blood from the external jugular vein is given below.

1. Wrap the infant in a small sheet to prevent movement of arms and legs.

2. Place the infant on the edge of a table or bed so that the head just hangs over the edge.

3. Now pin the sheet holding the baby to the table or bed.

4. Turn the baby's head to one side and locate the external jugular vein. If the baby cries—or can be induced to cry—the external jugular vein becomes quite prominent. You do not, of course, use a tourniquet to locate the vein.

5. Cleanse the area with a piece of cotton moistened with alcohol.

6. Attach a sterile needle to a syringe.

7. Hold the skin taut, insert the needle, and withdraw the blood.

8. Withdraw the needle and place the piece of cotton moistened with alcohol on the site of the puncture. Apply gentle pressure until bleeding has ceased.

9. Note: In obtaining blood from infants, it is always a good policy to double check the wound and make certain that bleeding has ceased before leaving the room or ward.

Chapter 3

Preparation of Blood

BEFORE the blood is tested, it usually undergoes some form of preparation. For example, in order to count the cells, the technologist dilutes the blood. In order to study the different types of cells, he makes a blood smear. For other tests, he may obtain plasma or serum.

The various preparations of blood are listed below and discussed on the following pages.

1. Diluted blood
2. Blood smear
3. Anticoagulated blood
4. Blood plasma
5. Blood serum
6. Cell suspension

DILUTED BLOOD

Quite often, the physician seeks information regarding the number of cells in a patient's blood. This information aids him considerably in the diagnosis and treatment of many diseases.

The red cells, white cells, and platelets are so highly concentrated, however, that the blood must be diluted in order to count them. The dilution is made by sucking a measured portion of blood and diluting fluid into a pipet. A pipet containing diluted blood is illustrated in Figure 44.

BLOOD AND
DILUTING FLUID

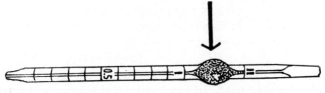

FIG. 44.—Pipet containing diluted blood.

Diluted blood is used in the following tests:

> White cell count
> Red cell count
> Hemoglobin determination
> Mean corpuscular values
> Red cell indexes
> Platelet count (direct method)
> Eosinophil count

Diluted blood is not very stable. For the platelet count, the diluted blood will only keep about 30 minutes. After this, the platelets begin to disintegrate. For the other tests listed above, however, the diluted blood will keep for about 2 hours.

BLOOD SMEAR

An examination of the type, maturity, and appearance of the red and white cells may furnish the physician with extremely significant information. To perform this test, it is necessary to make a blood smear.

The blood smear is made by placing a drop of blood on a glass slide and spreading or smearing the blood over the slide (Fig. 45).

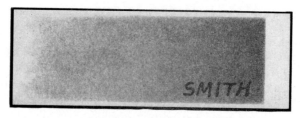

FIG. 45.—Blood smear.

A blood smear is used in the following tests:

> Differential white cell count
> Stained red cell examination
> Reticulocyte count
> Platelet count (indirect method)
> L. E. cell examination
> Bone marrow smears

After the blood smear has been made, it is stained. During the staining process, the cells are "fixed" or preserved. If the cells are not fixed, they may become distorted.

As a rule, the blood smear should be stained within 2 hours after it is made. This will fix the cells and prevent any distortion.*

When the blood smear has been stained, it will keep indefinitely. After about 2 years, however, the colors may begin to fade.

ANTICOAGULATED BLOOD

In many cases, the physician is interested in the volume occupied by the red cells and the speed of their fall. Since clotted blood can not be used to perform these tests, an agent is needed to prevent the blood from clotting. Such an agent is called an anticoagulant.

An anticoagulant prevents the blood from clotting by removing or inactivating one of the essential factors in coagulation. An example follows.

Calcium is one of the essential factors in coagulation. It is normally present in blood. When oxalate salts are added to blood, they react with the calcium. The reaction produces calcium oxalate. The calcium oxalate precipitates. And the blood, lacking calcium, can not clot.

Some of the more popular anticoagulants are: (1) a mixture of ammonium oxalate and potassium oxalate, (2) Sequestrene, (3) heparin, and (4) sodium citrate.

When the mixture of ammonium oxalate and potassium oxalate is used as the anticoagulant, the test tube containing the powdered oxalate is commonly referred to as an oxalated tube.

When Sequestrene is used as the anticoagulant, the test tube containing the Sequestrene is commonly referred to as a Sequestrenized tube. By a similar token, we may have a heparinized tube or a citrated tube.

Oxalated tubes and Sequestrenized tubes are used by most laboratories. These tubes are usually prepared in advance and set aside until needed. They do not deteriorate.

The term, anticoagulated tube, is a general term applying to an oxalated tube, Sequestrenized tube, heparinized tube, or citrated tube.

When blood is added to an oxalated tube, we call it oxalated blood. When blood is added to a Sequestrenized tube, we call it Sequestrenized blood. By a similar token, we may have heparinized blood or citrated blood.

Oxalated blood and Sequestrenized blood are used by most laboratories.

The term, anticoagulated blood, is a general term applying to oxalated blood, Sequestrenized blood, heparinized blood, and citrated blood.

Since questions concerning anticoagulants are frequently found on student examinations, the student should carefully study the anticoagulants in Table 1.

* The cells may also be fixed and thereby preserved by simply dipping the slide in methyl alcohol.

Table 1.

The Action, Function, and Preparation of Anticoagulants

1. Mixture of Ammonium Oxalate and Potassium Oxalate

The mixture of ammonium oxalate and potassium oxalate is also referred to by the following terms: Heller and Paul's mixture, double oxalate, balanced oxalate, and Wintrobe's anticoagulant.

The mixture of ammonium oxalate and potassium oxalate prevents the blood from clotting by removing and precipitating the calcium.

This anticoagulant prevents the blood cells from swelling or shrinking and it can therefore be used for examinations in hematology.

This anticoagulant, however, contains nitrogen (in the ammonium, NH_4). It also contains potassium (in the potassium oxalate). Therefore, blood containing this anticoagulant should not be used for such blood chemistry tests as urea nitrogen, nonprotein nitrogen, and potassium.

If it is used for the above blood chemistry tests, the nitrogen in the anticoagulant will make the urea nitrogen and nonprotein nitrogen values erroneously high. Likewise, the potassium in the anticoagulant will make the potassium values erroneously high.

The amount of anticoagulant required for 5 cc. (or less) of blood is 10 milligrams.

Preparation of mixture of ammonium oxalate and potassium oxalate solution: Using the rough balance, weigh out 12.0 grams of ammonium oxalate and 8.0 grams of potassium oxalate. Place them in a 1 liter volumetric flask and add distilled water to the 1 liter mark. Mix. Note: Some technologists add 4 or 5 cc. of formalin (40% formaldehyde) to the solution. This acts as a preservative.

Preparation of oxalated tubes: Place 0.5 cc. of the above solution in a test tube and evaporate to dryness either at room temperature or in an oven which is not over 80° C. (The oxalate decomposes at higher temperatures.) The powdered oxalate remaining in the test tube will serve as an anticoagulant for 5 cc. (or less) of blood.

2. Sequestrene

Sequestrene is also known as Versene and EDTA. It is the sodium or potassium salt of ethylenediamine tetraacetic acid.

Sequestrene prevents the blood from clotting by removing and "binding" the calcium.

Sequestrene may be used for both hematology and chemistry tests. It is considered an excellent anticoagulant and it is widely used.

The amount of Sequestrene required for 10 cc. (or less) of blood is 10 milligrams of the dry powder or 0.1 cc. of a 10% solution.

Preparation of 10% Sequestrene solution: Using the rough balance, weigh out 10 grams of Sequestrene. Place in a clean bottle and add 100 cc. of distilled water. Mix.

Preparation of Sequestrenized tubes: Put 0.1 cc. of the 10% Sequestrene solution in a test tube. The Sequestrene in the test tube does not have to be evaporated; it may be used in the liquid form. It does not deteriorate. The Sequestrenized tube will serve as an anticoagulant for 10 cc. (or less) of blood.

3. Heparin

Heparin is believed to prevent the blood from clotting by hindering the formation of thrombin.

Heparin is a good anticoagulant but it is expensive.

When heparin is used as an anticoagulant, blood smears stained with Wright's stain have a blue background.

The amount of heparin required for 10 cc. (or less) of blood is 0.2 cc. of a saturated solution or 2 milligrams of the dry powder.

Preparation of saturated heparin solution: Using the rough balance, weigh out 1.0 gram of powdered heparin. Place in a clean bottle and add 100 cc. of distilled water. Mix.

Preparation of heparinized tubes: Pipet 0.2 cc. of the saturated heparin solution into a test tube. The heparin in the test tube may be used in the liquid form or evaporated to dryness at room temperature (or in a 37° C. incubator or water bath). The heparinized tube will serve as an anticoagulant for 10 cc. (or less) of blood.

4. Sodium Citrate

Sodium citrate prevents the blood from clotting by removing and "binding" the calcium.

Sodium citrate is used mainly as an anticoagulant in the collection of blood for transfusions.

The blood is collected in a sterile ACD solution.

The sterile ACD solution contains the following ingredients: tri-sodium citrate (22.0 Gm.); citric acid (8.0 Gm.); dextrose (24.5 Gm.); and distilled water to make 1000 milliliters.

For each 100 milliliters of blood to be drawn, 15 milliliters of the above sterile ACD solution is used.

To prepare oxalated blood or Sequestrenized blood, proceed as follows:

1. Make a venipuncture and withdraw about 5 cc. (cubic centimeters) of blood.
2. Transfer to an oxalated tube (or Sequestrenized tube).
3. Mix the blood and anticoagulant *by completely inverting the test tube 10 to 12 times. Do not shake!*

Oxalated blood and Sequestrenized blood are used as blood preparations in the following tests: sedimentation rate, hematocrit reading, **ABO** grouping, and Rh typing.

When these tests are performed, the oxalated blood or Sequestrenized blood must be used within a specified time. Otherwise the blood undergoes changes which make the results inaccurate.

For the above tests, the oxalated blood and Sequestrenized blood have the following keeping time:

Test	Approximate Keeping Time of Oxalated Blood and Sequestrenized Blood
sedimentation rate	2 hr.
hematocrit reading	24 hr.
ABO grouping	48 hr.
Rh typing	48 hr.

In addition to being used as blood preparations for the above tests, oxalated blood and Sequestrenized blood have another very important function.

Although they themselves are blood preparations, they are used to make other blood preparations.

For example, oxalated blood and Sequestrenized blood may be used to make the *diluted blood* for a white cell count. Or they may be used to make the *blood smear* for a differential white cell count.

In view of the above, the following question arises: When oxalated blood or Sequestrenized blood is used to make other blood preparations, what is the keeping time?

For example, suppose oxalated blood is made this morning. Can it be used this afternoon to make the *diluted blood* for a white cell count?

The approximate keeping time of oxalated blood and Sequestrenized blood for the various tests is given in Table 2.

A few points to remember:

(1) When oxalated blood or Sequestrenized blood is being saved for future use, it should be stored in the refrigerator. Upon removal from the refrigerator, it should be thoroughly mixed by *completely* inverting the test tube 40 to 50 times.

(2) Oxalated blood should *not* be used for the following blood chemistry tests: urea nitrogen, nonprotein nitrogen, and potassium (see Table 1, page 78).

(3) Sequestrenized blood may be used for the above blood chemistry tests. It may also be used for most blood chemistry tests which call for an anticoagulant in the blood.

(4) When blood is drawn for blood chemistry tests, the patient must be fasting, that is, he must not have eaten for 8 hours prior to the withdrawal of blood. If the patient is not fasting, digested food material may interfere with the accuracy of the chemical test.

Table 2.

Approximate Keeping Time of Oxalated Blood and Sequestrenized Blood

Test	Keeping Time
White cell count	24 hr.
Red cell count	24 hr.
Hemoglobin determination	24 hr.
Differential white cell count	1 hr.
Stained red cell examination	1 hr.
Sedimentation rate	2 hr.
Hematocrit reading	24 hr.
Reticulocyte count	1 hr.
Mean corpuscular values	3 hr.
Red cell indexes	3 hr.
Platelet count	
Direct method	1 hr.
Indirect method	1 hr.
Eosinophil count	2 hr.
Abnormal hemoglobins	2 hr.
Bone marrow smears	1 hr.
ABO grouping	48 hr.
Rh typing	48 hr.
Coombs' test (direct test)	2 hr.
Malaria smears	1 hr.

BLOOD PLASMA

A centrifuge is an instrument which spins fluids at a high rate of speed. For example, the average centrifuge spins fluids at the rate of 3,000 RPM (revolutions per minute). This forces the solid material to the bottom and leaves the liquid portion above. A typical centrifuge, with the operating directions, is shown in Figure 46, page 82.

When anticoagulated blood is centrifuged, the cells go to the bottom of the test tube. The liquid portion above the cells is blood plasma.
Blood plasma is used in the following tests:

> Fibrinogen deficiency test
> Prothrombin time
> Partial thromboplastin time

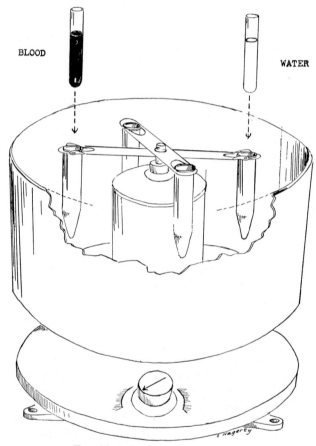

FIG. 46.—Operation of centrifuge.

1. Obtain a test tube of oxalated blood.
2. Get a test tube that is *exactly* the same size as the test tube containing the blood.
3. Add water to this test tube until the level of water is *exactly* equal to the level of blood in the other test tube.
4. Place the test tube containing the blood in one holder.
5. Place the test tube containing the water in the *opposite* holder. (This balances the centrifuge.)
6. Turn the operating dial to the desired speed (full speed unless otherwise specified).
7. Allow to spin for about 10 minutes.
8. Stop by turning the operating dial in the reverse direction.

The blood plasma used in the above tests, however, must be prepared with a special type and quantity of anticoagulant. The type and quantity of anticoagulant is specified in the procedure for each test.

To obtain blood plasma, proceed as follows:

1. Make a venipuncture and withdraw about 5 cc. of blood.
2. Transfer the blood to a test tube containing the specified type and quantity of anticoagulant.
3. Mix the blood and anticoagulant *by completely inverting the test tube 10 to 12 times. Do not shake!*
4. Centrifuge the blood at full speed for about 10 minutes.
5. Remove the blood from the centrifuge.
6. Using a medicine dropper or pipet, remove the plasma and transfer it to another test tube.
7. Blood plasma does not keep. As a general rule, the blood plasma should be prepared directly after the blood is withdrawn. Then it should be used immediately.

BLOOD SERUM

If blood is placed in a test tube, it forms a clot. The clot contracts and expresses a fluid known as serum. The serum differs from plasma in that it contains no fibrinogen—a substance used in the formation of the clot.

Blood serum is seldom used for examinations in hematology but it is frequently used for tests in serology and blood chemistry.

To obtain serum, proceed as follows:

1. Make a venipuncture and withdraw about 5 cc. of blood.
2. Transfer the blood to a serological tube (Fig. 47).
3. Place the test tube containing the blood in a beaker or test tube rack.
4. Let it stand for at least 30 minutes. This allows the blood to clot.

   Note: If you wish, you may let the blood stand for several hours before continuing to the next step.

5. Get a toothpick or applicator stick and gently loosen the clot so it does not stick to the walls of the test tube.
6. Centrifuge at full speed for about 10 minutes.
7. Remove the blood from the centrifuge.
8. Using a medicine dropper or pipet, remove the serum and transfer it to another test tube.
9. Serum will keep for several days. It is best, however, to keep it stored in the refrigerator.

CELL SUSPENSION

What happens when blood is placed in a salt solution?

If the salt concentration is less than 0.85%, water passes through the membrane covering the red cells. The red cells swell. Eventually they rupture or hemolyze. Such a salt solution is a *hypotonic solution* (see Fig. 48).

On the other hand, if the salt concentration is more than 0.85%, water leaves the red cells. The red cells shrink or crenate. Such a salt solution is a *hypertonic solution* (see Fig. 49).

However, if the salt concentration is exactly 0.85%, water neither enters nor leaves the red cells. The red cells neither swell nor shrink. Such a salt solution is an *isotonic solution*.

You may recall from your previous studies that the hypotonic and hypertonic solutions illustrate the principle of osmosis: When two liquids of

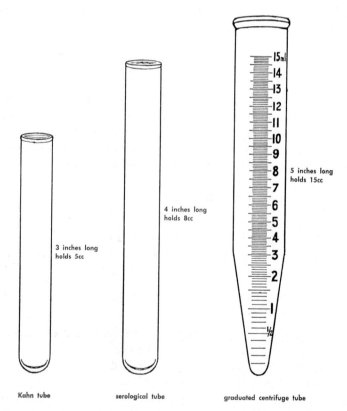

Kahn tube   serological tube   graduated centrifuge tube

FIG. 47.—Test tubes used in hematology. For all practical purposes, 1 cc. (cubic centimeter) equals 1 ml. (milliliter). Therefore, cc. may be used in place of ml. and vice versa.

different densities are separated by a semipermeable membrane (the membrane covering the red cells), *the flow of water is always toward the greater density.*

In the case of the isotonic solution, the density outside the red cells is the same as the density inside the red cells. Therefore, there is no flow of water.

Since isotonic solutions do not change the red cells, they can be used to preserve the red cells. This preservation of the red cells is essential in the performance of some tests.

An isotonic solution may be made with various types of salt: sodium chloride, calcium chloride, potassium chloride, etc.

If the isotonic solution is made with sodium chloride, the solution is called *physiological sodium chloride* or *physiological saline.*

Physiological saline is widely used in medical laboratories.

The physiological saline is often referred to as "normal" saline. This

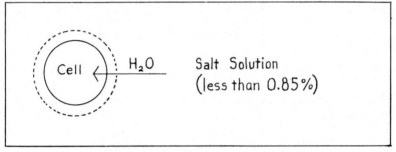

Red Cell in Hypotonic Solution

FIG. 48.—Water leaving hypotonic solution and entering red cell.

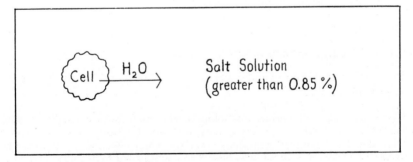

Red Cell in Hypertonic Solution

FIG. 49.—Water leaving red cell and entering hypertonic solution.

means that it is normal from a physiological point of view. It is not, however, normal from a chemical point of view.*

Physiological saline is prepared by placing 8.50 grams of sodium chloride in a 1 liter volumetric flask and adding distilled water to the 1 liter mark.

When physiological saline is poured into a test tube and a few drops of blood are added, the preparation is called a *cell suspension.*

A cell suspension is rarely used for examinations in hematology but it is occasionally used for tests in serology and blood banking.

The cell suspension should be used within 2 hours after it is prepared. Otherwise, the cells may lose their clumping or agglutinating power.

The cell suspension may be made by any of the methods given below. When a 2% cell suspension is called for, however, the second method is preferred. When a cell suspension in serum is called for, the third method is employed.

METHOD 1:

1. Pour about 4 cc. of physiological saline into a Kahn tube (Fig. 47, page 84).
2. Add a few drops of either finger tip blood or fresh anticoagulated blood.
3. Place a stopper in the mouth of the tube and invert several times to mix the cells.

METHOD 2 (2% cell suspension):

1. Using a 1 milliliter serological pipet, transfer 0.4 milliliter of fresh anticoagulated blood to a graduated centrifuge tube (Fig. 47, page 84).
2. Add physiological saline to the 10 milliliter mark.
3. Mix by inverting the tube several times.

METHOD 3 (cell suspension in serum):

1. Make a venipuncture and expel about 5 cc. of blood into a serological test tube.

---

* When we speak of normal physiological solutions, we are concerned with weight or density. When we speak of normal chemical solutions, however, we are concerned with ionic or electrical ability. There is quite a difference. For example, a normal physiological solution may have *8.50* grams of salt in one liter. Whereas a normal chemical solution may have *58.45* grams of salt in one liter.

2. Allow to clot (takes about 30 minutes).
3. Using a toothpick or applicator stick, gently loosen the clot so it does not stick to the walls of the test tube.
4. Centrifuge at full speed for about 10 minutes.
5. *Very gently* shake the tube so that some of the cells are shaken into the serum.
6. With a quick deliberate motion, pour about 1 cc. of the serum into another test tube.
7. Note: The serum containing the suspended cells may also be removed with a medicine dropper or pipet.

SUMMARY

This chapter concludes with 3 summaries:

A summary of the approximate keeping time of the six blood preparations is given in Table 3.

A summary of the most frequently performed examinations and the blood preparation required is given in Table 4, page 88.

A summary of the six blood preparations is given in Plate 1, page 88.

Table 3.

Approximate Keeping Time of the Six Blood Preparations

Blood Preparation	Approximate Keeping Time
Diluted blood	2 hours (except for platelet count which should be done within 30 minutes)
Blood smear	2 hours before staining 2 years after staining
Anticoagulated blood	varies with test; see Table 2, page 81
Blood plasma	should be prepared from fresh blood and should be used immediately
Blood serum	48 hours
Cell suspension	2 hours

Table 4.

Most Frequently Performed Examinations and the Blood Preparation Required*

Test	*Blood Preparation Required*
White cell count	Diluted blood
Red cell count	Diluted blood
Hemoglobin determination	Diluted blood or none
Differential white cell count	Blood smear
Stained red cell examination	Blood smear
Sedimentation rate	Anticoagulated blood
Hematocrit reading	Anticoagulated blood
Reticulocyte count	Blood smear
Sickle cell examination	Anticoagulated blood or none
Osmotic fragility test	None
Mean corpuscular values	Diluted blood and anticoagulated blood
Red cell indexes	Diluted blood and anticoagulated blood
Bleeding time	None
Coagulation time	None
Platelet count	Diluted blood or blood smear
Clot retraction time	None
Fibrinogen deficiency test	Blood plasma
Prothrombin time	Blood plasma
Partial thromboplastin time	Blood plasma
Eosinophil count	Diluted blood
Spinal cell count	(Spinal fluid)
L. E. cell examination	Blood clot and blood smear
Fetal hemoglobin determination	Anticoagulated blood
Hemoglobin electrophoretic separations	Anticoagulated blood
Bone marrow smears	Blood smear

* Note that several of the tests require no blood preparation. In these tests, the blood is used directly as it comes from the patient.

Some of the tests may be performed with one blood preparation or another blood preparation. For example, a platelet count may be performed with *diluted blood* or a *blood smear*. The type of blood preparation is governed by the method of performing the test.

Several of the tests require two different blood preparations. For example, the red cell indexes require diluted blood and anticoagulated blood.

PLATE 1

Summary of the Six Blood Preparations

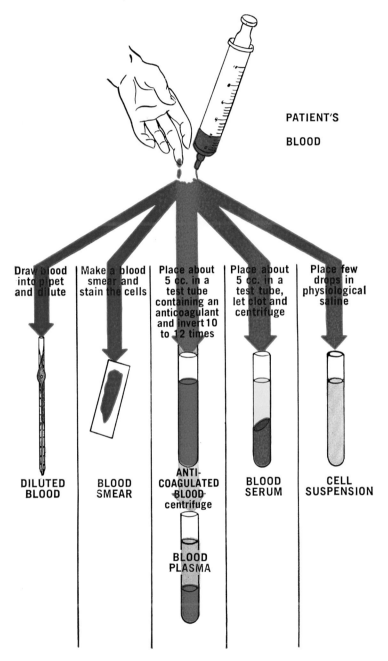

PATIENT'S BLOOD

| Draw blood into pipet and dilute | Make a blood smear and stain the cells | Place about 5 cc. in a test tube containing an anticoagulant and invert 10 to 12 times | Place about 5 cc. in a test tube, let clot and centrifuge | Place few drops in physiological saline |

DILUTED BLOOD

BLOOD SMEAR

ANTI-COAGULATED BLOOD
centrifuge

BLOOD SERUM

CELL SUSPENSION

BLOOD PLASMA

PART 2
Complete Blood Count

INTRODUCTION

THE complete blood count consists of 5 tests: white cell count, red cell count, hemoglobin determination, differential white cell count, and stained red cell examination.

In addition to the 5 tests listed above, the complete blood count usually consists of a color index and a platelet estimation.

The color index is a calculation which furnishes information relative to the amount of hemoglobin in the red cells. It will be discussed under the hemoglobin determination.

The platelet estimation is simply a very rough estimation of the number of platelets in the blood smear. It will be discussed under the differential white cell count.

The complete blood count is used in the diagnosis of many diseases and it is a popular series of tests. In fact, about half the requisitions coming into the hematology department call for a complete blood count. In view of this, the material of this section should be thoroughly mastered by the student.

A complete blood count is commonly referred to as a CBC. A sample CBC report, including the normal values, is given in Fig. 50.

The normal values for the various tests in a complete blood count may vary slightly from textbook to textbook.

For example, the following authors give the accompanying normal values for the red cell count in women.

Wintrobe	4.2 to 5.4 million per cu. mm.
Miale	3.6 to 5.0 million per cu. mm.
Goodale	4.6 to 4.8 million per cu. mm.

The above variations are no cause for alarm; similar variations may be found in any growing science.

The student may also find that the tests performed in a CBC may vary slightly from laboratory to laboratory. For example, some laboratories may omit the red cell count in their CBC. Other laboratories may include a hematocrit reading in their CBC.

Each of the 5 tests performed in our presentation of the complete blood count will be confined to a separate chapter, the material being presented as follows

7

Complete Blood Count

REPORT OF A COMPLETE BLOOD COUNT

Patient: Dickson, Miss Candice   85 006
Date: 7-7-72
Physician: Dr. Tom Maxwell

Test	Patient's Values	Normal Values
White Cell Count	6,800	5,000 to 10,000 per cu. mm.
Red Cell Count	5,000,000	women: 4.0 to 5.5 million per cu. mm.
		men: 4.5 to 6.0 million per cu. mm.
		infants: 5.0 to 6.5 million per cu. mm.
Hemoglobin Determination	15 Grams	women: 12 to 16 Gm. per 100 cc. (83% to 110%)
(Haden-Hausser method)	(97%)	men: 14 to 18 Gm. per 100 cc. (97% to 124%)
		infants: 14 to 20 Gm. per 100 cc. (97% to 138%)
Color Index	1.0	0.9 to 1.1
Differential White Cell Count		
Myeloblasts	0	0%
Progranulocytes	0	0%
Neutrophilic myelocytes	0	0%
Neutrophilic metamyelocytes	0	0%
Neutrophilic band cells	4	2% to 6%
Neutrophilic segmented cells	60	55% to 75%
Lymphocytes	30	20% to 35%
Monocytes	4	2% to 6%
Eosinophilic segmented cells	2	1% to 3%
Basophilic segmented cells	0	0% to 1%
Miscellaneous white cells		
abnormal lymphocytes	0	0%
plasmacytes	0	0%
disintegrated cells	0	0%
Platelet estimation	Normal	4 to 8 for every 100 red cells
Stained Red Cell Examination		
Nucleated Red Cells		
rubriblasts	0	0
prorubricytes	0	0
rubricytes	0	0
metarubricytes	0	0
total	0	0
Abnormal Erythrocytes		
hypochromia	absent	absent
anisocytosis	absent	absent
poikilocytosis	absent	absent
miscellaneous		
sickle cells	absent	absent
target cells	absent	absent
Cabot rings, etc.	absent	absent
		absent

Examinations performed by: *Sandra Frisbee*

FIG. 50.—Sample CBC report.

Chapter 4

White Cell Count

THE white cell count is also referred to as a white blood cell count, white blood count, WBC, w.b.c., leukocyte count, total leukocyte count, white corpuscle count, and white corpuscle enumeration.

The discussion of the white cell count will cover the following:

> Significance of the White Cell Count
> Discussion of Procedures for the White Cell Count
> Microscopic Method for the White Cell Count
> Coulter Counter Method for the White Cell Count

The student review questions for the white cell count are numbered 25–36 and begin on page 728 of the Appendix.

SIGNIFICANCE OF THE WHITE CELL COUNT

The white cell count is the number of white cells in 1 cubic millimeter of blood.

In health, the white cell count varies between 5,000 and 10,000 cells per cubic millimeter. For example, a person may have a white cell count of 6,000 in the morning and 8,000 in the afternoon. These variations are caused by baths, exercise, digestion, and similar activities.

Since the white cell count normally fluctuates between 5,000 and 10,000 cells per cubic millimeter, we can say that *the normal values for the white cell count are 5,000 to 10,000 cells per cubic millimeter of blood.*

In some diseases, the white cell count rises above the normal values. For example, in appendicitis, the white cell count may rise to 20,000 cells per cubic millimeter.

In other diseases, the white cell count drops below the normal values. For example, in measles, the white cell count may drop to 3,000 cells per cubic millimeter.

Quite often, the white cell count rises and falls—like a barometer—to indicate the course of a disease or the progress of infection.

What causes the white cell count to rise above the normal values?

A rise above the normal values is due to a stimulation of the white cell factories in the bone marrow. The stimulation may be caused by such factors as bacteria and invading organisms.

What causes the white cell count to drop below the normal values?

A drop below the normal values is due to a depression of the white cell factories in the bone marrow.   The depression may be caused by such agents as viruses and undesirable chemicals.

When the white cell count rises above the normal values, it is referred to as a leukocytosis (lu″ko-si-to′sis).

When the white cell count drops below the normal values, it is referred to as a leukopenia (lu″ko-pe′ne-ah).

Some conditions where these abnormalities may be expected are listed in Table 5.

Table 5.—Conditions Accompanied by Abnormal White Cell Counts

High White Cell Count (leukocytosis)	Low White Cell Count (leukopenia)
appendicitis	measles
pneumonia	influenza
leukemia	brucellosis
tonsillitis	typhoid fever
meningitis	agranulocytosis
abscesses	infectious hepatitis
rheumatic fever	lupus erythematosus
diphtheria	cirrhosis of liver
smallpox	paratyphoid fever
chickenpox	protein therapy
peritonitis	radiation
erythroblastosis fetalis	myxedema
uremia	psittacosis
ulcers	sandfly fever
newborn	scrub typhus
pregnancy	dengue
menstruation	rheumatoid arthritis

The white cell count is thus useful in diagnosis.

Suppose, for a moment, you have a pain in your right side.   Is the pain caused by a simple stomach-ache?   Or is it caused by something more serious, such as appendicitis?

A white cell count may be performed.   If the count is normal, it points to a simple stomach-ache.   If the count is above normal, it points to appendicitis.

The white cell count is one of the most frequently performed tests in the laboratory.   It is performed about 2,000 times a month by the average hospital laboratory and about 100 times a month by the average physician's office.

DISCUSSION OF PROCEDURES FOR THE WHITE CELL COUNT

The most commonly employed methods for performing the white cell count are:

1. Microscopic Method
2. Electronic Methods
    (1) Coulter Counter Method
    (2) SMA Counter Method
    (3) Fisher Autocytometer Method

The microscopic method is often referred to as the "manual" method, counting chamber method, or hemocytometer method.

The electronic methods are often referred to as the automatic methods or automated methods.

The methods listed above will now be discussed relative to the principle of the method and some relevant comments.

MICROSCOPIC METHOD

Principle

The microscopic method for the white cell count consists of diluting the blood and dissolving the red cells, transferring a small portion of the solution to a counting chamber, counting the white cells with a microscope, and making the calculations.

Comments

The microscopic method is direct, simple, and certainly accurate enough for diagnostic purposes.

With this method, a white cell count may be performed in about 5 minutes.

The microscopic method is used in most physicians' offices but it is being replaced by electronic methods in many hospital laboratories.

COULTER COUNTER METHOD

Principle

The white cells are suspended in a solution which is capable of conducting an electric current. This solution is then made to pass through a narrow opening between 2 electrodes. Since white cells do not conduct electricity, each passing white cell momentarily decreases a flow of current between the 2 electrodes. The decrease in current causes a voltage drop in the line. The number of voltage drops in the line is the key to the count.

Comments

With a Coulter Counter, a white cell count may be run in a matter of seconds.

A Coulter Counter is simple to operate; the operating procedure accompanies the instrument.

The Coulter Counter is illustrated in Fig. 78A, page 140.

Coulter Counters have been manufactured in several models and the price ranges between $5,000 and $70,000.

Complete information concerning the Coulter Counter may be obtained by writing Coulter Electronics, Hialeah, Florida.

SMA COUNTER METHOD

SMA stands for Sequential Multiple Analysis.

Principle

In this method, the white cells are suspended in a solution. This solution is made to pass through an optical system which causes each white cell to generate a light impulse. Each light impulse is then transformed into an electrical impulse. The number of electrical impulses are recorded and become the key to the count.

Comments

With an SMA Counter, a white cell count may also be run in a matter of seconds.

The SMA Counter is also simple to operate; the operating procedure accompanies the instrument.

SMA Counters may be purchased in a variety of models and the price ranges between $8,000 and $70,000.

Instruction manuals and further information concerning SMA Counters may be obtained by writing Technicon Corporation, Tarrytown, New York.

FISHER AUTOCYTOMETER METHOD

Principle

A bulletin published by the Fisher Scientific Company describes the principle of their instrument as follows.

"The Autocytometer utilizes an optical counting system, in which each cell or other particle in the diluted sample appears as a bright spot of light against a dark field, as it passes through a 'sensing zone' only 15 microns high. The flashes of light are picked up by a photomultiplier and converted to electrical impulses, which are totaled electronically and shown on the meter as the cell count in the original whole blood sample."

Comments

With the Fisher Autocytometer, a white cell count may also be run in a matter of seconds.

The Fisher Autocytometer costs about $3,000.

Instruction manuals and further information concerning the Fisher Autocytometer may be obtained by writing Fisher Instrument Manufacturing Division, Indiana, Pennsylvania.

MICROSCOPIC METHOD FOR THE WHITE CELL COUNT

The discussion will cover the necessary reagents and equipment, the procedure, and miscellaneous information.

NECESSARY REAGENTS AND EQUIPMENT

1. Anticoagulated blood or finger tip blood
2. White cell pipet (Fig. 51, page 96)
3. Rubber sucking tube (Fig. 52, page 98)
4. WBC diluting fluid. Note: The WBC diluting fluid is usually either 1% hydrochloric acid or 2% acetic acid. Preparations given in Appendix, page 692.
5. Counting chamber and coverglass (Fig. 57, page 105)
6. Small piece of clean cloth
7. Microscope

PROCEDURE

The procedure consists of 4 steps:

Step 1: Diluting the blood
Step 2: Charging the counting chamber
Step 3: Counting the cells
Step 4: Making the calculations

Each of the above 4 steps will be broken down into a *discussion* and a *procedure.*

The student should first read the *discussion* and then follow the directions in the *procedure.*

The student will save time if he follows the directions EXACTLY as they are given. He should not attempt to improvise. And, above all, he should not attempt to skip any steps.

STEP 1: DILUTING THE BLOOD

First read the *discussion;* then follow the directions in the *procedure.*

Discussion of Step 1

The dilution of the blood for the white cell count serves a dual purpose. First, it facilitates the counting process by suspending and dispersing the white cells. Second, it dissolves the mature red cells—the erythrocytes. This is essential since the erythrocytes greatly outnumber the white cells and would therefore interfere in the count.

The dilution for the count is made by sucking a measured portion of blood and diluting fluid into a pipet. The following equipment is needed: diluting fluid, white cell pipet, and rubber sucking tube.

The diluting fluid is usually referred to as WBC diluting fluid—the WBC standing for white blood count. The WBC diluting fluid may be any one of the following solutions: 1% hydrochloric acid solution, 2% acetic acid solution, or Türk's solution. The preparation of these solutions is given in the Appendix under preparation of solutions and reagents (page 692).

The white cell pipet attached to a rubber sucking tube is illustrated in Figure 51.

The stem of the pipet is the portion from 0.0 to 1.0. The mixing chamber is the bulb-like portion from 1.0 to 11.0.

The volume of the stem is exactly ten times less than the volume of the mixing chamber. Thus we can say that the *stem holds 1 unit of volume and the mixing chamber holds 10 units of volume.*

When we dilute the blood, we first suck up blood and then diluting fluid. The mixing chamber is thereby filled with a solution of blood and diluting fluid. The stem still contains diluting fluid but this is discarded later on in the procedure.

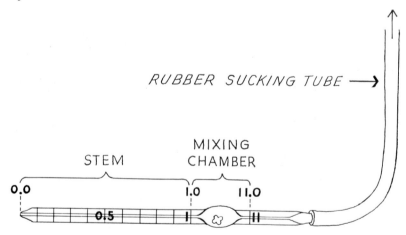

FIG. 51.—White cell pipet attached to rubber sucking tube.

Suppose blood is drawn to the 1.0 mark and diluting fluid to the 11.0 mark. The 10 units of the mixing chamber then contain 1 part blood and 9 parts diluting fluid. This is 1 part blood in 10 parts of solution (blood plus diluting fluid). Therefore, the blood has been diluted 1 in 10.

Suppose blood is drawn to the 0.5 mark and diluting fluid to the 11.0 mark. The 10 units of the mixing chamber then contain 0.5 part blood and 9.5 parts diluting fluid. This is 0.5 part blood in 10.0 parts of solution (blood plus diluting fluid). Therefore, the blood has been diluted 1 in 20.

In the 1 in 10 dilution, the number 10 is known as the dilution factor. Likewise, in the 1 in 20 dilution, the number 20 is known as the dilution factor. These dilution factors will be used later on in making the calculations.

The 1 in 10 dilution is sometimes used when the white cell count is very low. The 1 in 20 dilution, however, is used routinely. And this will be the dilution considered in our presentation of the white cell count.

The above dilutions usually give students some trouble. A good way to remember the 1 in 20 dilution is to recall that it is somewhat similar to a nickel being one-twentieth part of a dollar. Thus we may look upon the blood as a nickel, the diluting fluid 95 cents, and the entire solution one dollar.

You should note that the actual number of cubic centimeters contained in the pipet is unimportant. It is the ratio of blood to diluting fluid which is significant.

For example, 1 cc. of blood diluted with 19 cc. of diluting fluid is a dilution of 1 in 20. And the dilution factor is 20.

Also, 1 pint of blood diluted with 19 pints of diluting fluid is a dilution of 1 in 20. And the dilution factor is 20.

Thus, the exact quantity of diluted blood on hand is irrelevant. The significant point is the degree of dilution. This is expressed by the dilution factor.

You will note that if blood is drawn to the very first line and diluting fluid to the 11.0 mark, the blood has been diluted 0.1 in 10.0. This is a dilution of 1 in 100. Thus, the white cell pipet is said to have a dilution range of 1:10 to 1:100. Although this information is of little practical significance, it may be useful on student examinations.

A note of precaution before starting the procedure:

When you draw blood into the white cell pipet, you must adjust the blood so it is *exactly* on the 0.5 mark. Otherwise, a serious error is introduced into the count.

When you draw diluting fluid into the pipet, however, you may stop a little above or a little below the 11.0 mark without causing any serious error.

You may stop a little above or a little below the 11.0 mark because (1) the bore in this portion of the pipet is very small and (2) the solution in this portion of the pipet does not take part in the mixing process.

If you have trouble diluting the blood, do not get discouraged. The beginner usually has to make several attempts. The only answer is *practice*. Now follow the directions *exactly* as given in the Procedure for Step 1.

Procedure for Step 1

1. In diluting the blood, you may use anticoagulated blood or finger tip blood. However, you should use anticoagulated blood until you have completed about 6 white cell counts and somewhat mastered the technique of diluting the blood. Then you should make a finger puncture and use finger tip blood. The directions for making a finger puncture and obtaining finger tip blood are given on pages 6 to 23.

2. Assemble the following equipment: several cotton balls or gauze pads, WBC pipet, rubber sucking tube, WBC diluting fluid, test tube of anticoagulated blood, pencil, and small piece of paper.

   Note: Make sure that you have a WBC pipet and not an RBC pipet. The WBC pipet will have 11 marked just above the bulb whereas the RBC pipet will have 101 marked just above the bulb.

3. Place the above equipment within easy reach.

4. Attach the rubber sucking tube to the white cell pipet as illustrated in Figure 52.

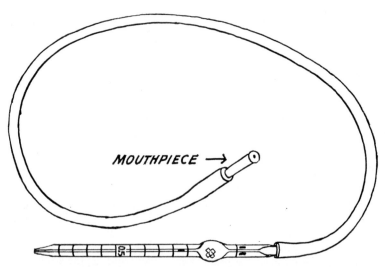

MOUTHPIECE →

Fig. 52.—Method of attaching rubber sucking tube to a white cell pipet.

5. If the rubber sucking tube has been used by someone else, dip the mouthpiece in a bottle of alcohol.

6. Then lay the pipet and rubber sucking tube on the table ready for use.

7. In the following steps, you will be sucking blood into the stem of the pipet. If you accidentally suck blood into the bulb of the pipet, immediately suck diluting fluid into the bulb until it is completely filled. Then put the pipet in the container for used pipets. Never let undiluted blood stand in the stem or bulb of a pipet because it will harden and may clog the pipet. If a pipet does become clogged with dried blood, it may be cleaned by following the directions on page 135.

8. Put a stopper in the mouth of the test tube and mix the blood by completely inverting the test tube 10 to 12 times. Do not shake the test tube.

Note: If you have a large test tube (about 4 inches long) which is less than half full of blood, it will be difficult for you to get the pipet in the blood. In such cases, after you have mixed the blood, transfer it to a small test tube (about 2 or 3 inches long).

9. After you have mixed the blood, place the test tube in a medicine glass or test tube rack. Then remove the stopper from the test tube.

10. Remove the cap from the bottle of WBC diluting fluid.

11. Study the method of sucking blood into the white cell pipet (Fig. 53).

12. Observe that the right hand holds the pipet so you can see the markings on the pipet (Fig. 53).

13. Observe that the tip of the pipet is braced against the lower inner wall of the test tube (Fig. 53).

Note: When you suck up blood, you must keep the tip of the pipet in the blood. If you momentarily lift the tip of the pipet out of the blood, you will suck an air bubble into the blood. Bracing the pipet as directed above helps to keep the pipet in the blood.

14. Now pick up your assembled white cell pipet and rubber sucking tube.

15. Put the mouthpiece of the rubber sucking tube in your mouth.

Note: Throughout the procedure, avoid getting a sharp bend or kink in the rubber sucking tube. A kink in the rubber sucking tube will cause the blood to be pushed or pulled in the stem of the pipet. (Somewhat like a sharp bend in a soda straw when you are sucking up a soda.)

16. With your right hand, hold the pipet so you can see the markings as illustrated in Figure 53.

17. With your left hand, pick up the test tube of blood.

18. Dip the pipet into the blood and brace the tip of the pipet against the lower inner wall of the test tube (Fig. 53).

19. Gently suck up blood until it is just a little bit past the 0.5 mark.

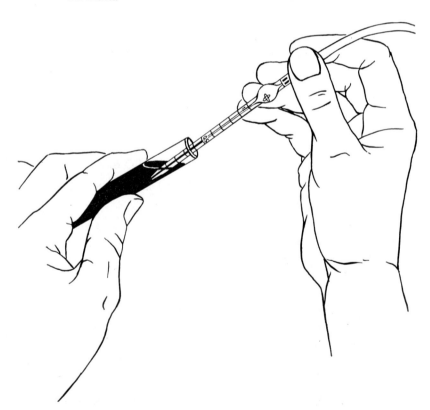

FIG. 53.—Sucking blood from a test tube into a white cell pipet.

20. Place the test tube back in the medicine glass or test tube rack.

21. Now hold the pipet as illustrated in Figure 54.

22. In the following manner, adjust the blood so it is <u>exactly</u> on the 0.5 mark:

23. Tease the blood out with your finger and blow <u>gently</u> on the rubber sucking tube.

    Note: If you remove too much blood, simply suck some blood back into the pipet.

24. When you have the blood <u>exactly</u> on the 0.5 mark, <u>press the tip of your tongue firmly against the opening in the rubber sucking tube.</u> This holds the blood in place.

    Note: You must get the blood <u>exactly</u> on the 0.5 mark. Otherwise, a serious error is introduced into the count.

25. Pick up a piece of cotton.

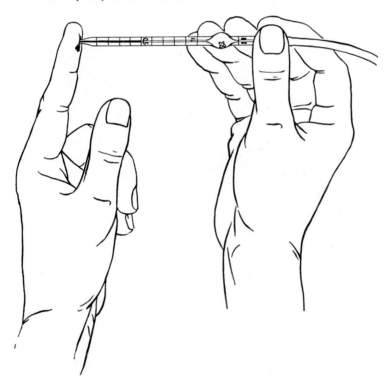

Fig. 54.—Adjusting the blood to the 0.5 mark. Note the solid column of blood. No empty spaces or air bubbles should be present in the column of blood.

26. Keeping your tongue firmly over the opening in the
    sucking tube, wipe off any blood adhering to the outside
    stem of the pipet.

27. Continue to keep your tongue over the opening in the
    sucking tube and proceed as follows:

28. Study the method of sucking WBC diluting fluid into the
    pipet (Fig. 55).

29. Observe that the right hand holds the pipet so you can
    see the 11.0 mark (Fig. 55).

30. Observe the angle of the pipet (Fig. 55).

    Note: The pipet must be held almost vertical. If the
    pipet is not held almost vertical, an air bubble will form
    in the bulb of the pipet.

31. Observe that the tip of the pipet is braced against the
    lower inner wall of the bottle (Fig. 55).

32. Hold the pipet in your right hand as illustrated in Figure
    55.

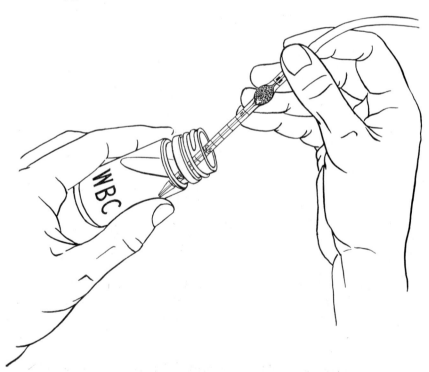

Fig. 55.—Sucking up WBC diluting fluid to the 11.0 mark.

33. With your left hand, pick up the bottle of WBC diluting fluid.

34. Check to see that the blood is <u>exactly</u> on the 0.5 mark.

35. Put the pipet in the bottle, suck up diluting fluid to the 11.0 mark, and press your tongue firmly against the opening in the sucking tube.

    Note: You may stop a little above or a little below the 11.0 mark without causing any serious error. If you go way past the 11.0 mark, however, you must detach the rubber sucking tube from the pipet. Then you must put the pipet in the container for used pipets, get another pipet, attach the pipet to the rubber sucking tube, and return to step 14.

36. Put the bottle of WBC diluting fluid on the table.

37. Now firmly hold the index finger of your left hand over the opening in the tip of the pipet. Keep this index finger of your left hand over the opening in the tip of the pipet until the next step is completed. This will prevent the loss of fluid and the formation of an air bubble in the bulb of the pipet.

38. With your right hand, detach the rubber sucking tube from the pipet.

39. Place the middle finger and thumb of your right hand over the ends of the pipet and shake for about 10 seconds. This prevents any clumping of the blood cells.

40. Air bubbles should <u>not</u> be present in the bulb of the pipet.

41. Air bubbles in the bulb of the pipet may be caused by any one of the following: (1) Failure to hold the pipet at the proper angle when diluting the blood. For example, if the pipet is held more toward the horizontal than the vertical, the level of fluid in the bulb may cause an air bubble to form in the bulb. The proper angle of the pipet is illustrated in Figure 55. (2) Momentarily lifting the pipet out of the diluting fluid when sucking up diluting fluid. (3) Failure to hold your index finger over the tip of the pipet when removing the rubber sucking tube.

42. Now check the bulb of your pipet for air bubbles.

    Note: A tiny air bubble (about the size of a pin head) is permissible.

43. If you have no air bubbles or only a tiny air bubble in the bulb of your pipet, proceed to step 45 below.

44. If you have a large air bubble in the bulb of your pipet, you must put the pipet in the container for used pipets and you must repeat steps 2 through 43.

45. Temporarily "store" the pipet as follows:

46. Holding the pipet in a horizontal position so the fluid will not run out, push it into a piece of paper as illustrated in Figure 56.

    Note: This prevents the tip of the pipet from touching anything with the subsequent drainage of fluid.

47. Write the patient's name on the piece of paper. (It is extremely important to correctly label all blood specimens. An unlabelled or mislabelled blood specimen in the blood bank department could cause the death of a patient! Therefore, get in the habit of correctly labelling all blood specimens.)

48. Now proceed to Step 2, Charging the Counting Chamber.

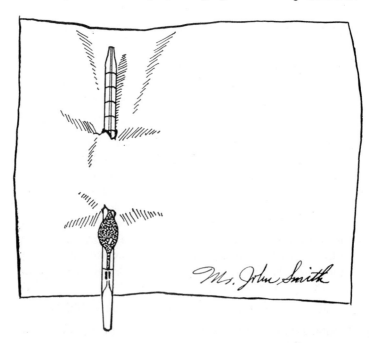

FIG. 56.—Method of "storing" and identifying a pipet containing diluted blood.

STEP 2: CHARGING THE COUNTING CHAMBER

First read the *discussion;* then follow the directions in the *procedure.*

Discussion of Step 2

A representative sample of the solution in the mixing chamber is to be transferred to a counting chamber. Therefore, two procedures should be considered. First, in order to insure a uniform distribution of cells, the blood and diluting fluid must be well mixed. Second, since the diluting fluid in the stem of the pipet did not take part in the dilution of the blood, it must be discarded. These two steps should be carefully performed, as illustrated below, for they are often major sources of error.

In addition to the pipet containing the diluted blood, this step calls for the following equipment: counting chamber and coverglass. These are illustrated in Figure 57.

In the counting chamber, ruled area 1 and ruled area 2 are tiny ruled areas. These ruled areas are so small that they can not be seen with the naked eye. Both ruled area 1 and ruled area 2 are identical. Ruled area 1, however, is usually used for the white cell count and ruled area 2 is usually used for the red cell count.

The two ruled areas are separated by an empty space or moat. When magnified by the microscope, each ruled area looks somewhat like a floor lined with white tile.

Raised ridge A and raised ridge B are elevated ridges (Fig. 57).

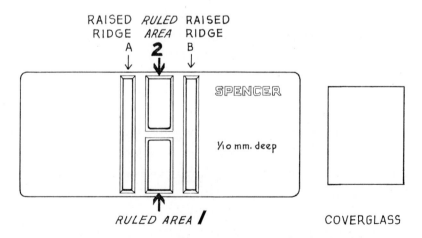

COUNTING CHAMBER

FIG. 57.—Counting chamber and coverglass. The counting chamber is technically known as a hemocytometer (he"mo-si-tom'e-ter).

8

When the coverglass is placed on these elevated ridges, it acts as a roof covering both ruled areas (see Fig. 58, upper illustration).

Between the coverglass and ruled areas, there is a tiny distance of 0.1 millimeter. This makes a small space between the coverglass and ruled areas (see Fig. 58, lower illustration).

This space between the coverglass and ruled areas will be filled with diluted blood (see Fig. 58, lower illustration).

In the white cell count, a tiny portion of the diluted blood flows beneath the roof of the coverglass and onto ruled area 1 (Fig. 59).

In the red cell count, a tiny portion of the diluted blood flows beneath the roof of the coverglass and onto ruled area 2 (Fig. 59).

The above two solutions do not mix because of the empty space or moat between ruled area 1 and ruled area 2.

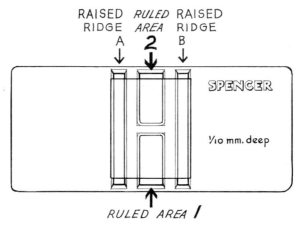

RAISED   *RULED*   RAISED
RIDGE   *AREA*   RIDGE
  A   **2**   B

SPENCER

¹⁄₁₀ mm. deep

RULED AREA **1**

COUNTING CHAMBER WITH COVERGLASS IN PLACE
Viewed from above

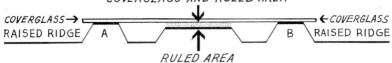

DILUTED BLOOD OCCUPIES SPACE BETWEEN
COVERGLASS AND RULED AREA

COVERGLASS→   ←COVERGLASS
RAISED RIDGE   A   B   RAISED RIDGE

RULED AREA

COUNTING CHAMBER WITH COVERGLASS IN PLACE
Viewed from the side (greatly enlarged)

Fig. 58.—Counting chamber with coverglass in place, viewed from above and from the side.

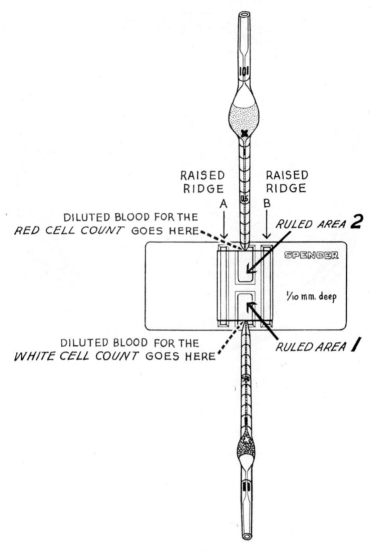

FIG. 59.—Adding diluted blood to the counting chamber.

When the counting chamber and coverglass are not in use, they are usually stored in a Petri dish. This protects them from dust and damage (Fig. 60).

The counting chamber and coverglass should be treated with respect, for they are easily broken. The counting chamber costs about $15.00, the coverglass about 50 cents.

Now follow the directions *exactly* as given in the Procedure for Step 2.

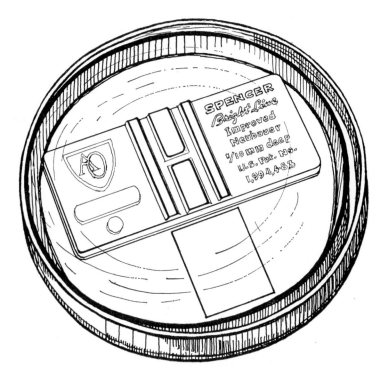

Fig. 60.—Counting chamber and coverglass stored in a Petri dish.

Procedure for Step 2

1. Get the counting chamber and coverglass (Fig. 61).

2. With a pencil, write the number 1 to the right of ruled area 1 as illustrated in Figure 61.

3. Now write the number 2 to the right of ruled area 2 as illustrated in Figure 61.

4. Get a clean piece of white cloth about half the size of a handkerchief. This cloth will be used to clean the counting chamber and coverglass. <u>Do not use this cloth for any other purpose.</u>

5. If the coverglass is on the counting chamber, remove it and place it on the table or a clean surface.

6. Using the cloth, clean the counting chamber by <u>thoroughly</u> rubbing ruled area 1 and ruled area 2.

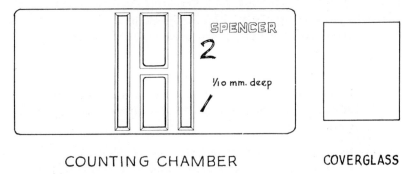

COUNTING CHAMBER   COVERGLASS

FIG. 61.—Counting chamber with the number *1* written opposite ruled area 1 and the number *2* written opposite ruled area 2.

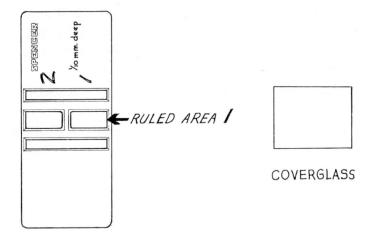

COVERGLASS

COUNTING CHAMBER

FIG. 62.—Position of the counting chamber prior to loading for the white cell count.

7. Now place the counting chamber so you can load ruled area 1 from your right (Fig. 62).

8. Pick up the coverglass. This must be kept perfectly clean and free from finger marks. Otherwise, you will have trouble seeing the cells.

   Note: Dirt or grease on the coverglass will cause the cells to look blurred. (Somewhat like grease on a pair of eye glasses will cause objects to look blurred.)

9. Now clean the coverglass as follows:

10. With your left hand, hold the coverglass <u>by the edges.</u>
    With your right hand, pick up the cloth. Now simultane-
    ously rub <u>both</u> sides of the coverglass. In other words,
    clean the coverglass as you would clean a pair of eye
    glasses.

    Note: When the coverglass is clean, handle it by the
    edges. This will keep your fingers from smearing the
    clean surface.

11. Holding the coverglass by the <u>longest</u> edges, place the
    <u>longest</u> edges on raised ridge A and raised ridge B of the
    counting chamber (Fig. 63).

12. Keeping your white cell pipet in a <u>horizontal position,</u>
    remove it from the storage place in the piece of paper.

13. Now put the thumb of your right hand over the tip of the
    pipet. Put the middle finger of your right hand over the
    other end or top of the pipet.

14. Observe the method of shaking a pipet which is illus-
    trated in Figure 64.

    Note: Mechanical shakers may be purchased for about
    $45.00.

RAISED RIDGE B →

RAISED RIDGE A →

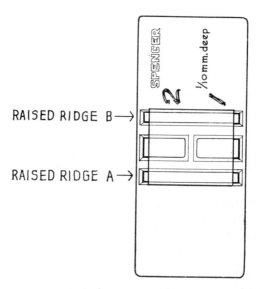

FIG. 63.—Counting chamber with <u>longest</u> edges of coverglass
placed on raised ridge A and raised ridge B.

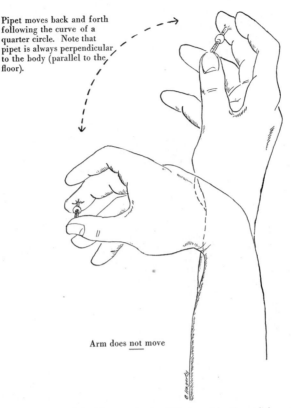

Pipet moves back and forth
following the curve of a
quarter circle. Note that
pipet is always perpendicular
to the body (parallel to the
floor).

Arm does not move

FIG. 64.—Proper method of shaking a pipet. The bead in the mixing chamber aids
in the mixing process by revolving in a circular direction.

15. Now shake your pipet <u>vigorously</u> for 2 to 3 minutes in the
manner illustrated in Figure 64.

Note: If the pipet is not <u>thoroughly</u> shaken, the distribution will be poor and the entire count will have to be
repeated. Failure to <u>thoroughly</u> shake the pipet is one
of the most frequent mistakes the beginner makes.

16. After you have <u>thoroughly</u> shaken the pipet for 2 to 3
minutes, observe the method of discarding the first 4
drops (Fig. 65).

17. Now place the index finger of your right hand over the
top of the pipet to control the flow of fluid.

18. And discard the first 4 or 5 drops onto a piece of cotton
(Fig. 65).

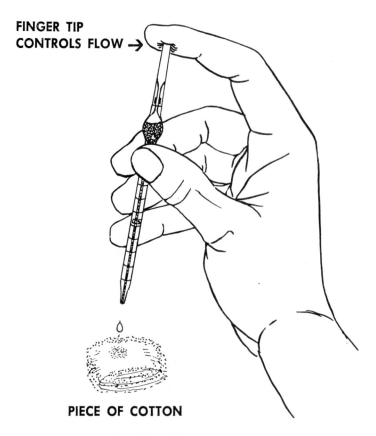

FINGER TIP
CONTROLS FLOW →

PIECE OF COTTON

Fig. 65.—Discarding the first 4 drops.

19. Then stop the flow by pressing down firmly with your index finger.

20. Now press your index finger firmly over the top of the pipet.

21. Then touch the tip of the pipet to a piece of cotton to remove any fluid.

22. Observe the manner of charging a counting chamber which is illustrated in Figure 66.

23. With your left hand, firmly hold the longest edges of the coverglass to keep it in place (Fig. 66).

24. Again touch the tip of the pipet to a piece of cotton to remove any fluid.

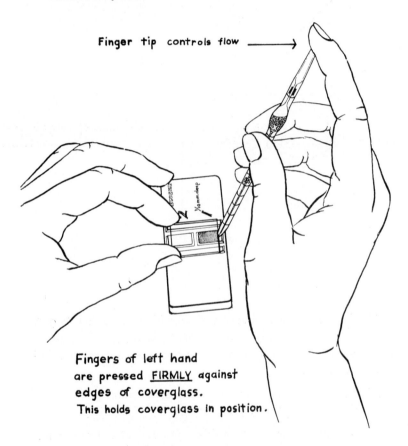

Finger tip controls flow ⟶

Fingers of left hand
are pressed FIRMLY against
edges of coverglass.
This holds coverglass in position.

FIG. 66.—Charging the counting chamber for the white cell count.

25. Place the tip of the pipet on the edge of ruled area 1 and push it flush against the coverglass (see below).

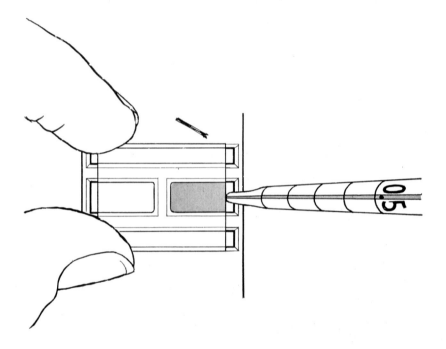

26. Carefully controlling the flow with your index finger, allow a very small portion of the solution to gradually seep under the coverglass and completely cover ruled area 1.

27. Then stop the flow with pressure from your index finger and pull the pipet away.

28. Lay the pipet on the table. Do not let the tip of the pipet touch anything because the fluid may drain out and you will then be unable to repeat the count or perform a hemoglobin determination (if you are using the Haden-Hausser method).

29. Carefully remove your left hand from the coverglass.

   Note: You may move the coverglass without causing any error or damage.

30. Observe the properly and improperly charged counting chambers in Figure 67.

31. Now inspect your counting chamber to see if it is flooded or contains air bubbles.

Properly Charged Counting Chamber

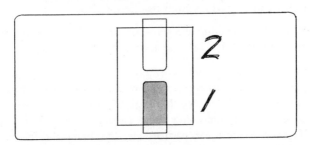

Note that the solution completely covers ruled area 1 and also that the solution is free from air bubbles.

Improperly Charged Counting Chambers

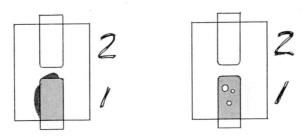

FLOODED Counting Chamber. Caused by allowing an excess of the solution to flow beneath the coverglass.

AIR BUBBLES in solution. Caused by air bubbles in pipet or unclean counting chamber or coverglass.

FIG. 67.—Properly and improperly charged counting chambers for the white cell count.

32. If your counting chamber is flooded or contains air bubbles, immediately clean the coverglass and counting chamber with the cloth. Then charge the counting chamber a second time.

    Note: You may use the same pipet without discarding the first 4 drops provided you use it within 2 or 3 minutes after the first attempt. Otherwise, you must shake the pipet again and discard the first 4 drops.

33. When the counting chamber is properly charged, proceed to Step 3, Counting the Cells.

    Note: Save the pipet containing the diluted blood, for you may have to repeat the count or use the remaining diluted blood for the hemoglobin determination. The diluted blood remaining in the pipet is used in the Haden-Hausser method of performing the hemoglobin determination.

STEP 3: COUNTING THE CELLS

First read the *discussion;* then follow the directions in the *procedure.*

Discussion of Step 3

The count is made by means of a microscope which is illustrated in Figure 68.

The microscope has 3 magnifying devices or objectives. These objectives are called the low power objective, the high power objective, and the oil immersion objective.

When the low power objective is used, the cells are magnified 100 times. This objective is used for the white cell count. It is usually labelled 10× or 16 mm.

When the high power objective is used, the cells are magnified 450 times, This objective is used for the red cell count. It is usually labelled 43×. 45×, or 4 mm.

When the oil immersion objective is used, the cells are magnified 950 times. This objective is used for the differential white cell count. It is usually labelled 95×, 97×, or *oil immersion.*

The 3 objectives are mounted on a revolving nosepiece which enables a particular objective to be swung into position directly over a specimen.

How is the magnification of a specimen determined?

The magnification of a specimen is determined by multiplying the magnification of the *objective* times the magnification of the *eyepiece.*

Thus, with a 10× objective and a 10× eyepiece, the white cells are magnified 100 times; and with a 45× objective and a 10× eyepiece, the red cells are magnified 450 times.

If the student is already familiar with the care and operation of a microscope, he should now go directly to the Procedure for Step 3 (page 120).

If the student is not familiar with the care and operation of a microscope, he should carefully study Figure 68 and the accompanying legend (pages 118–119) before going to the Procedure for Step 3 (page 120).

LEGEND FOR FIG. 68.—MICROSCOPE

This legend will discuss the following: (1) the labelling on the objectives, (2) instructions for cleaning the lens, and (3) instructions for the care of the microscope.

Labelling on the Objectives

1. N. A. on Objectives

N. A. stands for numerical aperture.

The numerical aperture is a figure designating the ability to reveal fine detail.

The higher the numerical aperture, the greater the ability to reveal fine detail.

Thus, the 10× objective might have an N. A. of .25, the 45× objective might have an N. A. of .66, and the 95× objective might have an N. A. of 1.25.

2. mm. on Objectives

mm. stands for millimeter.

Practically speaking, the mm. on the objective is an indication of the relative distance between the objective and the blood slide.

Thus, the 16 mm. objective is farthest from the blood slide, the 4 mm. objective is closer to the blood slide, and the 1.8 mm. objective is closest to the blood slide.

Technically speaking, however, the mm. on the objective refers to the equivalent focus (E. F.) of the objective.

3. Oil Immersion Objective

In the differential white cell count, a drop of oil is placed on a glass slide containing a blood smear and the oil immersion objective is immersed in this drop of oil.

What is the function of the oil?

Suppose, for a moment, that you see a stick which is half in water and half out. It appears bent. Why? Because light travels faster in air than in water.

Now, light travels at the same speed through both oil and glass. Therefore, the light rays are not bent. And the specimen does not appear distorted.

4. Achromatic Lens

An achromatic lens converges light rays of different colors to a single focus.

Instructions for Cleaning the Lens

1. If you see dirt when looking at the cells, get a piece of lens paper and moisten it with xylene. Then rub the lens paper on the following 3 places:
   a. the lens on top of the eyepiece
   b. the lens in the objective
   c. the lens on top of the condenser
2. Now take a piece of dry lens paper and rub it on the above 3 lenses.
3. Look through the eyepiece. If the dirt is still there, it is on the coverglass of your counting chamber. This, of course, is due to either improper cleaning of the coverglass or smearing the coverglass with your fingers.
4. *Note #1:*
   You can tell if the dirt is on the eyepiece by looking through the eyepiece and revolving the eyepiece with your fingers. If the dirt is on the eyepiece, it will move when you move the eyepiece.
5. *Note #2:*
   Sometimes dust or dirt may get on a second lens inside the eyepiece. To clean this lens, remove the eyepiece. Unscrew the lens. Now clean it with lens paper and xylene.

LEGEND FOR FIG. 68.—MICROSCOPE (Continued)

6. *Note #3:*
   When cleaning the lens, always use lens paper. Cloth or other material may scratch the lens. Also, do not use an excessive amount of xylene, for in time, it may dissolve the structure which houses the lens.

Instructions for Care of the Microscope

1. Occasionally clean the mirror with a soft cloth.
2. About once a week, clean the oil immersion objective with a piece of lens paper moistened with xylene.
3. When the microscope is not in use, keep it covered with a cloth or plastic cover to protect it from dust.
4. If it is necessary to move the microscope, proceed as follows: With your right hand, firmly grasp the curved arm just below the *fine adjustment*. Lift up. Now place your left hand under the base of the microscope. And move the microscope to the desired location.

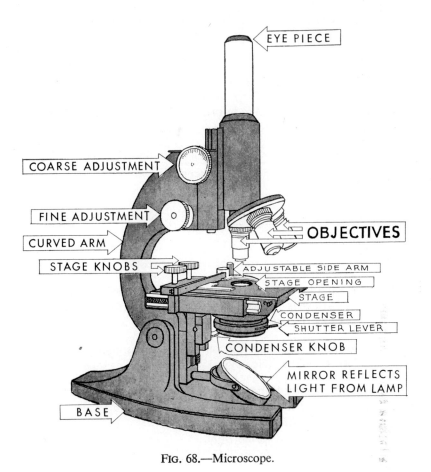

FIG. 68.—Microscope.

Procedure for Step 3

1. Turn to the microscope (Fig. 68).

2. The first step will be to get the 10× (16 mm.) objective in position <u>directly</u> over the opening in the stage.

3. If the 10× (16 mm.) objective is already in position directly over the opening in the stage, proceed to Step 7.

4. If the 10× (16 mm.) objective is not already in position <u>directly</u> over the opening in the stage, proceed as follows.

5. Observe that the 3 objectives are mounted on a turret or revolving nosepiece. This revolving nosepiece will revolve both to the left and to the right.

6. Now firmly grasp the 10× (16 mm.) objective and forcibly swing it into position directly over the opening in the stage.

   Note: When the 10× (16 mm.) objective reaches the proper position directly over the opening in the stage, a slight click is usually heard. Also, when the objective is in the proper position, it is difficult to move.

7. By turning the <u>coarse adjustment,</u> raise the 10× (16 mm.) objective about one or two inches above the opening in the stage.

8. By turning the <u>condenser knob,</u> raise the condenser <u>up as far as it will go.</u>

9. Turn on the light in front of the microscope.

10. Move the light (or microscope) so that the light is about 8 to 14 inches directly in front of the microscope and shines directly on the mirror.

11. To direct the proper light on the cells, it is necessary to adjust the mirror (Fig. 69).

12. The mirror may be moved in 4 directions:
    It may be rotated forward.
    It may be rotated backward.
    It may be turned to the right.
    It may be turned to the left.

13. Since it is extremely important to get the proper light on the cells, the student should complete the following exercise:

14. Place both hands on the mirror as illustrated in Figure 69.

15. Then move the mirror in the following 4 directions:
    (1) Rotate it slightly forward.
    (2) Rotate it slightly backward.
    (3) Turn it slightly to the right.
    (4) Turn it slightly to the left.

16. Now, with your naked eye, look at the opening in the stage and note the glass top of the condenser.

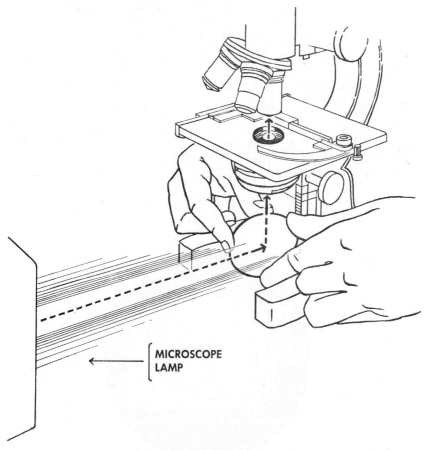

MICROSCOPE LAMP

FIG. 69.—Technologist using *both* hands to adjust the mirror and obtain the proper light.

17. Using your naked eye and both hands, adjust the mirror so a bright light comes directly up through the CENTER of the glass top of the condenser.

Note #1: Sometimes the shutter lever of the condenser may be closed or partially closed and a bright light can not come up through the condenser. In such cases, open the shutter with the shutter lever (Fig. 68, page 119). Note #2: Observe that the mirror has two faces, front and back. Use the face which reflects the most light.

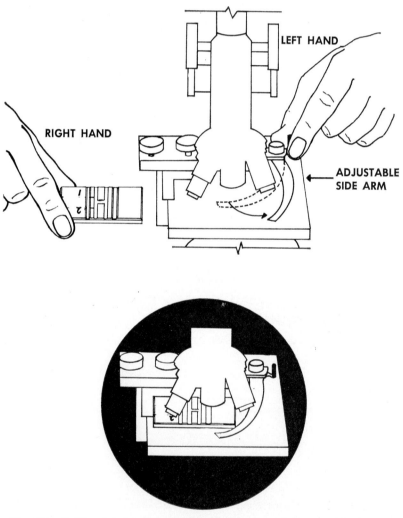

FIG. 70.—Putting the counting chamber in the jaws of the movable stage.

18. When you have the <u>bright</u> light coming up through the <u>center</u> of the condenser, proceed as follows:

19. Turn the <u>stage knobs</u> of the microscope and note that they move a portion of the stage. This portion of the stage is called the movable stage. The movable stage holds the counting chamber and allows it to be moved.

20. Now carefully pick up the counting chamber.

21. With your right hand, hold the counting chamber as illustrated in Figure 70.

22. With your left hand, pull back the <u>adjustable side arm</u> on the left portion of the movable stage (Fig. 70).

23. Now put the counting chamber into the jaws of the movable stage.

24. Now <u>gently</u> release the <u>adjustable side arm</u> and fit the counting chamber snugly into the jaws of the movable stage (Fig. 70).

25. In the next few steps, it is important to follow the directions exactly as given. Do <u>not</u> look into the eyepiece until the directions tell you to do so.

26. Turn the stage knobs and note that this moves the counting chamber.

27. By turning the <u>stage knobs</u>, move the counting chamber so the bright light comes directly up through the <u>CENTER</u> <u>of the solution in ruled area 1.</u> <u>This is important!</u>

28. Now lower the condenser by turning the <u>condenser knob</u> <u>one half turn.</u>

    Note: <u>The condenser knob must be turned at least one</u> <u>half turn. This diminishes the light. If the light is not</u> <u>diminished, you will not be able to see the cells.</u>

29. Look at the counting chamber from the side. And, by turning the <u>coarse adjustment</u>, carefully lower the 10× (16 mm.) objective until it is almost touching the cover-glass.

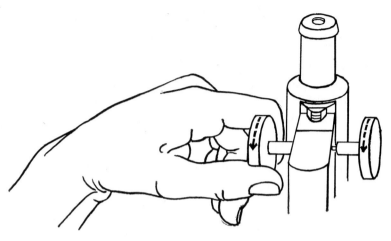

FIG. 71.—Rotating the *coarse adjustment toward* yourself (for the WBC).

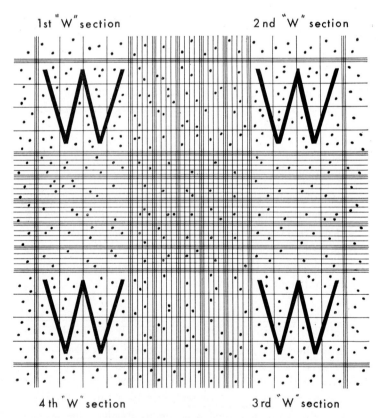

1st "W" section   2nd "W" section

4th "W" section   3rd "W" section

FIG. 72.—The 4 "W" sections of the counting chamber.
The black dots are white cells.

30. In the next step you must rotate the <u>coarse adjustment</u> <u>toward yourself</u> (see Fig. 71).

    Note: If you rotate the <u>coarse adjustment</u> in the opposite direction, you will break the coverglass.

31. Now, while continuously <u>looking through the eyepiece,</u> <u>proceed as follows:</u>

32. Slowly <u>rotate the coarse adjustment toward yourself until</u> <u>you see some faint lines.</u> These faint lines will have a gray or yellow background.

    Note: It will require one quarter to one half turn of the <u>coarse adjustment.</u>

33. The faint lines will be a small portion of a large ruled area. This large ruled area is illustrated in Figure 72.

34. If you do not see some faint lines after rotating the <u>coarse</u> <u>adjustment</u> one half turn, you did not make the light come directly up through the CENTER in step 17 or step 27. In such cases, you must remove the counting chamber from the stage of the microscope. Then you must repeat steps 9 to 33.

35. While looking in the eyepiece, <u>make any of the following</u> <u>adjustments:</u> If the light is too bright, turn the <u>condenser</u> <u>knob</u> and lower the condenser. If the light is too dim, turn the <u>condenser knob</u> and raise the condenser. If the lines have a black or hazy background, adjust the mirror.

    Note: When you look into the eyepiece, form the habit of keeping <u>both eyes open.</u> This will ease the strain on your eyes.

36. If your light has been properly reduced by lowering the condenser in step 28, you will also see some <u>small black</u> <u>dots.</u> These small black dots are white cells (see Fig. 73).

37. When you have some white cells in view, rock the <u>coarse</u> <u>adjustment</u> back and forth until you get the cells in good focus.

38. Then turn the <u>fine adjustment</u> back and forth and get the cells in perfect focus.

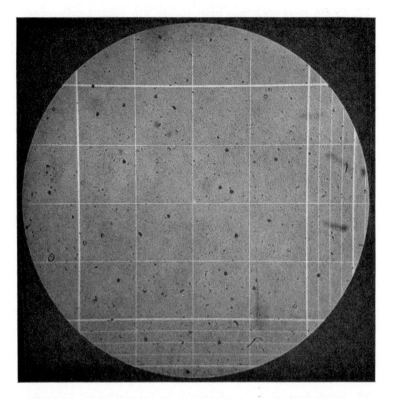

Fɪɢ. 73.—The 1st "W" section as seen through the 10× (16 mm.) objective of the microscope. The numerous small black dots are white cells. (Courtesy of Mr. Cecil Gilliam.)

39. Now, while looking at the cells, rock the <u>fine adjustment</u> back and forth and note that this gives you a more complete picture. It enables you to see the size of the white cells. And it will help you to distinguish between white cells and "junk" or artefacts in the solution.

40. Turn to Figure 72, page 124, and observe the following:
    a. Each "W" section is composed of 16 small squares.
    b. The 1st "W" section is in the upper left hand corner of the illustration.
    c. The 1st "W" section is identified as follows:
    d. The 1st "W" section is the only "W" section <u>which has no crossed lines or squares directly above it and directly to the left of it.</u>

41. Observe the view of the 1st "W" section as seen through the $10 \times$ (16 mm.) objective of the microscope (Fig. 73).

Note: Observe that the "W" section is composed of 16 small squares. Observe that there are no crossed lines or squares directly above the "W" section. Also observe that there are no crossed lines or squares directly to the left of the "W" section. These 2 features identify it as the 1st "W" section.

42. Look in the eyepiece and, by turning the stage knobs, bring the 1st "W" section into view.

43. When you have the 1st "W" section in view, observe the difference between good distribution and poor distribution of the white cells (Fig. 74).

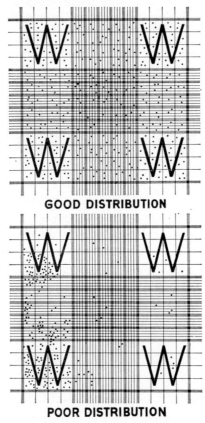

GOOD DISTRIBUTION

POOR DISTRIBUTION

FIG. 74.—Good and poor distribution of white cells. The cells must be evenly distributed as illustrated in the upper figure. If the cells are not evenly distributed, as illustrated in the lower figure, different "W" sections would give vastly different counts. This, of course, would yield an erroneous white cell count.

44. Look in the eyepiece and, by moving the stage knobs, make a survey of your 4 "W" sections to see if your cells are evenly distributed.

45. If your cells are not evenly distributed, it indicates faulty technique in mixing the cells or discarding the first 4 drops. In such cases, you must clean the counting chamber and coverglass with the cloth. Then you must repeat the mixing, discarding, and charging process (pages 108 to 128).

46. If your cells are evenly distributed, study the method of counting the white cells which is illustrated in Figure 75 and described in the accompanying legend below.

Note: You should actually make the practice count as directed in the legend before going to step 47, page 130.

LEGEND FOR FIG. 75.—
COUNTING THE WHITE CELLS IN THE 1ST "W" SECTION.

1. As you count, you should keep your left hand on the *fine adjustment* and *continuously* rotate this *fine adjustment* back and forth. Rotating the *fine adjustment* back and forth will enable you to see the various "layers" of objects.

2. The white cells are all the same size. If you see objects that are smaller than white cells, do not count them. If you see objects that are larger than white cells, do not count them. These objects are "junk" or artefacts in the diluting fluid or counting chamber.

3. The white cells are round. If you see objects that are not round, do not count them. Also, if you see objects that do not hold their round shape when you rock the fine adjustment back and forth, do not count them. These objects are also "junk" or artefacts in the diluting fluid or counting chamber.

4. In counting, you start in the upper left hand corner of the "W" section and follow the path of the arrow as illustrated in this figure.

5. You keep the count in your head and then write down the total count for the entire "W" section.

6. For practice, count the white cells in this figure, comparing your count with the accompanying score board.

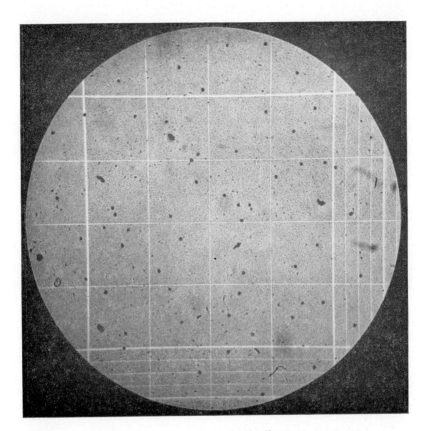

White cells in the 1st "W" section

START
HERE

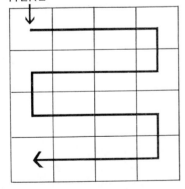

2	3	2	2
2	2	4	3
3	2	1	2
3	2	3	3

Start in the upper left hand
corner. Follow path of
arrow.

Score board for each small
square of above "W" section.
Total count is 39.

FIG. 75.—Counting the white cells in the 1st "W" section.
(Courtesy of Mr. Cecil Gilliam.)

47. After you have made the practice count in the above illustration, turn to the microscope and count the white cells in your 1st "W" section.

48. Write down the total number counted in your 1st "W" section.

49. Now move to the 2nd "W" section. You can be sure you have the 2nd "W" section if the lines above the "W" section and the lines to the right of the "W" section are not crossed or checkered (see Fig. 72, page 124).

50. Count the cells in this 2nd "W" section.

51. Write down the total number counted in your 2nd "W" section.

52. Now move to the 3rd "W" section (see Fig. 72, page 124).

53. Count the cells in this 3rd "W" section.

54. Write down the total number counted in your 3rd "W" section.

55. Now move to the 4th "W" section (see Fig. 72, page 124).

56. Count the cells in this 4th "W" section.

57. Write down the total number counted in your 4th "W" section.

58. Add the 4 counts.

59. Your total count is the total number of cells in the 4 "W" sections.

60. Example:

     26 cells in 1st "W" section
     22 cells in 2nd "W" section
     24 cells in 3rd "W" section
     28 cells in 4th "W" section

     100 total number of cells in 4 "W" sections

61. Note: Your count in any 2 "W" sections should not vary by more than 12 cells. For example, your count should not show 30 cells in one "W" section and 48 cells in another "W" section. If there is a variation of more than 12 cells in any 2 "W" sections, it means that your distribution was not good. In such cases, you must repeat the mixing, discarding, and charging process.

62. After you have added your 4 counts, remove the counting chamber from the microscope. Pick up the piece of cloth and thoroughly clean the coverglass and ruled areas of the counting chamber. Put the counting chamber and coverglass back in the Petri dish.

    Note: If ruled area 2 is loaded for the red cell count, you do not, of course, clean the ruled areas.

63. Proceed to Step 4, Making the Calculations.

    Note: Save the pipet containing the diluted blood for you may want to repeat the count.

STEP 4: MAKING THE CALCULATIONS

First read the *discussion;* then follow the directions in the *procedure.*

Discussion of Step 4

The white cell count is the number of white cells in *1.0* cubic millimeter of *undiluted* blood. But we diluted the blood! And we counted the cells in less than 1.0 cubic millimeter! Therefore, we must multiply our total number of cells by 2 correction factors.

The first correction factor compensates for the dilution of the blood. Since we diluted the blood 1 in 20, the dilution correction factor is 20. Of course, if we had diluted the blood 1 in 10, the dilution correction factor would be 10.

The second correction factor compensates for the volume in which the cells were counted. This is discussed below.

Each "W" section has an area of 1 square millimeter and a depth of 0.1 millimeter. The volume of 1 "W" section is found as follows:

$$\text{area} \quad \times \text{depth} \quad = \text{volume}$$

$$1 \text{ sq. mm.} \times 0.1 \text{ mm.} = 0.1 \text{ cu. mm.}$$

Thus, the volume of 1 "W" section is 0.1 cubic millimeter.
The volume of the 4 "W" sections is found as follows:

$$\begin{array}{ccc} \text{Number of} & \text{Volume of} & \text{Total vol. of} \\ \text{"W" sect.} \times 1 \text{ "W" sect.} & = 4 \text{ "W" sect.} \end{array}$$

$$4 \qquad \times 0.1 \text{ cu. mm.} = 0.4 \text{ cu. mm.}$$

Thus, the volume of the 4 "W" sections is 0.4 cubic millimeter.

Consequently, we have the following problem: When we counted the cells in the 4 "W" sections, we counted the cells in *0.4* cubic millimeter. Now we must report the number in 1.0 cubic millimeter.

To solve the problem, we must multiply our count by a volume correction factor. This is found as follows:

$$\text{Vol. cor. factor} = \frac{\text{volume desired}}{\text{volume used}} = \frac{1.0 \text{ cu. mm.}}{0.4 \text{ cu. mm.}} = 2.5$$

Thus, the volume correction factor is 2.5.

As previously stated, we have a dilution correction factor of 20. And now we also have a volume correction factor of 2.5.

When the total number of cells in the 4 "W" sections is multiplied by the above correction factors of 20 and 2.5, the number of cells in 1 cubic millimeter of blood is obtained. This is our white cell count.

To illustrate, if the total number of cells in the 4 "W" sections is 100, the calculation is made as follows.

Number of cells   Dil.   Vol.   Number of
in 0.4 cu. mm. $\times$ cor. $\times$ cor.   = cells in
(4 "W" sections)   factor   factor   1.0 cu. mm.

100            $\times$ 20 $\times$ 2.5   = 5,000

Since the product of the dilution and volume correction factors is 50 ($20 \times 2.5 = 50$), the calculation can be made by simply multiplying the total number of cells in the 4 "W" sections by 50   Thus,

Number of cells   Correction   Number of
in 0.4 cu. mm. $\times$ factors   = cells in
(4 "W" sections)   1.0 cu. mm.

100            $\times$ 50   =   5,000

Procedure for Step 4

1. To make the calculations for your white cell count, proceed as follows:

2. Multiply the total number of cells in the 4 "W" sections by 50.

3. Example:
   100 cells in 4 "W" sections
    50 correction factors
   ____
   5,000 cells in 1 cubic millimeter of blood

4. After you have made your calculation, make out your report as indicated in the sample report below.

5. Sample report:

Report of a White Cell Count

Patient: Dickson, Miss Candice   92053
Date: 7-7-72
Physician: Dr. Tom Maxwell

Patient's Values	Normal Values
5,000	5,000 to 10,000 per cu. mm.

Examination performed by: Sandra Frisbie

---

6. After you have signed your report, hand it in.

MISCELLANEOUS INFORMATION FOR
THE MICROSCOPIC METHOD

This section covers the following:

1. Summary of the Microscopic Method
2. Cleaning the Counting Chamber and Pipets
3. Sources of Error in the Microscopic Method
4. Short-cut Method for Counting and Calculating
5. Dilutions and Calculations for High Counts and Low Counts
6. Correction for Nucleated Red Cells

1. Summary of the Microscopic Method

After performing his first white cell count, the student may perform additional counts by skipping the *discussion* and going directly to the *procedure*.

For the convenience of the student, the steps and reference pages are summarized below.

Step 1. Diluting the blood
  a. Discussion: page 96
  b. Procedure: page 98

Step 2. Charging the counting chamber
  a. Discussion: page 105
  b. Procedure: page 108

Step 3. Counting the cells
  a. Discussion: page 117
  b. Procedure: page 120

Step 4. Making the calculations
  a. Discussion: page 132
  b. Procedure: page 133

2. Cleaning the Counting Chamber and Pipets

Immediately after use, clean the counting chamber and coverglass with a soft cloth. If the diluted blood has dried on the counting chamber, clean the counting chamber and coverglass with water. Then dry with the soft cloth.

After the white cell pipet and red cell pipet have been used, place them in a glass of water. The water should completely cover the pipets. This prevents the diluted blood from drying. Pipets stored in this manner may sit for hours before cleaning.

The white cell pipet and red cell pipet are cleaned by means of a suction or aspirator which is attached to a faucet. The procedure follows:

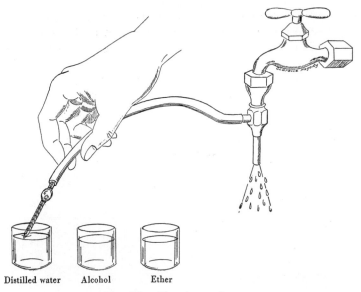

Distilled water   Alcohol   Ether

Fig. 76.—Cleaning a pipet.

1. Attach a suction or aspirator to a faucet as illustrated in Figure 76.

2. Insert the pipet in the rubber tube as illustrated.

3. Turn the faucet on to the point where there is sufficient force to produce a good suction.

4. Then use either method A or method B below.

   Method A: Allow the pipet to suck up 5 or 6 fillings of distilled water. Then place the pipet in a beaker and dry in a drying oven.

   Method B: Allow the pipet to suck up 4 fillings of distilled water, then 1 filling of rubbing alcohol, and finally 1 filling of either acetone or ether.

5. Note: Most large laboratories have a pipet washer capable of cleaning 18 pipets at a time. This pipet washer is illustrated in Figure 77, page 136.

If a pipet becomes stained or clogged with dried blood, clean it as follows:
First, get a stylet (a fine wire about 6 inches long). Run the stylet through the pipet several times.

Then get some 10% nitric acid. This acid should be handled with care for it could give you a burn.

Pour a little of the nitric acid into a medicine glass. Attach a rubber sucking tube to the pipet. *Carefully* suck up the acid into the pipet until it is filled. Detach the pipet from the rubber sucking tube. Then lay the pipet in a pan or basin for a few days.

At the end of a few days, pick up the pipet and let the acid drain into the sink. Then clean the pipet thoroughly with your suction device (Fig. 76).

PIPET WASHER

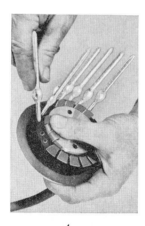 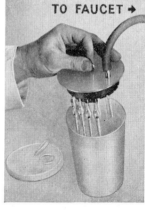

A   *B*

FIG. 77.—Cleaning many pipets. (Courtesy of Arthur H. Thomas Co.)
A, Showing washer flap valves lifted for insertion of pipets of various sizes; unused holes are automatically closed off.
B, Showing pipets being immersed in detergent or rinse.

3. Sources of Error in the Microscopic Method

The most frequent sources of error in the microscopic method are:

1. Failure to have the blood *exactly* on the 0.5 mark
2. Failure to shake the pipet thoroughly
3. Failure to discard the first 4 drops
4. Failure to properly charge the counting chamber

The least frequent sources of error are:

1. Inaccurate pipets or counting chamber
2. Moist or unclean pipets
3. Excessive pressure on finger when obtaining blood (this causes a slight dilution of the blood by the tissue juices)

4. Failure to mix the blood (if the blood is taken from a test tube)
5. Drawing up too little or too much diluting fluid
6. Slowness in manipulation, thus allowing the blood to clot
7. Air bubbles in the pipet (caused by failure to keep pipet submerged in the diluting fluid during the dilution process or detaching pipet from rubber sucking tube without holding finger over end of pipet)
8. Air bubbles in counting chamber (caused by air bubbles in pipet or unclean counting chamber or coverglass)
9. Presence of yeast or other contaminants in the diluting fluid
10. Presence of many nucleated red cells (found in erythroblastosis fetalis and thalassemia) causing a high white cell count
11. Mistakes in counting or calculations

4. Short-cut Method for Counting and Calculating

After some experience, many technologists use the following short-cut method for performing a white cell count. This method is *not* recommended for beginners.

1. *Carefully* check the distribution of the cells.
2. If distribution is good, proceed as follows:
3. Count the cells in 2 "W" sections which are kitty-corner to each other (either the 1st and 3rd "W" sections or the 2nd and 4th "W" sections in Figure 72, page 124).
4. Add the 2 counts.
5. Multiply by 100 or "add 2 zeros."
6. *Example:*
   1 "W" section had a count of 40. The other "W" section had a count of 50. Total is 90. Adding 2 zeros to 90 gives a count of 9,000.

5. Dilutions and Calculations for High Counts and Low Counts

High Counts

In leukemia, the white cell count may be extremely high, often as high as 100,000 to 500,000 cells per cubic millimeter. In such cases, the counting may be facilitated by making a greater dilution of the blood. This is accomplished by using a *red cell pipet*. The increased dilution, of course, must be compensated for in the calculation.

To increase the dilution and make the proper calculation, proceed as follows:

1. Using a *red cell pipet*, draw blood to the 1.0 mark.
2. Draw WBC diluting fluid to the 101 mark.
3. Now proceed exactly as in the normal white cell count: shake the pipet, discard the first 4 drops, charge the counting chamber, and count the cells in the 4 "W" sections.

10

4. Multiply the total number of cells in the 4 "W" sections by 250. The answer is the white cell count.
5. *Note:* Normally the blood is diluted 1 in 20. The dilution correction factor is therefore 20. However, in the above case, the blood is diluted 1 in 100. The dilution correction factor is therefore 100. Multiplying this dilution correction factor of 100 by the volume correction factor of 2.5, gives us the figure 250.

Low Counts

In agranulocytosis and many virus diseases, the white cell count may be extremely low, often varying between 500 and 3,000 cells per cubic millimeter. The accuracy of the count may be increased by making a lesser dilution of the blood. This decreased dilution, of course, must be compensated for in the calculation.

To decrease the dilution and make the proper calculation, proceed as follows:

1. Using the white cell pipet, draw blood to the 1.0 mark.
2. Draw WBC diluting fluid to the 11.0 mark.
3. Now proceed exactly as in the normal white cell count: shake the pipet, discard the first 4 drops, charge the counting chamber, and count the cells in the 4 "W" sections.
4. Multiply the total number of cells in the 4 "W" sections by 25. The answer is the white cell count.
5. *Note:* Normally the blood is diluted 1 in 20 and the dilution correction factor is 20. However, in the above case, the blood is diluted 1 in 10. Our dilution correction factor is therefore 10. Multiplying this dilution correction factor of 10 by the volume correction factor of 2.5, gives us the figure 25.

6. Correction for Nulceated Red Cells

In some anemias, such as thalassemia and erythroblastosis fetalis, many nucleated red cells may be found in the blood. Since these nucleated red cells are not dissolved by the white cell diluting fluid, they are counted as white cells. This would give us an erroneously high white cell count. Consequently, the count must be corrected.

If you find large numbers of nucleated red cells in the stained red cell examination, correct the white cell count with the formula given below:

Formula:

$$\text{corrected white cell count} = \text{uncorrected white cell count} \times \frac{100}{100 + A}$$

Where,

100 = white cells counted in the differential white cell count

A = number of nucleated red cells counted while counting the 100
     white cells of the differential white cell count

Example:

Suppose we had a white cell count of 15,000. And we counted 50 nucleated red cells while counting the 100 white cells of the differential white cell count.

Then our uncorrected white cell count would be 15,000. And A would equal 50.

Substituting these values in the formula, we have:

$$\text{corrected white cell count} = \text{uncorrected white cell count} \times \frac{100}{100 + A}$$

$$= 15,000 \quad \times \frac{100}{100 + 50}$$

$$= 15,000 \quad \times \frac{100}{150}$$

$$= 15,000 \quad \times \frac{2}{3}$$

$$= 10,000$$

COULTER COUNTER METHOD FOR THE WHITE CELL COUNT
(Courtesy of Coulter Electronics, Inc.)

For the white cell count, dilute the blood 1:500.
For the red cell count, dilute the blood 1:50,000.

ROUTINE COUNTING PROCEDURE WITH A 100μ APERTURE

1. Turn the power switch to the "ON" position (Fig. 78A, page 140).

2. Place a beaker of electrolyte containing sample particles in suspension on the sample stand making sure the aperture tube and external electrode are fully immersed; then open the vacuum control stopcock.

3. Adjust the sensitivity and positioning controls until the pattern looks like "A" of Figure 78B, and is centered on the oscilloscope screen.

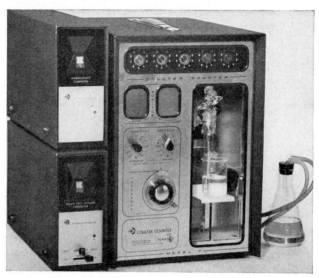

Fig. 78*A*.—The Model F Coulter Counter.
(Courtesy of Coulter Electronics, Inc.)

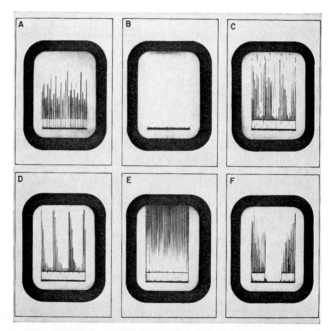

Fig. 78*B*.—Interpreting oscilloscope patterns.

A. Normal pattern when a sample is being counted.

B. Normal pattern showing aperture current "OFF" and at maximum gain.

C. Interference caused by hand on sample beaker.

D. Standing groups of pulses caused by electrical line interference.

E. Dense uniform pulse pattern seen when air is drawn through aperture tube.

F. Debris clogging orifice, causing gaps in pattern.

140

4. Adjust the threshold dial to brighten all blood cell pulses but no debris (small) pulses.

5. Close the vacuum control stopcock, isolating system from external vacuum. The mercury contacts the "start" electrode and the instrument begins to count, ceasing when the flow of mercury reaches the "stop" electrode. $\frac{1}{2}$ cc of mercury is measured between the start and stop electrodes, allowing the instrument to count particles in this same amount of suspension.

6. Observe the twin monitor system during counting to assure freedom from blockage and listen for an even rate of resonance from the sounder.

7. Read and record count shown on glow tubes.

8. Rinse the aperture tube three times with filtered saline and check background count on the filtered saline with all controls at the same settings. The background count is the count of the diluting fluid only and is generally disregarded in routine counting since it can normally be kept negligibly small with careful filtering and handling. For exacting work, refiltering may be necessary to eliminate excess dust particles. If high background counts are unavoidable after refiltering, these must be subtracted from the counts of the samples. When experience proves that filtering techniques are reliable, this step may be unnecessary.

9. If background count is truly negligible, correct the count obtained for coincidence loss according to Paragraph 3–2.2 of instruction and service manual. If desired, duplicate counts can be made on each sample by repeating the sequence from Step 2 through Step 10 until the confidence in precision of the technique warrants eliminating repetition.

10. If counting red blood cells, mltiuply the count by 100 to correct for the 1:50,000 dilution and measurement of $\frac{1}{2}$ cc instead of 1λ. The resultant figure is the number of red blood cells per cubic millimeter of whole blood.

11. If changing from white cell to red cell samples, flush the aperture tube thoroughly inside and out with clean saline, and repeat Steps 2 through 10.

Chapter 5

Red Cell Count

The red cell count is also referred to as a red blood cell count, red blood count, RBC, r.b.c., erythrocyte count, total erythrocyte count, red corpuscle count, and red corpuscle enumeration.

The discussion of the red cell count will cover the following:

> Significance of the Red Cell Count
> Discussion of Procedures for the Red Cell Count
> Microscopic Method for the Red Cell Count
> Coulter Counter Method for the Red Cell Count

The student review questions for the red cell count are numbered 37–48 and begin on page 730 of the Appendix.

SIGNIFICANCE OF THE RED CELL COUNT

The red cell count is the number of red cells in one cubic millimeter of blood.

The normal values for the red cell count are given in Table 6.

The red cell count may vary in health and disease. A few examples are given below.

When a man travels from a seacoast city to a mountainous city, the oxygen content of the air decreases. The decrease in oxygen stimulates the bone marrow to produce more red cells. Therefore, the red cell count rises.

For example, if a man travels from Los Angeles to Denver, his red cell count may rise from 5.0 to 5.5 million.

When a man travels from a mountainous city to a seacoast city, however, the oxygen content of the air increases. The increase in oxygen content causes the bone marrow to produce less red cells. Therefore, the red cell count drops.

Table 6.—Normal Values for the Red Cell Count

Women	4.0 to 5.5 million per cu. mm.
Men	4.5 to 6.0 million per cu. mm.
Newborn Infants	5.0 to 6.5 million per cu. mm.

For example, if a man travels from Denver to Los Angeles, his red cell count may drop from 5.5 to 5.0 million.

The red cell count also varies with changes in body fluid. To illustrate, consider pregnancy and a severe burn.

In pregnancy, the body gains fluid. The red cells become more dilute. Consequently, the red cell count drops below the normal values.

In a severe burn, however, the body loses fluid. The red cells thus become more concentrated. Consequently, the red cell count rises above the normal values.

The red cell count is useful in diagnosis. It drops below the normal values in anemia and leukemia. It rises above the normal values in polycythemia (pol"e-si-the'me-ah) vera and dehydration conditions.

A red cell count below the normal values may be referred to as oligocythemia (ol"ĭ-go-si-the'me-ah). However, this term is seldom used. A red cell count above the normal values is referred to as erythrocytosis (e-rith"ro-si-to'sis).

The red cell count is seldom performed in some laboratories and frequently performed in other laboratories. For example, only 10 red cell counts a month may be run by some laboratories whereas 1,000 red cell counts a month may be run by other laboratories

DISCUSSION OF PROCEDURES FOR THE RED CELL COUNT

The most commonly employed methods for performing the red cell count are:

1. Microscopic Method
2. Electronic Methods
   (1) Coulter Counter Method
   (2) SMA Counter Method
   (3) Fisher Autocytometer Method

The microscopic method is often referred to as the "manual" method, counting chamber method, or hemocytometer method.

The electronic methods are often referred to as the automatic methods or automated methods.

The methods listed above will now be discussed relative to the principle of the procedure and some relevant comments.

MICROSCOPIC METHOD

Principle

The microscopic method for the red cell count consists of diluting the blood, transferring a small portion of the solution to a counting chamber, counting the red cells with a microscope, and making the calculations.

Comments

With the microscopic method, a red cell count may be performed in about 5 minutes.

Unfortunately, the microscopic method for the red cell count is subject to an error of approximately 10%.

For example, suppose two experts are called upon to make a red cell count on the same sample of blood. Let us say that the actual red cell count on this blood is 5.0 million.

One expert could get 10% below the 5.0 million. This would be a count of 4.5 million.

The other expert could get 10% above the 5.0 million. This would be a count of 5.5 million.

In the above red cell count by the two experts, there is a difference of 1,000,000 cells!

This 10% error in the microscopic method is caused by differences in equipment, differences in measuring the sample of blood, the chance distribution of cells, and other similar factors.

The microscopic method for the red cell count is used in many physicians' offices but it is being replaced by electronic methods in many hospital laboratories.

COULTER COUNTER METHOD

Principle

In the Coulter Counter method, the red cells are suspended in a solution which is capable of conducting an electric current. This solution is then made to pass through a narrow opening between 2 electrodes. Since the red cells do not conduct electricity, each passing red cell momentarily decreases a flow of current between the 2 electrodes. The decrease in current causes a voltage drop in the line. The number of voltage drops in the line is the key to the count.

Comments

The Coulter Counter will run a red cell count in a matter of seconds.

A Coulter Counter is simple to operate; the operating procedure accompanies the instrument.

The Coulter Counter is illustrated in Fig. 78A, page 140.

SMA COUNTER METHOD

SMA stands for Sequential Multiple Analysis.

Principle

In this method, the red cells are suspended in a solution. This solution is made to pass through an optical system which makes each red cell generate a light impulse. Each light impulse is then transformed into an electrical impulse. The number of electrical impulses are recorded and become the key to the count.

Comments

The SMA Counter will also run a red cell count in a matter of seconds

The SMA Counter is also simple to operate; the operating procedure accompanies the instrument.

FISHER AUTOCYTOMETER METHOD

Principle

A bulletin published by the Fisher Scientific Company describes the principle of their instrument as follows.

"The Autocytometer utilizes an optical counting system, in which each cell or other particle in the diluted sample appears as a bright spot of light against a dark field, as it passes through a 'sensing zone' only 15 microns high. The flashes of light are picked up by a photomultiplier and converted to electrical impulses, which are totaled electronically and shown on the meter as the cell count in the original whole blood sample."

Comments

With the Fisher Autocytometer, a red cell count may also be run in a matter of seconds.

The Fisher Autocytometer is also simple to operate; the operating procedure accompanies the instrument.

MICROSCOPIC METHOD FOR THE RED CELL COUNT

The discussion will cover the necessary reagents and equipment, the procedure, and miscellaneous information.

NECESSARY REAGENTS AND EQUIPMENT

1. Anticoagulated blood or finger tip blood
2. Red cell pipet (Fig. 79)
3. Rubber sucking tube
4. RBC diluting fluid. Note: The RBC diluting fluid is usually either Hayem's solution or Gower's solution. The preparation of these solutions is given in the Appendix, page 696.
5. Counting chamber and coverglass
6. Small piece of clean cloth
7. Microscope

PROCEDURE

The procedure consists of 4 steps:

Step 1:   Diluting the blood
Step 2:   Charging the counting chamber
Step 3:   Counting the cells
Step 4:   Making the calculations

Each of the above 4 steps will be broken down into a *discussion* and a *procedure*.

The student should first read the *discussion* and then follow the directions in the *procedure*.

The student will save time if he follows the directions EXACTLY as they are given. He should not attempt to improvise. And, above all, he should not attempt to skip any steps.

STEP 1: DILUTING THE BLOOD

First read the *discussion;* then follow the directions in the *procedure.*

Discussion of Step 1

The dilution for the red cell count is made by sucking a measured portion of blood and diluting fluid into a pipet. The following equipment is needed: diluting fluid, red cell pipet, and rubber sucking tube.

The diluting fluid may be any one of the following solutions: Gower's solution, Hayem's solution, Toison's solution, Dacie's solution, or normal saline solution.

The preparation of the above diluting fluids is given in the Appendix (page 692).

The diluting fluid is commonly referred to as RBC diluting fluid—the RBC standing for red blood count.

The RBC diluting fluid is isotonic with the red cells, that is, it prevents the red cells from swelling or shrinking.

The red cell pipet, which is used to make the dilution, is illustrated in Figure 79.

The stem of the pipet is the portion from 0.0 to 1.0. This holds 1 unit of volume.

The mixing chamber is the bulb-like portion from 1.0 to 101. This holds 100 units of volume.

Suppose blood is drawn to the 0.5 mark and diluting fluid to the 101 mark. The 100 units of the mixing chamber then contain 0.5 part blood and 99.5 parts diluting fluid. This is 0.5 part blood in 100 parts of solution (blood plus diluting fluid). Therefore, the blood has been diluted 0.5 in 100.

The figure 0.5 may be written as $\frac{1}{2}$. Thus our dilution of 0.5 in 100 may be written as $\frac{1}{2}$ in 100.

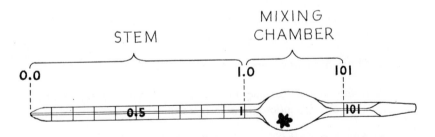

Fig. 79.—Red cell pipet. To distinguish the red cell pipet from the white cell pipet, note the following: The red cell pipet has 101 above the mixing chamber whereas the white cell pipet has 11 above the mixing chamber. Also, the red cell pipet has a red bead in the mixing chamber whereas the white cell pipet has a white bead in the mixing chamber.

When the dilution is $\frac{1}{2}$ in 100, the blood has been diluted 1 in 200. Consequently, the dilution correction factor for the red cell count is 200.

If blood were drawn to the 1.0 mark and diluting fluid to the 101 mark, the dilution would be 1 in 100. If blood were drawn to the 0.1 mark and diluting fluid to the 101 mark, the dilution would be 0.1 in 100 or 1 in 1,000. The dilution range of the red cell pipet is therefore said to be 1 in 100 to 1 in 1,000. However, the 1 in 200 dilution is the routine dilution and it is the only dilution of any practical importance.

A note of precaution before starting the procedure:

When you draw blood into the red cell pipet, you must get the blood *exactly* on the 0.5 mark. Otherwise, a serious error is introduced into the count. You may, of course, draw blood slightly past the 0.5 mark and then adjust it to the 0.5 mark.

When you draw diluting fluid into the pipet, however, you may stop a little above or a little below the 101 mark without causing any serious error.

If you have trouble diluting the blood, do not get discouraged. The beginner usually has to make several attempts. The only answer is *practice*.

Now follow the directions *exactly* as given in the Procedure for Step 1.

Procedure for Step 1

1. In diluting the blood, you can use either anticoagulated blood or finger tip blood. However, you should use anticoagulated blood until you have completed about 6 red cell counts and somewhat mastered the technique of diluting the blood. Then you should perform a finger puncture and make the dilution with finger tip blood (page 6).

2. Assemble the following equipment: several cotton balls or gauze pads, RBC pipet, rubber sucking tube, RBC diluting fluid, test tube of anticoagulated blood, pencil, and piece of paper.

3. Place the above equipment within easy reach.

4. If the rubber sucking tube has been used by someone else, dip the mouthpiece in a bottle of alcohol.

5. Attach the rubber sucking tube to that end of the pipet which is nearest the bulb.

6. Then put the pipet and rubber sucking tube on the table ready for use.

7. In the following steps, you will be sucking blood into the stem of the pipet. If you accidentally suck blood into the bulb of the pipet, immediately suck diluting fluid into the bulb until it is completely filled. Then put the pipet in the container for used pipets. Never let undiluted blood stand in the stem or bulb of a pipet because it will harden and may clog the pipet. If a pipet does become clogged with dried blood, you may clean it by following the directions on page 135.

8. Put a stopper in the mouth of the test tube and mix the blood by completely inverting the test tube 10 to 12 times. Do not shake!

   Note: If you have a large test tube (about 4 inches long) which is less than half full of blood, it will be difficult for you to get the pipet in the blood. In such cases, after you have mixed the blood, transfer it to a small test tube (about 2 or 3 inches long).

9. After you have mixed the blood, place the test tube in a medicine glass or test tube rack.

10. Then remove the stopper from the test tube.

11. Remove the cap from the bottle of RBC diluting fluid.

12. Pick up your red cell pipet and rubber sucking tube.

13. Put the mouthpiece of the rubber sucking tube in your mouth.

14. With your right hand, hold the pipet.

    Note: The red cell pipet has a much smaller bore than the white cell pipet. Consequently, the dilution procedure with the red cell pipet will require more gentle and controlled sucking.

15. With your left hand, pick up the test tube of blood.

16. Dip the pipet into the blood and brace the tip of the pipet against the lower inner wall of the test tube.

    Note: By bracing the pipet against the wall of the test tube, you steady the pipet. This makes it easier to keep the pipet in the blood. If you momentarily lift the pipet out of the blood, you will suck an air bubble into the pipet.

17. Being careful not to lift the pipet out of the blood, very gently suck up blood until it is a little bit past the 0.5 mark.

18. Then put the test tube back in the medicine glass or test tube rack.

19. Hold the pipet in a horizontal position.

20. Place the tip of the pipet against the index finger of your left hand.

21. In the following manner, adjust the blood so it is <u>exactly</u> on the 0.5 mark:

22. Tease the blood out with your index finger and blow gently on the rubber sucking tube.

    Note: If you remove too much blood, simply suck the blood back into the pipet.

23. When the blood is <u>exactly</u> on the 0.5 mark, press the tip of your tongue <u>firmly</u> against the opening in the sucking tube. This holds the blood in place.

24. Pick up a piece of cotton.

25. Keeping your tongue <u>firmly</u> over the opening in the sucking tube, wipe off any blood adhering to the outside stem of the pipet.

26. Observe the position of the hands in Figure 80.

    Note: You must hold the pipet almost straight up and down as shown in the illustration. If you hold the pipet toward the horizontal, you will get an air bubble in the bulb.

27. Pick up the bottle of RBC diluting fluid.

28. Check to see that the blood is <u>exactly</u> on the 0.5 mark.

29. Dip the pipet into the bottle, brace the tip of the pipet against the lower inner wall of the bottle, and suck up diluting fluid to the 101 mark.

    Note: You may stop a little below or a little above the 101 mark without causing any serious error. If you go way past the 101 mark, however, you must detach the rubber sucking tube from the pipet. Then you must put the pipet in the container for used pipets, get another pipet, attach it to the rubber sucking tube, and start again with step 12.

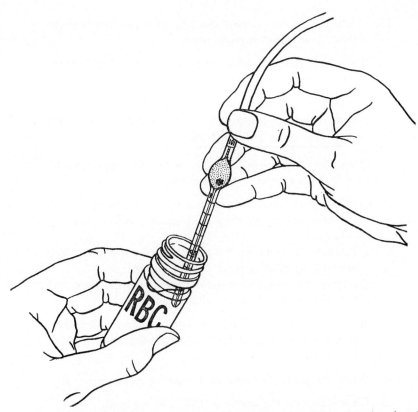

FIG. 80.—Sucking up RBC diluting fluid to the 101 mark. Note that the pipet is held almost vertical. It is *not* inclined toward the horizontal.

30. When the solution is on the 101 mark, press your tongue firmly against the opening in the sucking tube.

31. Put the bottle of RBC diluting fluid on the table.

32. Now firmly hold the index finger of your left hand over the opening in the tip of the pipet. Keep this index finger of your left hand over the opening in the tip of the pipet until the next step is completed. This will prevent the loss of fluid and the formation of an air bubble in the bulb of the pipet.

33. With your right hand, detach the rubber sucking tube from the pipet.

34. Place the middle finger and thumb of your right hand over the ends of the pipet and shake for about 10 seconds. This prevents any clumping of the blood cells.

35. A tiny air bubble (about the size of a pin head) in the bulb of your pipet is permissible.

36. If you have no air bubbles or only a tiny air bubble in the bulb of your pipet, proceed to step 38 below.

37. If you have a large air bubble in the bulb of your pipet, you <u>must</u> put the pipet in the container for used pipets and <u>repeat steps 2 through 36.</u>

   Note: An air bubble in the bulb of the pipet may be caused by any one of the following:

   (1) Failure to keep the pipet in an almost vertical position when sucking diluting fluid into the pipet (see Fig. 80, page 151).
   (2) Momentarily lifting the pipet out of the diluting fluid when sucking diluting fluid into the pipet.
   (3) Failure to keep your index finger over the tip of the pipet when detaching the rubber sucking tube.

38. Now hold the pipet in a horizontal position and push it into a piece of paper for temporary storage (Fig. 56, page 104).

39. Write the patient's name on the piece of paper.

40. Put the cap on the bottle of RBC diluting fluid.

41. Put the stopper back in the mouth of the test tube of blood.

42. Now proceed to Step 2, Charging the Counting Chamber.

STEP 2:   CHARGING THE COUNTING CHAMBER

First read the *discussion;* then follow the directions in the *procedure.*

Discussion of Step 2

In this step, the cells and diluting fluid are first mixed to insure an even distribution of cells. The diluting fluid in the stem of the pipet is then discarded because it did not take part in the dilution of the blood. Finally, a tiny portion of the solution is transferred to the counting chamber and the cells are given about 5 minutes to settle.

In a complete blood count, time can be saved by proceeding as follows:

1. Make the following dilutions:
    a. Dilute the blood for the white cell count.
    b. Dilute the blood for the red cell count.
    c. Dilute the blood for the hemoglobin determination.
2. Make the blood smear.
3. Start staining the blood smear.
4. Shake the red cell pipet and white cell pipet at the same time (**Fig. 82, page 155**).
5. Charge ruled area 1 for the white cell count.
6. Charge ruled area 2 for the red cell count.
7. Count the white cells in ruled area 1. Meanwhile, the red cells in ruled area 2 can be settling out.
8. Then count the red cells in ruled area 2.
9. Make the hemoglobin determination.
10. Calculate the color index.
11. Make the differential white cell count.
12. Make the platelet estimation.
13. Make the stained red cell examination.
14. Make out your report as illustrated in the sample CBC report of Figure 50, page 90.
15. Sign your report and hand it in.

Procedure for Step 2

1. Remove the counting chamber and coverglass from the Petri dish or similar container.

2. If the coverglass is covering the ruled areas, remove it and place it on the table.

3. Using a small cloth, clean the ruled areas by thoroughly rubbing them with the cloth.

11

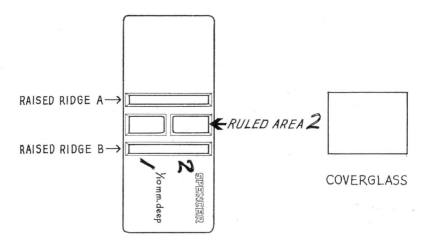

COUNTING CHAMBER

FIG. 81.—Position of the counting chamber prior to loading for the red cell count.

4. Now place the counting chamber so you can load ruled area 2 from your right (Fig. 81).

5. Pick up the coverglass. With your left hand, hold the coverglass by the edges. With your right hand, pick up the cloth. Now clean the coverglass by simultaneously rubbing both sides.

6. Hold the coverglass by the longest edges, taking care not to get your fingers on the clean surface. Then place the longest edges of the coverglass on the raised ridges of the counting chamber.

7. Now vigorously shake your pipet for 2 to 3 minutes.

   Note: After some experience, the white cell pipet and red cell pipet can be shaken together. This is done by holding the tips of the pipets against your thumb and the other ends against separate fingers (see Fig. 82).

8. While shaking the pipet, observe Figure 65 (page 112) and Figure 66 (page 113) and refresh your memory relative to discarding the first 4 drops and loading the counting chamber.

9. After you have thoroughly shaken the pipet for 2 to 3 minutes, hold your index finger over the opening in the top of the pipet.

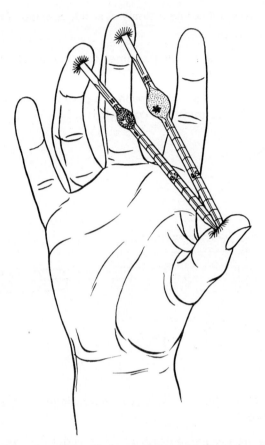

FIG. 82.—Shaking the white cell pipet and the red cell pipet at the same time.

10. Now, controlling the flow with your index finger, discard the first 4 or 5 drops onto a piece of cotton.

   Note: Sometimes the solution in the red cell pipet will not flow readily. In such cases, proceed as follows: Attach the rubber sucking tube to the pipet and blow <u>hard.</u> If the solution still does not flow, get a stylet (a <u>thin wire</u> about 6 inches long illustrated on page 62). Now run the stylet <u>completely</u> through the pipet.

11. After you have discarded the first 4 or 5 drops, stop the flow by pressure from your index finger.

12. With your left hand, firmly hold the <u>longest edges</u> of the coverglass to keep it in place.

13. Press your index finger <u>firmly</u> over the opening in the top of the pipet.

14. Then touch the tip of the pipet to a piece of cotton to remove any fluid.

15. Place the tip of the pipet on the edge of ruled area 2 and push it flush against the coverglass (see below).

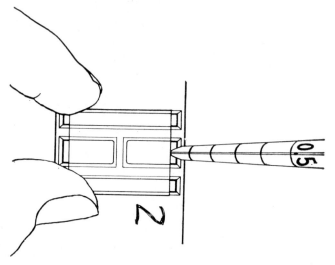

16. Controlling the flow with your index finger, proceed as follows:

17. Allow the solution to gradually seep under the coverglass and—

18. When the solution covers ruled area 2, quickly pull the pipet away.

19. Lay the pipet on the table.

20. <u>Carefully</u> remove your left hand from the coverglass.

    Note: In removing your left hand from the coverglass, you may move the coverglass without doing any harm.

21. Observe the properly and improperly charged counting chambers in Figure 83.

22. Now inspect your counting chamber to see if it is flooded or contains air bubbles.

23. If your counting chamber is flooded or contains air bubbles, immediately clean the coverglass and counting

chamber with the cloth. Then charge the counting chamber again.

Note: You may use the same pipet without shaking or discarding the first 4 drops <u>provided</u> you use it within 2 or 3 minutes after the first attempt. Otherwise, you must shake the pipet again and discard the first 4 drops.

24. When you have the counting chamber properly charged, proceed to Step 3, Counting the Cells.

Note: Save the pipet containing the diluted blood for you may want to repeat the count.

Properly Charged Counting Chamber

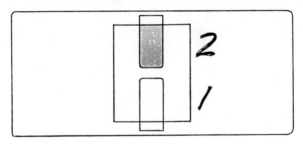

Note that the solution for the red cell count is much lighter than the solution for the white cell count. Note that the solution completely covers ruled area 2 and also that the solution is free from air bubbles

Improperly Charged Counting Chambers

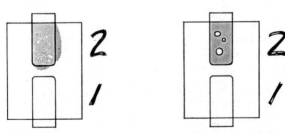

FLOODED Counting Chamber. Caused by allowing an excess of the solution to flow beneath the coverglass.

AIR BUBBLES in solution. Caused by air bubbles in pipet or unclean counting chamber or coverglass.

Fig. 83.—Properly and improperly charged counting chambers for the red cell count.

STEP 3:   COUNTING THE CELLS

First read the *discussion;* then follow the directions in the *procedure.*

Discussion of Step 3

In counting the red cells, some red cells, instead of lying flat, may be standing on end—like a coin. They will look like the 5 dark cells below:

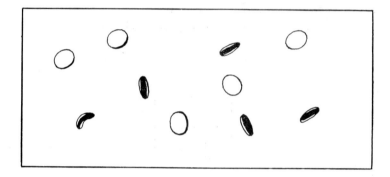

These cells, of course, should be counted.   In the above case, you would count 10 cells.

The above condition of red cells "standing on end" can usually be avoided if the red cells are given about 5 minutes to settle out.

With experience, you will be able to do a white cell count and red cell count together.   For example, you can charge ruled area 1 with the white cell pipet and ruled area 2 with the red cell pipet.   Then you can start counting the white cells.   Meanwhile, the red cells will be settling out. And, when you do start counting the red cells, you will find very few red cells "standing on end."

When you use the 10× (16 mm.) objective of the microscope, you can see an area the size of 1 "W" section in Figure 84.

When you use the 45× (4 mm.) objective of the microscope, you can see an area the size of 1 "R" section in Figure 84.

The red cells in the 1st "R" section, viewed with the 45× (4 mm.) objective, are shown in Fig. 85, page 161.

Carefully study this figure and legend, making the practice count as indicated and paying particular attention to the rules for counting red cells which touch boundary lines.

After you have completed the above practice count, follow the directions exactly as given in the Procedure for Step 3, page 162.

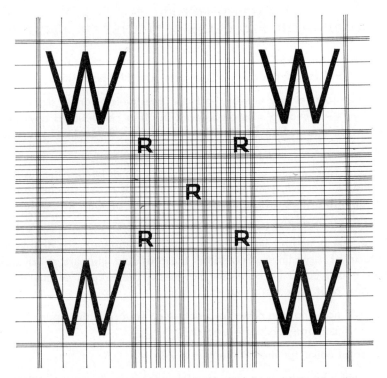

FIG. 84.—Position of the 5 "R" sections in the counting chamber.

This figure illustrates the Improved Neubauer ruling. It consists of 9 square millimeters.

Each "W" section is 1 square millimeter. Each "W" section is subdivided into 16 squares.

The central portion containing the 5 "R" sections is 1 square millimeter. Each "R" section is also subdivided into 16 squares.

You will note that the central square millimeter is really made up of 25 "R" sections. (But only 5 "R" sections are used in the red cell count.) Thus, each "R" section is $\frac{1}{25}$ or 0.04 square millimeter.

Since there are 25 "R" sections and each "R" section is subdivided into 16 small squares, the total number of small squares in the central square millimeter is $25 \times 16 = 400$.

LEGEND FOR FIG. 85.—
COUNTING THE RED CELLS IN THE 1ST "R" SECTION.

1. You keep the count in your head. You start in the upper left hand corner and follow the path of the arrow in the illustration.

2. If a cell touches *any one* of the triple lines which border the left side of the "R" section, you should count it. If a cell touches *any one* of the triple lines which border the top of the "R" section, you should count it.

3. If a cell touches *any one* of the triple lines which border the right side of the "R" section, you should not count it. If a cell touches *any one* of the triple lines which border the bottom of the "R" section, you should not count it.

4. Note: The boundary lines in some counting chambers are double lines instead of triple lines. Sometimes these double lines are so far apart that a cell could lie between the lines. These cells, of course, are treated as if they were touching a line.

5. You will note that the count for each small square in this figure is given in the accompanying score board.

6. The total count for the "R" section is 78.

7. You will also note that you start the count in the upper left hand corner and follow the path of the arrow.

8. For practice, count the cells in this figure.

9. Your total count does not have to exactly match the total count of 78 given in the illustration. But your total count should come within 1 or 2 cells of 78.

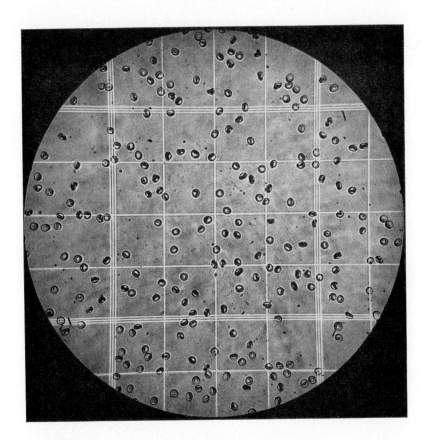

START
HERE

Red cells in the 1st "R" section

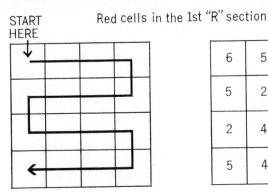

6	5	6	3
5	2	7	5
2	4	8	4
5	4	4	8

Start in the upper left hand
corner. Follow path of
arrow.

Score board for each small
square of above "R" section.
Total count is 78.

FIG. 85.—Counting the red cells in the 1st "R" section. (Photograph courtesy
of Mr. Cecil Gilliam.)

Procedure for Step 3

1. Turn on the light in front of the microscope.

2. Firmly grasp the 10× (16 mm.) objective and switch it into position directly over the opening in the stage.

   Note: A slight click is usually heard when the objective is in position.

3. By turning the coarse adjustment, raise the 10× (16 mm.) objective about 1 or 2 inches above the opening in the stage.

4. By turning the condenser knob, raise the condenser up as far as it will go.

5. Do not look in the eyepiece, but perform the following step with your naked eye:

6. By adjusting the mirror, make a bright light come directly up through the CENTER of the condenser and the opening in the stage.

7. With your right hand, grasp either end of the counting chamber. Pick up the counting chamber. Place the counting chamber on the stage of the microscope. Fit the counting chamber snugly into the jaws of the movable stage.

8. Do not look in the eyepiece but perform the following step with your naked eye:

9. By turning the stage knobs, move the counting chamber so the bright light comes directly up through the CENTER of the solution in ruled area 2. This is important!

10. Now lower the condenser by turning the condenser knob about one half turn.

11. Look at the counting chamber from the side. And, by turning the coarse adjustment, lower the 10× (16 mm.) objective until it is almost touching the coverglass.

12. In the next step, you will be rotating the coarse adjustment about one quarter turn toward yourself (see Fig. 86).

    Note: If you do not rotate the coarse adjustment toward yourself, you will break the coverglass.

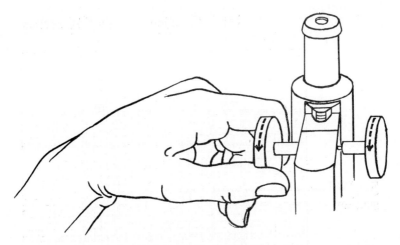

Fig. 86.—Rotating the coarse adjustment *toward* yourself (for the red cell count).

13. There is just one thin layer where the red cells will be in focus. This thin layer will appear with approximately one quarter turn of the <u>coarse adjustment</u>. The red cells will look like the red cells in Figure 88, page 165.

14. If you fail to continuously look through the eyepiece, however, you may go past the point where the cells appear. Consequently, in the next step, the important thing is keep your eye glued to the eyepiece and keep looking for red cells as you <u>slowly</u> turn the <u>coarse adjustment</u> toward yourself.

15. <u>Now, while continuously looking through the eyepiece, slowly rotate the coarse adjustment toward yourself until you see some red cells.</u>

16. If you do not see some red cells after rotating the <u>coarse adjustment</u> one half turn, you did not make the light come directly up through the CENTER in either step 6 or step 9. In such cases, you must remove the counting chamber from the stage of the microscope. Then you must repeat steps 3 through 15.

17. When the cells are in view, rock the <u>coarse adjustment</u> back and forth until you get the cells in good focus.

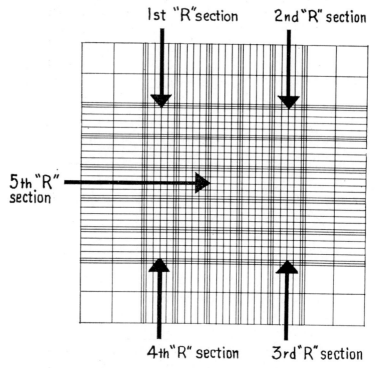

FIG. 87.—Heavily ruled area showing the 5 "R" sections.

18. Then make any of the following adjustments: If the light is too bright, lower the condenser. If the light is too dim, raise the condenser. If the cells have a dark or hazy background, adjust the mirror.

19. Observe the heavily ruled area containing the 5 "R" sections which is illustrated in Figure 87.

    Note: Since you are using the 10× (16 mm.) objective, this heavily ruled area containing the 5 "R" sections will occupy a single microscopic field.

20. When this heavily ruled area containing the 5 "R" sections is properly covered with red cells, it looks like the upper illustration in Figure 88, page 165.

21. Look in the eyepiece, turn the stage knobs, and bring into view the heavily ruled area containing the 5 "R" sections.

    Note: Rotating the fine adjustment back and forth helps to see the lines in their proper focus.

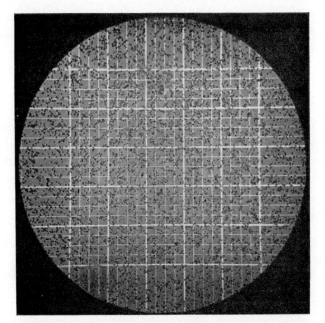

Good Distribution

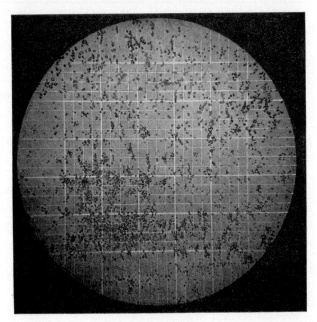

Poor Distribution

FIG. 88.—Good distribution and poor distribution of the red cells. The red cells must be evenly distributed as illustrated in the upper figure. If the red cells are not evenly distributed, as illustrated in the lower figure, different "R" sections would give vastly different counts. This, of course, would produce an error in the red cell count. (Photographs courtesy of Mr. Cecil Gilliam.)

22. When you have the heavily ruled area in view, turn to Figure 88, page 165, observe the illustrations, and read the legend below the illustrations.

23. Now look through the eyepiece and carefully check the distribution of your cells.

24. If your cells are not evenly distributed, it indicates faulty technique in mixing the cells or discarding the first 4 drops. In such cases, you <u>must</u> clean the counting chamber and coverglass with your cloth. Then you <u>must</u> repeat the shaking, discarding, and charging process (pages 153 through 166).

25. If your cells are evenly distributed, proceed as follows:

26 In the next step, <u>you must not move the counting chamber. You must not raise the objective. You may think that the objective is going to hit the coverglass. But the objective will not hit the coverglass. Therefore, to repeat, do not move the counting chamber! Do not raise the objective!</u>

Note: If you move the counting chamber or raise the objective in the next step, you will ruin the work of the past 24 steps. In such cases, you will have to take the counting chamber off the stage of the microscope and return to step 2, page 162.

27. Now, switch the $45\times$ (4 mm.) objective into position <u>directly</u> over the coverglass.

Note: When the objective reaches the proper position <u>directly</u> over the coverglass, a slight click will usually be heard. Also, when the objective is in the proper position, it will be difficult to move.

28. Now look through the eyepiece.

29. If the microscope is perfectly "geared," the cells will be in perfect focus.

30. If the microscope is not perfectly geared, the cells will not be in perfect focus. In such cases, proceed as follows:

31. Look through the eyepiece and turn the FINE adjustment either forward or backward until the cells appear in good focus.

   Note: If the cells start to disappear as you turn the fine adjustment in one direction, simply turn the fine adjustment in the opposite direction.

32. When you have the cells in perfect focus, turn to the illustration of the 1st "R" section (Fig. 85, page 161).

33. Observe that the lines to the left and above this 1st "R" section are not crossed or checkered. This absence of crossed lines to the left and above the "R" section identifies it as the 1st "R" section.

34. This 1st "R" section, composed of the 16 small squares, will occupy a single microscopic field.

35. Now, by turning the stage knobs, bring this 1st "R" section into view.

   Note: If you have trouble finding the 1st "R" section, use the following illustrations as guides: Figure 85, page 161, and Figure 87, page 164.

36. When you have the 1st "R" section in view, make any of the following adjustments:

37. If the light is too bright, lower the condenser. If the light is too dim, raise the condenser. If the cells have a dark or hazy background, adjust the mirror. If the cells are in poor focus, turn the fine adjustment and get them in good focus.

38. When your cells are properly focused and properly lighted, they should look like the cells in Figure 85, page 161.

39. Recall the method of counting the cells in 1 "R" section (Fig. 85, page 161).

40. Now count the cells in this 1st "R" section.

41. Then write down the total count for your 1st "R" section.

42. Now move to the 2nd "R" section. This 2nd "R" section will be 4 large squares to the right. You can be sure that you have the 2nd "R" section if the lines to the right and above the "R" section are not crossed or checkered (see Fig. 87, page 164).

43. Count the cells in this 2nd "R" section.

44. Write down the total count for your 2nd "R" section.

45. Move to the 3rd "R" section. It will be 4 large squares below. You can be sure you have the 3rd "R" section if the lines to the right and below the "R" section are not crossed or checkered (see Fig. 87, page 164).

46. Count the cells in this 3rd "R" section.

47. Write down the total count for your 3rd "R" section.

48. Now move to the 4th "R" section. It will be 4 large squares to the left (see Fig. 87, page 164).

49. Count the cells in this 4th "R" section.

50. Write down the total count for your 4th "R" section.

51. Now move to the 5th "R" section. It will be 2 large squares up and 2 large squares to the right. (See Fig. 87, page 164.)

52. Count the cells in this 5th "R" section.

53. Write down the total count for your 5th "R" section.

54. Add the 5 counts.

55. Example:

      92   count of 1st "R" section
   100   count of 2nd "R" section
    95   count of 3rd "R" section
   108   count of 4th "R" section
   105   count of 5th "R" section
   500   total number of cells in the 5 "R" sections

56. The sum of your 5 counts is the total number of cells in the 5 "R" sections.

57. Note: If there is a variation of more than 20 cells in any two "R" sections, your distribution was <u>not</u> good.   For example, you should not have 70 cells in one "R" section and 100 cells in another "R" section. If there is a variation of more than 20 cells in any two "R" sections, you must clean the counting chamber and coverglass.   Then you must re-shake the pipet, discard the first 4 drops, re-charge the counting chamber, and repeat the count.

58. After you have added your 5 counts, remove the counting chamber from the stage of the microscope.

59. Then clean the coverglass and ruled areas with a cloth.

60. Put the counting chamber and coverglass back in the Petri dish.

61. Then proceed to Step 4, Making the Calculations.

    Note: Save the pipet containing the diluted blood because you may want to repeat the count.

STEP 4:   MAKING THE CALCULATIONS

First read the *discussion;* then follow the directions in the *procedure.*

Discussion of Step 4

The red cell count is the number of red cells in 1.0 cubic millimeter of *undiluted* blood.   But we diluted the blood!   And we counted the cells in less than 1.0 cubic millimeter!   Therefore, we must multiply our total count by 2 correction factors.

The first correction factor compensates for the dilution of the blood. Since we diluted the blood 1 in 200, the dilution correction factor is 200.

The second correction factor compensates for the volume in which the cells were counted.   This is discussed below.

Each "R" section has an area of 0.04 square millimeter and a depth of 0.1 millimeter.   The volume of 1 "R" section is found as follows:

Area of 1	Depth of 1	Vol. of 1
"R" section	× "R" section =	"R" section
0.04 sq. mm.	× 0.1 mm.	= 0.004 cu. mm.

Thus, the volume of 1 "R" section is 0.004 cu. mm.

The total volume of the 5 "R" sections is found as follows:

Number of	Vol. of 1	Total vol. of
"R" sections	× "R" section	= 5 "R" sections
5	× 0.004 cu. mm.	= 0.02 cu. mm.

Thus, the total volume of the 5 "R" sections is 0.02 cubic millimeter.

Consequently, we have the following problem: When we counted the cells in the 5 "R" sections, we counted the cells in 0.02 cubic millimeter. Now we must report the number in 1.00 cubic millimeter.

The problem can be solved by multiplying by a volume correction factor. This is found as follows:

$$\text{Vol. cor. factor} = \frac{\text{volume desired}}{\text{volume used}} = \frac{1.00 \text{ cu. mm.}}{0.02 \text{ cu. mm.}} = 50$$

Thus, our volume correction factor is 50.

As previously stated, we have a dilution correction factor of 200.   And now we also have a volume correction factor of 50.

When the total number of cells in the 5 "R" sections is multiplied by the above correction factors of 200 and 50, the number of cells in 1 cubic millimeter of blood is obtained.   This is our red cell count.

To illustrate, if the total number of cells in the 5 "R" sections is 500, the calculation is made as follows:

Number of cells in 0.02 cu. mm. (5 "R" sections)	Dil. × cor. factor	Vol. × cor. factor	Number of = cells in 1.0 cu. mm.
500	× 200	× 50	= 5,000,000

Since the product of the dilution and volume correction factors is 10,000 (200 × 50 = 10,000), the calculation can be made by simply multiplying the total number of cells in the 5 "R" sections by 10,000. Thus,

Number of cells in 0.02 cu. mm. (5 "R" sections)	Correction × factors	Number of = cells in 1 cu. mm.
500	× 10,000	= 5,000,000

Now follow the directions in the Procedure for Step 4.

Procedure for Step 4

1. To make the calculations for your red cell count, proceed as follows:
2. Multiply the total number of cells in your 5 "R" sections by 10,000.
3. Example:

   500   total number of cells in 5 "R" sections
   10,000   correction factors
   5,000,000   cells in 1 cubic millimeter of blood

4. Note: The above calculation of multiplying by 10,000 is commonly referred to as "adding 4 zeros." Thus, by adding 4 zeros to 500, we get 5,000,000. This is usually written as 5.0 million.
5. After you have made your calculation, make out your report as indicated in the sample report below.
6. Sample report:

Report of a Red Cell Count

Patient: Dickson, Miss Candice   92053

Date: 7-7-72

Physician: Dr. Tom Maxwell

Patient's Values   **Normal Values**

5,000,000   women: 4.0 to 5.5 million per cu. mm.
                 men: 4.5 to 6.0 million per cu. mm.
                 infants: 5.0 to 6.5 million per cu. mm.

Examination performed by: Sandra Frisbie

---

7. After you have signed your report, hand it in.

MISCELLANEOUS INFORMATION FOR THE MICROSCOPIC METHOD

This section covers the following:

1. Summary of the Microscopic Method
2. Sources of Error in the Microscopic Method
3. Short-cut Method for Counting and Calculating
4. Correction for the Clumping of Red Cells

1. Summary of the Microscopic Method

After performing his first red cell count, the student may perform additional counts by skipping the *discussion* and going directly to the *procedure*.

For the convenience of the student, the steps and reference pages are summarized below.

Step 1. Diluting the blood
    a. Discussion: page 147
    b. Procedure: page 148
Step 2. Charging the counting chamber
    a. Discussion: page 153
    b. Procedure: page 153
Step 3. Counting the cells
    a. Discussion: page 158
    b. Procedure: page 162
Step 4. Making the calculations
    a. Discussion: page 170
    b. Procedure: page 171

2. Sources of Error in the Microscopic Method

The most frequent sources of error in the microscopic method are:
1. Failure to have the blood *exactly* on the 0.5 mark
2. Failure to shake the pipet thoroughly
3. Failure to discard the first 4 drops
4. Failure to properly charge the counting chamber

The least frequent sources of error are:
1. Inaccurate pipets or counting chambers
2. Moist or unclean pipets
3. Excessive pressure on finger when obtaining blood (this causes slight dilution of the blood by the tissue juices)
4. Failure to mix the blood (if the blood is taken from a test tube)

5. Drawing up too much or too little diluting fluid
6. Slowness in manipulation, thus allowing the blood to clot
7. Air bubbles in pipet (caused by failure to keep pipet submerged in the diluting fluid during the dilution process or detaching pipet from rubber sucking tube without holding finger over end of pipet)
8. Air bubbles in counting chamber (caused by air bubbles in pipet or unclean counting chamber or coverglass)
9. Presence of yeast or other contaminants in diluting fluid
10. Mistakes in counting or calculations

3. Short-cut Method for Counting and Calculating

After some experience, many technologists use the following short-cut method for performing a red cell count. This method is *not* recommended for beginners.

1. *Carefully* check the distribution of the cells.
2. If distribution is good, proceed as follows:
3. Count the cells in 2 "R" sections which are kitty-corner to each other. (Either the first and third "R" sections or the second and fourth "R" sections in Figure 87, page 164.)
4. Take the average of the 2 counts. For example, suppose one "R" section had 94 cells and the other "R" section had 98 cells. The average is the number which is half way between 94 and 98. This, of course, is 96. Consequently, the average of 94 and 98 is 96.
5. Now take half the average. For example, if the average is 96, half the average would be 48.
6. Now "add" 5 zeros to half the average. For example, suppose half the average was 48. You would "add" 5 zeros to 48. Thus, 4,800,000.
7. *Example #1:*
One "R" section had a count of 90. The other "R" section had a count of 98. The average is therefore 94. One half of 94 is 47. And "adding" 5 zeros to 47 gives a count of 4,700,000. This may be written as 4.7 million.
8. *Example #2:*
One "R" section had a count of 101. The other "R" section had a count of 110. The average is therefore 105.5 (or 106). One half of 106 is 53. And "adding" 5 zeros to 53 gives a count of 5,300,000. This may be written as 5.3 million.

4. Correction for the Clumping of Red Cells

On rare occasions, some of the red cells in the counting chamber may be clumped or agglutinated.

The clumping may be due to either of the following:

(1) The precipitation of certain proteins by the mercuric chloride in Hayem's diluting fluid. These proteins are present in multiple myeloma and kala-azar.

(2) The presence of cold agglutinins in the patient's blood. These cold agglutinins clump the red cells if the temperature drops below 20° C. (68° F.). The cold agglutinins may be found in atypical pneumonia and cirrhosis of the liver.

If the red cells show clumping, proceed as follows:

1. Obtain either Gower's solution or physiological saline solution (0.85% solution of sodium chloride).
2. Warm the solution to about 30° C. (86° F.).
3. Using the above solution as a diluting fluid, repeat the count.

COULTER COUNTER METHOD FOR THE RED CELL COUNT

The dilution for the white cell count is 1:500.

The dilution for the red cell count is 1:50,000.

With the exception of the above dilution, the procedure for the red cell count is similar to the procedure for the white cell count. See page 139.

Chapter 6

Hemoglobin Determination

Hemoglobin is pronounced he″mo-glo′bin. The word means blood globin or blood protein. It is often abbreviated Hb. or Hgb.

The hemoglobin determination will be discussed under the following headings:

Formation, Composition, and Function of Hemoglobin
Significance of the Hemoglobin Determination
Discussion of Procedures for the Hemoglobin Determination
Pitfalls to Avoid in the Hemoglobin Determination
Controls for the Hemoglobin Determination
Procedures for the Hemoglobin Determination
Preparation of a Standard Curve for the Hemoglobin Determination
Discussion of the Color Index

The student review questions for the hemoglobin determination are numbered 49–68 and begin on page 731 of the Appendix.

FORMATION, COMPOSITION, AND FUNCTION OF HEMOGLOBIN

Hemoglobin will be briefly discussed with respect to formation, composition, and function.

FORMATION OF HEMOGLOBIN

The formation of hemoglobin takes place in the developing red cells located in the bone marrow.

The manufacture of hemoglobin requires many materials. Among the essential materials are iron, protoporphyrin, amino acids, ribonucleic acid, and enzymes. Some of these materials are made by the red cell; others are received from the bone marrow.

In the formation of hemoglobin, the iron and protoporphyrin form heme. The amino acids and ribonucleic acid produce globin. And the heme and globin then unite to form hemoglobin.

The basic steps in the formation of hemoglobin are illustrated in Fig. 89.

175

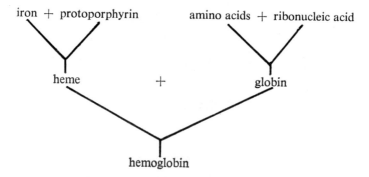

iron + protoporphyrin   amino acids + ribonucleic acid

heme   +   globin

hemoglobin

Fig. 89.—Basic steps in the formation of hemoglobin.

A relationship exists between the build-up of hemoglobin and the quantity of ribonucleic acid. As the build-up of hemoglobin increases, the quantity of ribonucleic acid decreases.

The formation of hemoglobin within the red cell requires about 1 week. When the task is completed, the hemoglobin occupies about ⅓ of the red cell. The other ⅔ of the red cell is mostly water.

COMPOSITION OF HEMOGLOBIN

You will recall that the molecular weight of water is about 18. The molecular weight of hemoglobin is about 67,000. Thus, hemoglobin is a very large molecule.

The hemoglobin molecule is made up of heme and globin.

Heme was formerly known as hematin. It is a pigment which contains iron. And it makes up about 4% of the hemoglobin molecule.

Globin is a colorless protein. It makes up about 96% of the hemoglobin molecule.

Thus, the hemoglobin molecule is 4% heme and 96% globin.

The hemoglobin molecule is illustrated in Figure 90.

FUNCTION OF HEMOGLOBIN

The function of hemoglobin is twofold. One, to carry oxygen from the lungs to the tissues. Two, to assist in the transport of carbon dioxide from the tissues to the lungs.

When hemoglobin is carrying oxygen, it is called oxyhemoglobin; when hemoglobin is conveying carbon dioxide, it is known as reduced hemoglobin.

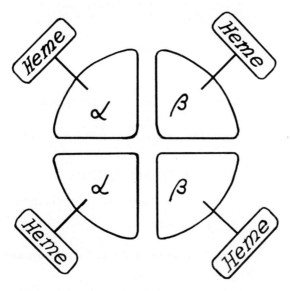

Fɪɢ. 90.—Diagrammatic representation of hemoglobin. The four polypeptide chains of globin are labelled α and β (from Wintrobe, *Clinical Hematology*, 6th edition).

One gram of hemoglobin is capable of combining with 1.34 milliliters of oxygen.

The iron in the heme is the key factor in hemoglobin. This iron is known as ferrous iron (Fe^{++}). The ferrous iron enables the hemoglobin to form a temporary union with oxygen.

In the lungs, the oxygen content is high and the ferrous iron forms the temporary union with oxygen.

In the tissues, the oxygen content is low and the ferrous iron releases the oxygen.

If the ferrous iron (Fe^{++}) in hemoglobin is ever oxidized to ferric iron (Fe^{+++}), a hemoglobin derivative known as methemoglobin is formed.

Normal blood contains about 0.1% methemoglobin. Increased amounts may be found in toxic conditions produced by oxidizing agents such as nitrates and chlorates.

The student should understand that oxyhemoglobin is oxygenated hemoglobin and not oxidized hemoglobin.

For example, a sponge will absorb and then give up water; neither the sponge nor water are changed.

The ferrous iron in hemoglobin temporarily holds and then gives up oxygen; neither the ferrous iron nor oxygen are changed.

If the ferrous iron in hemoglobin is oxidized, however, a transfer of an electron occurs and a different compound is formed.

Thus,

$$Fe^{++} \xrightarrow[\text{electron}]{\text{minus 1}} Fe^{+++}$$

(ferrous iron)　　　　　　　　　　　　　(ferric iron)

hemoglobin　　——————→　methemoglobin

SIGNIFICANCE OF THE HEMOGLOBIN DETERMINATION

The normal values for the hemoglobin determination are given in Table 7.

Table 7.—Normal Values for the Hemoglobin Determination

	Grams per 100 ml. blood	Percent
Women	12 to 16	83 to 110
Men	14 to 18	97 to 124
Newborn Infants . .	14 to 20	97 to 138

The hemoglobin values may be affected by age, sex, altitude, pregnancy, and disease. A brief discussion follows.

Newborn infants have higher hemoglobin values than adults. For example, the average newborn infant has a hemoglobin of about 17 grams per 100 milliliters of blood; and the average adult has a hemoglobin of about 15 grams per 100 milliliters of blood.

Men have higher hemoglobin values than women. For example, the average man has a hemoglobin of approximately 16 grams per 100 milliliters of blood; and the average woman has a hemoglobin of approximately 14 grams per 100 milliliters of blood.

The hemoglobin values may vary with changes in altitude. At a high altitude, the oxygen content of the air decreases and the red cell count and hemoglobin value increase. At a low altitude, the oxygen content of the air increases and the red cell count and hemoglobin value decrease. Thus, your hemoglobin may be 15 grams per 100 milliliters in the mountains and 14 grams per 100 milliliters at the seashore.

In pregnancy, the body gains fluid. Therefore, the red cells become less concentrated; consequently, the red cell count falls. Since the hemoglobin is contained in the red cells, the hemoglobin concentration also falls. Thus, the hemoglobin value may drop from 14 grams per 100 milliliters to 10–12 grams per 100 milliliters.

The above changes in the hemoglobin value—those changes due to age, sex, altitude, and pregnancy—are usually referred to as physiological changes.

Now let us consider the hemoglobin values in disease.

The hemoglobin values drop below normal in anemia and leukemia. For example, in iron deficiency anemia, the hemoglobin value may drop from a normal of 14 grams per 100 milliliters to 7 grams per 100 milliliters.

The hemoglobin values rise above the normal values in dehydration conditions and a disease known as polycythemia vera. For example, in a dehydration condition, such as a severe burn, the body loses fluid. The red cells become more concentrated and the red cell count rises. Since the hemoglobin is contained in the red cells, the hemoglobin value also rises.

By way of summary:

In health, the hemoglobin values are higher in newborn infants than in adults, higher in men than in women, higher in the mountains than at the seashore, and lower than usual in pregnancy.

In disease, the hemoglobin values are below normal in anemia and leukemia and above normal in dehydration conditions and polycythemia vera.

The hemoglobin determination is frequently performed. It is run about 2,000 times a month by the average hospital laboratory and about 100 times a month by the average physician's office.

DISCUSSION OF PROCEDURES FOR THE HEMOGLOBIN DETERMINATION

The procedures for the hemoglobin determination are many and varied. These procedures will be grouped and discussed under the following headings:

> Specific Gravity Method
> Gasometric Methods
> Chemical Methods
> Colorimetric Methods
> Summary

The above methods will now be discussed relative to the principle of the method and comments about the method.

SPECIFIC GRAVITY METHOD

The specific gravity method is also referred to as the copper sulfate method, the copper sulfate falling drop method, and the copper sulfate-specific gravity method.

Principle

Drops of blood are allowed to fall into 16 small bottles containing copper sulfate solutions of increasing specific gravity.

The results are read as follows.

(1) If the drop of blood falls in a few seconds, it has a greater specific gravity than the solution.

(2) If the drop of blood rises in a few seconds, it has a lesser specific gravity than the solution.

(3) If the drop of blood *remains suspended for about 15 seconds* (and then falls), it has the same specific gravity as the solution.

The bottles are labelled with the corresponding hemoglobin values.

Since all the drops of blood eventually fall and clear the solutions, the bottles can be used over and over again.

Comments

The specific gravity method has the following advantages: Fast. Simple. Inexpensive.

This method has the following disadvantage: Inaccurate.

The method is used mainly by blood banks as a screening test for blood donors.

GASOMETRIC METHODS

Either the oxygen method or the carbon monoxide method may be used. Both are quite similar. The oxygen method is discussed below.

Principle

Hemoglobin will combine with and liberate a fixed quantity of oxygen.

The blood is hemolyzed with saponin and the oxygen is collected and measured in a Van Slyke apparatus.

The volume of oxygen is corrected for temperature and pressure and the hemoglobin determined by the following formula:

$$\frac{\text{Volume of oxygen per 100 ml.}}{1.34} = \begin{array}{l}\text{grams of hemoglobin} \\ \text{per 100 ml.}\end{array}$$

Comments

The gasometric methods have the following advantage: None.

These methods have the following disadvantages: Time consuming. Involved technique. Expensive equipment. Inaccurate (fails to measure inactive hemoglobin such as methemoglobin and carboxyhemoglobin).

The methods were formerly used to calibrate instruments for determining the hemoglobin concentration.

CHEMICAL METHODS

The chemical methods are based on the fact that hemoglobin contains a fixed quantity of iron. This fixed quantity of iron is stated to be 0.34%. Thus, 1 gram or 1000 milligrams of hemoglobin contains 3.4 milligrams of iron.

The method of Wong for determining the iron content of blood and calculating the hemoglobin value is considered below.

Principle

Iron is detached from the hemoglobin by treating the blood with concentrated sulfuric acid in the presence of potassium persulfate. The proteins are precipitated with tungstic acid and filtered off. The iron content of the filtrate is determined in a colorimeter and the hemoglobin value calculated with the formula:

$$\frac{\text{mg. iron per 100 ml.}}{3.4} = \text{grams hemoglobin per 100 ml.}$$

Comments

The chemical methods have the following advantage: Accurate.

These methods have the following disadvantages: Time consuming. Involved technique.

The methods are used to calibrate various instruments for determining the hemoglobin concentration.

COLORIMETRIC METHODS

The colorimetric methods for the hemoglobin determination will be grouped and discussed as follows:

> Direct Matching Methods
> Acid Hematin Methods
> Alkali Hematin Method
> Oxyhemoglobin Method
> Cyanmethemoglobin Method

Direct Matching Methods

The direct matching methods which will be considered are: Tallqvist's procedure, Dare's procedure, and Spencer's procedure.

Principle

The color of blood is compared with a series of colored standards representing known quantities of hemoglobin.

Comments

The direct matching methods have the following advantages: Fast. Simple. Convenient.

Tallqvist's procedure and Dare's procedure are grossly inaccurate.

Spencer's procedure is accurate.

The direct matching methods are sometimes used at the bedside by the physician.

Spencer's procedure is a direct matching procedure but, since the blood is first hemolyzed by stirring with an applicator stick containing saponin, it may also be considered an oxyhemoglobin method.

Acid Hematin Methods

The acid hematin methods which will be considered are the Sahli-Hellige procedure and the Haden-Hausser procedure.

Principle

Blood is mixed with dilute hydrochloric acid. This hemolyzes the red cells and converts the hemoglobin to a brownish colored solution of acid hematin. The acid hematin solution is then compared with a colored glass standard or standards.

Comments

The acid hematin methods have the following advantages: Fast. Simple. Inexpensive.

These methods have the following disadvantage: Slightly inaccurate. (But not grossly inaccurate.)

The methods are used in many physicians' offices.

An acid hematin method using a photoelectric colorimeter is also employed in the handbook of procedures which accompanies some colorimeters.

Alkali Hematin Method

Principle

Blood is added to dilute sodium hydroxide. The solution is boiled. The hemoglobin is converted to a blue-green colored solution of alkali hematin.

The color of the solution is then either compared with known standards or measured in a colorimeter.

Comments

The alkali hematin method has the following advantage: Accurate.

This method has the following disadvantage: Will not accurately measure the hemoglobin of an infant. (An infant's blood contains alkali resistant fetal hemoglobin.)

The method is employed in the handbook of procedures which accompanies some colorimeters.

Oxyhemoglobin Method

Principle

Blood is mixed with a dilute solution of either sodium carbonate or ammonium hydroxide. This converts the hemoglobin to oxyhemoglobin. The depth of the resulting color is then measured in a photoelectric colorimeter.

Comments

The oxyhemoglobin method has the following advantages: Fast. Accurate.

This method has the following disadvantage: If traces of copper are present in the diluting fluid, they may convert oxyhemoglobin to methemoglobin and thereby slightly lower the values.

The method is employed in the handbook of procedures which accompanies some colorimeters.

Cyanmethemoglobin Method

Principle

Blood is mixed with Drabkin's solution which contains ferricyanide and cyanide. The ferricyanide oxidizes the iron in the hemoglobin, thereby changing hemoglobin to methemoglobin. The methemoglobin unites with the cyanide to form cyanmethemoglobin. The cyanmethemoglobin produces a color which is measured in a colorimeter.

Comments

The cyanmethemoglobin method has the following advantages: Fast. Accurate. Measures all forms of hemoglobin (except sulfhemoglobin).

This method has the following disadvantage:

To prepare Drabkin's solution, it is necessary to use a poison, cyanide; and the handling of a poison by inexperienced help in a busy laboratory can be dangerous.

The preparation of Drabkin's solution in the laboratory may be eliminated, however, by simply buying the prepared solution from a medical supply house.

The prepared Drabkin's solution is so dilute that the danger of cyanide poisoning is nil.

The cyanmethemoglobin method for the determination of hemoglobin is the method of choice in most hospital laboratories.

SUMMARY

The methods for the hemoglobin determination which we have just discussed are summarized below.

> Specific gravity method
> Gasometric methods
>   oxygen method
>   carbon monoxide method
> Chemical methods
>   Wong's iron content method
> Colorimetric methods
>   direct matching methods
>   Tallqvist's procedure
>   Dare's procedure
>   Spencer's procedure
>   acid hematin methods
>   Sahli-Hellige procedure
>   Haden-Hausser procedure
>   alkali hematin method
>   oxyhemoglobin method
>   cyanmethemoglobin method

The specific gravity method is used by blood banks as a screening test for blood donors, the gasometric and chemical methods are more or less of historical interest, and the colorimetric methods are the methods currently being used in medical laboratories.

PITFALLS TO AVOID IN THE HEMOGLOBIN DETERMINATION

The pitfalls in the hemoglobin determination may be avoided by good equipment and good technique.

The pitfalls to avoid in equipment and technique are discussed below.

PITFALLS TO AVOID IN EQUIPMENT

The discussion will cover pipet pitfalls, cuvet pitfalls, and colorimeter pitfalls.

Pipet Pitfalls

1. Use Sahli pipets which have been calibrated to meet specifications of less than $\pm 2\%$ error.

Cuvet Pitfalls

1. Use cuvets that are clean, free from scratches and flaws, and have been "matched" in the colorimeter.
2. The cuvets should not be washed with other glassware. They should be washed separately. Then they should be thoroughly rinsed with distilled water. And finally they should be allowed to drain dry.

Colorimeter Pitfalls

1. Make sure the colorimeter has been properly calibrated.
2. Make sure the calibration table or standard curve has been recently checked with a hemoglobin control.
3. Make sure that a new calibration table or standard curve is prepared if:
   (1) a new bulb is inserted in the colorimeter
   (2) a new photoelectric cell is inserted in the colorimeter
   (3) the colorimeter has been repaired
   (4) the colorimeter has been moved

PITFALLS TO AVOID IN TECHNIQUE

The discussion will deal with sample pitfalls, pipetting pitfalls, colorimeter operational pitfalls, and personal pitfalls.

Sample Pitfalls

1. Blood from a finger puncture may contain tissue juices and lymphatic fluid, especially if the finger is tightly squeezed, and these will dilute the blood. This dilution can be significant since only 0.02 milliliter of blood is used for the determination. Consequently, if it is at all possible, use blood from a venipuncture rather than blood from a finger puncture.
2. If the blood has been recently drawn, mix the blood in the test tube by *completely* inverting the test tube 10 to 12 times. If the blood has been sitting in the refrigerator several hours or overnight, mix the blood by *completely* inverting the test tube 40 to 50 times.

13

Pipetting Pitfalls

1. Dirt or moisture in a pipet will affect the results; therefore, make sure the pipet is clean and *dry*.
2. In drawing blood into a pipet, make sure you get the blood *EXACTLY* on the mark. This is the most critical point in the entire procedure!
3. Make sure to wipe off the blood on the outside stem of the pipet and then double check to see that the blood is still *exactly* on the mark.
4. After you have expelled the blood from a pipet into the diluting fluid, remove *all* the blood from the inside bore of the pipet by drawing the solution into the pipet and expelling it back into the solution 3 times.

Colorimeter Operational Pitfalls

1. In some procedures, the color of the final solution fades; therefore, do not delay the reading in the colorimeter.
2. If a colorimeter is not warmed up, allow about 5 minutes for it to warm up.
3. Make sure to use the proper filter or wave length in a colorimeter.
4. Make sure to thoroughly mix the blood and diluting fluid in a cuvet.
5. Before inserting a cuvet in a colorimeter, take a piece of tissue paper and thoroughly wipe off moisture and finger prints on the lower $\frac{3}{4}$ of the cuvet. (Moisture or finger prints on a cuvet will interfere with the passage of the light beam and this can greatly affect the results.)

Personal Pitfalls

1. Double check a colorimeter reading.
2. Double check a colorimeter reading with the corresponding value in the calibration table or standard curve.

CONTROLS FOR THE HEMOGLOBIN DETERMINATION

Any instrument which measures hemoglobin may be referred to as a hemoglobinometer.

Hemoglobinometers are used in the colorimetric methods for the hemoglobin determination.

Hemoglobinometers may be divided into visual hemoglobinometers and photoelectric hemoglobinometers.

With visual hemoglobinometers, the naked eye is used to measure color; with photoelectric hemoglobinometers, a photoelectric cell is used to measure color.

The discussion will cover controls for visual hemoglobinometers and controls for photoelectric hemoglobinometers.

CONTROLS FOR VISUAL HEMOGLOBINOMETERS

With visual hemoglobinometers, different persons may arrive at different hemoglobin values for the same specimen. This is due to the fact that different persons may make different color comparisons.

For example, three persons may look at the same specimen. The first person may make an evaluation of 13 grams. The second person may make an evaluation of 14 grams. And the third person may make an evaluation of 15 grams.

In using visual hemoglobinometers, such as the Haden-Hausser, use the following method of control for the personal difference involved in comparing colors.

Using your visual hemoglobinometer, run a hemoglobin determination on any sample of blood.

On this same sample of blood, have a hemoglobin determination run on a photoelectric hemoglobinometer that has been properly calibrated.

Compare your hemoglobin value on the visual hemoglobinometer with the hemoglobin value on the photoelectric hemoglobinometer.

If your hemoglobin value on the visual hemoglobinometer exactly matches the hemoglobin value on the photoelectric hemoglobinometer, you have no problem. However, if your hemoglobin value on the visual hemoglobinometer differs from the hemoglobin value on the photoelectric hemoglobinometer, you should make a correction on all your future readings. Two examples are given below.

If your hemoglobin value on the visual hemoglobinometer was 12 grams and the hemoglobin value on the photoelectric hemoglobinometer was 13 grams, you are "under-reading." Therefore, on all future hemoglobin determinations with the visual hemoglobinometer, you should add 1 gram to your reading.

If your hemoglobin value on the visual hemoglobinometer was 14 grams and the hemoglobin value on the photoelectric hemoglobinometer was 13 grams, you are "over-reading." On all future hemoglobin determinations with the visual hemoglobinometer, you should subtract 1 gram from your reading.

If you are using a visual hemoglobinometer, it is a wise policy to check your visual hemoglobinometer reading with a photoelectric hemoglobinometer reading every 2 or 3 months.

CONTROLS FOR PHOTOELECTRIC HEMOGLOBINOMETERS

Hemoglobin controls for photoelectric hemoglobinometers may be purchased from medical supply houses.

The names of several hemoglobin controls are: Hematrol, Hemachrome-Fe, Hycel hemoglobin control, and Hyland hemoglobin control.

These hemoglobin controls are solutions of known hemoglobin concentration which may be employed to check the reagents, equipment, and procedure in the determination of hemoglobin.

The majority of hemoglobin controls are accompanied by literature which gives directions for their use.

In most instances, the directions simply tell the technologist to treat the control as a sample of blood, run a hemoglobin determination, and compare the result with the value given on the control.

If the value obtained does not agree with the value given on the control, the technologist must find the "bug" in his procedure. This is accomplished by checking the diluting solution, pipets, cuvets, colorimeter, and standard curve. In some instances, this task can become quite involved.

Hemoglobin controls are run with different frequencies at different laboratories.

Some laboratories run a control with each hemoglobin determination, whereas other laboratories run a control only once a week.

In the majority of hospital laboratories, where inexperienced help, as well as students and interns, may use the solutions, glassware, and colorimeter, a control is run at the beginning and end of each working day.

Running a control only takes a few minutes and it can often save a lot of headaches and embarrassment.

PROCEDURES FOR THE HEMOGLOBIN DETERMINATION

The procedures for the hemoglobin determination may be divided into two groups: visual procedures and photoelectric procedures.

The visual procedures employ the use of a visual hemoglobinometer whereas the photoelectric procedures employ the use of a photoelectric hemoglobinometer.

Three visual procedures and five photoelectric procedures will be given in this text.

These procedures are listed below, the first 3 procedures being visual procedures and the last 5 procedures being photoelectric procedures.

1. Spencer Procedure
2. Sahli-Hellige Procedure
3. Haden-Hausser Procedure
4. Leitz Photrometer Procedure
5. Hellige CliniCol Procedure
6. Bausch & Lomb Spectronic 20 Procedure
7. Photovolt Lumetron Procedure
8. Coleman Spectrophotometer Procedure

Since the student in the average laboratory school will be using only one of the above procedures, he should ask the instructor which procedure he will use. When he learns the name of the procedure, he should make a careful study of this procedure and a superficial study of the other procedures.

The student will note that some procedures determine the grams of hemoglobin per 100 milliliters of blood and then refer to a conversion table to find the per cent hemoglobin.

Unfortunately, different instruments have different conversion tables. For example, one instrument may convert 10 grams of hemoglobin to 65%. Whereas another instrument may convert 10 grams of hemoglobin to 69%. These inconsistencies arose during the development of the various instruments.

Consequently, when you report the hemoglobin determination, you should report the procedure used, the number of grams, and the per cent.

If an instrument does not have a conversion table, you may convert grams to per cent by referring to Table 8.

Table 8.—Converting Grams to Per Cent in the Hemoglobin Determination
(Table based on 14.5 grams = 100%)

Gm.	%	Gm.	%	Gm.	%	Gm.	%
1.0	6.9	6.0	41	11.0	76	16.0	110
1.5	10	6.5	45	11.5	79	16.5	114
2.0	14	7.0	48	12.0	83	17.0	117
2.5	17	7.5	52	12.5	86	17.5	121
3.0	21	8.0	55	13.0	90	18.0	124
3.5	24	8.5	59	13.5	93	18.5	128
4.0	28	9.0	62	14.0	97	19.0	131
4.5	31	9.5	66	14.5	100	19.5	135
5.0	35	10.0	69	15.0	104	20.0	138
5.5	38	10.5	72	15.5	107	20.5	142

The reporting of hemoglobin in per cent is frowned upon by most medical research men but many practicing physicians prefer to have the report in per cent as well as grams.

The student should always find the per cent hemoglobin because it is used to calculate the color index. The color index is a calculation which enables the student to check his work. It will be discussed after the procedures for the hemoglobin determination (page 206).

A sample report for the hemoglobin determination is given in Fig. 91.

Report of a Hemoglobin Determination

Patient: Jones, Mrs. Betty

Date: 10-10-72

Physician: Dr. Charles Butterworth

Hemoglobin Determination
(Haden-Hausser method)

Patient's Values		*Normal Values*
15 grams (97%)	women:	12 to 16 Gm. per 100 ml. (83% to 110%)
	men:	14 to 18 Gm. per 100 ml. (97% to 124%)
	infants:	14 to 20 Gm. per 100 ml. (97% to 138%)

Examination performed by: Sandra Frisbie

FIG. 91.—Sample report of the hemoglobin determination.

1. SPENCER PROCEDURE

1. Get materials for a finger puncture and the Spencer hemoglobinometer (Fig. 92).

2. Make a finger puncture, wipe away the first drop of blood, and place a drop on the open chamber of the hemoglobinometer. Hemolyze the blood by stirring with the applicator, and close the chamber.

3. Press the illuminating switch, look through the eyepiece, match the colors, and take the reading.

4. Report the method used, the grams of hemoglobin per 100 cc. of blood, and the per cent.

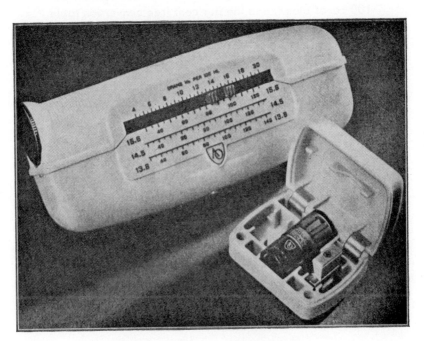

FIG. 92.—Spencer hemoglobinometer.

2.   SAHLI-HELLIGE PROCEDURE

1. Get materials for a finger puncture, a bottle of 1% (approximately 0.1 normal) hydrochloric acid, a pipet for measuring 20 cu. mm. of blood, and the Sahli-Hellige hemoglobinometer (Fig. 93).   Preparation of 1% hydrochloric acid is given in Appendix on page 696.

2. Fill the graduated tube of the hemoglobinometer to the 10 mark with the 1% hydrochloric acid.

3. Make a finger puncture, wipe away the first drop, and draw blood into the pipet to the 20 mark.   Wipe the tip of the pipet, and expel the blood into the graduated tube.   Rinse the pipet several times by first drawing the solution up and then expelling it back into the graduated tube.

4. Add distilled water drop by drop, mixing after each addition, until the color of the solution matches the color of the standard.   Take the reading corresponding to the height to which the solution has risen.

5. Report the method used, the grams of hemoglobin per 100 cc. of blood, and the per cent (see conversion table on opposite page).

Table 9.—The Sahli-Hellige Conversion Table

Gm.	1	2	3	4	5	6	7	8	9
%	6.5	13.0	19.5	26.0	32.5	39.0	45.5	51.9	58.4

Gm.	10	11	12	13	14	15	16	17	18
%	64.9	71.4	77.9	84.4	90.9	97.4	103.9	110.4	116.9

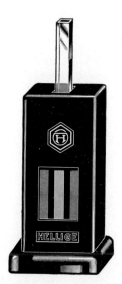

FIG. 93.—Sahli-Hellige hemoglobinometer.
(Courtesy of Hellige, Inc.)

3. HADEN-HAUSSER PROCEDURE

1. Get materials for a finger puncture, a white cell pipet, and a bottle of 1% hydrochloric acid (preparation given in Appendix on page 696).

2. Make the finger puncture, wipe away the first drop, draw blood to the 0.5 mark of the pipet, and the hydrochloric acid to the 11.0 mark. (This is the same as the usual 1 in 20 dilution for the white cell count. If the patient is anemic, make a 1 in 10 dilution by drawing blood to the 1.0 mark and diluting fluid to the 11.0 mark. The hemoglobin reading is then divided by 2 in order to compensate for this decreased dilution.)

3. Discard the first 4 drops, and fill the trough of the hemoglobinometer (Fig. 94). Match the color of the blood with the scale, and take the reading.

4. Report the method used, the grams of hemoglobin per 100 cc. of blood, and the per cent (see conversion table on opposite page).

Table 10.—The Haden-Hausser Conversion Table

Gm.	1	2	3	4	5	6	7	8	9
%	6.5	13.0	19.5	26.0	32.5	39.0	45.5	51.9	58.4
Gm.	10	11	12	13	14	15	16	17	18
%	64.9	71.4	77.9	84.4	90.9	97.4	103.9	110.4	116.9

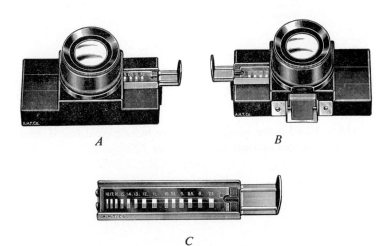

A   *B*

C

FIG. 94.—Haden-Hausser hemoglobinometer (clinical model). This instrument uses the same principles as the larger laboratory model but has no built-in light source. *A*, Front view showing comparator slide in position; *B*, rear view showing light filter in position; *C*, comparator slide with cover-glass in position. (From Haden, Principles of Hematology.)

4. LEITZ PHOTROMETER PROCEDURE (Courtesy E. Leitz Co.)

Hemoglobin

Sheard and Sanford; Peters and Van Slyke: Am. J. Clin. Path., 3, 412, 1933. Quantitative Clinical Chemistry, Vol. I—Interpretations, The Williams and Wilkins Co., Baltimore, 1932.

Draw finger-tip or oxalated blood to the first mark (0.025 cc.) on the hemoglobin pipet.

Dilute with 0.1% sodium carbonate to the 5.025 cc. graduation. Assist in accurately stopping at the meniscus by slight pressure of the finger on the rubber tubing at tip of pipet.

Expel directly into an absorption cell.

Let stand 5 minutes.

Read in Leitz-Photrometer (Fig. 95) with filter 550.

Determine concentration in grams from table.

Calculate per cent hemoglobin as follows:

$$\frac{\text{grams hemoglobin}}{\text{considered normal}} \times 100 = \text{per cent}$$

Example:

$$\frac{13.95}{15.5} \times 100 = 90\%$$

where 13.95 is the number of grams hemoglobin found, and 15.5 is the considered equivalent of 100%.

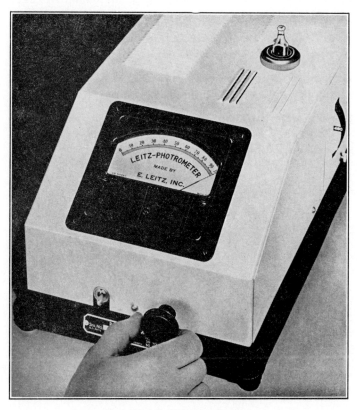

FIG. 95.—Leitz photrometer.

5. HELLIGE CLINICOL PROCEDURE (Courtesy Hellige, Inc.)

Hemoglobin (Oxyhemoglobin)

Sheard and Sanford: Am. J. Clin. Path., 3, 412, 1933.

1. Pipette exactly 4.0 ml. Sodium Carbonate, 0.1% (No. R-319), into a clean, dry absorption cell No. 904.

2. Add 20 cmm. fresh or oxalated blood. Rinse pipette by drawing up and expelling some of the mixture several times. If finger tip blood is used, the specimen must be obtained without pressure from a free-flowing incision.

3. Stir blood suspension thoroughly with a glass rod.

4. Place approximately 5 ml. distilled water in a second absorption cell for use as the blank.

5. Rotate filter selector of CliniCol (Fig. 96) to filter No. 520.

6. Insert absorption cell containing the blank and set meter to 100. Important: Absorption cells must always be inserted with a frosted side facing the operator.

7. Replace absorption cell containing the blank with absorption cell containing the unknown.

8. Note meter reading and obtain result in grams hemoglobin per 100 ml. blood directly from hemoglobin (oxyhemoglobin) calibration chart.

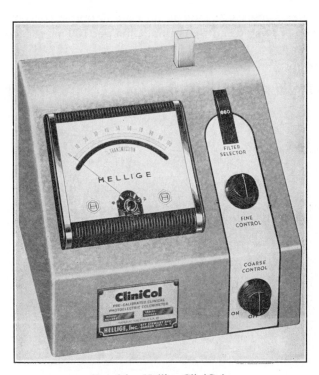

FIG. 96.—Hellige CliniCol.

6. BAUSCH & LOMB SPECTRONIC 20 PROCEDURE
(Courtesy Bausch & Lomb Co.)

Hemoglobin

Cyanmethemoglobin Method

1. Into 2 colorimeter tubes pipette exactly 5 ml. Drabkin's solution (for preparation, see Appendix, page 695).

2. In one tube add 0.02 ml. whole blood (unknown). Rinse pipette several times by drawing some of the liquid into the pipette and expelling.

3. Mix contents of tube by swirling.

4. The other tube is the "blank."

5. Allow tubes to stand for 10 minutes.

6. Set wavelength at 540 mμ and then place "blank" tube in instrument and set 100% T. (Fig. 97).

7. Replace "blank" with "unknown."

8. Refer transmission reading to table to obtain concentration of sample in grams hemoglobin per 100 ml. of blood.

Reference:

U. S. Armed Forces Medical Journal Vol. V., No. 5, 693 (May 1954).

Note:

1. Drabkin's solution contains cyanide.   When filling pipettes a suction bulb should be used.

2. Drabkin's solution should not be used after precipitate has formed on bottom of storage bottle.

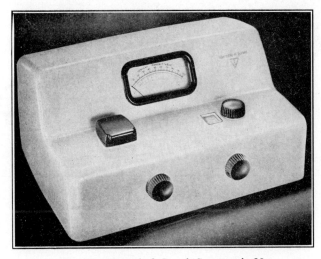

Fig. 97.—Bausch & Lomb Spectronic 20.

14

7. PHOTOVOLT LUMETRON PROCEDURE
(Courtesy Photovolt Corp.)

Hemoglobin (Acid Hematin)

Measure exactly 0.02 ml. blood in a pipette (to contain). Wipe off outside of pipette.

Blow the blood into exactly 10 ml. of 0.1 N HCl in a colorimeter tube.

Rinse the pipette by sucking up the solution and blowing it out.

Stopper and mix.

Read per cent transmission in Lumetron after 3 minutes using green filter 530, against water as the blank set at 100% transmission (Fig. 98).

With the transmission value as obtained, find result directly from Calibration Card which indicates "per cent of normal" opposite the transmission readings.

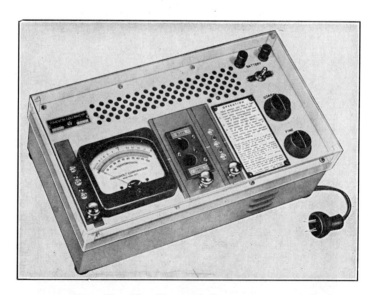

FIG. 98.—Photovolt Lumetron.

8. COLEMAN SPECTROPHOTOMETER PROCEDURE
(Courtesy Coleman Instruments)

Hemoglobin (Cyanmethemoglobin)

Reference:

Stadie, W. C.: J. Biol. Chem., *41*, 237, 1920.
Drabkin, D. L. and Austin, J. H.: J. Biol. Chem., *98*, 719, 1932; *112*, 51 (1935).
Crosby, Munn and Furth: U.S. Armed Forces Med. J., *5*, 693, 1954.

Procedure:

Measure exactly 5.0 ml. of Drabkin's Reagent (for preparation, see Appendix, page 695) into a test tube.

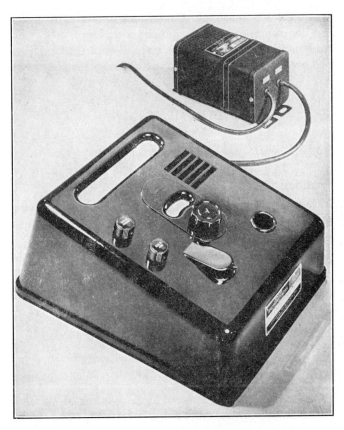

Fig. 99.—Coleman Spectrophotometer.

Mix the blood sample thoroughly and transfer exactly 0.02 ml. (Sahli pipette) into the reagent.

Rinse the pipette three times with the reagent in the test tube.

Allow the tube to stand for 10 minutes.

Transfer a portion of the contents of the tube to a 12 $\times$ 75 mm. cuvette and read in the Spectrophotometer at 540 mμ, using a cuvette of Drabkin's Reagent as a reference blank (Fig. 99).

Read the hemoglobin value in grams per cent from the table.

PREPARATION OF A STANDARD CURVE FOR THE HEMOGLOBIN DETERMINATION

The procedure for preparing a standard curve is usually given with the literature which accompanies the hemoglobin standard.

The directions which accompany the Hycel cyanmethemoglobin standard are given below and are hereby presented through the courtesy of Hycel, Inc.

INSTRUMENTS (1-9)

Instrument	Wave Length or Filter	Recommended Cuvette Size
1. Bausch and Lomb Spectronic "20"	540 mμ	13 mm. dia.
2. Beckman Model B	540 mμ	10 mm. (square)
3. Beckman Model DU	540 mμ	10 mm. (square)
4. Coleman Junior	540 mμ	12 mm. dia.
5. Coleman Universal	540 mμ	12 mm. dia.
6. Fisher Hemophotometer	-preset-	16 mm. dia.
7. Klett-Summerson	Filter "54"	14 mm. dia.
8. Leitz	Filter "530"	12 mm. (square)
9. Photovolt Lumetron	Filter "530"	14 mm. dia.

PREPARATION OF STANDARD CURVE: For instruments 1–9

The standard curve is set up by increasing dilutions of the Hycel Cyanmethemoglobin Standard. For the 5.0 ml. volume employed in the unknown samples the undiluted standard corresponds to 20.0 Gm % hemoglobin.

Dilutions are made to correspond to 15 Gm. %, 10 Gm. %, 5 Gm. % and zero. Dilutions must be made with the Hycel Cyanmethemoglobin Reagent—never with water.

Place five test tubes in a rack. Mark the tubes, 20, 15, 10, 5 and B. Dilutions should correspond to following table:

% Gm. Hemoglobin	20	15	10	5	Blank
Volume of Standard:	6.0 ml.	4.5 ml.	3.0 ml.	1.5 ml.	none
Volume of Reagent:	none	1.5 ml.	3.0 ml.	4.5 ml.	6.0 ml.

Transfer the dilutions to well matched cuvettes. Set the instrument to the proper wave length or filter. Adjust instrument so the *blank tube* has zero Optical Density or 100% Transmission. Take the readings for the standards and plot Optical Density on straight graph paper and % Transmission on semi-log graph paper.

DETERMINATION OF UNKNOWN SAMPLE
(Instruments 1-9)

Place 5.0 ml. of reagent in test tube. Add exactly 0.02 ml. of blood. Mix contents by inverting several times. Transfer contents to cuvette and read against Reagent Blank. Transfer reading to standard curve and obtain hemoglobin concentration in Gm. %.

INSTRUMENTS (10-15)

Instrument	Wave Length or Filter	Recommended Cuvette Size
10. Cenco-Sheard-Sanford Photelometer	Filter "B" or Filter No. 7	17 mm. dia.
11. Coleman Junior	540 mμ	19 mm. dia.
12. Coleman Junior II	540 mμ	19 mm. dia.
13. Coleman Universal	540 mμ	19 mm. dia.
14. Evelyn	Filter "530"	19 mm. dia.
15. Photovolt Lumetron	Filter "530"	18 mm. dia.

PREPARATION OF STANDARD CURVE: For instruments 10-15

The standard curve is set up by increasing dilutions of the Hycel Cyanmethemoglobin Standard. For the 6.0 ml. volume employed in the unknown samples the undiluted standard corresponds to 24.0 Gm. % hemoglobin. Dilutions are made to correspond to 18 Gm. %, 12 Gm. %, 6 Gm. % and zero. Dilutions must be made with the Hycel Cyanmethemoglobin Reagent— never with water.

Place five test tubes in a rack. Mark the tubes, 24, 18, 12, 6 and B. Dilutions should correspond to following table:

% Gm. Hemoglobin	24	18	12	6	Blank
Volume of Standard:	6.0 ml.	4.5 ml.	3.0 ml.	1.5 ml.	none
Volume of Reagent:	none	1.5 ml.	3.0 ml.	4.5 ml.	6.0 ml.

Transfer the dilutions to well matched cuvettes. Set the instrument to the proper wave length or filter. Adjust instrument so the *blank tube* has zero Optical Density or 100% Transmission. Take the readings for the standards and plot Optical Density on straight graph paper and % Transmission on semi-log graph paper.

DETERMINATION OF UNKNOWN SAMPLE
(Instruments 10-15)

Place 6.0 ml. of reagent in test tube. Add exactly 0.02 ml. of blood. Mix contents by inverting several times. Transfer contents to cuvette and read against Reagent Blank. Transfer reading to Standard Curve and obtain hemoglobin concentration in Gm. %.

DISCUSSION OF THE COLOR INDEX

One of the most difficult concepts for students to understand is a relationship between the hemoglobin determination and the red cell count. This relationship is known as the color index. A brief discussion follows.

The color index is a rough indication of the amount of hemoglobin in the red cells.

Since the color index is calculated with a formula, it is a stumbling block for those students who "can't get math."

In view of this, we will begin our discussion with two simple explanations and a visual illustration. Then we will proceed to the actual formula and present a few examples.

First of all, we should understand the following: One half may be expressed as 0.5 or $\frac{1}{2}$. And, one tenth may be expressed as 0.1 or $\frac{1}{10}$.

The word "about" means approximately. For example, when we say the color index is about 0.5, we simply mean it is approximately 0.5. Thus, it may be 0.4 or 0.6.

If the red cells are full of hemoglobin, the color index is about 1.0.

If the red cells are half full of hemoglobin, the color index is about 0.5.

If the red cells are one tenth full of hemoglobin, the color index is about 0.1.

In the above cases, the red cells would look something like the red cells in Figure 100, page 207.

You should understand that all the red cells would not look *exactly* alike. But, if the red cells were full of hemoglobin, all of them would look *approximately* like the cell on the left (Fig. 100).

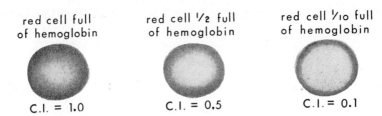

FIG. 100.—Red cells containing various amounts of hemoglobin.

If the red cells were half full of hemoglobin, all of them would look *approximately* like the cell in the center (Fig. 100).

If the red cells were one tenth full of hemoglobin, all of them would look *approximately* like the cell on the right (Fig. 100).

The color index has two functions: First, it tells the physician if he is dealing with a hypochromic (less color) anemia. Second, it tells the student or technologist if he has made a gross error in his red cell count or hemoglobin determination.

The color index is calculated immediately after performing the red cell count and hemoglobin determination.

The inspection of the red cells for their hemoglobin content is a separate examination. It is referred to as the stained red cell examination.

The stained red cell examination is performed *after* the red cell count, hemoglobin determination, and calculation of the color index.

For example, you do a red cell count and hemoglobin determination. From the information furnished by the red cell count and hemoglobin determination, you calculate the color index. This calculation tells you what the red cells should look like.

Then you perform the stained red cell examination. This examination shows you what the red cells actually do look like.

And, if your work has been properly performed, there should be no discrepancy between what the red cells should look like and what they actually do look like.

In the formula for the color index, the following abbreviations are used:

color index = C. I.

red blood count = RBC

hemoglobin = Hb.

grams = Gm.

Now, here is the monster formula itself.*

$$\text{C. I.} = \frac{\text{Hb. in \%}}{\text{First 2 figures of RBC} \times 2}$$

* The derivation of this formula is given on page 378.

The significance of the color index will be apparent from the following 4 examples.

Example #1

Suppose you did an RBC and Hb. and obtained the following results:

$$RBC = 5,000,000$$
$$Hb. = 14.5 \text{ Gm. } (100\%)$$

Your color index would be

$$C.\ I. = \frac{\text{Hb. in } \%}{\text{First 2 figures of RBC} \times 2}$$

$$= \frac{100}{50 \times 2}$$

$$= \frac{100}{100}$$

$$= 1.0$$

Since the normal values for the color index are 0.9 to 1.1, the above color index is normal.

When the color index is normal, the red cells should be full of hemoglobin.

When you did your stained red cell examination, you would expect the red cells to look something like the red cells in Figure 101.

If your red cells did not look like the red cells in Figure 101, you would know that you had made a mistake in your red cell count or hemoglobin determination. And you would repeat these tests.

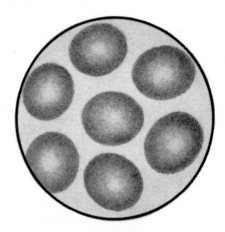

FIG. 101.—Red cells full of hemoglobin.

Example #2

Suppose you did an RBC and Hb. and obtained the following results:

$$RBC \doteq 5,000,000$$
$$Hb. \ = 7 \ Gm. \ (48\%)$$

Your color index would be

$$\text{C. I. } = \frac{\text{Hb. in } \%}{\text{First 2 figures of RBC} \times 2}$$

$$= \frac{48}{50 \times 2}$$

$$= \frac{48}{100}$$

$$= 0.48*$$

$$= 0.5$$

This color index is one-half normal.

When the color index is one-half normal, the red cells should be about one-half full of hemoglobin.

When you did your stained red cell examination, you would expect the red cells to look something like the red cells in Figure 102.

If your red cells did not look like the red cells in Figure 102, you would know that you had made a mistake in your red cell count or hemoglobin determination. And you would repeat these tests.

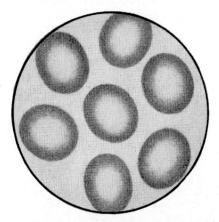

FIG. 102.—Red cells half full of hemoglobin.

* If the 2nd figure after the decimal point is 5 or above, the number is rounded off to the next higher number. Thus, 0.45, 0.46, 0.47, 0.48, and 0.49 would become 0.5.

If the 2nd figure after the decimal point is less than 5, this 2nd figure is simply dropped. Thus, 0.44, 0.43, 0.42, and 0.41 would become 0.4.

Example #3

Suppose you did an RBC and Hb. and obtained the following results:

$$RBC = 4,000,000$$
$$Hb. = 1.5 \text{ Gm. } (10\%)$$

Your color index would be

$$C. I = \frac{Hb. \text{ in } \%}{\text{First 2 figures of RBC} \times 2}$$

$$= \frac{10}{40 \times 2}$$

$$= \frac{10}{80}$$

$$= 0.13$$

$$= 0.1$$

This color index is $\frac{1}{10}$ normal.

When the color index is $\frac{1}{10}$ normal, the red cells should be about $\frac{1}{10}$ full of hemoglobin.

When you did your stained red cell examination, you would expect the red cells to look something like the red cells in Figure 103.

If your red cells did not look like the red cells in Figure 103, you would know that you had made a mistake in your red cell count or hemoglobin determination. And you would repeat these tests.

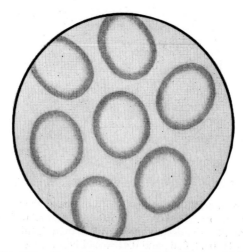

Fig. 103.—Red cells one-tenth full of hemoglobin.

Example #4

Suppose you did an RBC and Hb. and obtained the following results:

$$RBC = 2,500,000$$
$$Hb. = 14.5 \text{ Gm. } (100\%)$$

Your color index would be

$$C. I. = \frac{\text{Hb. in } \%}{\text{First 2 figures of RBC} \times 2}$$

$$= \frac{100}{25 \times 2}$$

$$= \frac{100}{50}$$

$$= 2.0$$

Now the normal values for the color index are 0.9 to 1.1.

Would the above color index of 2.0 be possible?

No. It would not. In effect, you would be saying that you could fill a water glass double the amount it would hold.

In the above case, of course, *you would realize that you had made a mistake in your red cell count or hemoglobin determination. And you would repeat these tests.**

The color index is included as part of a complete blood count in many laboratories. It should always be calculated by the student for, as indicated above, it enables him to detect any gross errors in his red cell count or hemoglobin determination.

The student is strongly advised to solve the 3 problems given below. The answers are given directly after the problems.

Problem 1:

A patient's red cell count is 4,800,000.

His hemoglobin determination is 13 grams (90%).†

What is his color index?

In the stained red cell examination, would his red cells look like the red cells in Figures 101, 102, or 103?

Problem 2:

A patient's red cell count is 3,500,000.

His hemoglobin is 6 grams (41%).

What is his color index?

In the stained red cell examination, would his red cells look like the red cells in Figures 101, 102, or 103?

* On very rare occasions, such as in pernicious anemia, it is possible to have a color index above the normal values of 0.9 to 1.1. This is caused by the presence of extra large red cells well packed with hemoglobin (page 589).

† A table for converting grams to per cent may be found on page 189.

Problem 3:

A patient's red cell count is 4,300,000.
His hemoglobin is 2 grams (14%).
What is his color index?
In the stained red cell examination, would his red cells look like the red cells in Figures 101, 102, or 103?

Answers to the above problems:

	Color Index	Figure
Problem 1	0.9	Fig. 101
Problem 2	0.6	Fig. 102
Problem 3	0.2	Fig. 103

When the student performs his first hemoglobin determination and color index, he will usually perform a white cell count and red cell count. After he completes these tests, he should make out his report as indicated in the sample report shown in Figure 104.

Report of a WBC, RBC, Hb., and C. I.

Patient: Dickson, Miss Candice

Date: 7-7-72

Physician: Dr. Tom Maxwell

Test	Patient's Values	Normal Values
White Cell Count	6,800	5,000 to 10,000 per cu. mm.
Red Cell Count	5,000,000	women: 4.0 to 5.5 million per cu. mm. men: 4.5 to 6.0 million per cu. mm. infants: 5.0 to 6.5 million per cu. mm.
Hemoglobin Determination (Haden-Hausser method)	15 grams (97%)	women: 12 to 16 Gm. per 100 ml. (83% to 110%) men: 14 to 18 Gm. per 100 ml. (97% to 124%) infants: 14 to 20 Gm. per 100 ml. (97% to 138%)
Color Index	1.0	0.9 to 1.1

Examinations performed by: Sandra Frisbie

FIG. 104.—Sample report for a white cell count, red cell count, hemoglobin determination, and color index.

Chapter 7

Differential White Cell Count

The differential white cell count is also referred to by the following terms: Diff., differential, differential w. c. c., and differential leukocyte count.

The discussion will cover the significance of the differential white cell count and the procedure for the differential white cell count.

The student review questions for the differential white cell count are numbered 69–119 and begin on page 733 of the Appendix.

SIGNIFICANCE OF THE DIFFERENTIAL WHITE CELL COUNT

The differential white cell count is a determination of the different white cells in a patient's blood. The report often plays a large part in the diagnosis of disease. A brief discussion follows.

We classify men as to race. Thus we have the following races: white, yellow, and black.

In a similar manner, we classify the white cells as to series. Thus we have the following series:

granulocytic	gran″u-lo-sit′ik
monocytic	mon″o-sit′ik
lymphocytic	lim″fo-sit′ik
plasmacytic	plas″mah-sit′ik

The white race may be divided into three branches: Americans, Europeans, and Asiatics.

In a similar vein, the granulocytic series may be divided into three branches:

eosinophils	e″o-sin′o-fils
neutrophils	nu′tro-fils
basophils	ba′so-fils

The monocytic, lymphocytic, and plasmacytic series do not have any branches.

We may therefore picture four series of white cells, with one series being divided into three branches. Thus,

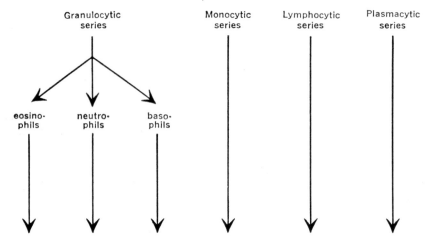

The people of each race go through various stages of development. We designate these stages with such names as infant, child, juvenile, and adult. In a similar manner, the cells of each series go through various stages of development. We designate these stages with such terms as blast, pro, and meta.

Now, we frequently take pictures of people at various stages of life. And, in a similar manner, we can make drawings of cells at various stages of development.

Suppose we place the infant cell of each series at the top of a page. Then show how the cell changes as it grows older. This has been done in Plate 2.

The cells above the dotted lines are the very young cells—the infants and children. These cells are usually confined to their birthplace in the bone marrow.

The cells below the dotted lines are the older cells—the adults. These cells, with the exception of the plasmacyte, are found in the blood stream.

Thus, normal blood contains only 6 different types of white cells. The names of these cells, together with their pronunciation, are listed below.

Cell	Pronunciation
Neutrophilic band cell	Nu″tro-fil′ik band cell
Neutrophilic segmented cell	Nu″tro-fil′ik segmented cell
Lymphocyte	Lim′fo-sīt
Monocyte	Mon′o-sīt
Eosinophilic segmented cell	E″o-sin″o-fil′ik segmented cell
Basophilic segmented cell	Ba-so-fil′ik segmented cell

The student should memorize the names and pronunciation of the above 6 cells. He should also study their various features. These are illustrated in Plate 2.

PLATE 2   STAGES IN THE DEVELOPMENT OF

GRANULOCYCTIC SERIES

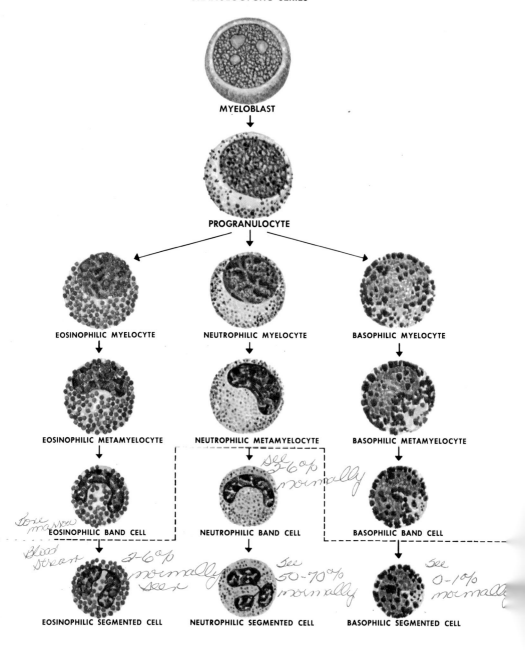

MYELOBLAST

PROGRANULOCYTE

EOSINOPHILIC MYELOCYTE   NEUTROPHILIC MYELOCYTE   BASOPHILIC MYELOCYTE

EOSINOPHILIC METAMYELOCYTE   NEUTROPHILIC METAMYELOCYTE   BASOPHILIC METAMYELOCYTE

bone marrow   EOSINOPHILIC BAND CELL   *See 2-6% normally*   NEUTROPHILIC BAND CELL   BASOPHILIC BAND CELL

Blood stream   *2-6% normally See*   EOSINOPHILIC SEGMENTED CELL   *See 50-70% normally*   NEUTROPHILIC SEGMENTED CELL   *See 0-1% normally*   BASOPHILIC SEGMENTED CELL

WHITE CELLS (Stain: Wright's; Magnification: × 1500)

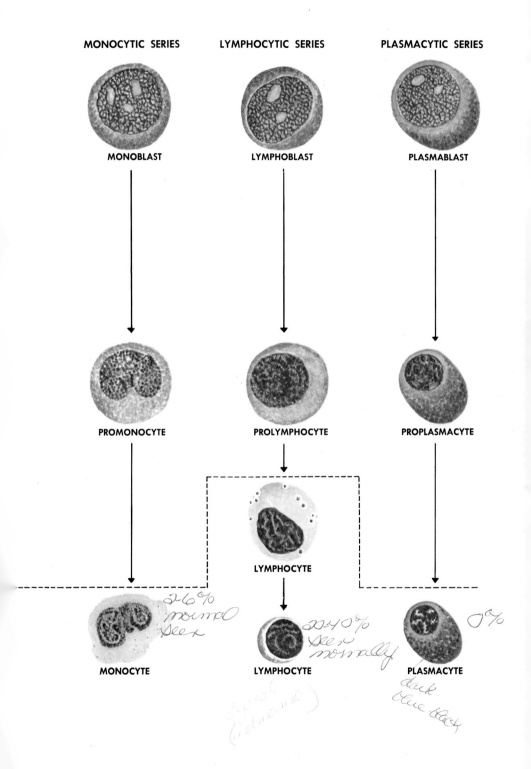

MONOCYTIC SERIES

LYMPHOCYTIC SERIES

PLASMACYTIC SERIES

MONOBLAST

LYMPHOBLAST

PLASMABLAST

PROMONOCYTE

PROLYMPHOCYTE

PROPLASMACYTE

LYMPHOCYTE

MONOCYTE

LYMPHOCYTE

PLASMACYTE

2-6%
normal
seen

20-40%
seen
normally

0%

dark
blue black

The 6 cells in normal blood are not present in equal numbers. For example, the blood contains more lymphocytes than monocytes. When we count 100 white cells and report the number of each type present, we perform a differential white cell count.

Since we count 100 cells, the report is given in per cent. For example, suppose our count shows 30 monocytes and 70 lymphocytes. We would then report 30% monocytes and 70% lymphocytes.

The normal percentages for the differential white cell count are given in Table 11.

Table 11.—Normal Percentages for the Differential White Cell Count*

Cell	Per Cent
Neutrophilic band cells	2 to 6
Neutrophilic segmented cells	55 to 75
Lymphocytes	20 to 35
Monocytes	2 to 6
Eosinophilic segmented cells	1 to 3
Basophilic segmented cells	0 to 1

* Infants and children of pre-school age are an exception to these values. They usually have more lymphocytes than neutrophilic segmented cells.

In disease, a particular cell may show an increased percentage. For example, in lymphocytic leukemia, we may find 80% to 100% lymphocytes. Thus, our differential might show 95% lymphocytes, 5% neutrophilic segmented cells, and none of the other cells.

The increased cell percentage which is found in the more common diseases is given in Table 12.

Table 12.—Increased Cell Percentage Found in the More Common Diseases

Increased Per Cent of Eosinophilic Cells	Increased Per Cent of Neutrophilic Cells	Increased Per Cent of Basophilic Cells
asthma	appendicitis	chronic granulocytic leukemia
hay fever	pneumonia	polycythemia vera
skin diseases	tonsillitis	irradiation (x-ray)
brucellosis	meningitis	hemolytic anemia
parasitic infestations	abscesses	removal of spleen
allergic eczema	granulocytic leukemia	

Increased Per Cent of Monocytes	Increased Per Cent of Lymphocytes	Increased Per Cent of Plasmacytes
tuberculosis	mumps	measles
typhus fever	whooping cough	chicken pox
Rocky Mountain spotted fever	German measles	scarlet fever
monocytic leukemia	infectious mononucleosis	multiple myeloma
subacute bacterial endocarditis	lymphocytic leukemia	serum sickness
	acute infectious lymphocytosis	plasmacytic leukemia

Consequently, the differential white cell count may serve as a straw in the wind of diagnosis.

Suppose, for a moment, the physician has a problem: Does this patient have a simple stomach ache or appendicitis?

A normal differential points to a simple stomach ache. But this differential

| Neutrophilic band cells | 15% |
| Neutrophilic segmented cells | 85% |

makes the diagnosis—appendicitis!

Why are the neutrophilic band cells and neutrophilic segmented cells increased in appendicitis?

Because the body needs—and produces—these cells to ingest the invading bacteria.

The other cells of the differential white cell count have similar callings:

The monocytes destroy bacteria, foreign particles, and protozoa.

The eosinophilic segmented cells aid in detoxification; they also break down and remove protein material.

The function of the lymphocytes is uncertain. It is believed, however, that the lymphocytes (1) produce antibodies and (2) destroy the toxic products of protein metabolism.

The function of the basophilic segmented cells is also uncertain. It is believed, however, that the basophilic segmented cells keep the blood from clotting in inflamed tissue.

The function of the plasmacytes is to produce antibodies.

Where are the white cells produced?

The cells of the granulocytic series and monocytic series are produced in the bone marrow.

The cells of the lymphocytic series are produced in the bone marrow and also in the spleen and lymphatic tissue.

The cells of the plasmacytic series are believed to be derived from either primitive lymphocytes or primitive reticulum cells.

How long do the white cells live?

The average white cell lives 5 days in the bone marrow and 10 days in the blood stream. Some lymphocytes, however, have a much longer life span. Some lymphocytes live as long as 200 days.

Now for some terminology.

Leuko means white and *cyte* means cell. Thus, a leukocyte is a white cell. The word is pronounced lu′ko-sīt.

The suffix *-osis* on the end of a word means an *increase in*. Thus, a leukocytosis is an increase in white cells. It is pronounced lu″ko-si-to′sis.

When the percentage of eosinophilic cells is increased, the condition is referred to as an eosinophilic leukocytosis.

When the percentage of neutrophilic cells is increased, we have a neutrophilic leukocytosis.

When the percentage of basophilic cells is increased, we have a basophilic leukocytosis.

When the percentage of monocytes is increased, we have a monocytosis.

When the percentage of lymphocytes is increased, we have a lymphocytosis.

And when the percentage of plasmacytes is increased, we have a plasmacytosis.

Now let us study the white cells seen in the more common types of leukocytosis.

A white cell is made up of a nucleus and cytoplasm. The nucleus is the central portion. The cytoplasm is the outer portion.

Thus,

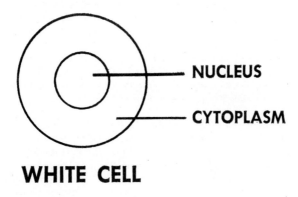

WHITE CELL

In identifying the various types of white cells, the following three factors should always be kept in mind:

1. The size of the cell
2. The features of the nucleus
3. The features of the cytoplasm

In Plate 3, which we will study next, the cells have been stained with Wright's stain and magnified about 800 times. The numerous small pink objects surrounding the white cells are red cells. In actual practice, so many white cells would seldom be seen in one field. They have been put there for the purpose of illustration.

Now carefully read the legend to Plate 3 and, as directed, study the cells in Plate 3.

15

LEGEND FOR PLATE 3.—
VARIOUS TYPES OF LEUKOCYTOSIS

First, turn to the illustration labelled *Lymphocytosis.*

The illustration labelled *Lymphocytosis* contains 1 neutrophilic segmented cell and 8 lymphocytes. Note that some lymphocytes are small and some are large. Consequently, in this case, the size of the cell does not help to identify the cell.

Turn to the illustration labelled *Monocytosis.* This illustration contains 1 neutrophilic segmented cell, 1 lymphocyte, and 3 monocytes. Notice that the monocytes are large cells. They are the largest cells found in normal blood. Consequently, the size of the monocyte is an aid in identification.

Monocytes are sometimes confused with large lymphocytes. The two cells can usually be distinguished by the features of their nucleus. Notice that the nucleus of the monocyte is spongy and sprawling. Whereas the nucleus of the lymphocyte is closely knit and (usually) round.

Now turn to the illustration labelled *Neutrophilic Leukocytosis.* This illustrates the difference between neutrophilic band cells and neutrophilic segmented cells.

What is the difference between a neutrophilic band cell and a neutrophilic segmented cell?

In a neutrophilic band cell, the nucleus is shaped like a band. The nucleus is not broken up into pieces or segments. Note the band cell at 1 o'clock in the illustration.

In a neutrophilic segmented cell, however, the nucleus is broken up into two or more segments. These segments are connected by a fine filament which is usually visible. Note the segmented cell at 12 o'clock in the illustration.

Quite often, it is difficult to tell whether a cell is a band cell or a segmented cell. In such cases, the accepted policy is to call the cell a segmented cell.

Now carefully study the illustration and note that it contains 3 neutrophilic band cells and 4 neutrophilic segmented cells. The neutrophilic band cells are located at 1, 4, and 9 o'clock in the illustration.

Turn to the illustration labelled *Eosinophilic Leukocytosis.* This contains 1 neutrophilic segmented cell, 1 lymphocyte, 3 eosinophilic segmented cells, and 1 ruptured eosinophilic segmented cell. The identifying characteristic of the eosinophil is the large red granules in the cytoplasm. Notice the difference between the large red granules in the eosinophilic segmented cells and the small pink granules in the neutrophilic segmented cell.

The question arises: "Do we count ruptured cells such as the ruptured eosinophilic segmented cell mentioned above?"

These ruptured cells are seldom seen. They should not be counted as a cell. But they should be recorded and reported as *disintegrated cells.*

Turn to the illustration labelled *Plasmacytosis.* This contains 1 neutrophilic segmented cell, 1 lymphocyte, and 2 plasmacytes. Notice that the nucleus of the plasmacyte is located near the edge of the cell. The cytoplasm of the plasmacyte is deep blue, usually a deeper blue than that shown in the illustration.

Turn to the illustration labelled *Infectious Mononucleosis* (infectious mon"o-nu"kle-o'sis).

Notice the two cells on the left. They are abnormal lymphocytes. If you look closely, you may see the "moth-eaten" appearance of the cytoplasm. These cells are seen in a disease known as infectious mononucleosis. The cells will be more fully discussed and illustrated in a later section (page 245 and page 661).

PLATE 3

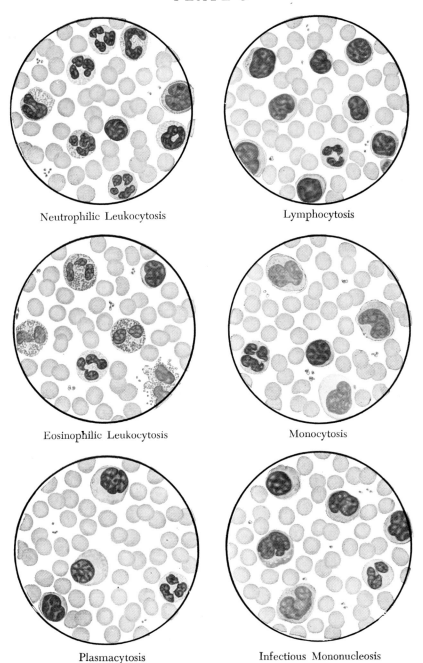

Neutrophilic Leukocytosis

Lymphocytosis

Eosinophilic Leukocytosis

Monocytosis

Plasmacytosis

Infectious Mononucleosis

VARIOUS TYPES OF LEUKOCYTOSIS

(From Miller, Seward E., *A Textbook of Clinical Pathology*, 7th edition,
The Williams & Wilkins Company.)

After reading the legend to Plate 3 and studying the cells in Plate 3, the student should answer the 3 questions listed below.

1. What is the difference between a monocyte and a lymphocyte?
2. What is the difference between a neutrophilic band cell and a neutrophilic segmented cell?
3. What is the difference between an eosinophilic segmented cell and a neutrophilic segmented cell?

The student is strongly advised to answer the above 3 questions before continuing. If necessary, he should carefully re-read the legend to Plate 3 and re-study the cells in Plate 3.

In conclusion to the study of Plate 3, note that the cells in the same "family" have similar features but differ slightly.

For example, in the illustration labelled *Neutrophilic Leukocytosis*, the neutrophilic segmented cells have similar features. But, like people in the same family, these cells differ slightly from cell to cell.

In the illustration labelled *Lymphocytosis*, note the similar features but slight differences among the 8 lymphocytes. *Also note that in some lymphocytes, the cytoplasm is sparse and barely visible.*

Consequently, when you see the cells in the microscope, you should expect to see slight variations among cells in the same "family."

Is the differential white cell count usually run as part of a complete blood count and how often is it run?

The differential white cell count is usually run as one of the five tests in a complete blood count. It is performed about 2,000 times a month in the average hospital laboratory and about 100 times a month in the average physician's office.

Before turning to the procedure for the differential white cell count, we will discuss 3 questions that are frequently asked by students.

Question 1:

Are abnormal differential white cell counts accompanied by abnormal white cell counts? For example, if the differential shows 100% lymphocytes, would you expect the white cell count to be abnormal?

Abnormal differentials are usually, but not always, accompanied by abnormal white cell counts. For example, consider appendicitis and infectious mononucleosis.

In appendicitis, the differential is abnormal and the white cell count is also abnormal. Thus, the differential may show 88% neutrophilic segmented cells and 12% neutrophilic band cells. And the white cell count may be 18,000 cells per cubic millimeter.

In infectious mononucleosis, however, the differential is abnormal but the white cell count may be normal. Thus, the differential may show 70% lymphocytes and 30% neutrophilic segmented cells. But the white cell count may be a normal count of 8,000 cells per cubic millimeter.

Question 2:

What is a "poly" or polymorphonuclear cell? What is a "stab" cell? What is a "juv" or juvenile cell?

Before 1948, a cell had many names. For example, a neutrophilic segmented cell was called a filamented cell, a lobocyte, a polymorphonuclear cell, etc.

To stem the tide of confusion, certain recommendations were made by the American Society of Clinical Pathologists and the American Medical Association. These recommendations are used throughout this text. A brief discussion follows.

All white cells belong to the leukocytic series. This series is further broken down into 4 series: lymphocytic series, monocytic series, granulocytic series, and plasmacytic series.

The new name and old names for each cell in the above 4 series is given in Table 13.

All red cells belong to the erythrocytic series. The new name and old names for each cell in the erythrocytic series is given in the discussion of red cells (Table 17, page 269).

All platelets belong to the thrombocytic series. The new name and old name for each cell in the thrombocytic series is given in the discussion of platelets (Table 29, page 416).

Question 3:

What is meant by relative counts and absolute counts?

Suppose a patient's differential showed 30% monocytes and 70% lymphocytes; and his white cell count was 10,000 cells per cubic millimeter.

His *relative* monocyte count would be 30%. His *absolute* monocyte count would be 30% × 10,000 = 3,000 cells per cu. mm.

His *relative* lymphocyte count would be 70%. His *absolute* lymphocyte count would be 70% × 10,000 = 7,000 cells per cu. mm.

In actual practice, the technologist is seldom asked to calculate absolute counts. Student examinations, however, may sometimes be seasoned with questions concerning these counts.

Of what value are relative counts and absolute counts?

Relative counts and absolute counts may be of value to the physician if a patient has a differential which is abnormal but a white cell count which is normal or below normal. An illustration follows.

Table 13.—New Name and Old Names for the White Cells

Name of Series	New Name for Cell	Old Names for Cell
Lymphocytic	Lymphoblast	Myeloblast, hemocytoblast, lymphoidocyte, stem cell, lymphocyte
	Prolymphocyte	Large lymphocyte, pathologic large lymphocyte, atypical leukocytic lymphocyte, monocyte, immature lymphocyte
	Lymphocyte	Small, medium or large lymphocyte, normal lymphocyte, small, medium or large mononuclear
Monocytic	Monoblast	Myeloblast, hemocytoblast, lymphoidocyte, lymphocyte, stem cell, immature monocyte
	Promonocyte	Premonocyte, hemohistioblast, immature monocyte, Ferrata cell
	Monocyte	Large mononuclear, transitional, plasmatocyte, endothelial leukocyte, histiocyte, resting wandering cell
Granulocytic	Myeloblast	Granuloblast, hemocytoblast, lymphoidocyte, lymphocyte, stem cell
	Progranulocyte	Promyelocyte II, leukoblast, myeloblast, premyelocyte, promyelocyte, progranulocyte A
	Myelocyte*	Granulocyte, myelocyte B, non-filament, class I
	Metamyelocyte*	Metagranulocyte, juvenile, juv, myelocyte C, non-filament, class I
	Band Cell*	Staff cell, stab cell, non-filament, class I, rod nuclear, polymorphonuclear, stab-kernige, rhabdocyte, non-segmented.
	Segmented*	Poly, polymorphonuclear, PMN, filamented, class II, III, IV, or V, lobocyte
Plasmacytic	Plasmablast	Myeloblast, hemocytoblast, lymphoidocyte, lymphocyte, stem cell, lymphoblastic plasma cell, myeloma cell
	Proplasmacyte	Türk cell, Türk irritation form, lymphoblastic or myeloblastic plasma cell, myeloma cell
	Plasmacyte	Plasma cell, Unna's plasma cell, Marschalko's plasma cell, plasmacytic lymphocyte, myeloma cell

* A cell in the granulocytic series which is older than the progranulocyte shows specific granules. It was suggested that the type of granules be specified. Thus, we have
   eosinophilic, neutrophilic, and basophilic myelocytes
   eosinophilic, neutrophilic, and basophilic metamyelocytes
   eosinophilic, neutrophilic, and basophilic band cells
   eosinophilic, neutrophilic, and basophilic segmented cells

For example, suppose the differential shows 70% lymphocytes and the white cell count is 3,000.

The percentage of lymphocytes is above normal and, standing by itself, would point to a disorder involving the lymphocytes.

But, when you calculate the absolute lymphocyte count:

$$70\% \times 3,000 = 2,100$$

(normal values are 1,000 to 3,500 per cu. mm.)

You find that the absolute lymphocyte count is normal.

Thus, you discover that (1) although the lymphocytes are increased in *per cent*, (2) they are not increased in *number*.

Therefore, the disorder does not involve the lymphocytes.

But why is the percentage of lymphocytes increased?

The percentage of lymphocytes is *increased* because some other cell in the differential is *decreased*.

By way of analogy: In a class of 10 boys and 10 girls, the *percentage* of boys increases if some of the girls stay home. (But the *number* of boys does not increase.)

How do you determine the normal values for absolute counts?

The normal values for absolute counts are determined as follows:

(1) Multiply the lower limit of the normal values for the differential times the lower limit of the normal values for the white cell count.

(2) Multiply the upper limit of the normal values for the differential times the upper limit of the normal values for the white cell count.

For example, let us find the normal values for the absolute count of lymphocytes.

You will recall that the normal values for lymphocytes in the differential are 20% to 35% and the normal values for the white cell count are 5,000 to 10,000 cells per cubic millimeter.

The lower limit of the normal values for the differential are therefore 20% and the lower limit of the normal values for the white cell count are 5,000. And,

$$20\% \times 5,000 = 1,000$$

The upper limit of the normal values for the differential are 35% and the upper limit of the normal values for the white cell count are 10,000. And,

$$35\% \times 10,000 = 3,500$$

Therefore, for lymphocytes, the normal values for the absolute count are 1,000 to 3,500 cells per cubic millimeter.

The normal values for the absolute counts of other white cells are found in a similar manner.

However, as previously stated, the medical technologist seldom receives a request to calculate an absolute count.

PROCEDURE FOR THE DIFFERENTIAL WHITE CELL COUNT

NECESSARY REAGENTS AND EQUIPMENT

1. *fresh* anticoagulated blood or finger tip blood
2. round wooden applicator sticks (Fig. 106, page 226)
3. glass slides
4. staining dish (Fig. 110, page 235)
5. Wright's stain

   A small bottle of Wright's stain is usually kept on the work bench. A large bottle is usually kept in the store room. When it is necessary to fill the small bottle, *the stain should be filtered as it is added to the small bottle. The filtering process is absolutely necessary because it removes precipitated stain, crystals, fungi, and debris.*
6. buffer solution for Wright's stain

   A small bottle of buffer solution is also usually kept on the work bench. A large bottle is usually kept in the refrigerator. The refrigerator temperature prevents the growth of bacteria and fungi.
7. distilled water
8. immersion oil
9. microscope

PROCEDURE

The procedure for the differential white cell count is broken down into 4 steps:

Step 1: Making the blood smear
Step 2: Staining the cells
Step 3: Counting the cells
Step 4: Reporting the count

Each of the above 4 steps will be broken down into a *discussion* and a *procedure.*

The student should first read the *discussion* and then follow the directions in the *procedure.*

The student will save time if he follows the directions EXACTLY as they are given. He should not attempt to improvise. And, above all, he should not attempt to skip any steps.

STEP 1: MAKING THE BLOOD SMEAR

First read the *discussion;* then follow the directions in the *procedure.*

Discussion of Step 1

The simplest way to count a handful of pennies, nickels, and dimes is to spread them out on a table. And the simplest way to count the different types of white cells is to spread them out on a glass slide. The preparation is called a blood smear.

A blood smear is also referred to by the following terms: blood film, blood slide, and peripheral blood smear.

The importance of making a good blood smear can not be over emphasized. If it is poorly made, the cells may be so distorted that it is impossible to recognize them. This is particularly true in noting changes in the size, shape, and hemoglobin content of the red cells.

There are two methods of making a blood smear: the slide method and the coverglass method. The slide method is the simplest and the most popular.

The student should make his blood smear by the slide method unless he is instructed to use the coverglass method.

The procedure for the slide method begins on page 226 and the procedure for the coverglass method is given in Figure 105.

Now follow the directions in the Procedure for Step 1, page 226.

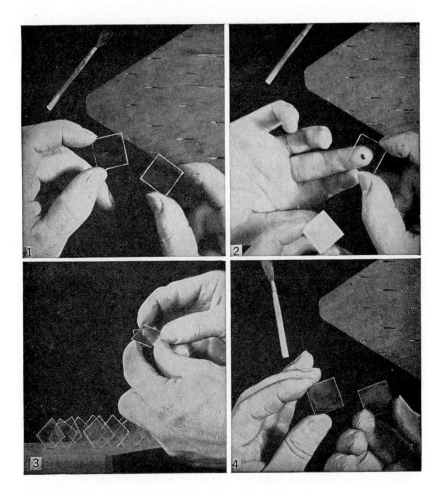

Fig. 105.—Coverglass method of making a blood smear.

1. Coverglass ($\frac{7}{8}$ inch, No. 2) is held at the adjacent corners with the thumb and forefinger of each hand; 2, the drop of blood is touched with the coverglass held in the right hand; 3, the coverglass carrying the drop of blood is quickly placed parallel on the coverglass held in the left hand; 4, after the blood has spread by capillary attraction, the coverglasses are drawn apart with a steady motion, care being taken to keep them parallel. After drying in the air, the films are ready for staining. The drop of blood must be globoid and just large enough to cover the coverglass when properly spread. (Haden, *Clinical Laboratory Methods:* courtesy of C. V. Mosby Company.)

Procedure for Step 1

1. In making a blood smear, you may use anticoagulated blood or finger tip blood. You should use anticoagulated blood, however, until you have completed about 3 differentials and somewhat mastered the technique of making a blood smear. Then you should perform a finger puncture and make the blood smear with finger tip blood (page 6).

2. Fresh anticoagulated blood must be used, that is, the anticoagulated blood must not be over 1 hour old. If the anticoagulated blood is more than 1 hour old, the anticoagulant may greatly distort the white cells.

3. Assemble the following and place within easy reach: test tube of fresh anticoagulated blood, 10 glass slides, and 2 wooden applicator sticks (Fig. 106).

4. Mix the blood by completely inverting the test tube 10 to 12 times. Then remove the stopper.

5. Hold the 2 wooden applicator sticks together and dip them into the test tube of blood.

6. Keeping the 2 sticks together, remove them from the test tube.

7. Note the position of the drop of blood on the slide in Figure 106.

8. Now touch the 2 bloody sticks to a slide so a small drop adheres to the slide as illustrated in Figure 106.

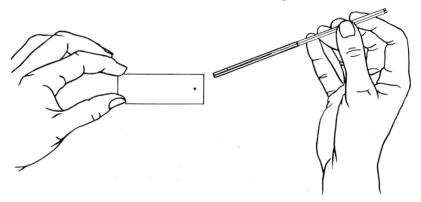

FIG. 106.—Using two wooden applicator sticks to place a drop of blood on a glass slide.

9. Put the sticks back in the test tube of blood.

10. After you have the small drop of blood on the slide, place the slide on a table or flat surface in the position illustrated below.

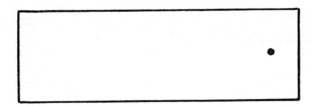

11. With your left hand, hold the edges of the slide as illustrated below.

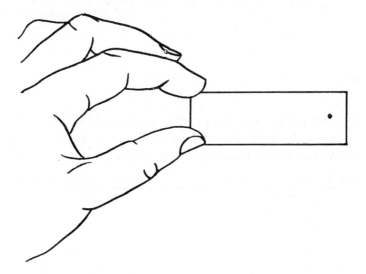

12. With your right hand, pick up another slide. This slide will be used as a spreader.

13. In the illustration below, note that the spreader is placed on the slide so that it makes about a 25 degree angle with the slide.

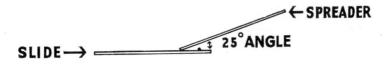

SLIDE→   ←SPREADER
                         25° ANGLE

14. Note: It is extremely important to place the spreader at the above angle of 25 degrees. THE SPREADER MUST BE MAINTAINED AT THIS 25 DEGREE ANGLE THROUGHOUT THE REMAINDER OF THE PROCEDURE.

15. Now hold the spreader in your right hand as shown below and place it on the slide so that it makes about a 25 degree angle with the slide.

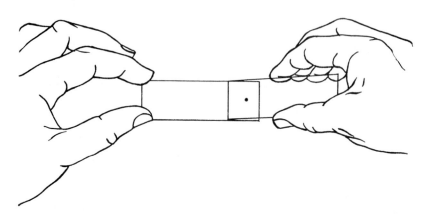

16. Note: When you have a 25 degree angle between the spreader and slide, the raised edge of the spreader will be about 1 inch above the table.

17. Keeping the spreader at this 25 degree angle, proceed as follows:

18. Draw the spreader toward the drop of blood and contact the blood. Thus,

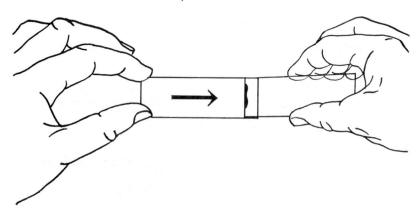

19. The blood should fan out to the edges of the spreader as shown above. If the blood does not fan out to the edges of the spreader, wiggle the spreader a little to make it do so.

20. Note: Do not let the blood get ahead of the spreader because it may cut or distort the cells.

21. In the next step, you must do 3 things simultaneously:

  (1) Keep the spreader constantly at the 25 degree angle.

  (2) Keep the edge of the spreader pressed firmly against the slide.

  (3) Push the spreader smoothly and RAPIDLY over the entire length of the slide (see below).

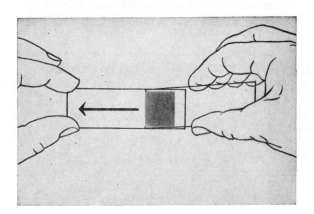

22. Now, keeping the spreader constantly at the 25 degree angle, press the edge of the spreader firmly against the slide, and push the spreader smoothly and RAPIDLY over the entire length of the slide.

23. The completed blood smear is illustrated below:

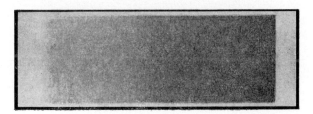

24. These are the criteria of a good blood smear:

(1) The thick area makes a gradual transition to the thin area (Fig. 107).

(2) The blood on the thin area does not extend to the end of the slide. (The blood may even cover only half the slide, provided the thick area makes a gradual transition to the thin area.)

25. Now compare your blood smear with the good smear and poor smear illustrated in Figure 107.

26. These are the usual causes of a poor blood smear:

(1) The drop of blood is too large.
(2) The spreader is pushed with a jerky motion.
(3) The spreader is not pushed rapidly enough. The spreader should be pushed with almost the same speed that you use to strike a match.

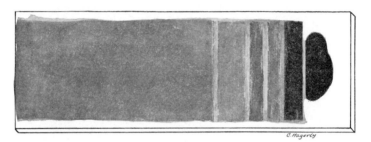

POOR SMEAR

Thin area for counting

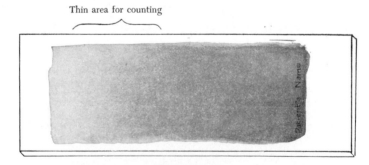

GOOD SMEAR

FIG. 107.—Good and poor blood smears.

27. Note: If the drop of blood is too large, you can take a portion of the drop by using the technique illustrated in Figure 108.

28. Now, for practice, make at least 6 more blood smears, using a clean slide and a clean spreader for each smear.

Note: It takes practice to make good blood smears.

29. After you have made at least 6 more blood smears, select two of your best smears.

30. Put these two smears aside. One of these smears will be stained. The other smear will be kept in reserve in case you make a mistake.

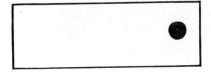

Slide with too large a drop

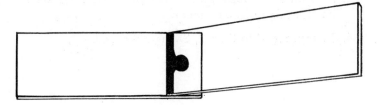

Taking a portion of the drop
with the spreader

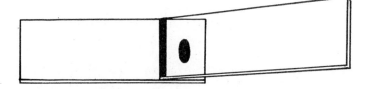

Lifting the spreader off the
slide and putting the spreader
on another portion of the slide

FIG. 108.—Technique of taking a portion of a drop of blood.

31. The poor smears are worthless. Either throw the slides away or put them in a cleaning jar and clean them at a later date.*

32. Let the blood smears dry (takes a few minutes). The drying process may be hastened by waving the smears rapidly in the air. When the drying process is hastened, as mentioned above, there is less distortion of the cells.

33. As illustrated below, the smear is labelled by writing the patient's name on the <u>blood</u> portion of the smear. This, of course, <u>etches the patient's name into</u> the blood.

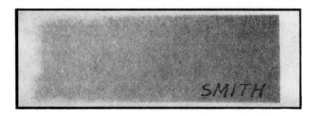

34. Now get an ordinary pen or pencil.

35. As illustrated above, write the patient's name on the bottom edge of each smear.

36. Then proceed to Step 2, Staining the Cells.

---

* Some laboratories use the slides only once and then throw them away. Other laboratories clean the slides and use them over and over. Directions for cleaning the slides are given on page 297.

STEP 2: STAINING THE CELLS

First read the *discussion;* then follow the directions in the *procedure.*

Discussion of Step 2

Poly means many. *Chrome* means color. Consequently, a stain of many colors is a *polychrome stain.*

The original polychrome stain was discovered by the Russian physician, Romanowsky.

Among the many modifications of Romanowsky's stain are the following: Wright's stain, Giemsa stain, Jenner's stain, May-Grünwald stain, and May-Grünwald-Giemsa stain.

For all practical purposes, these 5 modifications of Romanowsky's stain do not vary to any great extent in composition and staining qualities. In fact, the difference in staining qualities can probably only be recognized by an expert. Of these 5 stains, the most popular is Wright's.

Wright's stain is a methyl alcohol solution of an acid dye and a basic dye. The acid dye is known as eosin; it is red in color. The basic dye is known as methylene blue; it is blue in color.

The white cells are largely identified by their preference for the above dyes. And, in some cases, the cells are even named for the dye which they prefer. For example, cells which prefer the acid dye (eosin) are called eosinophils—meaning love of eosin. Whereas cells which prefer the basic dye are called basophils. And cells which prefer a mixture of the acid dye and basic dye are called neutrophils.

In the staining process, a buffer solution is used to control the acid-base balance of the stain. This is a most important function. If the buffer solution is too acid, it makes the acid dye too bright and the basic dye too faint. On the other hand, if the buffer solution is too basic, it makes the basic dye too bright and the acid dye too faint. In either case, the result is a poorly stained slide.

The acid-base balance of a solution is measured by the pH value. The pH value of a solution may be anywhere from 0 to 14. The lower the pH value, the more acid the solution; the higher the pH value, the more basic the solution.

The buffer solution used with Wright's stain should have a pH value of 6.4, 6.5, 6.6, 6.7, or 6.8. These pH values make the best color contrast between the acid dye and basic dye. The directions for preparing the buffer solution and Wright's stain are given in the Appendix on page 699.

In an emergency, distilled water may be used as a buffer solution. It is not advisable to use distilled water routinely, however, because the pH of distilled water varies with the absorption of carbon dioxide. Thus, the pH may be 6.9 one week and 6.5 the next week.

16

The staining process may be performed by any of the following methods:

1. Staining dish method
2. Staining jar or "dip" method
3. Automatic method

The staining dish method involves placing the blood smear on the rack of a staining dish and adding stain and buffer solution. This method will be used in our procedure.

The staining jar or "dip" method involves dipping the blood smear into several solutions.

The automatic method involves staining the blood smear by a unique and ingenious machine.

Among the automatic staining machines on the market are the Lipshaw Automatic Stainer and the Ames Automatic Stainer.

The price of the above automatic stainers is about $1500.

The Ames Automatic Stainer is illustrated in Figure 109.

Now follow the directions in the Procedure for Step 2.

Procedure for Step 2

1. From the smears that you made, choose your best smear.

2. Place the blood smear on the rack of the staining dish (Fig. 110).

   Note: Make sure that you have the bloody portion facing up.

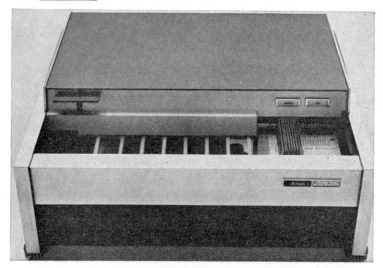

Fig. 109.—Ames Automatic Stainer.

3. Using either a medicine dropper or dropper bottle, distribute 50 drops of Wright's stain evenly over the entire slide (Fig. 111, page 236).

Note: The 50 drops of Wright's stain should spread itself evenly over the slide. If the stain does not spread itself evenly over the slide, the staining dish is not level. Correct the situation by placing a glass slide or two under the appropriate edge of the staining dish.

4. When the 50 drops of Wright's stain have been evenly distributed over the entire slide, let it stand for about 1 minute.

Note: Leaving the Wright's stain on the slide for a little more than 1 minute before adding the buffer solution will not affect the stain. It should not be left much longer than 2 minutes, however, because the alcohol in the stain will start to evaporate and may leave a precipitate on the slide.

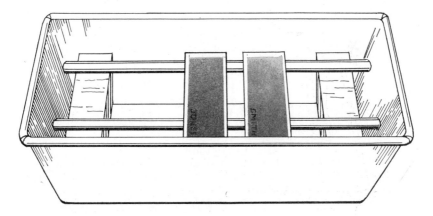

FIG. 110.—Staining dish. Note that the slides are placed on the rack so that a small space separates the slides. If the slides are placed too close together, the stain will run from one slide to the other.

5. Look at Figure 112 and observe that the buffer solution may be added with either a medicine dropper or dropper bottle and that <u>the solution is being evenly distributed over the stain.</u>

METHOD USING MEDICINE DROPPER

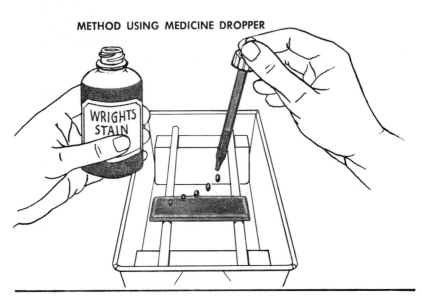

METHOD USING DROPPER BOTTLE

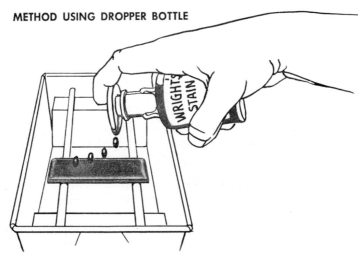

FIG. 111.—Methods of distributing Wright's stain evenly over the entire slide. Note that the stain is being *evenly distributed* over the entire slide.

6. After the Wright's stain has been on your slide for about 1 minute, add 25 drops of buffer solution so that it is evenly distributed over the stain. (Fig. 112)

METHOD USING MEDICINE DROPPER

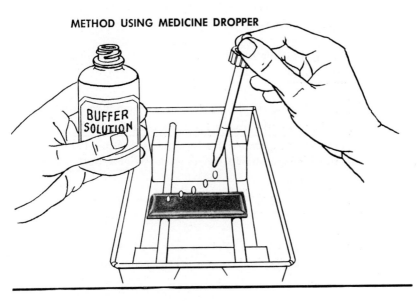

METHOD USING DROPPER BOTTLE

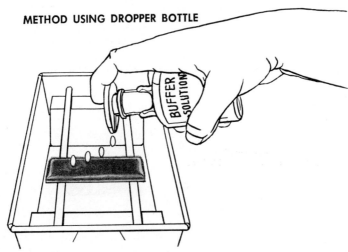

Fig. 112.—Methods of adding buffer solution to Wright's stain. Note that the buffer solution is being *evenly distributed* over the stain.

7. Now the stain and buffer solution must be thoroughly mixed. If these solutions are not thoroughly mixed, the cells will be poorly stained. These poorly stained cells will be difficult or even impossible to identify.

8. The method of mixing the stain and buffer solution is described in the next step. Carefully study the directions and accompanying illustration.

9. In mixing the stain and buffer solution, the following must be observed:

   (1) The blowing should be done from a position about 4 inches directly above the slide (see Fig. 113).
   (2) The blowing should be forceful (see Fig. 113).
   (3) The blowing should be done on several portions of the slide.
   (4) The blowing should last for 1 minute or longer.
   (5) The solution, of course, should not be blown off the slide.
   (6) Note: When the solutions are well mixed, a shiny scum usually floats on top of the solution.

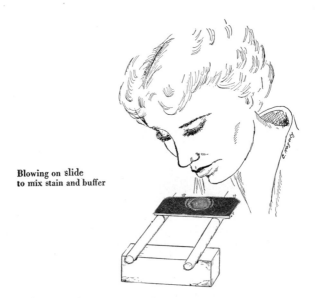

Blowing on slide
to mix stain and buffer

FIG. 113.—Mixing the stain and buffer solution by blowing on the slide.

10. Now mix the stain and buffer solution as explained in the last step and illustrated in Figure 113.

11. When the stain and buffer have been well mixed, allow them to set for 8 to 12 minutes. The best staining time can be determined by simply trying different staining times.

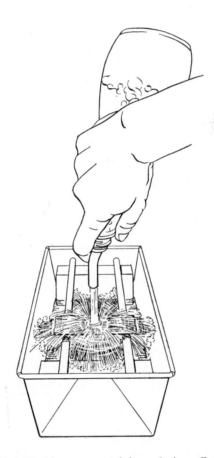

FIG. 114.—Flushing excess staining solution off the slide.

Note that a *heavy*, *forceful* stream of distilled water is used to flush off the excess staining solution.

12. <u>Note:</u> Should you ever forget and leave the stain and buffer solution on too long, say for 20 to 30 minutes, the cells may be over-stained. In such cases, the stain may be completely removed and the slide restained. To remove the stain: (If you have put immersion oil on the slide, first take a piece of lens paper and wipe off the oil.) Soak the slide for about 10 minutes in a glass of methyl, isopropyl, or rubbing alcohol. Then remove the slide, allow to dry, and stain in the usual manner.

13. After the staining solution has set for 8 to 12 minutes, the excess staining solution must be <u>flushed off</u> the slide. If the slide is removed from the staining rack without the flushing off process, some of the shiny scum and precipitated stain will settle on the slide. These will look like dots and clusters of debris when the smear is examined with the microscope.

14. Observe the manner of flushing off the excess staining solution which is illustrated in Figure 114, page 239.

15. Now, <u>while the slide is still sitting on the staining rack,</u> pour a heavy forceful stream of distilled water (about $\frac{3}{4}$ of a cup) directly over the center of the slide.

16. After the excess staining solution has been flushed off the slide, remove the slide from the staining rack.

17. With a small towel, wipe off the bottom or <u>unstained side</u> of the slide.

    <u>Note</u> if you are in doubt as to which is the <u>unstained side,</u> hold the smear up to the light and look for the patient's name. The patient's name is written on the <u>stained side.</u> You should therefore wipe off the <u>opposite side,</u> that is, the <u>unstained side.</u>

18. Put a piece of paper under the slide and lean it against the staining dish or some support so it will drain and dry (takes about 4 minutes).

19. Now proceed to Step 3, Counting the Cells.

STEP 3: COUNTING THE CELLS

First read the *discussion;* then follow the directions in the *procedure.*

Discussion of Step 3

The discussion will cover normal differentials, abnormal differentials, summary, and conclusions.

Normal Differentials

The neutrophilic segmented cell may be used to compare the size of the other white cells.

For example, we can say that the neutrophilic segmented cell is medium. In comparison, a small lymphocyte would be small. And a monocyte would be large.

Thus,

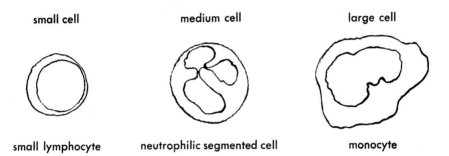

small cell   medium cell   large cell

small lymphocyte   neutrophilic segmented cell   monocyte

But what is the actual size of the white cells?

The neutrophilic segmented cells range between 10 and 15 microns in diameter.

Thus, the small lymphocytes would be about 8 microns in diameter and the monocytes would be about 17 microns in diameter.

You will recall that there are two parts to each white cell: the nucleus or central portion, the cytoplasm or outer portion.

And, if a cell is not readily identified, you should ask yourself these 3 questions:

    1. What is the size of this cell?
    2. What are the features of the nucleus?
    3. What are the features of the cytoplasm?

The above three questions are developed in greater detail in Table 14.*

* Many instructors require their students to copy Table 14 by hand and place the copy alongside their microscopes. The actual writing out of the questions reinforces the learning of the student. And this, in turn, saves wear and tear on the instructor.

17

Table 14.—Running Down the Identity of a White Cell

A. What is the size of this cell?
1. Is this cell medium in size like a segmented cell?
2. Is this cell small like some lymphocytes (which may be only slightly larger than a red cell)?
3. Is this cell large like a monocyte?

B. What are the features of the nucleus?
1. Is the nucleus segmented like a segmented cell?
2. Is the nucleus band shaped like a band cell?
3. Is the nucleus round and closely knit like a lymphocyte?
4. Is the nucleus spongy and sprawling like a monocyte?
5. Is the nucleus covered with large purple or purplish-black granules like a basophilic segmented cell?

C. What are the features of the cytoplasm?
1. Does the cytoplasm have small pink or brownish granules like a neutrophilic segmented cell and a neutrophilic band cell?
2. Does the cytoplasm have large red granules like an eosinophilic segmented cell?
3. Does the cytoplasm have large purple or purplish-black granules like a basophilic segmented cell?
4. Is the cytoplasm light blue like a lymphocyte?
5. Is the cytoplasm light gray like a monocyte?

You should carefully study the above table so that you will be able to run down the identity of a white cell which may seem difficult to identify.

In identifying some cells, you may have to ask yourself all of the questions in Table 14.

You will find that some cells, like people, may lack certain identifying features. But you should be able to identify most cells by the features which are present.

For example, you may not be able to see the granules in a segmented cell. Thus, the segmented cell could be an eosinophilic segmented cell, a basophilic segmented cell, or a neutrophilic segmented cell.

If you can not see the granules in a segmented cell, however, you are safe in calling the segmented cell a *neutrophilic* segmented cell.

Why?

If the segmented cell were an *eosinophilic* segmented cell, the granules would be large and red. In other words, the granules would be easily recognized. Consequently, there would be no question about the identity of the cell.

If the segmented cell were a *basophilic* segmented cell, the granules would be large and purple or purplish-black. Again, the granules would be easily recognized. And there would be no question about the identity of the cell.

In a neutrophilic segmented cell, however, the granules are not easily recognized. This is due to the small size of the granules and their light pink or brownish staining characteristics.

Consequently, in a case where you can not see the granules in a segmented cell, you are safe in calling the cell a *neutrophilic* segmented cell.

In the above instance, you have first identified the cell as a segmented cell. Then, by the process of elimination, you have further identified the segmented cell as a *neutrophilic* segmented cell. In identifying other questionable cells, you may use a similar approach.

The 6 white cells found in a normal differential white cell count are: neutrophilic band cell, neutrophilic segmented cell, lymphocyte, monocyte, eosinophilic segmented cell, and basophilic segmented cell.

These cells will be illustrated in the forthcoming Plate 4 and discussed in the accompanying legend.

Abnormal Differentials

As previously mentioned, the 6 white cells discussed above may deviate from their normal percentages. For example, you will recall that the percentage of neutrophils is increased in appendicitis and the percentage of lymphocytes is increased in infectious mononucleosis. These deviations from the normal percentages are a common occurrence in disease.

Another common occurrence in disease is the appearance of plasmacytes, abnormal white cells, and immature white cells.

The plasmacytes, abnormal white cells, and immature white cells will now be discussed.

Plasmacytes may be seen in measles, chickenpox, scarlet fever, multiple myeloma, serum sickness, and plasmacytic leukemia.

Measles, chickenpox, and scarlet fever are usually diagnosed without the aid of a differential white cell count. Multiple myeloma, serum sickness, and plasmacytic leukemia are extremely rare. Consequently, plasmacytes are seldom seen by the average technologist.

A plasmacyte will be illustrated in the forthcoming Plate 5 and discussed in the accompanying legend.

The abnormal white cell most frequently encountered is the abnormal lymphocyte seen in infectious mononucleosis. This cell will also be illustrated in the forthcoming Plate 5 and discussed in the accompanying legend.

How do you report abnormal lymphocytes?

Abnormal lymphocytes should be reported as abnormal lymphocytes. For example, if the differential white cell count showed 10 neutrophilic segmented cells, 75 normal lymphocytes, and 15 abnormal lymphocytes, the report would be made as follows: neutrophilic segmented cells 10, normal lymphocytes 75, and abnormal lymphocytes 15.

Now, let us consider the immature white cells which may be seen in abnormal differentials.

(discussion continued on page 246)

PLATE 4

White Cells Found in a Normal Differential White Cell Count

Stain: Wright's   Magnification: X1500

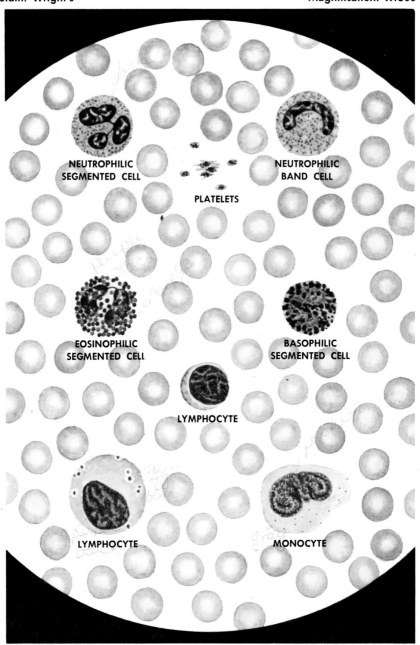

NEUTROPHILIC SEGMENTED CELL

PLATELETS

NEUTROPHILIC BAND CELL

EOSINOPHILIC SEGMENTED CELL

BASOPHILIC SEGMENTED CELL

LYMPHOCYTE

LYMPHOCYTE

MONOCYTE

Legend for Plate 4

White Cells Found in a Normal Differential White Cell Count

Neutrophilic Segmented Cell
Size: medium
Nucleus: broken up into segments
Cytoplasm: contains small pink or brownish granules
Comments: May be confused with a neutrophilic band cell. When in doubt, call cell a neutrophilic segmented cell
When found: 55% to 75% in normal blood; increased in appendicitis; pneumonia, and many other diseases

Neutrophilic Band Cell
Size: medium
Nucleus: shaped like a band
Cytoplasm: contains small pink or brownish granules
Comments: May be confused with neutrophilic segmented cell. When in doubt, call cell a neutrophilic segmented cell
When found: 2% to 6% in normal blood; increased in appendicitis, pneumonia, and many other diseases

Eosinophilic Segmented Cell
Size: medium
Nucleus: usually has 2 lobes or segments
Cytoplasm: contains large red granules
Comments: Eosinophilic segmented cell may be confused with neutrophilic segmented cell. Eosinophilic segmented cell has large red granules whereas neutrophilic segmented cell has small pink or brownish granules
When found: 1% to 3% in normal blood; increased in asthma, hay fever, and many other diseases

Basophilic Segmented Cell
Size: small or medium
Nucleus: usually indistinct; appears buried under large purple or purplish-black granules
Cytoplasm: contains large purple or purplish-black granules
Comments: Easily identified by the large purple or purplish-black granules scattered throughout the cell.
When found: 0% to 1% in normal blood

Lymphocyte
Size: small, medium, or large
Nucleus: closely knit and usually round
Cytoplasm: light blue; may contain a few reddish granules (azurophilic granules); cytoplasm may be sparse and even absent in some small lymphocytes
Comments: Large lymphocyte may be confused with monocyte. Nucleus of large lymphocyte is closely knit and usually round. Nucleus of monocyte is spongy and sprawling. The illustration shows a small lymphocyte and a large lymphocyte. The size of the lymphocyte is not reported. All small, medium, and large lymphocytes are simply reported as lymphocytes
When found: 20% to 35% in normal blood; increased in infectious mononucleosis, lymphocytic leukemia, and many other diseases

Monocyte
Size: large
Nucleus: spongy and sprawling
Cytoplasm: light gray; may contain very tiny reddish granules
Comments: Monocyte may be confused with large lymphocyte. Nucleus of monocyte is spongy and sprawling. Nucleus of lymphocyte is closely knit and usually round.
When found: 2% to 6% in normal blood; increased in tuberculosis and monocytic leukemia

Legend for Plate 5

White Cells Most Frequently Encountered in Abnormal Differential
White Cell Counts

Myeloblast

Size: large

Nucleus: round; usually contains 1 to 3 "holes" or nucleoli

Cytoplasm: deep blue; no granules

Comments: If myeloblasts are found in the smear, progranulocytes and myelocytes should also be present. If progranulocytes and myelocytes are not present, the "myeloblast" is not a myeloblast

When found: none in normal blood; 0% to 3% in granulocytic leukemia

Plasmacyte

Size: small, medium, or large

Nucleus: small; round or oval; usually located near edge of cell; sometimes resembles spokes of a wheel

Cytoplasm: deep blue

Comments: The small nucleus usually located near the edge of the cell and the deep blue cytoplasm make this cell fairly easy to identify

When found: none in normal blood; 0% to 15% in measles, chickenpox, scarlet fever, multiple myeloma, serum sickness, and plasmacytic leukemia

---

Progranulocyte

Size: large

Nucleus: round or oval

Cytoplasm: light blue; may or may not have granules; if granules are present, they are purplish red in color

Comments: If progranulocytes are found in the smear, myelocytes should also be present. If no myelocytes are present, the "progranulocyte" is not a progranulocyte

When found: none in normal blood; 0% to 8% in granulocytic leukemia

Abnormal Lymphocyte

Size: large

Nucleus: round, oval, or irregular

Cytoplasm: gray or light blue; cytoplasm has "moth-eaten" or vacuolated appearance

Comments: This abnormal lymphocyte is often referred to as an "I.M." cell. The "moth-eaten" appearance of the cytoplasm distinguishes it from the normal lymphocyte and monocyte

When found: none in normal blood; 5% to 35% seen in infectious mononucleosis

---

Neutrophilic Myelocyte

Size: large

Nucleus: round or oval

Cytoplasm: contains small pink or brownish granules

Comments: If neutrophilic myelocytes are found in the smear, neutrophilic metamyelocytes and neutrophilic band cells should also be present. If the latter 2 cells are not present, the "neutrophilic myelocyte" is not a neutrophilic myelocyte

When found: none in normal blood; 0% to 35% in severe infections and granulocytic leukemia

Neutrophilic Metamyelocyte

Size: large

Nucleus: indented or bean shaped

Cytoplasm: contains small pink or brownish granules

Comments: If neutrophilic metamyelocytes are found in the smear, many neutrophilic band cells should also be present. The neutrophilic metamyelocyte may be confused with a monocyte. The cytoplasm of the neutrophilic metamyelocyte is pink whereas the cytoplasm of the monocyte is gray

When found: none in normal blood; 0% to 25% in severe infections and granulocytic leukemia

PLATE 5
White Cells Most Frequently Encountered in
Abnormal Differential White Cell Counts

Stain: Wright's   Magnification: X1500

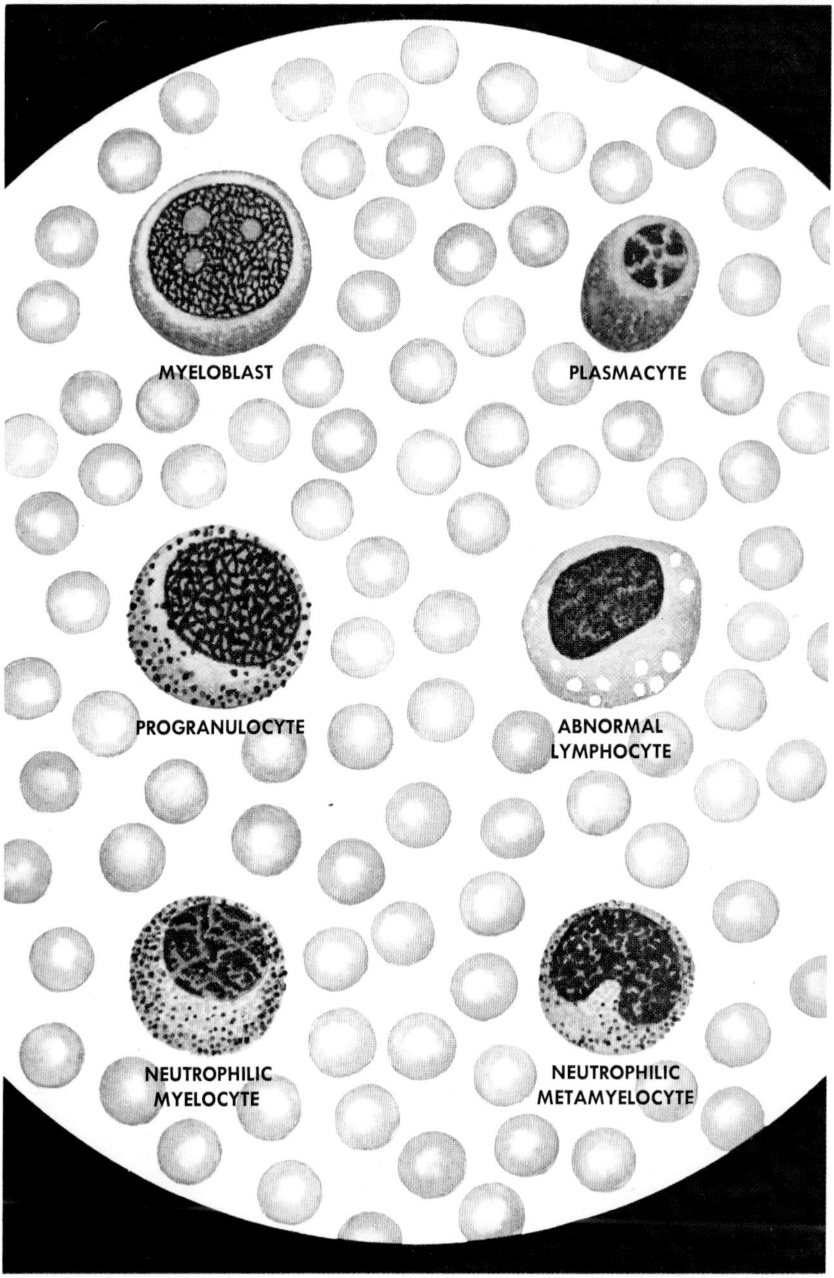

MYELOBLAST

PLASMACYTE

PROGRANULOCYTE

ABNORMAL
LYMPHOCYTE

NEUTROPHILIC
MYELOCYTE

NEUTROPHILIC
METAMYELOCYTE

The immature white cells most frequently encountered in abnormal differentials are listed below:

Cell	Pronunciation
myeloblast	mi′ĕ-lo-blast
progranulocyte	pro-gran′u-lo-sīt
neutrophilic myelocyte	nu″tro-fil′ik mi′ĕ-lo-sīt
neutrophilic metamyelocyte	nu″tro-fil′ik met″ah-mi′ĕ-lo-sīt

You will recall that the above 4 cells are immature cells of the granulocytic series (Plate 2, page 214).

The myeloblast is the infant cell. This cell develops into a progranulocyte.

The progranulocyte may develop into an eosinophilic myelocyte, neutrophilic myelocyte, or basophilic myelocyte. (See Plate 2, page 214.)

About 95 per cent of the progranulocytes, however, become neutrophilic myelocytes. And, in diagnosis, the neutrophilic myelocyte is the only cell of significance. Consequently, the neutrophilic myelocyte is the only cell which we will consider.

The neutrophilic myelocyte develops into a neutrophilic metamyelocyte.

The neutrophilic metamyelocyte becomes a neutrophilic band cell and thence a neutrophilic segmented cell.

Thus, we have the development illustrated in Figure 115.

What happens to the cell as it goes from a neutrophilic myelocyte to a neutrophilic segmented cell?

As the cell goes from a neutrophilic myelocyte to a neutrophilic segmented cell, *the only significant change occurs in the nucleus.*

At first, the nucleus is round, then it becomes indented, then it becomes band shaped, and then it becomes segmented (Fig. 115).

Thus, the changes in the nucleus become the key to the identity of the cell. To illustrate, consider the following questions and answers:

What is the difference between a neutrophilic myelocyte and a neutrophilic metamyelocyte?

The neutrophilic myelocyte has a round or oval nucleus and the neutrophilic metamyelocyte has an indented nucleus (Fig. 115).

What is the difference between a neutrophilic metamyelocyte and a neutrophilic band cell?

The neutrophilic metamyelocyte has an indented nucleus and the neutrophilic band cell has a band shaped nucleus (Fig. 115).

What is the difference between a neutrophilic band cell and a neutrophilic segmented cell?

The neutrophilic band cell has a band shaped nucleus and the neutrophilic segmented cell has a segmented nucleus (Fig. 115).

Sometimes the difference between the above cells may be so slight that it is difficult to make the classification.   In such cases, *the accepted policy is to call the cell the more mature form.*

For example, if the nucleus is very slightly indented, the cell could be called a neutrophilic myelocyte or a neutrophilic metamyelocyte.   By adhering to the accepted policy of calling the cell the more mature form, we would call the cell a neutrophilic metamyelocyte.

Try to remember that cells are like people: Their features change as they grow older.   And, as you know, it is often difficult to tell whether a person is 39 years old or 45 years old.

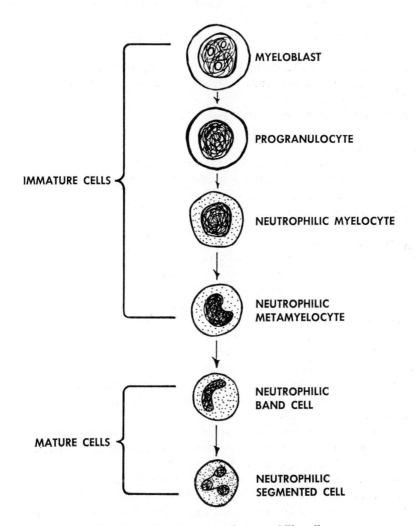

FIG. 115.—Development of neutrophilic cells.

The above 4 immature white cells are also illustrated in Plate 5 and further discussed in the accompanying legend.

The student should realize that these 4 immature white cells are normal white cells. But, when these cells are seen in the blood stream, their presence indicates stress, injury, or insult to the body.

Summary

Now let us summarize what we have learned about normal and abnormal differential white cell counts.

In normal differentials, that is, in health, 6 different white cells may be seen. These white cells are the neutrophilic band cell, neutrophilic segmented cell, lymphocyte, monocyte, eosinophilic segmented cell, and basophilic segmented cell.

In abnormal differentials, that is, in disease, the following may occur:

a. The above 6 white cells may deviate from their normal percentages.

b. Plasmacytes may be seen.

c. Abnormal white cells may be seen. (The most frequently encountered abnormal white cell is the abnormal lymphocyte seen in infectious mononucleosis.)

d. Immature white cells may be seen. (The most frequently encountered immature white cells are the myeloblast, progranulocyte, neutrophilic myelocyte, and neutrophilic metamyelocyte.)

Conclusions

For the present, you should make a careful examination of Plate 4 and a superficial examination of Plate 5.

When you begin your study of blood diseases, however, you should make a careful examination of both plates, comparing the white cells in Plate 4 with the white cells in Plate 5.

In studying the above plates, the student should also note the following: (1) The numerous small round objects are red cells and (2) the tiny objects in the upper part of Plate 4 are platelets.

Both the red cells and platelets will be frequently seen during the differential white cell count. In fact, about 500 red cells and about 30 platelets will be seen for every 1 white cell.

After making a differential white cell count, it is customary to make a rough estimation of the platelets, recording them as normal, decreased, or increased.

Thus, the student finds that he must be able to identify only 12 different white cells. These are the 6 white cells found in a normal differential white cell count and the 6 white cells most frequently encountered in abnormal differential white cell counts (Plates 4 and 5).

What about the other white cells which we first met in the development of white cells (Plate 2, page 214)?

These white cells are rarely seen or of little significance in diagnosis.

For example, the following white cells are rarely seen:

lymphoblast	monoblast	plasmablast
prolymphocyte	promonocyte	proplasmacyte

And the white cells which follow are not only rarely seen but of little (if any) significance in diagnosis:

eosinophilic myelocyte	basophilic myelocyte
eosinophilic metamyelocyte	basophilic metamyelocyte
eosinophilic band cell	basophilic band cell

In learning the features of the 6 white cells found in a normal differential white cell count, it is a decided advantage to obtain some color crayons and actually draw the cells shown in Plate 4.

These drawings, of course, should be made after you have seen the cells under the microscope.

When you begin your study of blood diseases, also draw the 6 white cells in Plate 5.

In your drawings, make sure you illustrate the differences between the white cells in Plate 4 and the white cells in Plate 5.

For example, pay particular attention to any differences in size, any differences in the nucleus, and any differences in the cytoplasm.

Before turning to the procedure for identifying and tabulating the white cells in the blood smear, you should understand that the color of a cell in a blood smear may vary slightly from the color of a cell in a book.

These differences in color, of course, are due to various factors:

(1) The color of a cell in a blood smear may vary with different batches of stain and buffer solution.

(2) The color of a cell in a blood smear may vary with the technique of staining the smear.

(3) The color of a cell in a blood smear can not be exactly reproduced in any textbook.

In our color presentation of the white cells, we have purposely accented the differences among the various white cells. This has been done so the student may have a vivid mental picture of each individual white cell.

After you have made a careful study of Plate 4 and the accompanying legend (page 244), follow the directions in the Procedure for Step 3 (page 250).

Procedure for Step 3

1. Observe the sample work-sheet for the differential white cell count which is illustrated in Figure 116.

2. In this illustration, you will note that the cells have been recorded by making a / mark, the ⊬⊬⊦ meaning that 5 cells have been recorded.

3. Get a piece of paper and write down the names of the cells as illustrated in Figure 116.

4. Now turn to the microscope.

5. Switch the oil immersion (95×) objective into position directly over the opening in the stage.

6. By turning the coarse adjustment, raise the oil immersion (95×) objective about 1 inch above the opening in the stage.

7. By turning the condenser knob, raise the condenser up as far as it will go.

Note: Moving the condenser up as far as it will go helps to insure the maximum amount of light. This is absolutely essential in the identification of some cells. Therefore, make sure that you have raised the condenser up as far as it will go.

Cell	Count	Total Number
Neutrophilic band cells . .	||||	4
Neutrophilic segmented cells	⊬⊬⊦ ⊬⊬⊦ ⊬⊬⊦ ⊬⊬⊦ ⊬⊬⊦ ⊬⊬⊦ ⊬⊬⊦ ⊬⊬⊦ ⊬⊬⊦ ⊬⊬⊦ ⊬⊬⊦ ⊬⊬⊦	60
Lymphocytes	⊬⊬⊦ ⊬⊬⊦ ⊬⊬⊦ ⊬⊬⊦ ⊬⊬⊦ ||||	29
Monocytes	⊬⊬⊦	5
Eosinophilic segmented cells	||	2
Basophilic segmented cells .	0	0
		100

Fig. 116.—Sample work-sheet for the differential white cell count.

8. Next, turn on the microscope light.

9. Do not look in the eyepiece but perform the following step with your naked eye:

10. Adjust the mirror so a BRIGHT light comes directly up through the center of the condenser and the opening in the stage.

    Note: Sometimes the shutter lever of the condenser may be closed or partially closed and a bright light can not come up through the condenser. In such cases, open the shutter with the shutter lever (Fig. 68, page 119).

11. Get your stained blood smear. Make sure it is dry. Place a large drop of immersion oil on the thin area of the smear (Fig. 117).

12. Hold the slide so the thin area is on your left. Then fix the slide firmly in the jaws of the movable stage.

13. By turning the stage knobs, move the slide so the drop of oil is directly over the bright light coming up through the condenser.

14. Look at the slide from the side and put your hand on the coarse adjustment.

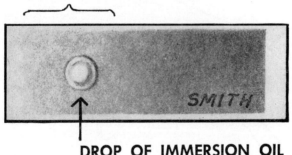

THIS THIN AREA OF THE BLOOD SMEAR IS FOR IDENTIFYING THE CELLS

DROP OF IMMERSION OIL

FIG. 117.—Position of the drop of immersion oil on the stained blood smear.

15. Now turn the coarse adjustment and lower the oil immersion (95×) objective INTO the drop of oil.

Note: You may, of course, have to move the slide to get the drop of oil under the objective. The slide is moved by turning the stage knobs.

16. When you have the oil immersion (95×) objective in the drop of oil, continue turning the coarse adjustment until the oil immersion (95×) objective is touching the glass slide.

17. In the next step, you will be rotating the coarse adjustment about $\frac{1}{16}$ turn toward yourself (see Fig. 118).

Note: There is just one thin layer where the cells will be in view. Therefore, in the next step, keep your eye glued to the eyepiece so you do not go past this point.

18. Now, while continually looking through the eyepiece, VERY SLOWLY rotate the coarse adjustment toward yourself until you see some cells.

Note #1: The oil immersion objective, of course, should not rise out of the drop of oil.

Note #2: If you fail to see some cells after rotating the coarse adjustment about $\frac{2}{16}$ turn, repeat steps 14, 15, 16, 17, and 18.

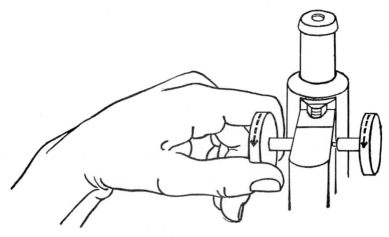

Fig. 118.—Rotating the coarse adjustment *toward* yourself (for the differential white cell count.)

19. After you have brought the cells into view with the coarse adjustment, bring the cells into perfect focus by rotating the fine adjustment.

20. When the cells are in perfect focus, place the index finger and thumb of both hands on the mirror.

21. Now, look through the eyepiece and adjust the mirror so the maximum amount of light shines on the cells. This is important!

22. Study the method of operating the microscope for this examination (Fig. 119, page 254).

    Note: In identifying a cell, you should always rotate the fine adjustment back and forth. This enables you to see the various "layers" of the cell and thereby aids in identification.

23. Now look through the eyepiece and turn the stage knob on your right until you see a white cell. You should average about 1 white cell to every 7 microscopic fields.

    Note: The round pink objects are red cells. The white cells, of course, are two or three times larger than red cells.

24. When you have a white cell in view, again adjust the mirror and make sure you have the maximum amount of light shining on the white cell. This is important!

25. Then rotate the fine adjustment back and forth so you see the various "layers" of the white cell.

26. Identify the white cell and record it with a mark on your work-sheet.

27. Observe the method of examining the blood smear (Fig. 120, page 255).

    Note: In this illustration, note that you are gradually moving the smear toward the thick portion of the smear. When you look in your microscope, however, it will appear that you are moving the smear in the opposite direction. This illusion is due to the optical system of the microscope.

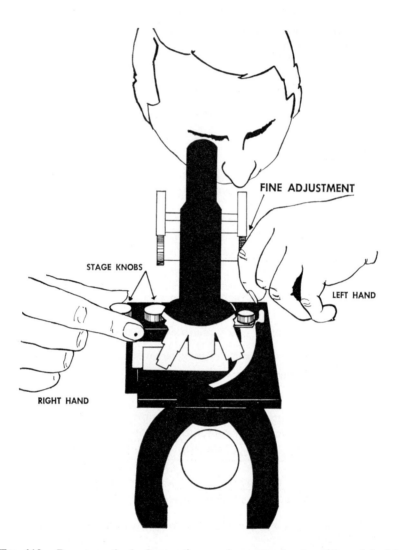

Fɪɢ. 119.—Proper method of operating a microscope for the differential white cell count.

1. The right hand turns the *stage knobs.*
2. The left hand rocks or rotates the *fine adjustment* back and forth.
3. Note: In identifying a cell, you should always rock the fine adjustment back and forth. Rocking the fine adjustment back and forth enables you to see the various "layers" of the cell. In other words, it helps you to see the cell in 3 dimensions. This is very important in the identification of an immature or abnormal cell.

28. You may start at any part of the arrow in Figure 120.

29. Now <u>roughly</u> following the path of the arrow, look for another white cell.

30. When you find another white cell, rotate the <u>fine adjust-ment</u> back and forth and identify the cell.

   <u>Note:</u> You will find that neutrophilic segmented cells come in various sizes, shapes, and shades. Do not expect all neutrophilic segmented cells to look exactly alike. This also applies to lymphocytes, monocytes, etc.

31. When you have identified your second white cell, record the cell with a mark on your work-sheet.

32. After you have recorded your second white cell, proceed to steps 33, 34, 35, etc.

33. Some abnormalities and irregularities found in blood smears are illustrated in Plate 6 and Plate 7 and described in the accompanying legends.

thin area for counting

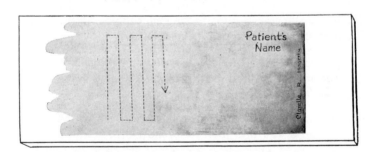

FIG. 120.—Method of examining the blood smear for the differential white cell count. When a blood smear is made, the large cells tend to accumulate on the edge of the smear, whereas the small cells tend to stay in the middle of the smear. If the cells are counted only on the edges or only in the middle of the smear, it would not be a true representative sample of the patient's cells. Therefore, the smear is examined by following the path of the arrow shown above. In following the path of the arrow, note that you are moving toward the *thicker* end of the smear. When you look in the microscope, however, it will appear that you are moving in the opposite direction. As you move the smear, of course, the oil is dragged along on the smear.

256   Complete Blood Count

34. In these illustrations, the abnormalities and irregularities listed below are most frequently encountered. The other abnormalities and irregularities are rarely seen.

> 1. Distorted lymphocytes
> 2. Accumulated white cells
> 3. Smudge cells
> 4. Disintegrated cell
> 5. Poorly stained eosinophils
> 6. Precipitated stain

35. Therefore, before continuing, study Plate 6 (page 257) and the accompanying legend so you will not have to call your instructor and ask: "What's this?"

36. If you see any of the abnormalities shown in the above illustrations, you should treat them as directed in the legends opposite the plates.

37. In performing your differential white cell count, do not skip any cells.

38. If you see a cell you are not sure of, remember to ask yourself the 3 questions in Table 14, page 242:

> What is the size of this cell?
> What are the features of the nucleus?
> What are the features of the cytoplasm?

39. If you still cannot identify the cell, ask your instructor for help or record the cell as unidentified.

Note: Unidentified cells are mentioned in the report but are not counted as part of the 100 cells in the differential white cell count.

40. Now, continue to roughly follow the path of the arrow in Figure 120 and look for white cells.

Note: The white cells should be looked for only in those THIN AREAS of the blood smear where the red cells are spread out as illustrated in Plate 4, page 244. If you get up into those thick areas of the blood smear where the red cells are bunched together, the white cells will be shriveled up. And you will have extreme difficulty in identifying them.

41. Every time you see a white cell, identify the cell, and record it with a mark on your work-sheet.

(continued on page 259)

PLATE 6
Abnormalities and Irregularities Found in Blood Smears

Stain: Wright's

Magnification: X1500

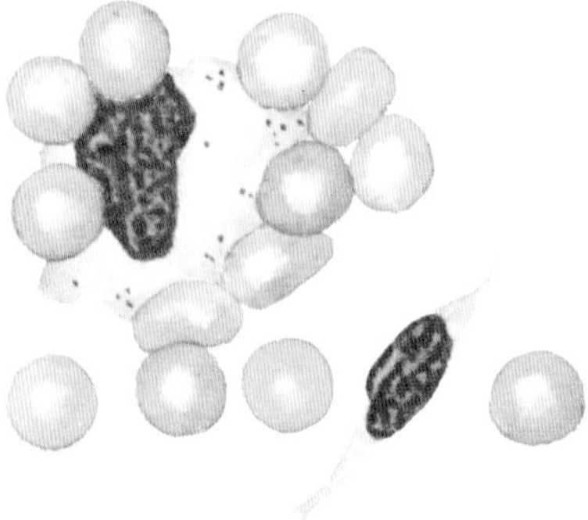

1. Distorted lymphocytes

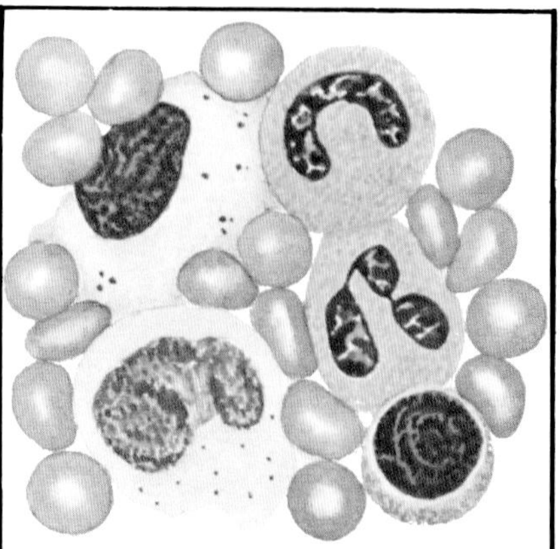

2. Accumulated white cells

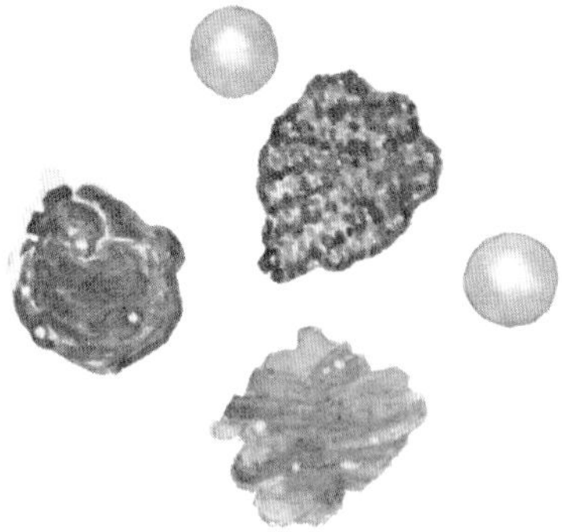

3. Smudge cells

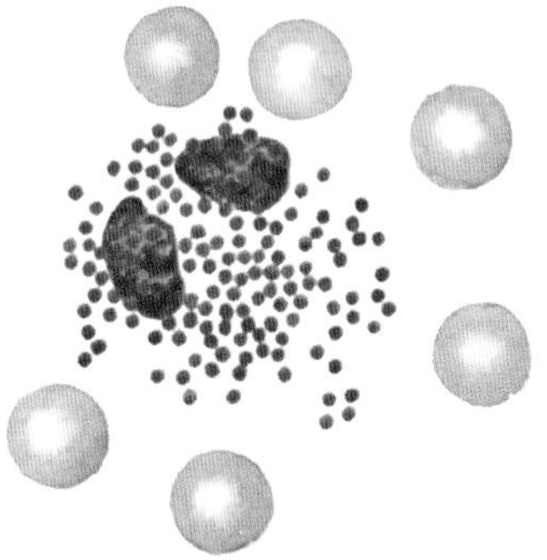

4. Disintegrated cell (eosinophil)

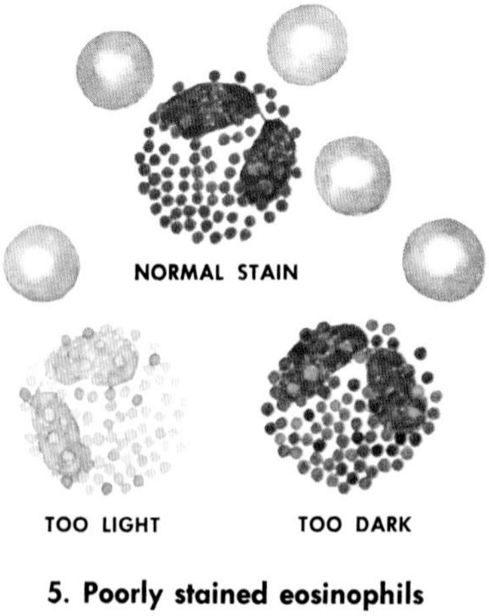

NORMAL STAIN

TOO LIGHT

TOO DARK

5. Poorly stained eosinophils

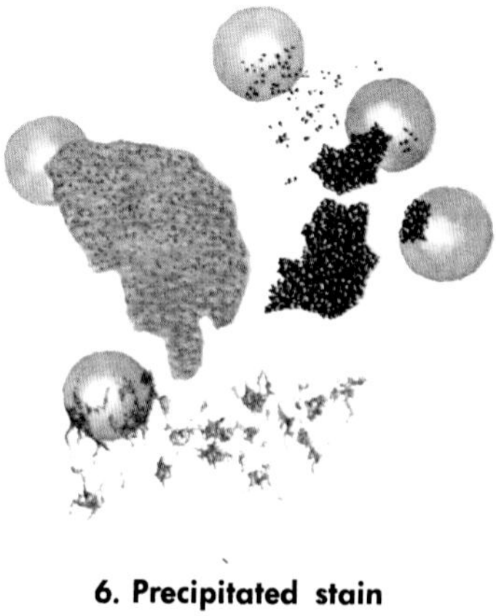

6. Precipitated stain

Legend for Plate 6

Abnormalities and Irregularities Found in Blood Smears

1 . Distorted Lymphocytes

Squashed or distorted lymphocytes are sometimes seen. They are caused by excessive pressure on the cells during the process of making the smear. Distorted lymphocytes should be recorded as normal lymphocytes.

2. Accumulated White Cells

A bunch of white cells may sometimes be seen on the edge of a blood smear. They are caused by improper spreading during the process of making the smear. They should not be counted or recorded.

3. Smudge Cells

A smudge cell is the bare nucleus of a ruptured white cell.

A few smudge cells may be found in a normal blood smear. They may be caused by heavy pressure on the cells during the process of making the smear.

A large number of smudge cells may be seen in leukemia. Their presence may indicate an increase in the fragility of the cells or abnormal destruction of the cells.

Smudge cells should neither be counted nor recorded.

4. Disintegrated Cell

Disintegrated cells are ruptured cells. As shown in the illustration, both the nucleus and the cytoplasm are seen. Disintegrated cells should not be counted as one of the 100 cells of a differential white cell count. But they should be recorded and reported as *Disintegrated Cells.*

Disintegrated cells may be found in blood smears which have been improperly prepared. For example, excessive pressure on the cells may cause the cells to rupture.

Disintegrated cells may be found in blood smears which have been made from old anticoagulated blood, that is, anticoagulated blood which is over two hours old.

Disintegrated cells may also be seen in the blood of patients having various toxic conditions.

5. Poorly Stained Eosinophils

Poorly stained eosinophils are occasionally seen. They may be caused by the following (1) incorrect pH of buffer solution, (2) improper mixing of stain and buffer solution, or (3) too short a staining time.

Poorly stained eosinophils should be counted and recorded as normal eosinophils.

6. Precipitated Stain

Precipitated stain is occasionally seen. It is caused by failure to properly flush the excess stain off the slide during the staining process (see page 240).

Precipitated stain has no significance and, of course, should not be reported.

Legend for Plate 7

Abnormalities and Irregularities Found in Blood Smears

7. Neutrophil With Toxic Granules

Toxic granules are large, coarse granules in the cytoplasm. In color, they are dark blue, purple, or black.

Neutrophils with toxic granules are sometimes seen in normal blood smears. They are caused by over-staining the smear or using a buffer solution with a pH value above 6.8.

Neutrophils with toxic granules may also be seen in severe infections, chemical poisoning, and malignant neutropenia (agranulocytosis).

The number of neutrophils with toxic granules should be recorded and reported under *Miscellaneous White Cells.*

8. Hypersegmented Neutrophil

The nucleus of a normal neutro-philic segmented cell is broken up into 3 segments. The nucleus of the hypersegmented cell, however, is broken up into 5 to 10 segments. This hypersegmented neutrophil is usually larger than the normal neu-trophilic segmented cell.

The hypersegmented neutrophil is often referred to as a "P. A. poly" cell. It may be seen in pernicious anemia. The number of hyperseg-mented neutrophils in the differen-tial white cell count should be re-corded and reported under *Miscel-laneous White Cells.*

9. Vacuolated Cell

A vacuolated cell has holes or vacuoles in the cytoplasm. The vac-uoles are a sign of degeneration.

Vacuolated cells may be found in normal blood if the smear is made from oxalated blood which is over two hours old.

Vacuolated cells may also be seen in severe infections, chemical poison-ing, and leukemia.

If the blood smear was made from fresh blood, the number of vacuo-lated cells should be reported under *Miscellaneous White Cells.*

10. Tissue Cells

Tissue cells may be squeezed out of the tissue during the finger puncture. They resemble a monocyte. Tissue cells and monocytes can usually be distinguished on the following basis.

In a tissue cell, the outer edges of the cytoplasm are usually raveled or fragmentary. Often a "tail" is pres-ent. In a monocyte, however, the outer edges of the cytoplasm are usually clearcut and definite.

Tissue cells are rarely seen. They should be recorded and reported, however, so that they are not mis-taken for other cells.

11. Basket Cell

A basket cell is a net-like nucleus from a ruptured white cell.

A few basket cells may be found in a normal blood smear. They are probably older forms of the smudge cell.

Basket cells should not be recorded or reported.

12. Crescent Bodies

Crescent bodies are also known as semilunar bodies, selenoid bodies, and achromocytes. They are be-lieved to be the remains of old erythrocytes.

Crescent bodies are sometimes seen in normal blood smears. They are also seen in malaria and hemolytic anemias.

Crescent bodies should not be re-corded or reported.

PLATE 7
Abnormalities and Irregularities Found in Blood Smears

Stain: Wright's   Magnification: X1500

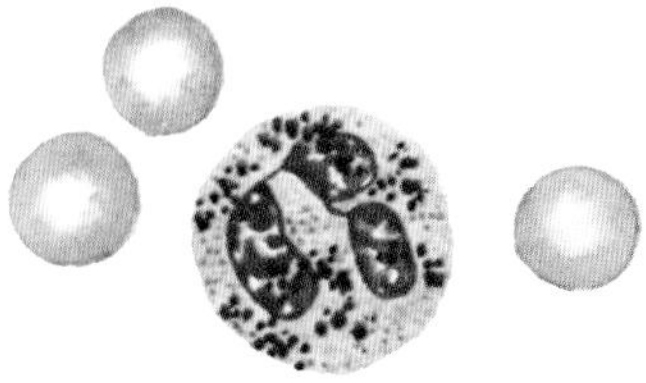

7. Neutrophil with toxic granules

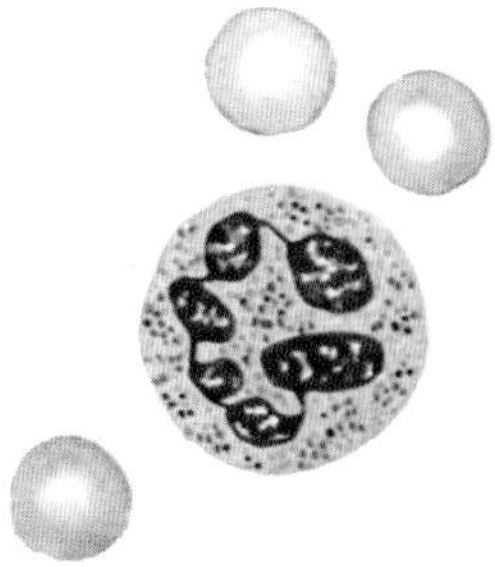

8. Hypersegmented neutrophil

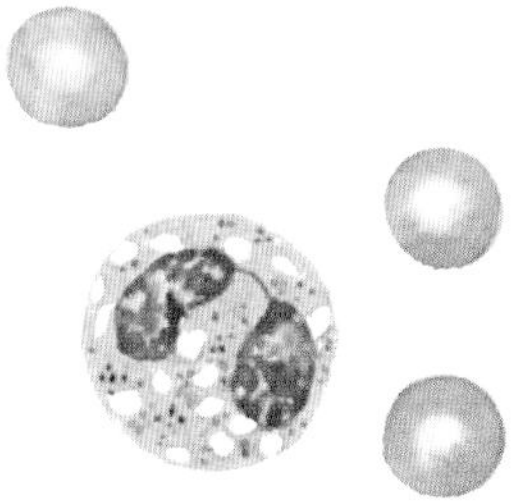

9. Vacuolated cell

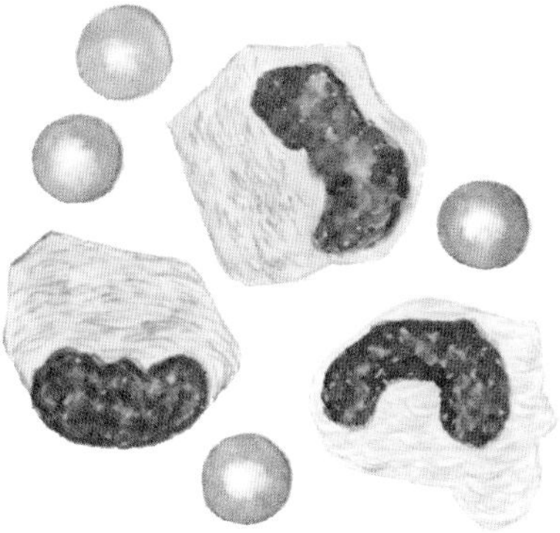

10. Tissue cells

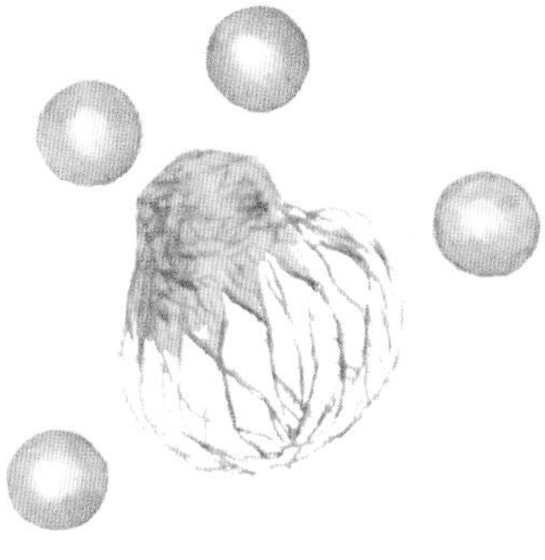

11. Basket cell

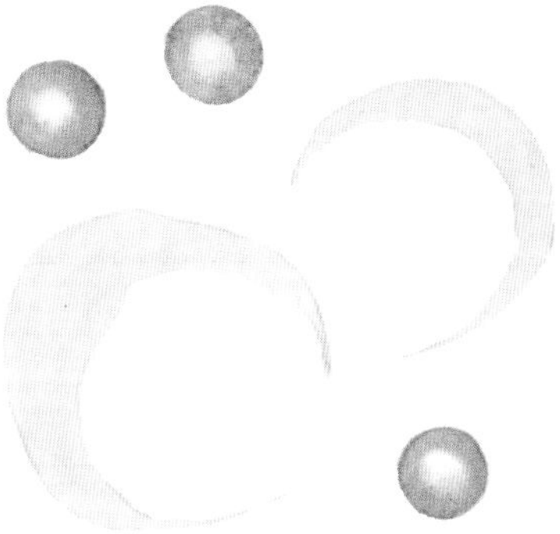

12. Crescent bodies

42. When you have identified and recorded 100 white cells, write down the total number for each cell (see Fig. 116, page 250).

    Note: If you have counted several more than 100 cells, say 105, take 3 off your highest total and 2 off your next highest total.

43. After you have written down the total number for each white cell, you must make a rough estimate of the number of platelets.

44. Platelets usually come in groups of 3, 4, or 5.

45. Note that 7 platelets are illustrated in Plate 4, page 244.

46. If the platelets are normal, you should have about 4 to 8 platelets for every 100 red cells.

47. Now scan 25 to 30 microscopic fields and roughly estimate if the platelets are normal, decreased, or increased.

48. On your work-sheet, write down your platelet estimation as normal, decreased, or increased.

    Note: A good platelet estimation will require some practice and experience.

49. When you have finished the above, let your stained blood smear remain on the stage of the microscope for it will be used in the stained red cell examination (page 267).

50. Then proceed to Step 4, Reporting the Count.

51. Note: After you have attained some confidence in identifying the white cells, you may increase your speed by doing the following:
    Carefully identify and record about 12 cells on the thin area of the smear. If the cells appear normal, move up to the thick area of the smear. Here the cells are closer together and the count can be made in less time. You should never go immediately to the thick area, however, because the cells in this area are not "spread out" and any abnormalities may be completely over-looked.

STEP 4:   REPORTING THE COUNT

First read the *discussion;* then follow the directions in the *procedure.*

Discussion of Step 4

A report of the differential white cell count is sometimes referred to as a *hemogram.*

When 100 white cells have been identified and recorded, the report of the differential white cell count is given according to either of the following: one, the Schilling classification; two, the filament and non-filament classification.   An explanation of each method follows.

Schilling Classification

Schilling was one of the first to notice that in many diseases there is an increase in the precentage of immature neutrophils of the granulocytic series.   His blood chart reported the percentages of the various cell types and—in part—was arranged in the following manner:

	Neutrophilic Myelo-cytes	*Neutrophilic Metamyelo-cytes*	*Neutrophilic Band Cells*	*Neutrophilic Segmented Cells*
Normal values	0%	0%	2 to 6%	55 to 75%

Note that the immature cells are on the left side of the chart.   If the percentage of these immature cells became increased, Schilling called it a "shift to the left."

When the shift to the left was accompanied by a low white cell count, Schilling called it a *degenerative shift to the left.*

A degenerative shift to the left is seen in such diseases as typhoid fever. It is caused by a depression of the cell factories in the bone marrow.

When the shift to the left was accompanied by a high white cell count, Schilling called it a *regenerative shift to the left.*

A regenerative shift to the left is seen in such diseases as pneumonia. It is caused by a stimulus of the cell factories in the bone marrow.

A "shift to the right" implies an increase in hypersegmented neutrophils. It may be seen in pernicious anemia.

The Schilling classification of the differential white cell count has become quite popular.   The cell types which are reported and the normal percentages are given in Table 15.

Table 15.—Schilling Classification of the Differential White Cell Count

Cell	Normal Percentages
Neutrophilic myelocytes	0
Neutrophilic metamyelocytes	0
Neutrophilic band cells.	2 to 6
Neutrophilic segmented cells	55 to 75
Lymphocytes	20 to 35
Monocytes	2 to 6
Eosinophilic segmented cells	1 to 3
Basophilic segmented cells	0 to 1

Filament and Non-Filament Classification

The filament and non-filament classification reports the percentage of each cell with the exception of the neutrophils of the granulocytic series. The neutrophils of the granulocytic series are divided into two groups: a mature group and an immature group. A brief discussion follows.

According to the filament and non-filament classification, the mature cells of the granulocytic series are the neutrophilic segmented cells. These cells have a nucleus which is broken up into segments, the segments being connected by a fine filament. Hence they are called *filamented cells*.

According to the filament and non-filament classification, the immature cells of the granulocytic series are the neutrophilic myelocytes, neutrophilic metamyelocytes, and neutrophilic band cells. These cells do not have filaments in their nucleus. Hence they are called *non-filamented cells*.

The neutrophilic segmented cells are therefore the *filamented cells*. And the neutrophilic myelocytes, neutrophilic metamyelocytes, and neutrophilic band cells are the *non-filamented cells*.

To illustrate the filament and non-filament classification, consider the following differential:

Cell	Per Cent
Neutrophilic myelocytes	0
Neutrophilic metamyelocytes. . .	1
Neutrophilic band cells	14
Neutrophilic segmented cells . .	80
Lymphocytes	4
Monocytes	1

The 80 per cent neutrophilic segmented cells gives us 80 per cent *filamented cells*. And, by adding the neutrophilic myelocytes, neutrophilic metamyelocytes, and neutrophilic band cells, we obtain 15 per cent *non-filamented cells*.

Thus, the above differential would be reported as follows:

Non-filamented cells	15%
Filamented cells	80%
Lymphocytes	4%
Monocytes	1%

The cells reported and the normal percentages for the filament and non-filament classification are given in Table 16.

Table 16.—Filament and Non-Filament Classification of the Differential White Cell Count

Cell	Normal Percentages
Non-filamented cells { Neutrophilic myelocytes / Neutrophilic metamyelocytes / Neutrophilic band cells }	2 to 6
Filamented cells { Neutrophilic segmented cells } . .	55 to 75
Lymphocytes	20 to 35
Monocytes	2 to 6
Eosinophilic segmented cells	1 to 3
Basophilic segmented cells	0 to 1

Note

The Schilling classification is the simplest and also the most popular. Unless the physician requests otherwise, use the Schilling classification.

In the report of the differential white cell count, it is also customary to include a rough estimation of the number of platelets, reporting them as *normal, decreased,* or *increased.*

Now follow the directions in the Procedure for Step 4.

Procedure for Step 4

1. Obtain a piece of paper and write out a report form as illustrated in Figure 121.

2. Fill in the name of the patient, the date, and the name of the physician.

   <u>Note:</u> Students in private schools and colleges, of course, can simply fill in fictitious names for the patient and physician.

3. Now obtain your work-sheet for the differential white cell count.

REPORT OF A DIFFERENTIAL WHITE CELL COUNT

Patient:

Date:

Physician:

White Cells	Patient's Values	Normal Values
Myeloblasts	_____	0%
Progranulocytes	_____	0%
Neutrophilic myelocytes	_____	0%
Neutrophilic metamyelocytes . . .	_____	0%
Neutrophilic band cells	_____	2% to 6%
Neutrophilic segmented cells . . .	_____	55% to 75%
Lymphocytes.	_____	20% to 35%
Monocytes	_____	2% to 6%
Eosinophilic segmented cells . . .	_____	1% to 3%
Basophilic segmented cells	_____	0% to 1%
Miscellaneous white cells		
abnormal lymphocytes	_____	0%
plasmacytes	_____	0%
disintegrated cells.	_____	0%
_____	_____	0%
_____	_____	0%
Platelets:	_____	4 to 8 for every 100 red cells

Examination performed by:

Fig. 121.—Sample report form for the differential white cell count.

REPORT OF A DIFFERENTIAL WHITE CELL COUNT

Patient: **Masters, Mrs. Betty**

Date: **2-2-72**

Physician: **Dr. Paul Ehrlich**

White Cells	Patient's Values	Normal Values
Myeloblasts	0	0%
Progranulocytes	0	0%
Neutrophilic myelocytes	0	0%
Neutrophilic metamyelocytes . . .	0	0%
Neutrophilic band cells	4	2% to 6%
Neutrophilic segmented cells . . .	60	55% to 75%
Lymphocytes.	30	20% to 35%
Monocytes	4	2% to 6%
Eosinophilic segmented cells . . .	2	1% to 3%
Basophilic segmented cells	0	0% to 1%
Miscellaneous white cells		
abnormal lymphocytes		0%
plasmacytes		0%
disintegrated cells.	1	0%
		0%
		0%
Platelets:	**normal**	4 to 8 for every 100 red cells

Examination performed by:

Sandra Frisbie

FIG. 122.—Report of a normal differential white cell count.

4. Transfer the figures from your work-sheet to your report form.

   Note: If you have no myeloblasts, progranulocytes, etc. simply put a 0 in the space.

5. Check to see that your total number of cells equals 100.

   Note: Any abnormal lymphocytes, plasmacytes, etc. are considered part of the 100. Any disintegrated cells are reported but not considered as part of the 100.

6. In the space opposite the word Platelets, write in the result of your platelet estimation, using the terms normal, decreased, or increased.

7. A completed report of a normal differential white cell count is illustrated in Figure 122.

8. Now sign your report and hand it in.

9. In most laboratories, the usual procedure is to do a stained red cell examination immediately after the differential white cell count. The stained red cell examination is done on the same blood smear as the differential white cell count.

10. If you are going to do a stained red cell examination at this time, let the blood smear remain on the stage of the microscope and turn to the stained red cell examination (page 267).

11. If you are not going to perform your stained red cell examination at this time, remove the blood smear from the microscope. Using a piece of lens paper, wipe off the immersion oil. (This does not injure the cells or blood smear in any way.) Now "store" the blood smear in a safe place. If you are "storing" unstained blood smears, put them face down if you have cockroaches or other live stock in the area.

SUMMARY OF THE DIFFERENTIAL WHITE CELL COUNT

After completing his first differential white cell count, the student may perform additional counts by simply following the procedure in each step.

For the convenience of the student, the steps and reference pages are summarized below:

Chapter 8

Stained Red Cell Examination

The stained red cell examination is also referred to as the red cell morphology, red blood cell morphology, and RBC morphology.

The stained red cell examination is performed on the same blood smear as the differential white cell count. Because of this, the stained red cell examination is often considered as part of the differential white cell count. This is a most unfortunate misconception.

The stained red cell examination is not a part of the differential white cell count. The stained red cell examination is a separate and distinct examination.

This chapter will consider the stained red cell examination and some related material. The discussion covers the following:

Significance of the Stained Red Cell Examination
Discussion of the Procedure for the Stained Red Cell Examination
Procedure for the Stained Red Cell Examination
Time Saving Method of Performing a Complete Blood Count
Directions for Cleaning Slides

The student review questions for the stained red cell examination are numbered 120–148 and begin on page 739 of the Appendix.

SIGNIFICANCE OF THE STAINED RED CELL EXAMINATION

The stained red cell examination is the fifth and final test in a complete blood count. It is run about 2,000 times a month in the average hospital laboratory and about 100 times a month in the average physician's office.

The stained red cell examination is an examination for nucleated red cells and abnormal erythrocytes. These are discussed below.

NUCLEATED RED CELLS

In going from birth to death, the red cell goes through 6 stages of development. As the cell goes from one stage to another, it is given a new name. Thus,

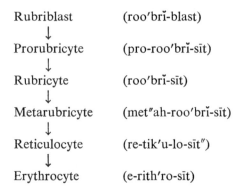

Rubriblast	(roo′brĭ-blast)
↓	
Prorubricyte	(pro-roo′brĭ-sīt)
↓	
Rubricyte	(roo′brĭ-sīt)
↓	
Metarubricyte	(met″ah-roo′brĭ-sīt)
↓	
Reticulocyte	(re-tik′u-lo-sīt″)
↓	
Erythrocyte	(e-rith′ro-sīt)

The first 4 cells contain a nucleus. Consequently, they are called nucleated red cells.

The nucleated red cells are often referred to as young red cells or immature red cells.

The nucleated red cells are normally confined to their home in the bone marrow. They may be seen in the blood stream, however, in some anemias and leukemias.

Nucleated red cells in the blood stream act as a veiled warning of some abnormality in the life of the red cells; and this, in turn, usually foreshadows some form of anemia.

The oldest nucleated red cell is the metarubricyte. As the metarubricyte grows and develops, it loses its nucleus and becomes a reticulocyte. The reticulocyte has a net-like substance, a reticulum, in place of a nucleus.

Most of the reticulocytes remain at home in the bone marrow; a few, however, slip into the blood stream.

As the red cell completes its development, the reticulocyte loses its reticulum. In so doing, it becomes an erythrocyte. This is the mature red cell.

Thus, we find that the red cell is born and brought up in the bone marrow. This period of life is brief, lasting only one week. Then the mature red cell—the erythrocyte—is nudged into the blood stream.

Now let us consider some terminology.

As stated previously, the blood cells have recently undergone a change in terminology.

The new name and old names for the red cells are given in Table 17.

Table 17.—New Name and Old Names for the Red Cells

Erythrocytic Series of Cells

New Name	Old Names
Rubriblast	pronormoblast, erythroblast, megaloblast, promegaloblast, normoblast, hemocytoblast, stem cell, myeloblast, lymphoidocyte, karyoblast
Prorubricyte	basophilic normoblast, erythroblast, megaloblast, pronormoblast, normoblast, macronormoblast, macroblast, prokaryocyte
Rubricyte	polychromatophilic normoblast, normoblast, pronormoblast, macronormoblast, erythroblast, karyocyte
Metarubricyte	orthochromic normoblast, normoblast, erythroblast, metakaryocyte
Reticulocyte	immature erythrocyte, juvenile red cell
Erythrocyte	red blood cell, erythroplastid, normocyte, akaryocyte

As you see, in Table 17, the red cells belong to the erythrocytic series of cells.

The erythrocytic series is often referred to by the old name *normoblastic series*.

And the nucleated red cells also are often referred to by their old names.

The new name and most frequently used old name for the nucleated red cells is given below:

New Name for Nucleated Red Cells	Old Name Most Often Used
rubriblast	pronormoblast
prorubricyte	basophilic normoblast
rubricyte	polychromatophilic normoblast
metarubricyte	orthochromic normoblast

Due to the "die hards" and immaturity in the field, the student should learn both names for the nucleated red cells, that is, the new name and old name most often used.

(The red cells could have been numbered. For example, a rubriblast could be called red cell #1, a prorubricyte could be called red cell #2, etc. But such terms probably would have been too simple and too practical.)

The student should carefully study the following Plate 8 and the accompanying legend; he should then continue with the heading *Abnormal Erythrocytes* which follows this plate.

Legend for Plate 8

Development of a Red Cell (erythrocytic series)

1. Rubriblast

Size: a little larger than a neutrophilic segmented cell

Nucleus: large; round; usually contains a few "holes" or nucleoli

Cytoplasm: deep blue

When Found: none in normal blood; 0% to 3% in leukemia, erythroblastosis fetalis, and many severe anemias

Comments: This is the infant cell of the erythrocytic series. If this cell is present, many older cells (prorubricyte and rubricyte) should also be present in the smear. If these older cells are not present, the "rubriblast" is not a rubriblast.

2. Prorubricyte

Size: about the size of a neutrophilic segmented cell

Nucleus: large; round; usually located in dead center of cell

Cytoplasm: blue

When Found: none in normal blood; 0% to 6% in leukemia, erythroblastosis fetalis, and many severe anemias

Comments: May be mistaken for a plasmacyte or lymphocyte. When in doubt, use "the company they keep" method of identification. For example, if several nucleated red cells are present in the smear, call the cell in question a prorubricyte. If several plasmacytes are present, call the cell a plasmacyte.

3. Rubricyte

Size: a little smaller than a neutrophilic segmented cell

Nucleus: round; usually located in dead center of cell

Cytoplasm: light gray

When Found: none in normal blood; 0% to 10% in leukemia, erythroblastosis fetalis, and many severe anemias

Comments: This cell may be mistaken for a lymphocyte. When in doubt, use "the company they keep" method of identification. If other nucleated red cells are present, call cell a rubricyte. If no other nucleated red cells are present, call cell a lymphocyte.

4. Metarubricyte

Size: a little larger than an erythrocyte

Nucleus: small; round

Cytoplasm: light brown or reddish brown

When Found: none in normal blood; 0% to 25% in leukemia, erythroblastosis fetalis, and many severe anemias

Comments: The small round nucleus and light brown or reddish brown cytoplasm make this cell easy to identify.

5. Reticulocyte

Size: about the size of a large erythrocyte

Nucleus: none; after a special stain, center of cell shows a net-like substance or reticulum

Cytoplasm: pink or reddish brown

When Found: 1% to 2% in normal blood; increased in hereditary spherocytic anemia; decreased in aplastic anemia

Comments: With the normal blood stain (Wright's), the reticulocyte appears as an erythrocyte. The reticulocyte can only be identified with a special stain. The reticulocyte in the illustration has been stained with brilliant cresyl blue.

6. Erythrocyte

Size: 7.0 to 8.0 microns in diameter

Nucleus: none

Cytoplasm: pink or reddish brown

When Found: thousands in normal and abnormal blood smears

Comments: easy to identify.

PLATE 8
DEVELOPMENT OF A RED CELL
(Erythrocytic Series)

Stain: Wright's

Magnification: X1500

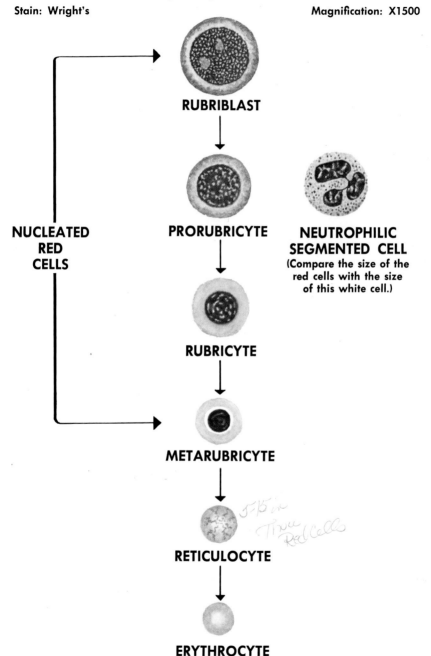

RUBRIBLAST

NUCLEATED
RED
CELLS

PRORUBRICYTE

NEUTROPHILIC
SEGMENTED CELL
(Compare the size of the
red cells with the size
of this white cell.)

RUBRICYTE

METARUBRICYTE

RETICULOCYTE

ERYTHROCYTE

ABNORMAL ERYTHROCYTES

The abnormal erythrocytes differ from normal erythrocytes in size, shape, or content. These differences are significant in distinguishing the various anemias.

For example, if the erythrocytes are unusually large, it may indicate pernicious anemia. If the erythrocytes are shaped like a sickle or crescent, it may point to sickle cell anemia. And, if the erythrocytes are pale or hollow, it may indicate hypochromic anemia.

The abnormal erythrocytes fall into 4 groups: (1) differences in size, (2) differences in shape, (3) differences in content, and (4) miscellaneous differences.

Each of the 4 groups is broken down into several categories as shown in Table 18.

Table 18.—Abnormal Erythrocytes

Group 1. Differences in size
1. anisocytosis
2. microcytosis
3. macrocytosis

Group 2. Differences in shape
1. poikilocytosis
2. spherocytosis
3. ovalocytosis
4. target cells
5. sickle cells
6. burr cells
7. acanthrocytes

Group 3. Differences in content
1. hypochromia
2. polychromatophilia
3. basophilic stippling
4. Cabot rings and Howell-Jolly bodies
5. siderocytes
6. Heinz bodies
7. malaria parasites

Group 4. Miscellaneous differences
1. rouleau formation
2. crenated erythrocytes
3. partially hemolyzed erythrocytes
4. design formation of erythrocytes
5. acid stain of erythrocytes
6. alkaline stain of erythrocytes

The abnormal erythrocytes listed in the above table will be illustrated in 4 color plates.

Each color plate will be accompanied by a legend which discusses the abnormal erythrocyte with respect to pronunciation, synonyms, definition, cause, and associated disease.

The student should carefully study the following 4 color plates and accompanying legends. He should then continue with the heading *Discussion of the Procedure for the Stained Red Cell Examination.* This discussion follows the last color plate.

Legend for Plate 9

Abnormal Erythrocytes: Differences in Size

Diameter and Thickness of an Erythrocyte

If you were to press a rounded piece of dough between your thumb and middle finger, it would take the shape of an erythrocyte. Thus, an erythrocyte is a biconcave disk.

The average erythrocyte has a diameter of 7.5 microns, the normal range being 7.0 to 8.0 microns.

The average erythrocyte has a thickness of 2.0 microns, the normal range being 1.8 to 2.2 microns.

The diameter and thickness of an erythrocyte are illustrated on the right.

Note: There are about 25,000 microns in 1 inch.

Normal Erythrocytes

There is a slight variation in the size of normal erythrocytes. For example, a healthy person may have some erythrocytes measuring 7.2 microns in diameter, other erythrocytes measuring 7.4 microns in diameter, and still other erythrocytes measuring 7.9 microns in diameter.

This slight variation in the size of normal erythrocytes is illustrated on the right.

Anisocytosis (an-i-so-si-to′sis)

Anisocytosis is a marked variation in the size of erythrocytes. It is illustrated on the right.

Anisocytosis is caused by an abnormality in the development of red cells. It may be seen in leukemia, pernicious anemia, and many other anemias.

Microcytosis (mi″kro-si-to′sis)

Microcytosis is a decrease in the size of erythrocytes. It is illustrated on the right.

Microcytosis may be caused by a deficiency of the raw materials needed to manufacture red cells. This occurs in iron deficiency anemia.

In this anemia, not only are the erythrocytes smaller than normal, but they are usually deficient in hemoglobin.

Macrocystosis (mak″ro-si-to′sis)

Macrocytosis is an increase in the size of erythrocytes. It is illustrated on the right.

Macrocytosis may be found in a healthy newborn infant. Here it is a normal occurrence.

Macrocytosis may also be seen in pernicious anemia. Here it indicates a deficiency in the materials needed to manufacture red cells.

PLATE 9
Abnormal Erythrocytes: Differences in Size

Stain: Wright's

Magnification: X1000

NORMAL ERYTHROCYTE
VIEWED FROM ABOVE

7.5 MICRONS

7.5 MICRONS IN DIAMETER

NORMAL ERYTHROCYTE
VIEWED FROM THE SIDE

live upts 120 days

2 MICRONS

2 MICRONS IN THICKNESS

DIAMETER AND THICKNESS OF AN ERYTHROCYTE

(normocytic)   *variation in size*

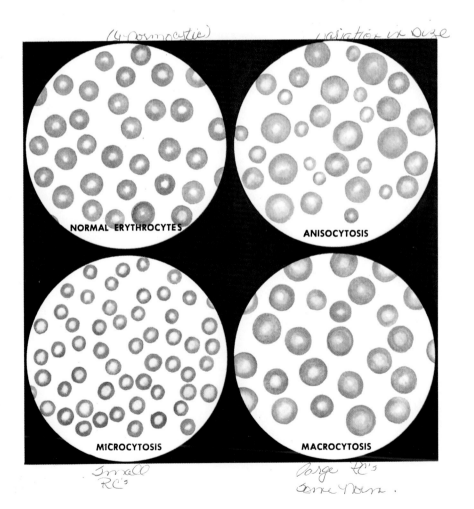

NORMAL ERYTHROCYTES

ANISOCYTOSIS

MICROCYTOSIS

MACROCYTOSIS

small RC's

large RC's come down.

Legend for Plate 10

Abnormal Erythrocytes: Differences in Shape

Poikilocytosis (poi″ki-lo-si-to′sis)

Poikilocytosis is a variation in the shape of erythrocytes. It is illustrated on the right.

Poikilocytosis is caused by a defect in the formation of red cells. It may be seen in pernicious anemia, iron deficiency anemia, and many other types of anemia.

Spherocytosis (sfe″ro-si-to′sis)

Spherocytosis is the presence of sphere shaped erythrocytes. These sphere shaped erythrocytes are thicker than the normal disk shaped erythrocytes. Because of this greater thickness, they take a much darker stain. This is illustrated on the right.

Spherocytosis is usually an inherited abnormality. It may be seen in hereditary spherocytic anemia.

Ovalocytosis (o-val″o-si-to′sis)

Ovalocytosis is also referred to as elliptocytosis.

Ovalocytosis is the presence of oval shaped erythrocytes. They are illustrated on the right.

Ovalocytosis is an inherited abnormality. It may be found in hereditary elliptocytosis; and it may sometimes be seen in thalassemia and sickle cell anemia.

Target Cells

Target cells are also known as Mexican hat cells and leptocytes. These cells resemble a target. They are illustrated on the right.

Target cells are an inherited abnormality. They may be found in thalassemia.

Sickle Cells

Sickle cells are also called drepanocytes and meniscocytes.

Sickle cells are shaped like a sickle or crescent. They are illustrated on the right.

Sickle cells are an inherited abnormality. They may be seen in sickle cell anemia, a disease confined mainly to members of the Negro race.

Burr Cells and Acanthrocytes

Burr cells have blunt projections on their outer edges. They are illustrated on the right.

Burr cells have no known significance. They may be seen in uremia, carcinoma of the stomach, and bleeding peptic ulcer.

Acanthrocytes are also known as acanthocytes.

Acanthrocytes are "thorny" cells. They have sharp thorn-like projections on their outer edges. They are illustrated on the right.

Acanthrocytes are an inherited abnormality. They may be seen in retinitis pigmentosa.

PLATE 10
Abnormal Erythrocytes: Differences in Shape

Stain: Wright's   Magnification: X1000

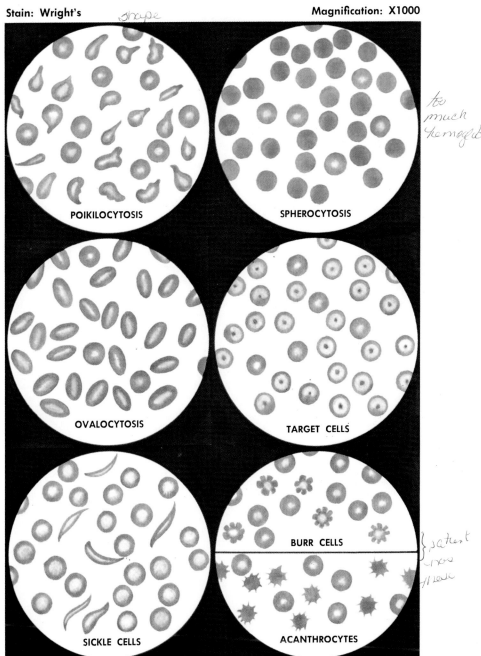

POIKILOCYTOSIS

SPHEROCYTOSIS

OVALOCYTOSIS

TARGET CELLS

SICKLE CELLS

BURR CELLS

ACANTHROCYTES

Abnormal Erythrocytes: Differences in Content

Hypochromia (hi-po-kro′me-ah)

Hypochromia is also referred to as hypochromasia.

Hypochromia means less color. It is a condition showing pale or hollow erythrocytes. They are illustrated on the right.

Hypochromia is caused by a deficiency of hemoglobin. It may be seen in iron deficiency anemia, chronic posthemorrhagic anemia, and many other anemias.

Polychromatophilia (pol″e-kro″mah-to-fil′e-ah)

Polychromatophilia is also referred to as polychromasia or diffuse basophilia.

Polychromatophilia means love of many colors. The many colors are various shades of blue combined with tinges of pink.

The erythrocytes in the blood smear are colored a dirty blue. They are illustrated on the right.

Polychromatophilia indicates the presence of undeveloped erythrocytes. It may be seen in pernicious anemia and many other anemias.

Basophilic Stippling

Basophilic stippling is also referred to as punctate basophilia.

Basophilic stippling is a coarse granulation which is sometimes found in erythrocytes. The granules are blue, gray, or brown in color. They are illustrated on the right.

Basophilic stippling indicates the presence of undeveloped erythrocytes. It may be seen in lead poisoning, leukemia, and many types of anemia.

Cabot Rings and Howell-Jolly Bodies

Cabot rings are ring-like bodies which may be present in erythrocytes. The rings are blue, purple, brown, or reddish in color. They are illustrated on the right.

Howell-Jolly bodies appear as single or double dots on erythrocytes. The dots are blue, purple, brown, or reddish in color. They are illustrated on the right.

Cabot rings and Howell-Jolly bodies are thought to be nuclear fragments. They may be seen in severe anemias.

Siderocytes (sid′er-o-sits)

Siderocytes are erythrocytes containing free iron. When stained with a special stain, the free iron appears as very faint bluish specks. This is illustrated on the right.

Siderocytes may be seen in hemolytic anemia.

Heinz Bodies

Heinz bodies are not visible with Wright's stain, they require a special stain.

With a methyl violet stain, Heinz bodies appear as deep purple particles. In shape, they are round or irregular. In size, they are usually about as large as Howell-Jolly bodies. They usually lie near the edge of the erythrocyte.

Heinz bodies are believed to be precipitated hemoglobin and their presence is thought to indicate some injury to the erythrocytes.

They may be found in some forms of hemolytic anemia.

Malaria Parasites

Malaria parasites appear in various forms. The most common form is the ring form. This may be seen in erythrocytes.

The ring form of the malaria parasite consists of a red dot and a blue ring. It should not be confused with a platelet lying upon an erythrocyte.

The ring forms of the malaria parasite are illustrated in the upper half of the Plate on the right. Whereas platelets superimposed upon erythrocytes are illustrated in the lower half of the Plate on the right.

Erythrocytes containing malaria parasites may be found in malaria.

PLATE 11
Abnormal Erythrocytes: Differences in Content

Stain: Wright's   Magnification: X1000

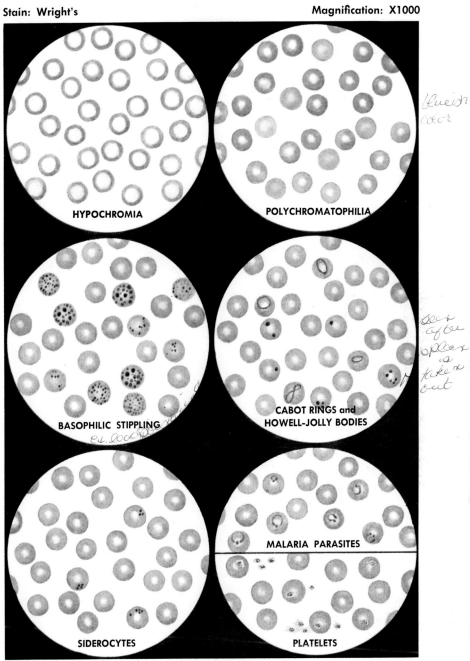

HYPOCHROMIA

POLYCHROMATOPHILIA

BASOPHILIC STIPPLING

CABOT RINGS and
HOWELL-JOLLY BODIES

SIDEROCYTES

MALARIA PARASITES

PLATELETS

Legend for Plate 12

Abnormal Erythrocytes: Miscellaneous Differences

Rouleau Formation (roo-lo' formation)

Rouleau formation is the arrangement of erythrocytes in rolls or stacks. It is illustrated on the right.

Rouleau formation has no known cause. It is sometimes seen in a normal blood smear, possibly due to the cells being away from their natural environment and subject to the pressure of a blood smear. It is often seen in multiple myeloma, a disease associated with an increase in plasma globulin.

If rouleau formation is seen in only a few microscopic fields, it should not be reported. If it is seen in many microscopic fields, however, it should be reported.

Crenated Erythrocytes

Crenated erythrocytes have puckered outer edges. They are illustrated on the right.

Crenated erythrocytes may be produced in a blood smear which dries slowly. In the drying process, fluid leaves the cell and the cell shrinks.

Crenated erythrocytes are often found in various portions of the blood smear. They have no diagnostic significance.

Partially Hemolyzed Erythrocytes

Partially hemolyzed erythrocytes are lightly colored and malformed. They are illustrated on the right.

Partially hemolyzed erythrocytes may be caused by moisture on the slide prior to making the smear. They may be seen in various portions of the smear. They have no significance.

Design Formation of Erythrocytes

Design formation is the presence of erythrocytes in various designs or patterns. It is illustrated on the right.

Design formation may be caused by fat or oil on the slide. It may also be caused by getting the blood ahead of the spreader during the process of making the smear. This puts pressure on the erythrocytes and results in design formation.

Design formation is sometimes found on the edge of a blood smear. It has no significance.

Acid Stain of Erythrocytes

The buffer solution used with Wright's stain should have a pH value between 6.4 and 6.8.

If the buffer solution is too acid (pH 6.3, 6.2, 6.1, *etc.*), the erythrocytes are colored a reddish color. This is illustrated on the right.

An acid stain greatly changes the normal staining characteristics of the blood cells—especially the white cells. These cells will then be difficult to identify. Consequently, an acid stain should be avoided.

Alkaline Stain of Erythrocytes

The buffer solution used with Wright's stain should have a pH value between 6.4 and 6.8.

If the buffer solution is too alkaline (pH 6.9, 7.0, *etc.*), the erythrocytes are colored a dirty gray. This is illustrated on the right.

An alkaline stain greatly changes the normal staining characteristics of the blood cells—especially the white cells. These cells will then be difficult to identify. Consequently, an alkaline stain should be avoided.

PLATE 12
Abnormal Erythrocytes: Miscellaneous Differences

Stain: Wright's   Magnification: X1000

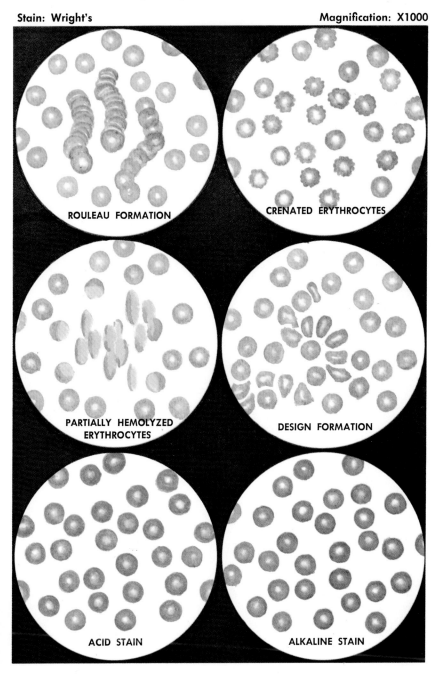

ROULEAU FORMATION

CRENATED ERYTHROCYTES

PARTIALLY HEMOLYZED ERYTHROCYTES

DESIGN FORMATION

ACID STAIN

ALKALINE STAIN

DISCUSSION OF THE PROCEDURE FOR THE STAINED RED CELL EXAMINATION

The discussion will cover (1) the method of examining and reporting nucleated red cells and (2) the method of examining and reporting abnormal erythrocytes.

METHOD OF EXAMINING AND REPORTING NUCLEATED RED CELLS

The usual procedure is to tabulate the nucleated red cells that are seen while counting the 100 white cells for the differential white cell count.

For example, suppose you saw 40 nucleated red cells while counting your 100 white cells for the differential white cell count.

You would then record and report these 40 nucleated red cells.

These nucleated red cells are recorded and reported in either one of the following ways.

Some laboratories make a differential nucleated red cell count, that is, they identify and report each individual nucleated red cell. For example, their report might read something like this:

nucleated red cells

rubriblasts	1
prorubricytes	3
rubricytes	11
metarubricytes	25
total	40

The above cells, of course, would have been seen and recorded while making the differential white cell count.

Other laboratories do not bother to identify the type of nucleated red cell. When a nucleated red cell is seen, they simply record it as a nucleated red cell. For example, if 1 rubricyte and 2 metarubricytes were seen in a microscopic field, they would record 3 nucleated red cells.

If 40 nucleated red cells were seen and recorded during the differential white cell count, their report would read like this:

nucleated red cells

rubriblasts	
prorubricytes	
rubricytes	
metarubricytes	
total	40

(discussion continued on page 287)

Legend for Plate 13

THE MOST FREQUENTLY ENCOUNTERED ABNORMALITIES IN THE STAINED RED CELL EXAMINATION

The discussion will cover nucleated red cells, normal and abnormal erythrocytes, and malaria parasites and platelets.

Nucleated Red Cells

1. In the upper portion of Plate 13, note the difference between the nucleated red cells and the lymphocytes. The 3 lymphocytes have been put there for the purpose of comparison.

2. In the upper right hand corner of the plate, note the two nucleated red cells with the clover-leaf shaped nucleus. The nucleus of these cells is rupturing, the process being known as karyorrhexis (kar"e-o-rek'sis). This condition may be seen in some severe anemias.

3. The 1 nucleated red cell with the blue cytoplasm is a prorubricyte. The 2 nucleated red cells with the gray cytoplasm are rubricytes. And the 3 nucleated red cells with the brown cytoplasm are metarubricytes.

4. Sometimes it is difficult to tell whether a cell is a nucleated red cell or a lymphocyte. When such a situation arises, use the "company they keep" method of identification. For example, if several easily identified nucleated red cells are present, call the cell in question a nucleated red cell. However, if no easily identified nucleated red cells are present, call the cell in question a lymphocyte.

Normal and Abnormal Erythrocytes

In the dead center of the plate, there are 6 normal erythrocytes. They have been put there for the purpose of comparison. Surrounding these 6 normal erythrocytes are various types of abnormal erythrocytes. These abnormal erythrocytes show a *moderate* degree of hypochromia, anisocytosis, and poikilocytosis.

Malaria Parasites and Platelets

In the lower portion of the plate, note the difference between the malaria parasites and the platelets. The malaria parasite is *in* the red cell; it is never in the space between two red cells. The platelet, however, is usually in the space between two red cells. When a platelet gets *on* a red cell, the confusion may arise, for it may resemble a malaria parasite. The malaria parasite, however, is a sharp clear red dot and blue ring. Whereas a platelet is a fuzzy bluish red dot.

PLATE 13
The Most Frequently Encountered Abnormalities in the Stained Red Cell Examination

Stain: Wright's   Magnification: X1500

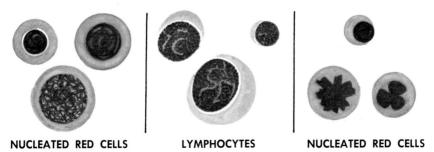

NUCLEATED RED CELLS   LYMPHOCYTES   NUCLEATED RED CELLS

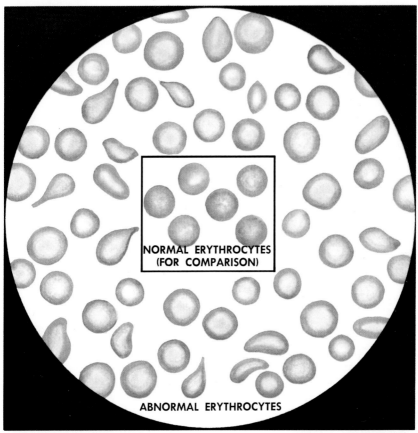

NORMAL ERYTHROCYTES
(FOR COMPARISON)

ABNORMAL ERYTHROCYTES

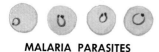

MALARIA PARASITES

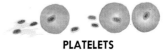

PLATELETS

The latter method of reporting nucleated red cells is certainly the simplest. To be on the safe side, however, use the method recommended by your particular school or laboratory.

You may have some trouble identifying nucleated red cells. You will find that some nucleated red cells look like small lymphocytes. You can usually distinguish the two cells on the following basis.

If it is a nucleated red cell, (1) the nucleus will usually be centrally located and completely surrounded by cytoplasm and (2) the patient will have some form of anemia.

The anemia will usually be apparent from the red cell count and hemoglobin determination. However, these tests may not always indicate the presence of anemia. For example, if a patient with leukemia has just received a transfusion, his red cell count and hemoglobin may be normal. But nucleated red cells may be found in the blood smear.

METHOD OF EXAMINING AND REPORTING
ABNORMAL ERYTHROCYTES

In making this examination, you must look on the thin area of the blood smear where the erythrocytes are spread out. It is impossible to perform this examination on the thick area of the blood smear where the erythrocytes are bunched together.

In looking for abnormal erythrocytes, you should look particularly for the 3 forms which are most commonly found: hypochromia, anisocytosis, and poikilocytosis. Most of the other abnormal erythrocytes fall into one of the following categories:

1. Rarely seen unless accompanied by hypochromia, anisocytosis, or poikilocytosis.
   For example, Cabot rings, Howell-Jolly bodies, polychromatophilia, etc. are rarely seen unless accompanied by hypochromia, anisocytosis, or poikilocytosis.
2. Usually suspected by the physician and identified more readily with special tests.
   For example, if the physician suspects sickle cell anemia, he orders a special test for sickle cells.

How do you report hypochromia, anisocytosis, and poikilocytosis?

The above abnormalities in erythrocytes may be reported in one of two ways:

(1) The abnormalities in erythrocytes may be reported as *slight, moderate,* or *marked.*

(2) The abnormalities in erythrocytes may be reported as either *present* or *absent.*

A brief discussion of the above methods of reporting abnormal erythrocytes is given below.

21

When hypochromia is found, some laboratories report it as slight, moderate, or marked. The slight, moderate, or marked, of course, refer to the degree of hypochromia. Such a sharp breakdown in the degree of hypochromia, however, seems unnecessary.

First, the degree of hypochromia may be more accurately determined from the color index or mean corpuscular hemoglobin. Second, the degree of hypochromia is often difficult to establish—especially for the beginner.

In view of this, we suggest that hypochromia be reported as either *present* or *absent*. We also suggest that anisocytosis and poikilocytosis be reported as either *present* or *absent*.

For those students who must report the red cell abnormalities as *slight*, *moderate* or *marked* we offer the following guide:

We have presented a *moderate* degree of hypochromia, anisocytosis, and poikilocytosis in Plate 13, page 284.

If the above abnormalities—hypochromia, anisocytosis, and poikilocytosis—were less pronounced, you would report a *slight* degree of hypochromia, anisocytosis, or poikilocytosis.

If the above abnormalities were more pronounced, you would report a *marked* degree of hypochromia, anisocytosis, or poikilocytosis.

A note of precaution before turning to the procedure:

Sometimes normal erythrocytes may become so distorted that they may be mistaken for hypochromia, anisocytosis, or poikilocytosis.

For example, if the blood smear is made on a glass slide which contains moisture, dirt, or grease, the erythrocytes may become greatly distorted. And, if the blood is pushed ahead of the spreader during the process of making the smear, the erythrocytes may become greatly distorted.

These distorted erythrocytes may be mistaken for hypochromia, anisocytosis, or poikilocytosis.

To avoid reporting these distorted erythrocytes as abnormal erythrocytes, follow this rule:

If you see hypochromia or anisocytosis or poikilocytosis in only a few microscopic fields, you should ignore it.

But, if you see hypochromia or anisocytosis or poikilocytosis in every microscopic field you examine, you should report it.

Since the student will be practicing on normal blood, he should expect to find normal erythrocytes. He should carefully study these normal erythrocytes, however, and note the slight variation in their size, shape, and content.

By studying this slight difference in normal erythrocytes, the student is less likely to make *the common mistake of reporting abnormal erythrocytes in normal blood*.

Now carefully study Plate 13 and the accompanying legend, page 284.

After you have studied the above plate and legend, turn to the procedure for the stained red cell examination.

PROCEDURE FOR THE STAINED RED CELL EXAMINATION

1. Obtain a piece of paper and write out a report form for the stained red cell examination (Fig. 124, page 290).

2. If you have just completed the differential white cell count, the stained blood smear will already be on the stage of the microscope. And the oil immersion objective will already be lowered into the drop of oil. In such cases, (1) turn on the microscope light, (2) move the blood smear to the THIN AREA of the smear as shown in Figure 123, and (3) proceed to step 16.

3. If you have not just completed the differential white cell count and are starting from scratch, proceed as follows:

4. Turn on the microscope light.

5. Raise the condenser up as far as it will go.

   Note: Make sure that you have the condenser up as far as it will go.

6. Place both hands on the mirror.

7. Now adjust the mirror so a bright light comes directly up through the glass top of the condenser and the opening in the stage.

8. Look at the blood smear illustrated in Figure 123 and note that the THIN AREA of the blood smear is used for the examination.

9. Now place a drop of immersion oil on the THIN AREA of your stained blood smear.

THIN AREA used for examination

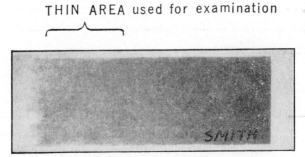

FIG. 123.—Thin area of the blood smear used in the stained red cell examination.

REPORT OF A STAINED RED CELL EXAMINATION

Patient:

Date:

Physician:

	Patient's Values	Normal Values
Nucleated Red Cells		
rubriblasts	_____	___0___
prorubricytes	_____	___0___
rubricytes	_____	___0___
metarubricytes	_____	___0___
total	_____	___0___
Abnormal Erythrocytes		
hypochromia	_____	___absent___
anisocytosis	_____	___absent___
poikilocytosis	_____	___absent___
miscellaneous		
sickle cells	_____	___absent___
target cells	_____	___absent___
Cabot rings, etc.	_____	___absent___
_____	_____	___absent___
_____	_____	___absent___

Examination performed by:

FIG. 124.—Sample report form for the stained red cell examination.

10. Put the stained blood smear in the jaws of the movable stage.

11. By turning the stage knobs, bring the drop of oil directly over the opening in the stage.

12. Switch the oil immersion (95×) objective into position directly over the smear.

13. Look at the slide from the side. Turn the coarse adjustment and lower the oil immersion (95×) objective into the drop of oil.

14. Now continue turning the coarse adjustment until the oil immersion (95×) objective is touching the glass slide.

15. Now, while continually looking in the eyepiece, VERY SLOWLY rotate the coarse adjustment toward yourself until you see some cells.

    Note: The oil immersion objective must remain in the drop of oil. The cells should come into view when you rotate the coarse adjustment about $\frac{1}{16}$ turn toward yourself. If the cells do not come into view, repeat steps 13, 14, and 15.

16. When you have the cells in view, rock the fine adjustment back and forth and bring the cells into perfect focus.

17. Now place both hands on the mirror.

18. Look in the eyepiece and adjust the mirror so the maximum amount of light shines on the cells. This is important!

19. Look at the red cells in Figure 125 and observe the following:

    a. The red cells are evenly distributed.
    b. The red cells are not scattered, over-lapping, or bunched together.

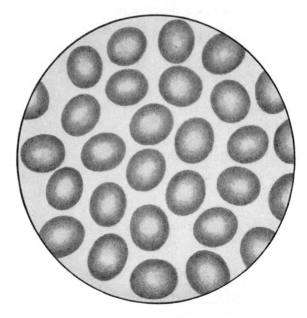

Fig. 125.—Even distribution of the red cells in the stained red cell examination. Note that the red cells are evenly distributed; they are not scattered, over-lapping, or bunched together.

20. Now look in the eyepiece to see if your red cells are evenly distributed.

21. If your red cells are evenly distributed, proceed to step 23.

    Note: The red cells must be evenly distributed. This is important!

22. If your red cells are not evenly distributed, look in the eyepiece and turn the stage knobs until you find an area where the red cells are evenly distributed.

23. When you have an area where the red cells are evenly distributed, briefly review the normal erythrocytes and abnormal erythrocytes in Plate 13, page 284.

24. A microscopic field is the area which can be seen by looking in the eyepiece.

25. Now examine about 15 microscopic fields and look for nucleated red cells and abnormal erythrocytes.

Note to Students: You will be practicing on normal blood. Therefore, you will not see any nucleated red cells and the erythrocytes will be normal. You should carefully examine these normal erythrocytes, however, and note the slight variation in their size, shape, and hemoglobin content. This slight variation, of course, is normal. And you should make out your report as illustrated in Figure 126, page 294.

26. If the red cells are normal, make out the report as illustrated in Figure 126, page 294.

27. When you have filled in your report, sign it and hand it in.

28. If your blood smear does not have to be saved, put it in a cleaning jar which contains "bleach" and soapy water.

Note: When a batch of used slides has accumulated, clean them as directed below (page 297).

29. Now carefully read the following Steps 30–35.

30. If you were examining an abnormal blood smear or a smear from a patient, you would have proceeded as follows.

31. If nucleated red cells were present, you would have recorded the number seen while counting the 100 white cells of the differential white cell count.

Note: If it were the practice in your laboratory to classify each nucleated red cell, you would, of course, have done so. Otherwise, you would simply have recorded the total number seen.

32. After you had completed the above, you would have made a platelet estimation and then turned to the THIN AREA of the blood smear and carefully examined the erythrocytes.

(continued on page 296)

REPORT OF A STAINED RED CELL EXAMINATION

Patient: Jones, Mrs. Betty   54361

Date: 7 - 7 - 72

Physician: Dr. Joseph Conrad

	Patient's Values	Normal Values
Nucleated Red Cells		
rubriblasts		0
prorubricytes		0
rubricytes		0
metarubricytes		0
total	0	0
Abnormal Erythrocytes		
hypochromia	absent	absent
anisocytosis	absent	absent
poikilocytosis	absent	absent
miscellaneous		
sickle cells	absent	absent
target cells	absent	absent
Cabot rings, etc.	absent	absent
		absent
		absent
Examination performed by:	Sandra Frisbie	

FIG. 126.—Sample report of normal red cells in the stained red cell examination.

REPORT OF A STAINED RED CELL EXAMINATION

Patient: Doe, Mr. John   95467

Date: 7-7-72

Physician: Dr. Tom Maxwell

	Patient's Values	Normal Values
Nucleated Red Cells		
rubriblasts	1	0
prorubricytes.	4	0
rubricytes	10	0
metarubricytes	29	0
total	44	0
Abnormal Erythrocytes		
hypochromia	slight	absent
anisocytosis	moderate	absent
poikilocytosis	marked	absent
miscellaneous		
sickle cells	absent	absent
target cells	absent	absent
Cabot rings, etc.	absent	absent
polychromatophilia	slight	absent
		absent

Examination performed by: *Sandra Frisbee*

FIG. 127.—Sample report of abnormal red cells in the stained red cell examination. As stated in the text, some laboratories do not classify the nucleated red cells. They report only the total number present. Thus, these laboratories would simply write 44 in the space for total nucleated red cells.

Also, as stated in the text, some laboratories do not report the degree of hypochromia, anisocytosis, poikilocytosis, etc. Thus, these laboratories would simply write *present* for hypochromia, anisocytosis, poikilocytosis, etc.

33. If hypochromia, anisocytosis, poikilocytosis, etc. were present, you would have recorded them as present.

Note: If it were the practice in your laboratory to qualify these abnormalities as slight, moderate, or marked, you would, of course, have done so. Otherwise, you would simply have recorded them as present.

34. After recording any nucleated red cells and abnormal erythrocytes, you would have made out your report as illustrated in the sample report of Figure 127, page 295.

35. Note: In most laboratories, if the differential white cell count or stained red cell examination is abnormal, the stained blood smear is saved for the inspection of the chief technologist or physician.

TIME SAVING METHOD OF PERFORMING A COMPLETE BLOOD COUNT

As previously stated, a CBC or complete blood count consists of 5 tests plus the color index and platelet estimation. Thus,

white cell count
red cell count
hemoglobin determination
color index
differential white cell count
platelet estimation
stained red cell examination

After you have once performed the above individual tests, you may per-form a CBC in the following time saving manner.

1. Dilute the blood for the white cell count.

2. Dilute the blood for the red cell count.

3. Dilute the blood for the hemoglobin determination.
   (If you are using the Haden-Hausser method of perform-ing the hemoglobin determination, you will use the con-tents of the white cell pipet. Therefore, you will not have to make this dilution.)

4. Make the blood smear.

5. Start staining the blood smear.

6. Shake the white cell pipet and red cell pipet at the same time.

7. Charge ruled area 1 for the white cell count.

8. Charge ruled area 2 for the red cell count

9. Count the white cells in ruled area 1.

10. Count the red cells in ruled area 2.

11. Make the hemoglobin determination.

12. Calculate the color index.

13. Perform the differential white cell count on the blood smear, recording any nucleated red cells seen.

14. Make a platelet estimation on the blood smear.

15. Examine the thin area of the blood smear for abnormal erythrocytes.

16. Make out your report for the complete blood count as illustrated in Figure 50, page 90.

17. Sign your name to the report.

18. Give the report to your instructor or follow the usual procedure in your laboratory.

DIRECTIONS FOR CLEANING SLIDES

After use, the slides should be soaked in a solution of "bleach" and soap powder. They may soak for a few hours or a few days. The usual practice is to allow them to soak until a good batch has accumulated.

To clean the slides, proceed as follows:

1. Using soapy water and a hand brush, thoroughly scrub both sides of the slides.

2. Now thoroughly rinse the slides 4 or 5 times in clear water.

3. Dry both sides of the slides with a clean lint-free towel.

4. Light a Bunsen burner.

5. Pick up a slide with your hand and hold it by a corner. Now place the slide directly in the flame so that one side receives the full force of the flame. Hold it there for about 5 seconds. Turn the slide over so the other side receives the full force of the flame. Hold it there for about 5 seconds.

   Note: This flaming process is absolutely essential, for it removes the last traces of moisture and debris. These could distort the cells when the smear is made.

6. Place the slide in a box. It is now ready for use.

PART 3
Further Red Cell Examinations

INTRODUCTION

IN a complete blood count, we performed a red cell count and a stained red cell examination. The information which these tests furnish, however, is not sufficient for the diagnosis and treatment of many types of anemia. Consequently, we must perform further red cell examinations.

Part 3 deals with further red cell examinations; it is made up of the following:

With the exception of the sedimentation rate, all the above examinations are used in the diagnosis and treatment of the anemias.

Chapter 9

Sedimentation Rate

THE sedimentation rate is also referred to by the following terms: sed. rate, erythrocyte sedimentation rate, E S R or E. S. R., sedimenttaion rate of erythrocytes, sedimentation rate of blood, blood sedimentation test, suspension stability of erythrocytes, and suspension stability of blood.

The discussion of the sedimentation rate will cover the following:

> Significance of the Sedimentation Rate
> Discussion of Procedures for the Sedimentation Rate
> Westergren Method for the Sedimentation Rate
> Wintrobe Method for the Sedimentation Rate
> Cutler Method for the Sedimentation Rate
> Landau Method for the Sedimentation Rate
> Sources of Error in the Sedimentation Rate

The student review questions for the sedimentation rate are numbered 149–156 and begin on page 742 of the Appendix.

SIGNIFICANCE OF THE SEDIMENTATION RATE

When the red cells are allowed to settle out from their plasma, the speed of their fall is known as the sedimentation rate.

The sedimentation rate is measured in millimeters per hour. For example, if the red cells fall 25 millimeters in one hour, the sedimentation rate is 25 millimeters per hour.

The sedimentation rate may be performed by various methods. The more commonly employed methods and their normal values are listed in Table 19

Table 19.—Methods and Normal Values for the Sedimentation Rate

Methods	Normal Values	
	Men (*mm. per hr.*)	*Women* (*mm. per hr.*)
Westergren	0 to 15	0 to 20
Wintrobe	0 to 10	0 to 20
Cutler	0 to 8	0 to 10
Landau	0 to 5	0 to 8

300

Why do the normal values vary from method to method?

The sedimentation rate is partly governed by the length and diameter of the test tube. Since the length and diameter of the test tubes vary from method to method, the normal values vary from method to method.

The sedimentation rate is not specific for any particular disease. But it is useful in diagnosing and treating many diseases. It is increased in those conditions listed in Table 20.

Table 20.—Conditions Accompanied by an Increased
Sedimentation Rate

rheumatic fever	metallic poisoning
rheumatoid arthritis	syphilis
coronary thrombosis	tuberculosis
pneumonia	anemia
nephritis	leukemia
nephrosis	menstruation
cancer	pregnancy (after 3rd month)
multiple myeloma	agranulocytosis

Why is the sedimentation rate increased in disease?

Although the cause is unknown, speculation points to the plasma proteins: albumin, globulin, and fibrinogen.

In many diseases, these proteins deviate from their normal ratio or percentage. These deviations may be responsible for the increased sedimentation rate.

In addition to disease, what other factors will affect the sedimentation rate?

The sedimentation rate will increase with the following:

1. tilting the sedimentation rate tube
2. length of the sedimentation rate tube
3. rouleau formation of the red cells
4. temperature increase above ordinary room temperature (27° C.)

The sedimentation rate will decrease with the following:

1. decrease in diameter of sedimentation rate tube
2. if blood is not used within 2 hours
3. temperature decrease below 20° C. (example: blood just removed from refrigerator)

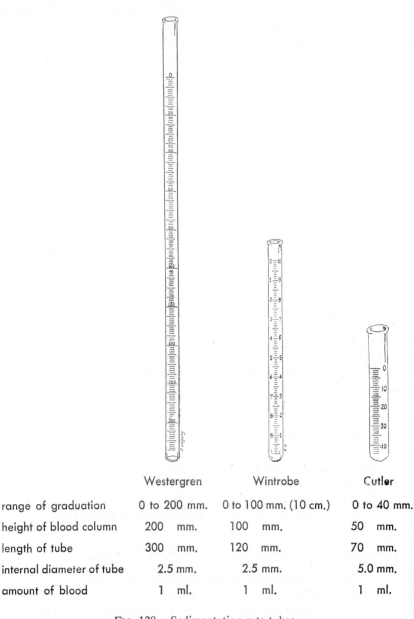

	Westergren	Wintrobe	Cutler
range of graduation	0 to 200 mm.	0 to 100 mm. (10 cm.)	0 to 40 mm.
height of blood column	200 mm.	100 mm.	50 mm.
length of tube	300 mm.	120 mm.	70 mm.
internal diameter of tube	2.5 mm.	2.5 mm.	5.0 mm.
amount of blood	1 ml.	1 ml.	1 ml.

FIG. 128.—Sedimentation rate tubes.

DISCUSSION OF PROCEDURES FOR THE
SEDIMENTATION RATE

The sedimentation rate is performed by filling a graduated tube with anticoagulated blood and recording the rate at which the red cells settle out from their plasma.

The sedimentation rate may be performed by the following methods:

Macro Methods
1. Westergren
2. Wintrobe
3. Cutler
4. Rourke-Ernstene
Micro Methods
1. Landau
2. Hellige-Vollmer
3. Cresta

The macro methods use 1 to 2 cubic centimeters of blood whereas the micro methods use about 1 drop of blood.

The Westergren method is the simplest and most widely used method of performing the sedimentation rate.

The Westergren, Wintrobe, Cutler, and Landau methods will be given in this text.

The sedimentation rate tubes used in the Westergren, Wintrobe, and Cutler methods are illustrated in Figure 128.

22

WESTERGREN METHOD FOR THE SEDIMENTATION RATE

NECESSARY REAGENTS AND EQUIPMENT

1. Materials for a venipuncture.
2. Oxalated tube or Sequestrenized tube. These tubes containing the anticoagulant are usually prepared in advance and set aside until needed. Consequently, some of these tubes should be sitting on the laboratory shelf. If none are available, prepare one of them by following the directions on page 78 or page 79.
3. Westergren tube (Fig. 128, page 302).
4. Westergren rack (Fig. 129, page 305).

Procedure

1. Obtain the requisition slip giving the patient's name, date, and tests requested.
2. Obtain the materials for a venipuncture: sterile 20 gauge needle, 10 cc. syringe, tourniquet, 70% alcohol, cotton or gauze pads, and a wax marking pencil.
3. Obtain an oxalated tube or a Sequestrenized tube.
   Note: The above anticoagulants have proven satisfactory. The original Westergren method uses a 3.8% solution of sodium citrate as the anticoagulant. One part of this liquid anticoagulant is mixed with 4 parts of blood. This dilution makes the results slightly higher.
4. Using the wax marking pencil, write the patient's name on the oxalated or Sequestrenized tube.
5. Make a venipuncture and withdraw about 5 cc. of blood.
   Note: Only about 2 cc. of blood are needed for the sedimentation rate; the remainder may be used for other tests.
6. Remove the needle from the syringe and transfer the blood to the oxalated or Sequestrenized tube.
7. Place a stopper in the mouth of the test tube and mix the blood and anticoagulant by completely inverting the test tube 10 to 12 times.
8. The test may be set up immediately or there may be a short delay. If there is a delay, it should not exceed 2 hours. If the delay exceeds 2 hours, the results will be inaccurate.
   Note: A marked delay causes a decrease in the sedimentation rate.

9. Obtain a Westergren tube (Fig. 128, page 302).

10. Mix the blood by completely inverting the test tube 10 to 12 times.

11. Observe the method of sucking blood into the Westergren tube (Fig. 129).

    Note: The beginner sometimes sucks blood into his mouth. To avoid this, he should practice beforehand, using water instead of blood.

12. Now suck blood into the Westergren tube until the blood is slightly above the 0 mark. Then quickly put your index finger over the opening in the top of the tube.

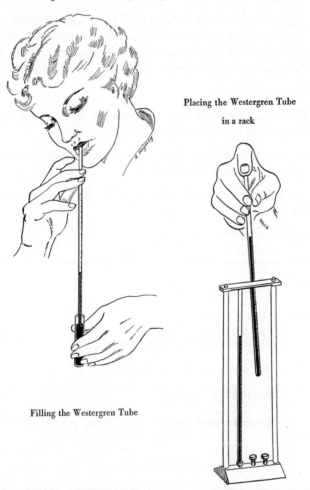

Placing the Westergren Tube

in a rack

Filling the Westergren Tube

FIG. 129.—Filling the Westergren tube and placing it in a rack.

13. Controlling the flow with your index finger, allow the blood to drain to the 0 mark.

14. When the blood is exactly on the 0 mark, press your index finger firmly over the opening in the top of the tube. This holds the blood in place.

15. Then pick up a piece of cotton and wipe the blood off the bottom of the tube.

16. Observe the method of setting the Westergren tube in the rack (Fig. 129).

17. Now place the Westergren tube in the rack so that it is exactly vertical.

    Note: The Westergren tube must be exactly vertical. If the tube is not vertical, the cells will pile up on the wall of the tube and fall faster. The reading, of course, will then be erroneously high.

18. Record the time.

19. Note that each line or mark on the Westergren tube represents 1 millimeter (Fig. 130).

20. In exactly 1 hour, record the number of millimeters the cells have fallen (Fig. 130).

21. Make your report as illustrated in the sample report below.

22. Sample report:

Patient: Doe, Mr. John

Date: 7-7-72

Physician: Dr. Joseph Conrad

Sedimentation rate: 8 mm. per hr.

Method: Westergren

Normal values: men: 0 to 15 mm. per hr.
                      women: 0 to 20 mm. per hr.

Technologist: Sandra Frisbie

23. Clean the Westergren tube with the suction device used for cleaning volumetric and serological pipets.

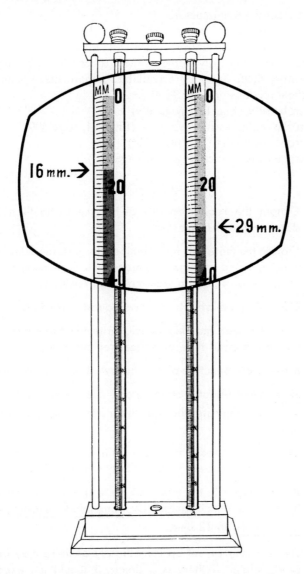

FIG. 130.—Reading the sedimentation rate in a Westergren tube. In the circled inset, the upper very light portion of each tube is plasma. The lower darker portion is red cells.

WINTROBE METHOD FOR THE SEDIMENTATION RATE

NECESSARY REAGENTS AND EQUIPMENT

1. Materials for a venipuncture
2. Oxalated tube or Sequestrenized tube. These tubes containing the anticoagulant are usually prepared in advance and set aside until needed. Consequently, some of these tubes should be sitting on the laboratory shelf. If none are available, prepare one of them by following the directions on page 78 or page 79.
3. Wintrobe tube (Fig. 131, page 309)
4. Wintrobe sedimentation rate rack (Fig. 131, page 309)
5. Wintrobe pipet (Fig. 131, page 309)
6. Wintrobe tube cleaner (Fig. 134, page 313)

Procedure

1. Obtain the requisition slip giving the patient's name, date, and tests requested.

2. Obtain the materials for a venipuncture: sterile 20 gauge needle, 10 cc. syringe, tourniquet, 70% alcohol, cotton or gauze pads, and a wax marking pencil.

3. Obtain an oxalated tube or a Sequestrenized tube.

4. Using the wax marking pencil, write the patient's name on the oxalated tube or Sequestrenized tube.

5. Make a venipuncture and withdraw about 5 cc. of blood.

   Note: Only about 2 cc. of blood are necessary for the sedimentation rate; the remainder can be used for other tests.

6. Remove the needle from the syringe and transfer the blood to the oxalated tube or Sequestrenized tube.

7. Put a stopper in the mouth of the test tube and mix the blood and anticoagulant by completely inverting the test tube 10 to 12 times.

8. The test may be set up immediately or there may be a short delay. If there is a delay, it should not exceed 2 hours. If the delay exceeds 2 hours, the results will be inaccurate.

   Note: A marked delay causes a decrease in the sedimentation rate.

9. Obtain a Wintrobe tube (Fig. 131).

10. Obtain a Wintrobe sedimentation rate rack (Fig. 131).

11. Obtain a Wintrobe pipet consisting of a long needle and a suction device (Fig. 131).

12. Mix the blood by completely inverting the test tube 10 to 12 times.

13. Assemble the Wintrobe pipet by attaching the long needle to the suction device.

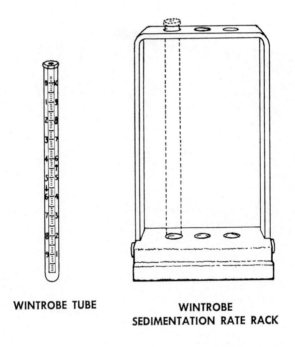

WINTROBE TUBE   WINTROBE
SEDIMENTATION RATE RACK

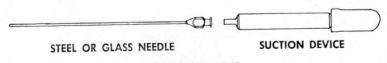

STEEL OR GLASS NEEDLE   SUCTION DEVICE

WINTROBE PIPET

FIG. 131.—Wintrobe tube, Wintrobe sedimentation rate rack, and Wintrobe pipet.

14. Exclude the air from the pipet by pressing the bulb.

15. Keep the bulb pressed down and put the needle in the test tube of blood.

16. Gradually release your pressure on the bulb and allow the blood to be drawn into the pipet until the pipet is about half full.

17. Put the long needle of the pipet in the Wintrobe tube until the needle touches the bottom of the tube as illustrated in Figure 132.

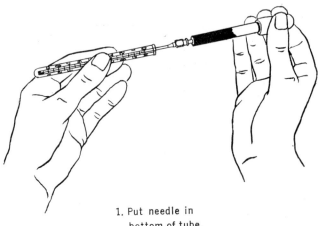

1. Put needle in
bottom of tube.

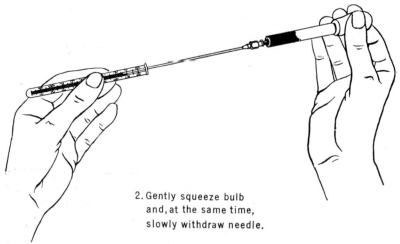

2. Gently squeeze bulb
and, at the same time,
slowly withdraw needle.

FIG. 132.—Filling the Wintrobe tube.

18. Now, when you once start to press the bulb, you must keep a continuous pressure on it. Otherwise, you will force air bubbles into the blood.

19. Gently squeeze the bulb so that blood starts to come out of the needle.

20. When blood starts to come out of the needle, continue your pressure on the bulb and slowly withdraw the needle.

21. Continue the above procedure until the Wintrobe tube is filled to the 0 mark.

    Note: The blood should not be above the "0" mark. No air bubbles should be present in the tube. Filling the tube may take a little practice and patience.

22. When you have the Wintrobe tube filled to the 0 mark, set the tube in the Wintrobe rack in an exact vertical position (Fig. 131, page 309).

    Note: The Wintrobe tube should be exactly vertical. If it is not exactly vertical, the cells will pile up on the wall of the tube and fall faster. The reading, of course, will then be erroneously high.

23. Record the time.

24. The sedimentation rate is read from the scale on the left side of the Wintrobe tube. This scale reads downward. It is 10 centimeters or 100 millimeters in length.

25. Thus, each number on the Wintrobe tube represents 1 centimeter. Whereas each line or mark on the Wintrobe tube represents 1 millimeter (Fig. 133).

The MARKINGS on the LEFT SIDE
of the tube are for the
SEDIMENTATION RATE

The MARKINGS on
the RIGHT SIDE of
the tube are for the
HEMATOCRIT
READING

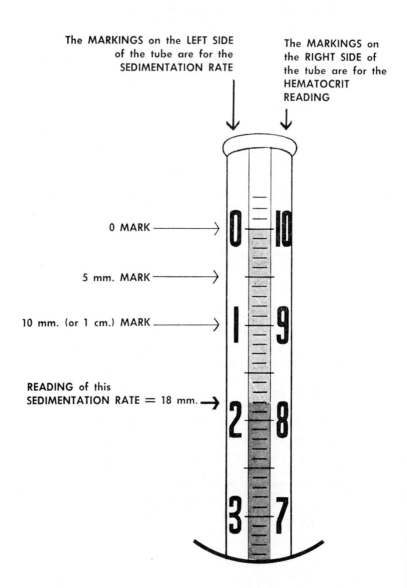

0 MARK ⟶

5 mm. MARK ⟶

10 mm. (or 1 cm.) MARK ⟶

READING of this
SEDIMENTATION RATE = 18 mm. ➤

FIG. 133.—Reading the sedimentation rate in a Wintrobe tube. The upper lighter portion of the tube is plasma; the lower darker portion is red cells.

26. The sedimentation rate is reported in mm. (millimeters).

27. Since each line or mark on the Wintrobe tube represents 1 millimeter, you can simply count the number of lines the cells fall.

28. In <u>exactly</u> 1 hour, count the number of lines or marks the cells have fallen. This will be the number of millimeters (Fig. 133).

29. Record your reading and make your report as indicated in the sample report below.

30. Sample report:

Patient: Doe, Mr. John

Date: 7-7-72

Physician: Dr. James Jenkins

Sedimentation rate: 18 mm. per hr.

Method: Wintrobe

Normal values:
             men: 0 to 10 mm. per hr.
             women: 0 to 20 mm. per hr.

Examination performed by: Sandra Frisbie

---

31. If you are also doing a hematocrit reading by the Wintrobe method, save the Wintrobe tube and turn to the Wintrobe method for the hematocrit reading on page 323.

32. When you have completed the above, clean the Wintrobe tube as directed in Figure 134, page 314.

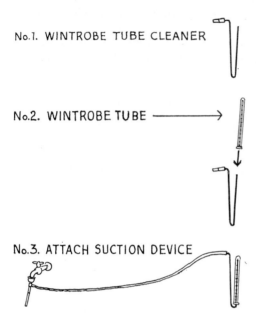

No.1. WINTROBE TUBE CLEANER

No.2. WINTROBE TUBE ──────→

No.3. ATTACH SUCTION DEVICE

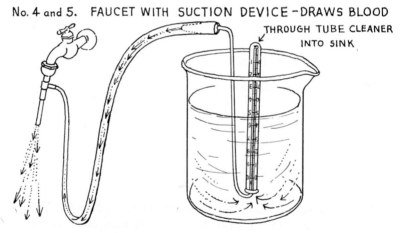

No. 4 and 5. FAUCET WITH SUCTION DEVICE–DRAWS BLOOD
THROUGH TUBE CLEANER
INTO SINK

FIG. 134.—Directions for cleaning a Wintrobe tube.

No. 1. Obtain a Wintrobe tube cleaner.

No. 2. Invert the Wintrobe tube and put it over the open end of the Wintrobe tube cleaner.

No. 3. Attach the Wintrobe tube cleaner to a suction device.

No. 4. Put the Wintrobe tube cleaner and Wintrobe tube in a beaker of water.

and 5. Turn on the faucet and allow the suction to draw the blood out of the Wintrobe tube.

Note: When the Wintrobe tube is clean, dry it in an oven.

CUTLER METHOD FOR THE SEDIMENTATION RATE

NECESSARY REAGENTS AND EQUIPMENT

1. Materials for a venipuncture
2. Oxalated tube or Sequestrenized tube. These tubes containing the anticoagulant are usually prepared in advance and set aside until needed. Consequently, some of these tubes should be sitting on the laboratory shelf. If none are available, prepare one of them by following the directions on page 78 and page 79
3. Cutler tube (Fig. 128, page 302).
4. Cutler sedimentation rate graph (Fig. 135)

Procedure

1. Obtain the requisition slip giving the patient's name, date, and tests requested.

2. Obtain the materials for a venipuncture: sterile 20 gauge needle, 10 cc. syringe, tourniquet, alcohol, cotton or gauze pads, and a wax marking pencil.

3. Obtain an oxalated tube or a Sequestrenized tube.

4. Using the wax marking pencil, write the patient's name on the oxalated tube or Sequestrenized tube.

5. Make a venipuncture and withdraw about 5 cc. of blood.

6. Remove the needle from the syringe and transfer the blood to the oxalated or Sequestrenized tube.

7. Put a stopper in the mouth of the test tube and mix the blood and anticoagulant by completely inverting the test tube 10 to 12 times.

8. The test may be set up immediately or there may be a short delay. If there is a delay, it should not exceed 2 hours. If the delay exceeds 2 hours, the resuts will be inaccurate because a delay of over 2 hours causes a decrease in the sedimentation rate.

9. Obtain a Cutler tube (Fig. 128, page 302).
10. Mix the blood by completely inverting the test tube 10 to 12 times.
11. Fill the Cutler tube to the 0 (zero) mark.
12. Set the Cutler tube in a rack so it is exactly vertical.
13. Note that each line or mark on the Cutler tube represents 1 millimeter.
14. In 5 minutes, read off the number of millimeters the red cells have fallen.
15. Obtain a Cutler sedimentation rate graph (Fig. 135).
16. Plot your reading on the Cutler sedimentation rate graph (Fig. 135).
17. Continue to make readings and plottings at 5 minute intervals until you have made 12 readings and plottings.
18. Write the patient's name and date on the sedimentation rate graph and hand in the report.

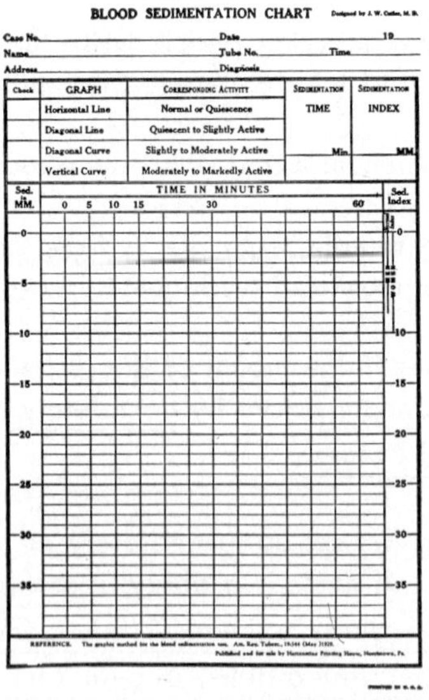
BLOOD SEDIMENTATION CHART

Case No. ______ Date ______ 19__
Name ______ Tube No. ______ Time ______
Address ______ Diagnosis ______

Check	GRAPH	Corresponding Activity	Sedimentation TIME	Sedimentation INDEX
	Horizontal Line	Normal or Quiescence		
	Diagonal Line	Quiescent to Slightly Active		
	Diagonal Curve	Slightly to Moderately Active	Min.	MM.
	Vertical Curve	Moderately to Markedly Active		

FIG. 135.—Cutler sedimentation rate graph.

LANDAU METHOD FOR THE SEDIMENTATION RATE

NECESSARY REAGENTS AND EQUIPMENT

1. Materials for a finger puncture
2. Bottle of 5% sodium citrate solution
3. Landau micro sedimentation pipet
4. Suction device for filling the pipet
5. A stand for holding the pipet

Procedure

1. Obtain the requisition slip giving the patient's name, date, and tests requested.

2. Obtain a Landau micro sedimentation pipet, a suction device for filling the pipet, and a stand for holding the pipet.

3. Obtain a bottle of 5% sodium citrate solution.

4. Obtain the materials for a finger puncture: sterile lancet, alcohol, and cotton or gauze pads.

5. Attach the suction device to the Landau pipet.

6. Put the tip of the pipet in the bottle of 5% sodium citrate.

7. By turning the top screw to the left, draw up the 5% sodium citrate solution to the first mark on the stem of the pipet.

8. Make a finger puncture. Wipe away the first drop. Produce a rounded drop of blood.

9. Put the tip of the pipet in the drop of blood.

10. By turning the top screw to the left, draw up blood until the mixture reaches the 2nd line on the stem of the pipet.

11. With a piece of cotton, wipe off the tip of the pipet.

12. Draw most of the mixture into the bulb but leave a little bit in the stem to prevent air bubbles.

13. Carefully shake the pipet to mix the blood and sodium citrate solution.

14. Slowly force the mixture back into the stem. Then draw most of the mixture back into the bulb, leaving a little bit in the stem to prevent the formation of air bubbles.

15. Again carefully shake the pipet to mix the blood and sodium citrate solution.

16. Repeat steps 14 and 15.

17. Now force the mixture back into the stem of the pipet. This mixture may hang at any place in the stem of the pipet but it should not touch the bottom or tip of the pipet.

18. Place a finger firmly over the tip of the pipet and detach the suction device.

19. Place the pipet in the stand for holding pipets.

20. In exactly 60 minutes, read off the results.

21. Make the report as illustrated in the sample report below

22. Sample report:

Patient: Betty Jo Smith (infant)

Date: 7-7-72

Physician: Dr. James Gilmore

Sedimentation rate: 4 mm. per hr.

Method: Landau

Normal values:

              men: 0 to 5 mm. per hr.
              women: 0 to 8 mm. per hr.

Technologist: Sandra Frisbie

---

23. Clean the pipet with the same suction device used in cleaning the white cell pipets. Then thoroughly dry in an oven.

SOURCES OF ERROR IN THE SEDIMENTATION RATE

1. Unclean sedimentation rate tubes

   Dirt, water, alcohol, ether, etc. will cause hemolysis and decrease the sedimentation rate.

2. Excessive anticoagulant

   Excessive anticoagulant will decrease the sedimentation rate.

3. Partially clotted blood

   The use of partially clotted blood will decrease the sedimentation rate.

4. Old blood

   The blood must be fresh, that is, it must be used within 2 hours after withdrawal. As blood stands, the red cells become more spherical and thus less inclined to assume rouleau formation. This decrease in rouleau formation decreases the sedimentation rate.

5. Failure to mix the blood

   The test tube containing the blood should be completely inverted 10 to 12 times before filling the sedimentation rate tube.

6. Use of cold unmixed blood

   Blood removed from the refrigerator should be allowed to return to room temperature (takes about 30 minutes) and then thoroughly mixed (tube inverted 30 to 40 times).

7. Air bubbles in column of blood

8. Inclined sedimentation rate tube

   The sedimentation rate tube must be placed in an *exact* vertical position. If the tube is not exactly vertical, the red cells will pile up on the inside wall of the tube and fall faster.

9. Miscellaneous

   The sedimentation rate increases with a decrease in the number of red cells. This condition exists in many anemias. And it was formerly the custom to make a correction for the sedimentation rate in anemia. However, this correction is no longer being made because it is now considered "an unnecessary refinement to a very crude test."

23

Chapter 10

Hematocrit Reading

THE word hematocrit is pronounced he-mat′o-krit. It comes from the Greek words for *blood* and *separate*. When translated freely, hematocrit means to separate the components of blood.

The hematocrit reading is often referred to by the following terms: Hct. reading, hematocrit, Hct., cell pack, packed cell volume, PCV, packed red cell volume, volume of erythrocytes, volume of packed red cells, and reading of packed red cells.

The discussion of the hematocrit reading will cover the following:

> Significance of the Hematocrit Reading
> Discussion of Procedures for the Hematocrit Reading
> Wintrobe Method for the Hematocrit Reading
> Adams Micro-Hematocrit Method
> Sources of Error in the Hematocrit Reading

The student review questions for the hematocrit reading are numbered 157–162 and begin on page 743 of the Appendix.

SIGNIFICANCE OF THE HEMATOCRIT READING

When blood is centifuged, the per cent occupied by the packed red cells is known as the hematocrit reading. For example, if 10 cc. of blood are centrifuged and the packed red cells occupy 5 cc., the hematocrit reading is 50 per cent.

The normal values for the hematocrit reading are:

men	40% to 54%
women	37% to 47%

When the red cell count or hemoglobin determination drops below the normal values, the hematocrit reading also drops below the normal values. Consequently, the hematocrit reading drops below the normal values in anemia and leukemia.

In a marked case of anemia, the hematocrit reading may drop to 20 per cent (Fig. 136).

320

The hematocrit reading may rise above the normal values. For example, consider polycythemia vera and dehydration conditions.

In polycythemia vera, the bone marrow produces an excessive amount of red cells. Consequently, the hematocrit reading rises above the normal values.

In dehydration conditions, the body loses fluid. The red cells become more concentrated. Consequently, the hematocrit reading rises above the normal values.

In some dehydration conditions, such as a severe burn case, the hematocrit reading may rise to 60 per cent (Fig. 136).

To summarize: The hematocrit reading is low in anemia and leukemia and high in polycythemia vera and dehydration conditions.

The hematocrit reading is frequently requested. It is performed about 3000 times a month by the average hospital laboratory and about 10 times a month by the average physician's office.

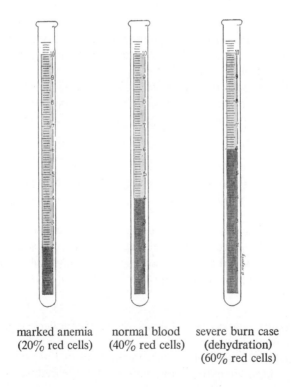

marked anemia   normal blood   severe burn case
(20% red cells)   (40% red cells)   (dehydration)
(60% red cells)

FIG. 136.—Low, normal, and high hematocrit readings. The upper lighter portion of each tube is plasma. The lower darker portion is red cells.

DISCUSSION OF PROCEDURES FOR THE HEMATOCRIT READING

The hematocrit reading may be performed by the following methods:

Macro Method
  1. Wintrobe
Micro Methods
  1. Adams Micro-Hematocrit
  2. Drummond Micro-Hematocrit
  3. International Micro-Hematocrit
  4. Lab-Line Micro-Hematocrit
  5. Schuco Scientific Micro-Hematocrit
Electronic Methods
  1. Coulter Counter
  2. AutoAnalyzer
  3. Yellow Springs Instrument (YSI)

The Wintrobe method was the pioneer in the field, but this method has practically been replaced by the faster micro methods which, in turn, are doomed to be replaced by the electronic methods.

The macro method and the micro methods call for the blood to be centrifuged and the percentage of packed red cells to be found by calculation.

The electronic methods are usually based on one of the following principles:

(1) The average red cell volume is determined, the red cell count is made, and the hematocrit found by calculation. (Example: Coulter Counter)

(2) The red cells will not conduct an electric current whereas the serum or plasma will conduct an electric current. Thus, the greater the percentage of red cells, the lesser the conduction of the electric current. (Example: Yellow Springs Instrument)

The Wintrobe method and Adams Micro-Hematocrit method will be presented in this text.

The procedures for the other micro methods listed above are similar to the Adams Micro-Hematocrit procedure. The procedures for the electronic methods come with the electronic instrument; most of the electronic procedures simply involve the pushing of a few buttons.

WINTROBE METHOD FOR THE HEMATOCRIT READING

NECESSARY REAGENTS AND EQUIPMENT

1. Materials for a venipuncture
2. Oxalated tube or Sequestrenized tube. These tubes containing the anticoagulant are usually prepared in advance and set aside until needed. Consequently, some of them should be sitting on the laboratory shelf. If none are available, prepare one of them by following the directions on page 78 or 79.
3. Two (2) Wintrobe tubes (Fig. 131, page 309)
4. Wintrobe pipet (Fig. 131, page 309)
5. Centrifuge

Procedure

1. If you have just completed a sedimentation rate in a Wintrobe tube, get the Wintrobe tube and proceed to step 14.

2. If you have about 2 cc. of the patient's blood, it is not necessary to withdraw any more blood. In such cases, proceed to step 11.

3. If you are starting from scratch, proceed as follows:

4. Obtain the requisition slip giving the patient's name, date, and request for laboratory tests.

5. Obtain the materials for a venipuncture: sterile 20 gauge needle, 10 cc. syringe, tourniquet, alcohol, cotton or gauze pads, and a wax marking pencil.

6. Obtain an oxalated or Sequestrenized tube.

7. Using the wax marking pencil, write the patient's name on the oxalated or Sequestrenized tube.

8. Make a venipuncture and withdraw about 5 cc. of blood

9. Remove the needle from the syringe and transfer the blood to the oxalated or Sequestrenized tube.

10. Put a stopper in the mouth of the test tube and mix the blood and anticoagulant by completely inverting the test tube 10 to 12 times.

11. Get a Wintrobe tube and a Wintrobe pipet consisting of a long needle and suction device (see Fig. 131, page 309).

12. Mix the blood by completely inverting the test tube 10 to 12 times.

13. Fill the Wintrobe tube with blood as illustrated in Figure 132, page 310.

14. Fill another Wintrobe tube with water or blood. This 2nd tube will be used to balance the centrifuge.

    Note: If you fill the 2nd Wintrobe tube with blood from another patient, make sure you label the Wintrobe tubes.

15. Put the Wintrobe tubes in opposite holders in the centrifuge. This balances the centrifuge.

    Note: Directions for operating a centrifuge are given on page 82.

16. Turn the operating dial or knob as far as it will go (full speed) and allow the blood to spin for 30 minutes.

17. At the end of 30 minutes, stop the centrifuge. Then remove the Wintrobe tubes from the centrifuge.

18. Observe the scale on the right side of the Wintrobe tube (Fig. 137).

19. Note that this scale starts at the bottom of the tube and reads upwards: 1, 2, 3, etc.

20. Also note that this scale is 10 centimeters in length.

21. Since the centimeters are divided into tenths, we may have readings of 4.0 centimeters, 4.2 centimeters, 4.7 centimeters, etc.

22. Now, starting at the bottom of your Wintrobe tube and reading upward, read off the number of centimeters corresponding to your level of packed red cells (Fig. 137).

    Note: You will see a very fine white layer on top of the packed red cells. This fine white layer is white cells and platelets.

23. Write down your reading and calculate the per cent as illustrated below:

    Example:

    $$\frac{4.2 \text{ cm. (packed cells)}}{10.0 \text{ cm. (blood used)}} \times 100 = 42\%$$

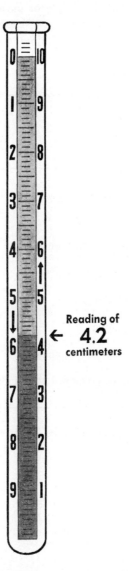

Reading of
← **4.2**
centimeters

FIG. 137.—Making the hematocrit reading in a Wintrobe tube.
The upper lighter portion of the tube is plasma.
The lower darker portion is the packed red cells.

24. <u>Note:</u> You may eliminate the above calculation by proceeding as follows: Each line or mark on the Wintrobe tube represents 1%. Therefore, simply count the number of lines from the bottom of the tube to the level of packed red cells. The total number of lines is the value of your hematocrit reading.

25. Make your report as illustrated in the sample report below.

26. Sample report:

Patient: Doe, Mr. John

Date: 7-7-72

Physician: Dr. Robert Rodgers

Hematocrit reading: 42%

Method: Wintrobe

Normal values:
                  men: 40% to 54%
                  women: 37% to 47%

Examination performed by: Sandra Frisbie

---

27. Clean the Wintrobe tube as illustrated in Figure 134, page 314.

ADAMS MICRO-HEMATOCRIT METHOD

NECESSARY REAGENTS AND EQUIPMENT

1. Capillary tube
   a. plain capillary tube if anticoagulated blood is going to be used
   b. anticoagulated capillary tube if finger tip blood is going to be used
2. Clay for sealing capillary tube (Fig. 138, page 328)
3. Micro-hematocrit centrifuge (Fig. 138, page 328)
4. Micro-hematocrit reader (Fig. 138, page 328)
5. Note: The above equipment is sold by various manufacturers. It may be obtained from your local medical supply house.

Procedure

1. Assemble the equipment listed above.

2. You may use either anticoagulated blood or finger tip blood.

3. If anticoagulated blood is to be used, proceed as follows: Mix the blood by completely inverting the test tube 10 to 12 times. Then carefully draw blood into a plain capillary tube until the tube is about $\frac{3}{4}$ full. Now proceed to step 5 below.

4. If finger tip blood is to be used, proceed as follows: Get an anticoagulated capillary tube and the materials for a finger puncture: cotton or gauze pads, 70% alcohol, and a sterile blood lancet. Make a finger puncture and produce a rounded drop of blood. Hold the capillary tube in a horizontal position. Put one end of the capillary tube in the drop of blood. Tilt the other end of the capillary tube downward so the blood flows into the tube. Fill the capillary tube about $\frac{3}{4}$ full.

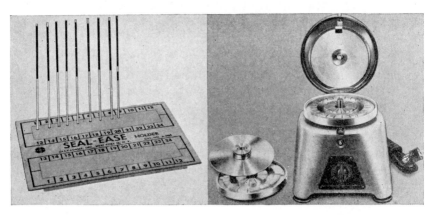

A   B

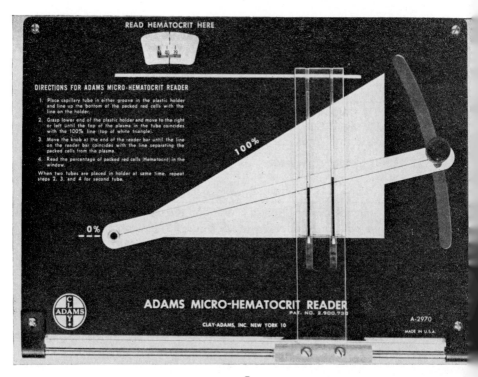

C

FIG. 138.—Equipment for the micro hematocrit. *A.* Clay for sealing capillary tubes. *B.* Centrifuge. *C.* Micro-hematocrit reader. (Courtesy of Clay-Adams Company.)

5. Seal off one end of the capillary tube by sticking one end in the clay for sealing capillary tubes (Fig. 138).

6. Put the capillary tube in the micro-hematocrit centrifuge so the open end of the capillary tube is nearest the center of the centrifuge (Fig. 138).

7. Centrifuge at full speed for 10 minutes.

8. Remove the capillary tube from the centrifuge.

9. By following the directions on your micro-hematocrit reader, make the reading (Fig. 138).

10. Make your report as indicated in the sample report below.

11. Sample report:

Patient: Mr. John Doe

Date: 7-7-72

Physician: Dr. John Jones

Hematocrit reading: 40%

Method: micro method

Normal values: 40% to 54% for men
                             37% to 47% for women

Technologist: Sandra Frisbie

SOURCES OF ERROR IN THE HEMATOCRIT READING

±10% margin of error

1. Obtaining blood sample after acute hemorrhage

Immediately after acute hemorrhage, the blood vessels are constricted. Hence, the red cells are more concentrated. Consequently, the hematocrit reading will be erroneously high.

Several hours after acute hemorrhage, however, fluids leave the tissues and enter the blood stream. Hence, the red cells are less concentrated. Consequently, the hematocrit reading will be erroneously low.

Thus, immediately after acute hemorrhage, the hematocrit reading is erroneously high; several hours after acute hemorrhage, the hematocrit reading is erroneously low.

2. Excessive anticoagulant

Excessive anticoagulant causes the red cells to shrink and therefore lowers the hematocrit reading.

Excessive anticoagulant may unknowingly be introduced into the procedure by only putting about 1 cc. of blood into a test tube containing anticoagulant for 5 cc. of blood.

3. Failure to thoroughly mix the blood

Before filling the hematocrit tube, the test tube of blood should be completely inverted 10 to 12 times (30 to 40 times if blood has stood for any length of time in the refrigerator).

4. Failure to centrifuge blood at the required speed (usually full speed)

5. Failure to centrifuge blood for the designated time

The blood should be centrifuged 30 minutes for the Wintrobe method and 5 to 10 minutes for the micro methods.

6. Leakage of blood from capillary tube in micro methods

7. Mistakes in making the reading or making the calculation

Chapter 11

Reticulocyte Count

The reticulocyte count is often referred to as a retic count.
The discussion of the reticulocyte count will cover the following:

Significance of the Reticulocyte Count
Discussion of Procedures for the Reticulocyte Count
Dry Method for the Reticulocyte Count
Wet Method for the Reticulocyte Count

The student review questions for the reticulocyte count are numbered
163–167 and begin on page 743 of the Appendix.

SIGNIFICANCE OF THE RETICULOCYTE COUNT

You will recall that the red cell goes through six different stages of
development:

rubriblast
prorubricyte
rubricyte
metarubricyte
reticulocyte
erythrocyte

The first 4 cells are confined to the bone marrow; the last 2 cells are found
in both the bone marrow and the blood stream.
Thus, both reticulocytes and erythrocytes are present in the blood.
The reticulocyte count is made by taking a sample of blood and comparing the number of reticulocytes with the number of erythrocytes. For
example, if there is 1 reticulocyte to 99 erythrocytes, the reticulocyte count
is 1%.
The normal values for the reticulocyte count are 1% to 2%, with newborn
infants having slightly higher values.
What is the significance of the reticulocyte count?
You will recall that the red cells are produced in the cell factories of the
bone marrow. When these factories are producing the normal quota of
red cells, the reticulocyte count stays within the normal values of 1% to 2%.

If there is trouble in the factories, such as a sudden "strike," the reticulo-cyte count drops below the normal values. If the strike can be ended—by means of medication—the reticulocyte count returns to the normal values and may even temporarily rise above the normal values.

Thus, the reticulocyte count indicates the conditions in the bone marrow. When the red cell production decreases, the reticulocyte count drops. When the red cell production increases, the reticulocyte count rises.

Can the reticulocyte count be useful in diagnosis and treatment?

The reticulocyte count is useful in diagnosing several types of anemia. For example, the reticulocyte count drops below normal in aplastic anemia and rises above normal during a relapse in hereditary spherocytic anemia.

The reticulocyte count is also useful in treating some types of anemia. For example, if a prescribed treatment is effective, the reticulocyte count will rise; if a prescribed treatment is not effective, the reticulocyte count will remain constant.

When the reticulocyte count drops below normal, it is referred to as a reticulocytopenia; when the reticulocyte count rises above normal, it is referred to as a reticulocytosis.

Some conditions where these abnormalities may be expected are listed in Table 21.

The reticulocyte count is performed about 60 times a month by the average hospital laboratory and about 3 times a month by the average physician's office.

Table 21.
Conditions Accompanied by Abnormal Reticulocyte Counts

Reticulocytopenia (below normal)	Reticulocytosis (above normal)
aplastic anemia	hereditary spherocytic anemia
pernicious anemia	sickle cell anemia
	thalassemia major
	paroxysmal noctural hemoglobinuria
	acquired autoimmune hemolytic anemia
	erythroblastosis fetalis
	acute posthemorrhagic anemia

DISCUSSION OF PROCEDURES FOR THE
RETICULOCYTE COUNT

Reticulocytes are slightly larger than erythrocytes and contain a granular net-like substance (Fig. 139).

In order to stain the granular net-like substance in the reticulocyte, the blood must be fresh and a special dye must be used.

After the cells have been stained, the reticulocytes and erythrocytes are counted until 1000 red cells have been tabulated. Then the percentage of reticulocytes is calculated.

Thus,

$$\frac{\text{number of reticulocytes counted}}{1000 \text{ red cells (reticulocytes \& erythrocytes)}} \times 100 = \% \text{ reticulocytes}$$

The reticulocyte count can be made by either the dry method or the wet method.

The dry method consists of mixing blood and a special staining solution to stain the reticulocytes, using the mixture to make a smear, counter staining the smear with Wright's stain, counting 1,000 red cells with the microscope, and calculating the percentage of reticulocytes.

The wet method consists of spreading a film of stain on a glass slide, adding a drop of blood, covering the preparation with a coverglass, counting 1,000 red cells with the microscope, and calculating the percentage of reticulocytes.

The dry method is usually preferred to the wet method because the blood smear in the dry method is a permanent preparation. Consequently, the blood smear may be stored and kept for future reference.

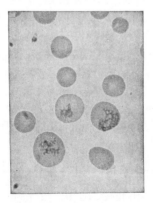

FIG. 139.—Reticulocytes. (Haden, Principles of Hematology.)

DRY METHOD FOR THE RETICULOCYTE COUNT

NECESSARY REAGENTS AND EQUIPMENT

1. Any one of the following staining solutions:
   a. 1% physiological saline solution of brilliant cresyl blue
   b. new methylene blue N solution
   c. 1% methyl alcohol solution of brilliant cresyl blue
   Note: One of the above staining solutions is usually sitting on the laboratory shelf. If none are available, one of them may be purchased from your local medical supply house or prepared by following the directions in the section on solutions and reagents which is given in the Appendix (page 695).
2. glass slides
3. finger tip blood or *fresh* anticoagulated blood
4. Wright's stain
5. microscope

Procedure

1. Obtain one of the following staining solutions:

   a. 1% physiological saline solution of brilliant cresyl blue
   b. new methylene blue N solution
   c. 1% methyl alcohol solution of brilliant cresyl blue

2. Filter about 1 cc. of the staining solution.

3. Put 3 drops of the filtered staining solution in a small test tube.

4. Either finger tip blood or fresh anticoagulated blood may be used. If anticoagulated blood is used, it must not be over 1 hour old because the number of reticulocytes decrease as the blood stands.

5. If finger tip blood is to be used, obtain the materials for a finger puncture: sterile lancet, alcohol, and cotton or gauze pads. Get the test tube containing the 3 drops of staining solution. Make a finger puncture and wipe away the first drop of blood. Then proceed to step 7 below.

6. If fresh anticoagulated blood is to be used, obtain the anticoagulated blood. Mix the blood by completely inverting the test tube 10 to 12 times. Get a clean medicine dropper. Then proceed to step 7 below.

7. Add 3 drops of blood to the test tube containing the 3 drops of filtered staining solution.

8. Mix the blood and staining solution as follows: Hold the top of the test tube with your left hand. Tap the bottom of test tube with your right hand.

9. Allow about 5 minutes to elapse. This gives the cells time to accept the stain.

10. After the 5 minutes have elapsed, gently mix again by tapping the bottom of the test tube.

11. Place a small drop on a glass slide and make a blood smear.

12. Allow the smear to dry. (It takes a few minutes.)

13. Stain the smear in the usual manner with Wright's stain and buffer solution. (This is called a counterstain.)

    Note: Make sure you flush the excess stain off the slide because precipitated stain on an erythrocyte may make the erythrocyte appear like a reticulocyte.

14. Observe the reticulocytes which are illustrated in Figure 139 an page 333 and Plate 8 on page 270.

15. Place a drop of immersion oil on the thin area of the slide, put the slide on the stage of the microscope, and lower the oil immersion (95✕) objective into the drop of oil.

16. Bring the cells into view and select an area where the red cells are evenly distributed.

    Note: In the area selected, the red cells should be evenly distributed. They should not be too far apart, overlapping, or bunched together.

17. In order to decrease the microscopic field and thus make it easier to count the cells, some technologists place a piece of paper containing a "window" in the eyepiece of the microscope. Thus,

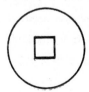

18. To make and insert this "window," proceed as follows: Remove the eyepiece from the microscope by simply lifting it up. Get a piece of paper and a scissors. Cut out a round piece of paper the same diameter as the eyepiece. Then cut the "window" in the piece of paper. Unscrew the top lens of the eyepiece. Put the piece of paper on the shelf of the eyepiece. Screw the top lens back on the eyepiece. And return the eyepiece to the microscope.

    Note: An eyepiece crossline disc which divides a microscopic field into 4 sections may be purchased from your local medical supply house.

19. Now the problem is to count 1000 red cells (erythrocytes and reticulocytes).

20. Therefore, count the 1000 red cells, making a written notation every time you see a reticulocyte.

21. Note: If you wish to increase the accuracy of your report, you may count 2000 cells. If you do count 2000 cells, however, substitute the number 2000 for 1000 in the calculation below.

22. Calculate the per cent of reticulocytes as illustrated below.

23. Example:

    If 10 reticulocytes were recorded while counting the 1000 red cells, the calculation is made as follows:

$$\frac{10 \text{ reticulocytes}}{1000 \text{ red cells (erythrocytes plus reticulocytes)}} \times 100 = 1\%$$

24. Make your report as indicated in the sample report below.

25. Sample report:

Patient:	Mr. John Doe
Date:	7-7-72
Physician:	Dr. John Jones
Reticulocyte count: 1%	
Method: dry method	
Normal values: 1% to 2%	
Technologist: Carol Moffatt	

WET METHOD FOR THE RETICULOCYTE COUNT

NECESSARY REAGENTS AND EQUIPMENT

1. Any one of the following staining solutions:
   a. 1% physiological saline solution of brilliant cresyl blue
   b. new methylene blue N solution
   c. 1% methyl alcohol solution of brilliant cresyl blue
   NOTE: One of the above staining solutions is usually sitting on the laboratory shelf. If none are available, one of them may be purchased from your local medical supply house or prepared by following the directions in the section on solutions and reagents which is given in the Appendix (page 695).
2. glass slides
3. coverglasses (These coverglasses come in a small box. They are *not* the same coverglasses used on the counting chamber in the white cell count.)
4. finger tip blood or *fresh* anticoagulated blood
5. microscope

Procedure

1. Obtain one of the following staining solutions:

   a. 1% physiological saline solution of brilliant cresyl blue
   b. new methylene blue N solution
   c. 1% methyl alcohol solution of brilliant cresyl blue

2. Filter about 1 cc. of the staining solution.

3. Put 1 drop of the filtered staining solution on a glass slide.

4. With the same technique used in making a blood smear, spread the solution over the slide. This slide now contains a thin film of stain. It will receive a drop of blood later on in the procedure.

5. Either finger tip blood or fresh anticoagulated blood may be used. If anticoagulated blood is used, it must not be over 1 hour old because the number of reticulocytes decrease as the blood stands.

6. If finger tip blood is to be used, obtain a few coverglasses and materials for a finger puncture: sterile lancet, alcohol, and cotton or gauze pads. Get the slide containing the thin film of stain which you prepared in step 4. Make a finger puncture and wipe away the first drop of blood. Then proceed to step 8 below.

7. If fresh anticoagulated blood is to be used, obtain the anticoagulated blood. Mix the blood by completely inverting the test tube 10 to 12 times. Get 2 wooden applicator sticks. Put the 2 wooden applicator sticks in the test tube of blood. Obtain a few coverglasses. Then proceed to step 8 below.

8. Place a small drop of blood on the slide containing the stain.

9. Put a coverglass on the small drop of blood. Then press down gently on the coverglass so the blood spreads out to the edges of the coverglass.

   Note: If you prefer, you may rim the edges of the cover-glass with petroleum jelly before placing it over the drop of blood. For directions, see page 342.

10. Let stand 10 minutes. This gives the cells time to accept the stain.

11. Observe the reticulocytes which are illustrated in Figure 139, page 333 and Plate 8, page 270.

12. After the 10 minutes have elapsed, place a drop of immersion oil on the coverglass. Then place the slide on the stage of the microscope and carefully lower the oil immersion (95×) objective into the drop of oil.

13. Bring the cells into view and select an area where the red cells are evenly distributed.

   Note: In the area selected, the red cells should be evenly distributed. They should not be too far apart, over-lapping, or bunched together.

14. In order to decrease the microscopic field and thus make it easier to count the cells, some technologists place a piece of paper containing a "window" in the eyepiece of the microscope. Thus,

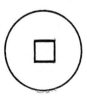

15. To make and insert this "window," proceed as follows: Remove the eyepiece from the microscope by simply lifting it up. Get a piece of paper and a scissors. Cut out a round piece of paper the same diameter as the eyepiece. Then cut the "window" in the piece of paper. Unscrew the top lens of the eyepiece. Put the piece of paper on the shelf of the eyepiece. Screw the top lens back on the eyepiece. And return the eyepiece to the microscope.

16. Now the problem is to count 1000 red cells (erythrocytes and reticulocytes).

17. Therefore, count the 1000 red cells, making a written notation every time you see a reticulocyte.

18. Note: If you wish to increase the accuracy of your count, you may count 2000 cells. If you do count 2000 cells, however, substitute the figure 2000 for 1000 in the calculation below.

19. Calculate the per cent of reticulocytes as illustrated below.

20. Example:

    If 10 reticulocytes were recorded while counting the 1000 red cells, the calculation is made as follows:

    $$\frac{10 \text{ reticulocytes}}{1000 \text{ red cells (erythrocytes plus reticulocytes)}} \times 100 = 1\%$$

21. Make your report as indicated in the sample report below.

22. Sample report:

Patient:	Mr. John Doe
Date:	7-7-72
Physician:	Dr. John Jones
Reticulocyte count:	1%
Method:	wet method
Normal values:	1% to 2%
Technologist:	Sandra Frisbie

Chapter 12

Sickle Cell Examination

THE sickle cell examination is also referred to as a sickling examination, sickling of erythrocytes examination, RBC sickling test, and sickle cell phenomenon demonstration.

The discussion of the sickle cell examination will cover the following:

Significance of the Sickle Cell Examination
Discussion of Procedures for the Sickle Cell Examination
Scriver and Waugh Method for the Sickle Cell Examination
Bisulfite Method for the Sickle Cell Examination
Sickledex Method for the Sickle Cell Examination

The student review questions for the sickle cell examination are numbered 168–172 and begin on page 744 of the Appendix.

SIGNIFICANCE OF THE SICKLE CELL EXAMINATION

A sickle cell is an erythrocyte which is shaped like a sickle or crescent. Thus,

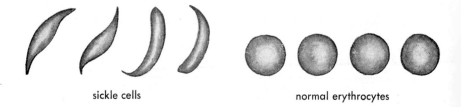

sickle cells   normal erythrocytes

Sickle cells may be found in sickle cell anemia and sickle cell trait.

Sickle cell anemia and sickle cell trait are usually confined to Negroes or persons of Negro ancestry.

Sickle cell anemia affects about 1% of all Negroes and sickle cell trait is found in about 10% of all Negroes.

Sickle cell anemia and sickle cell trait will be further discussed under blood diseases (page 603).

340

The sickle cell examination is frequently requested in those areas which have a large Negro population. In other areas, of course, it is rarely requested.

It should be understood that the sickle cell examination is a simple screening examination which indicates the presence or absence of sickle cells. This examination does not distinguish between sickle cell anemia and sickle cell trait.

To distinguish between sickle cell anemia and sickle cell trait, more complicated examinations are employed. The most commonly employed examination is known as hemoglobin electrophoresis. This examination will be discussed in a later section (page 518).

DISCUSSION OF PROCEDURES FOR THE SICKLE CELL EXAMINATION

If the oxygen is removed from the erythrocytes of a healthy person, the erythrocytes do not lose their normal shape. If the oxygen is removed from the erythrocytes of a person with sickle cell anemia or sickle cell trait, the erythrocytes become sickle shaped.

Why do the erythrocytes become sickle shaped under reduced oxygen tension?

The erythrocytes become sickled shaped under reduced oxygen tension because of the presence of an abnormal hemoglobin, Hb S.

Under reduced oxygen tension, this Hb S forms tactoids or fluid crystals that are rigid and distort the shape of the erythrocyte.

The sickling of erythrocytes may be demonstrated by the following methods:

> Scriver and Waugh Method
> Bisulfite Method
> Sickledex Method

In the Scriver and Waugh method, a rubber band is put tightly around the patient's finger. This stops the circulation; oxygen fails to enter the finger. The available oxygen in the finger is decreased by the metabolic activity of the cells. Then a finger puncture is made. A drop of blood is put on a glass slide and sealed from the air. The preparation is then inspected with the microscope.

The bisulfite method is performed by putting a drop of blood on a glass slide, adding a bisulfite reducing agent to remove the oxygen, covering the preparation with a coverglass, and then inspecting the preparation with a microscope.

The Sickledex method is performed by adding blood to a test solution and then inspecting the solution for turbidity.

The Scriver and Waugh method, bisulfite method, and Sickledex method are given on the following pages.

SCRIVER AND WAUGH METHOD FOR THE SICKLE CELL EXAMINATION

NECESSARY REAGENTS AND EQUIPMENT

1. a few small rubber bands
2. glass slides
3. coverglasses (These coverglasses come in a little box containing about 100 coverglasses. They are *not* the same as the coverglass used on the counting chamber in the white cell count.)
4. petroleum jelly
5. materials for a finger puncture
6. microscope

Procedure

1. Assemble the following: a few small rubber bands, a glass slide, several coverglasses, and some petroleum jelly.

2. Obtain the materials for a finger puncture: sterile lancet, alcohol, and cotton or gauze pads.

3. Apply a rubber band so it fits tightly around the base of the patient's middle finger (Illustration 1, Fig. 140).

   Note: The rubber band must fit tightly enough to stop the circulation.

4. Let the rubber band remain in this tight position for 5 minutes.

5. While the rubber band is still on the finger, make a finger puncture and place a small drop of blood on the middle of the glass slide (Illustration 2, Fig. 140).

6. On the fleshy portion of the palm of your left hand, just below the little finger, rub some petroleum jelly (Illustration 3, Fig. 140).

7. Pick up a coverglass.

8. Rim the edges of the coverglass with the petroleum jelly by scraping the petroleum jelly off your hand (Illustration 4, Fig. 140).

9. Now place the coverglass over the drop of blood so the blood is sealed under the coverglass (Illustration 5, Fig. 140).

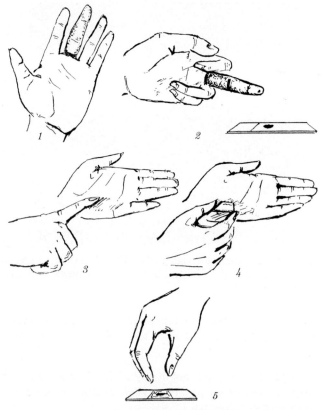

Fig. 140.—Preparing the blood specimen for a sickle cell examination. (Scriver and Waugh method.)

10. Press down gently on the coverglass so the blood spreads out to the edges of the coverglass.

11. Observe the sickle cells that are illustrated in Figure 141.

12. Place a drop of immersion oil on the coverglass and carefully examine the preparation with the oil immersion (95×) objective of the microscope.

13. If sickle cells are present, report the test as positive.

14. If sickle cells are not present in this first inspection, you must make additional inspections at certain time intervals. This is necessary because the reaction is sometimes delayed. If sickle cells are present in any of these additional inspections, you report the test as positive. Further inspections, of course, are then discontinued.

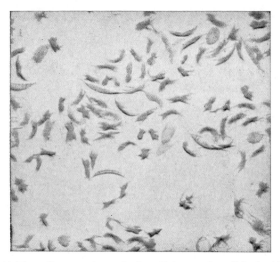

FIG. 141.—Sickle cells seen through the oil immersion (95×) objective of the microscope.   Magnification: 950×.   Scriver and Waugh method.   (Haden, *Principles of Hematology.*)

15. If sickle cells were not present in the first inspection, examine the preparation at the end of 1, 6, 12, and 24 hours.

16. If sickle cells are present in any of the above inspections, report the test as positive.   And, of course, discontinue any further inspections.

17. If it is necessary to make the 24 hour inspection and no sickle cells are present, report the test as negative.

18. A sample report is given below.

19. Sample report:

> **Patient:**   Doe, Mr. John
>
> **Date:**   7-7-72
>
> **Physician:**   Dr. Tom Maxwell
>
> **Sickle cell examination:** negative at the end of 24 hours
>
> **Method:** Scriver and Waugh
>
> **Examination performed by:** Sandra Frisbie

BISULFITE METHOD FOR THE SICKLE CELL EXAMINATION

(Daland and Castle)

NECESSARY REAGENTS AND EQUIPMENT

1. *fresh* preparation of bisulfite reagent (see step 1 below)
2. glass slides
3. toothpicks or wooden applicator stick
4. coverglasses (These coverglasses come in a box containing about 100 coverglasses. They are *not* the same as the coverglass used on the counting chamber in the white cell count.)
5. microscope

Procedure

1. You will need a fresh 2% solution of a bisulfite reagent. Prepare this solution by following either Method A or Method B below:

   Method A:
   Obtain some tablets containing 0.2 gram of sodium metabisulfite ($Na_2S_2O_5$). These tablets may be sitting on your laboratory shelf. If not, they may be obtained from your local medical supply house. Put 1 tablet in 10 cc. of distilled water. Mix. Pour the solution into a bottle which is equipped with a medicine dropper. Label the bottle 2% solution of sodium metabisulfite. This solution keeps only 1 day; therefore, discard at the end of the day.

   Method B:
   Using the rough balance, weigh out 0.5 gram of sodium metabisulfite ($Na_2S_2O_5$). Dissolve in 25 milliliters of distilled water. Label the bottle 2% solution of sodium metabisulfite. This reagent keeps only 1 day; therefore, discard at the end of the day.

2. You may use either finger tip blood or anticoagulated blood.

3. If you are going to use finger tip blood, obtain the following: a glass slide, a coverglass, one wooden applicator stick, and the fresh 2% solution of the bisulfite reagent. Get the materials for a finger puncture: sterile lancet, alcohol, and cotton or gauze pads. Make a finger puncture and wipe away the first drop of blood. Then proceed to step 5 below.

4. If you are going to use <u>anticoagulated blood,</u> obtain the following: the test tube of anticoagulated blood, 3 wooden applicator sticks, a glass slide, a coverglass, and the fresh 2% solution of the bisulfite reagent. Mix the blood. Put 2 of the wooden applicator sticks in the test tube. Then proceed to step 5 below.

5. Place a <u>small</u> drop of blood on the middle of the glass slide.

6. Add a drop of the bisulfite reagent.

7. Mix well with the applicator stick.

8. Place the coverglass on the preparation.

9. Press down gently on the coverglass so the mixture spreads out to the edges of the coverglass.

10. Allow 30 minutes to elapse. This gives the bisulfite reagent an opportunity to remove the oxygen.

11. Observe the sickle cells which are illustrated in Figure 141, page 344.

    <u>Note:</u> In your preparation, the sickle cells will appear smaller because you will be using the $45\times$ (4 mm.) objective.

12. In the next step, you do <u>not</u> remove the coverglass.

13. Using the $45\times$ (4 mm.) objective of the microscope, examine your preparation for sickle cells, paying particular attention to the erythrocytes near the edges of the coverglass.

14. If any sickle cells are present, report the test as positive.

15. If no sickle cells are present, report the test as negative.

16. A sample report is given below.

17. Sample report:

Patient: Doe, Mr. John

Date: 7-7-72

Physician: Dr. Charles Butterworth

Sickle cell examination: positive

Method: bisulfite method

Examination performed by: Jane Adams

SICKLEDEX METHOD FOR THE SICKLE
CELL EXAMINATION

NECESSARY REAGENTS AND EQUIPMENT

The necessary reagents and equipment which are listed below may be obtained in a single package from your local medical supply house.

1. Sickledex reagent powder
2. Sickledex test solution
3. test tubes
4. pipets
5. test tube holder
6. piece of newspaper or cardboard containing printed matter

The above reagents should be stored in the refrigerator at a temperature of 2° – 8° C.

Procedure

1. Remove the Sickledex reagent powder and Sickledex test solution from the refrigerator and allow the reagents to come to room temperature. (Takes about 30 minutes.)

2. Take 1 vial of Sickledex reagent powder and transfer the contents to a bottle of Sickledex test solution.

3. Shake the mixture vigorously for a few seconds.

4. Label the bottle Sickledex Working Solution.

5. Also put the date on the bottle of Sickledex Working Solution.

   Note: When not in use, this solution should be stored in the refrigerator at 2° – 8° C. Upon removal from the refrigerator, it should be allowed to come to room temperature before it is used. The solution may contain a slight sediment but this will not interfere with the test This solution keeps 1 month.

6. Pipet 2.0 ml. of the Sickledex Working Solution into a test tube.

7. You may use either finger tip blood or anticoagulated blood for this test.

8. Now, using a pipet, add 0.02 ml. of blood to the test tube containing the 2.0 ml. of Sickledex Working Solution.

   Note: If the patient is markedly anemic (below 7 grams), use 0.04 ml. of blood.

9. Invert the test tube several times to mix the blood and solution.

10. Allow the mixture to stand at room temperature for 3 minutes.

11. When the 3 minutes have elapsed, hold the piece of newspaper or cardboard containing printed matter about 1 inch behind the test tube.

12. If the solution is so cloudy that you can not see through the solution and observe the printed matter, report the test as positive.

13. If the solution is so clear that you can see through the solution and observe the printed matter, report the test as negative.

14. Note: Until you have become familiar with this test, it is strongly advisable to run a positive control by using blood from a known case of sickle cell anemia and a negative control by using blood from a normal Caucasian.

Chapter 13

Osmotic Fragility Test

The osmotic fragility test is also referred to by the following terms: fragility test, F. T., RBC frag test, red cell fragility test, erythrocyte fragility test, red cell osmotic fragility test, and erythrocyte osmotic fragility test. The discussion of the osmotic fragility test will cover the following:

> Significance of the Osmotic Fragility Test
> Discussion of Procedures for the Osmotic Fragility Test
> Screening Procedure for the Osmotic Fragility Test
> Sanford Method for the Osmotic Fragility Test

The student review questions for the osmotic fragility test are numbered 173–179 and begin on page 744 of the Appendix.

SIGNIFICANCE OF THE OSMOTIC FRAGILITY TEST

If blood is placed in an 0.85% salt solution, water neither enters nor leaves the red cells. The red cells neither swell nor shrink.

If blood is placed in an 0.30% salt solution, water enters the red cells. The red cells swell and eventually rupture or hemolyze.

The rate of hemolysis is governed by the structure of the red cells.

For example, consider the fate of 2 red cells: cell A and cell B.

Cell A is round and cell B has pinched in sides.

Both cells are put in an 0.30% salt solution.

Water starts to enter the cells.

Which cell will be the first to rupture or hemolyze?

Since cell A is round, it is already nearer the breaking point. Consequently, cell A will be the first to rupture or hemolyze.

Thus, the rate of hemolysis is governed by the structure of the red cells.

Now, what is the connection between this rate of hemolysis and the fragility of the red cells?

When the rate of hemolysis is increased, the fragility of the red cells is said to be increased.

When the rate of hemolysis is decreased, the fragility of the red cells is said to be decreased.

The fragility of the red cells is increased in some anemias and decreased in other anemias. A few examples follow.

349

The fragility of the red cells is increased in an anemia in which the red cells are almost round rather than disk shaped. Unfortunately for the student, this anemia has many names. Among the more commonly used names are: hereditary spherocytic anemia, hereditary spherocytosis, congenital hemolytic anemia, and congenital hemolytic jaundice.

The fragility of the red cells is decreased in those anemias in which the red cells are partially empty, thin, or sickle shaped. Among these anemias are severe iron deficiency anemia, thalassemia major, and sickle cell anemia.

The osmotic fragility test shows increased or decreased values in those conditions summarized in Table 22.

The osmotic fragility test is seldom requested. It is only performed about once a month in the average hospital laboratory and about once a year in the average physician's office.

Table 22.—Conditions Accompanied by Increased or Decreased Osmotic Fragility

Increased Osmotic Fragility	*Decreased Osmotic Fragility*
hereditary spherocytic anemia (also called hereditary spherocytosis, congenital hemolytic anemia, and congenital hemolytic jaundice)	iron deficiency anemia (severe cases)
acquired autoimmune hemolytic anemia	thalassemia major
erythroblastosis fetalis (ABO incompatibility)	sickle cell anemia
chemical poisons	obstructive jaundice
burns	polycythemia vera
	hemoglobin C disease

DISCUSSION OF PROCEDURES FOR THE OSMOTIC FRAGILITY TEST

The osmotic fragility test is performed by adding blood to salt solutions and recording the degree of hemolysis.

The osmotic fragility test may be performed by the following methods:

Screening Procedure
Sanford Method
Dacie Method
Incubation Method
Fragiligraph Method

The screening procedure is performed by adding blood to 0.50% and 0.85% sodium chloride, centrifuging, and inspecting the solutions for hemolysis.

The Sanford method is performed by adding blood to a graded series of 12 hypotonic salt solutions and noting the extent of hemolysis after a period of two hours.

The Dacie method is performed by adding heparinized blood to a graded series of 12 hypotonic salt solutions buffered to a pH of 7.4, allowing the preparations to stand at room temperature for 30 minutes, centrifuging, reading the degree of hemolysis in a colorimeter, and plotting the per cent hemolysis against the per cent salt concentration.

The incubation method is performed by obtaining sterile blood, removing the fibrinogen from the sterile blood in order to prevent clotting, incubating the sterile defibrinated blood at 37° C. for 24 hours, and then following the same procedure used in the above Dacie method.

The Fragiligraph method employs an electronic instrument. In this instrument, the blood is allowed to hemolyze in a solution as a beam of light continuously passes through the solution. The greater the hemolysis, the greater the transmission of light. Readings are automatically made at various time intervals, a fragility curve is automatically plotted, and the results are automatically printed.

The screening procedure and the Sanford method for the osmotic fragility test are given on the following pages.

SCREENING PROCEDURE FOR THE
OSMOTIC FRAGILITY TEST

The screening procedure for the osmotic fragility test is sometimes referred to as the presumptive osmotic fragility test.

NECESSARY REAGENTS AND EQUIPMENT

The reagents listed below may be sitting on your laboratory shelf or stored in the refrigerator. If not, they may either be purchased from your local medical supply house or prepared by following the directions in the section on solutions and reagents which is given in the Appendix (page 697).

1. 0.85% sodium chloride
2. 0.50% sodium chloride
3. 4 small test tubes
4. wax marking pencil
5. serological pipets
6. centrifuge

Procedure

1. Assemble the necessary reagents and equipment listed above.

2. Obtain anticoagulated blood from the patient and anticoagulated blood from a normal person.

3. Label the patient's blood Patient and the normal person's blood Control.

4. Label a test tube Patient 0.85%. Label another test tube Patient 0.50%.

5. Label a test tube Control 0.85%. Label another test tube Control 0.50%.

6. Add 5 ml. of 0.85% sodium chloride to the test tube labelled Patient 0.85%.

7. Add 5 ml. of 0.85% sodium chloride to the test tube labelled Control 0.85%.

8. Add 5 ml. of 0.50% sodium chloride to the test tube labelled Patient 0.50%.

9. Add 5 ml. of 0.50% sodium chloride to the test tube labelled Control 0.50%.

10. Add 0.5 ml. of the patient's anticoagulated blood to the test tube labelled Patient 0.85%.

11. Add 0.5 ml. of the patient's anticoagulated blood to the test tube labelled Patient 0.50%.

12. Add 0.5 ml. of the control's anticoagulated blood to the test tube labelled Control 0.85%.

13. Add 0.5 ml. of the control's anticoagulated blood to the test tube labelled Control 0.50%.

14. Gently invert each test tube to mix the contents. Do not shake!

15. Centrifuge the 4 test tubes at full speed for 5 minutes.

16. Remove the test tubes from the centrifuge and read as follows.

17. The solutions in both control tubes should be clear and colorless.

18. If the solutions in both control tubes are not clear and colorless, the salt solutions are inaccurate. This is usually due to contamination of the salt solutions by bacteria or fungi which alter the salt concentration. The growth of bacteria and fungi can be hindered by storing the salt solutions in the refrigerator.

19. If both control tubes are not clear and colorless, obtain new salt solutions and repeat the test.

20. If both control tubes are clear and colorless, inspect the two patient's tubes.

21. If both of the patient's tubes are clear and colorless, report the screen test as negative.

22. If the test tube labelled Patient 0.50% shows a very faint pink tinge, the screening test is positive and a quantitative method is indicated.

SANFORD METHOD FOR THE OSMOTIC
FRAGILITY TEST

NECESSARY REAGENTS AND EQUIPMENT

1. 0.50% solution of sodium chloride (for preparation, see step 1 below; this solution may also be purchased from your local medical supply house)
2. distilled water
3. 24 small test tubes (Kahn tubes)
4. 2 test tube racks (Kahn racks)
5. materials for a venipuncture

Procedure

1. Dry some chemically pure sodium chloride in an oven, and make an accurate 0.5% solution as follows: Using the analytical balance, weigh out 0.50 grams of the salt. Place in a 100 cc. volumetric flask, and add distilled water to the 100 cc. mark. Mix.

2. Get 2 test tube racks. Label one Control and the other Patient.

3. Place 12 small test tubes in each rack.

4. Label the tubes in each rack as follows: 25, 24, 23, 22, 21, 20, 19, 18, 17, 16, 15, and 14 (see Fig. 142).

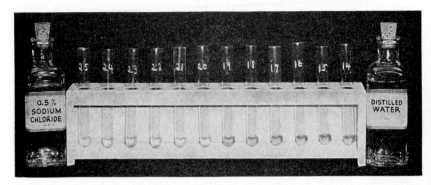

FIG. 142.—Set-up for a fragility test. (Giffen and Sanford)

5. Get the <u>Control</u> rack. Using the chart below, add to each test tube the number of drops of 0.5% sodium chloride and distilled water indicated. Thus, the test tube labelled 25 gets 25 drops of 0.5% sodium chloride solution and 0.0 drops of distilled water. The per cent salt solution, obtained by this dilution process, is given in the bottom row of the chart. Note that the per cent salt solution in any test tube may be obtained by multiplying the test tube number by 0.02. For example, test tube number 25 has a salt solution of $25 \times 0.02 = 0.50\%$.

Number on test tube	25	24	23	22	21	20	19	18	17	16	15	14
Number drops 0.5% NaCl	25	24	23	22	21	20	19	18	17	16	15	14
Number drops dist. water	0	1	2	3	4	5	6	7	8	9	10	11
% salt sol. obtained	.50	.48	.46	.44	.42	.40	.38	.36	.34	.32	.30	.28

6. Get the <u>Patient's</u> rack. Using the chart above, add to each test tube the number of drops of 0.5% sodium chloride and distilled water indicated. Thus, the test tube labelled 25 gets 25 drops of the 0.5% sodium chloride solution and 0.0 drops of distilled water. The per cent salt solution, obtained by this dilution process, is given in the bottom row of the chart. Note that the per cent salt solution in any test tube may be obtained by multiplying the test tube number by 0.02. For example, test tube number 25 has a salt solution of $25 \times 0.02 = 0.50\%$.

7. Take the patient's rack and materials for a venipuncture to the patient. Make a venipuncture and withdraw a few cc. of blood. Leave the needle on the syringe, and add one drop of blood to each tube. Shake the test tube rack to mix the contents of the test tubes.

8. In order to get blood for the control rack, make a venipuncture on a normal person, and withdraw a few cc. of blood. Leave the needle on the syringe, and add one drop to each tube of the control rack. Shake the test tube rack to mix the contents of the test tubes.

9. Let both test tube racks stand at room temperature for 2 hours.

10. Study Figure 143, noting the following: In normal blood, hemolysis begins in tube 22. This is denoted by the sediment of cells in the bottom of the test tube and the black dots in the liquid above the sediment. As you go to the right, the sediment of cells in the bottom of each tube decreases and the hemolysis in the liquid increases. Hemolysis is complete in tube 17 and, of course, all further tubes to the right.

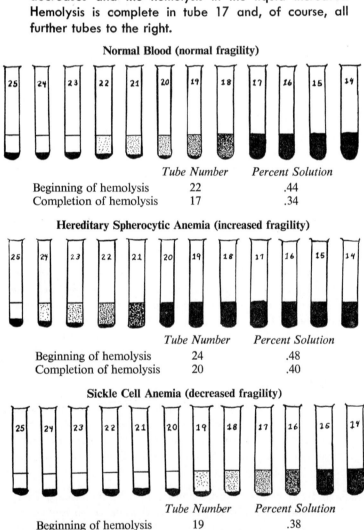

Normal Blood (normal fragility)

	Tube Number	Percent Solution
Beginning of hemolysis	22	.44
Completion of hemolysis	17	.34

Hereditary Spherocytic Anemia (increased fragility)

	Tube Number	Percent Solution
Beginning of hemolysis	24	.48
Completion of hemolysis	20	.40

Sickle Cell Anemia (decreased fragility)

	Tube Number	Percent Solution
Beginning of hemolysis	19	.38
Completion of hemolysis	15	.30

FIG. 143.—Normal and abnormal results of the osmotic fragility test. In hereditary spherocytic anemia, the rate of hemolysis is increased, indicating increased fragility. In sickle cell anemia, the rate of hemolysis is decreased, indicating decreased fragility.

11. After the 2 hours have elapsed, take the control rack and starting with the tube number 25 and going to the right toward the lower numbered tubes, note the test tube which contains the first faint pink tinge. This is the beginning of hemolysis (Fig. 143). Record the test tube number and the per cent salt solution. Continue going to the right toward the lower numbered tubes, and note the first tube which contains no sediment of cells. This is the completion of hemolysis (Fig. 143). Record the test tube number and the per cent salt solution.

12. Now take the patient's rack and, in the same manner, record the readings for the beginning and completion of hemolysis.

13. Report the beginning and completion of hemolysis for both the control and the patient.

14. Also report whether the patient's blood shows normal fragility, increased fragility, or decreased fragility.

   Note: Any hemolysis to the left of tube 22 means increased fragility.

15. A sample report is given below.

16. Sample report:

Patient: Doe, Mr. John

Date: 7-7-72

Physician: Dr. James Madison

Osmotic fragility test:

	Control	Patient
Beginning of hemolysis	.44%	.50%
Completion of hemolysis	.34%	.42%

Patient's blood shows increased fragility

Method: Sanford method

Examination performed by: Carol Moffatt

---

17. Note: The original Sanford method given above has undergone various changes. For example, some laboratories use a higher salt concentration than the 0.50% recommended by Sanford and some laboratories make the final readings in a colorimeter.

Chapter 14

Mean Corpuscular Values

The mean corpuscular values are often referred to as the mean corpuscular constants or average cell values.

The discussion of the mean corpuscular values will cover the following:

Significance of the Mean Corpuscular Values
Introduction to the Calculations
Calculation of the Mean Corpuscular Volume
Calculation of the Mean Corpuscular Hemoglobin
Calculation of the Mean Corpuscular Hemoglobin Concentration
Summary of Abbreviations, Normal Values, and Short Methods

The student review questions for the mean corpuscular values are numbered 180–187 and begin on page 745 of the Appendix.

SIGNIFICANCE OF THE MEAN CORPUSCULAR VALUES

The mean corpuscular values are concerned with the volume of the average erythrocyte and the amount of hemoglobin in the average erythrocyte. There are 3 mean corpuscular values:

Mean corpuscular volume
Mean corpuscular hemoglobin
Mean corpuscular hemoglobin concentration

The mean corpuscular volume is the volume of the average erythrocyte. The normal values are 80 to 90 cubic microns. Decreased values may be found in iron deficiency anemia and increased values may be found in pernicious anemia.

The mean corpuscular hemoglobin is the weight of hemoglobin in the average erythrocyte. The normal values are 27 to 32 micromicrograms. Decreased values may be found in iron deficiency anemia and increased values may be found in pernicious anemia.

The mean corpuscular hemoglobin concentration is the per cent of hemoglobin in the patient's packed red cell volume. The normal values are 33 to 38%. Decreased values may be found in iron deficiency anemia.

358

Increased values for the mean corpuscular hemoglobin concentration are considered to be an impossibility because of the hemoglobin saturation limits of the erythrocyte. For example, the *percentage* of hemoglobin in an erythrocyte can never exceed a certain limit designated by nature. Thus, we have the summary indicated in Table 23.

Table 23.—Normal Values for the Mean Corpuscular Values

	Normal Values	*When Decreased*	*When Increased*
Mean corpuscular volume . .	80 to 90 cubic microns	iron deficiency anemia	pernicious anemia
Mean corpuscular hemoglobin .	27 to 32 micro- micrograms	iron deficiency anemia	pernicious anemia
Mean corpuscular hemoglobin concentration	33 to 38 per cent	iron deficiency anemia	

The mean corpuscular values are usually abbreviated as follows:

mean corpuscular volume	M. C. V. or MCV
mean corpuscular hemoglobin	M. C. H. or MCH
mean corpuscular hemoglobin concentration	M. C. H. C. or MCHC

The mean corpuscular values are calculated about 15 times a month in the average hospital laboratory and about once a month in the average physician's office.

The calculation of the mean corpuscular values is frequently encountered on student examinations.

INTRODUCTION TO THE CALCULATIONS

In order to follow the forthcoming calculations, the student should thoroughly understand the material which is outlined and discussed below.

Recognition of large whole numbers
Multiplication of large whole numbers
Division of large whole numbers
Abbreviations of measures and weights
Equivalents of measures and weights
Accuracy of laboratory examinations

RECOGNITION OF LARGE WHOLE NUMBERS

By using mathematical shorthand, the figure 1,000 may be written as 10^3. Likewise, the figure 1,000,000 may be written as 10^6.

The mathematical shorthand which will be used in the forthcoming calculations is listed below.

$$10^1 = 10$$
$$10^2 = 100$$
$$10^3 = 1,000$$
$$10^4 = 10,000$$
$$10^5 = 100,000$$
$$10^6 = 1,000,000$$
$$10^{12} = 1,000,000,000,000$$

MULTIPLICATION OF LARGE WHOLE NUMBERS

When 10^a is multiplied by 10^b (a and b stand for any number), the rule is: Add the exponents.

Thus,

$$10^a \times 10^b = 10^{a+b}$$

For example,

$$10^2 \times 10^3 = 10^{2+3} = 10^5$$

and,

$$10^6 \times 10^6 = 10^{6+6} = 10^{12}$$

DIVISION OF LARGE WHOLE NUMBERS

When 10^a is divided by 10^b (a and b stand for any number), the rule is: Subtract the exponents.

Thus,

$$\frac{10^a}{10^b} = 10^{a-b}$$

For example,

$$\frac{10^{12}}{10^5} = 10^{12-5} = 10^7$$

and,

$$\frac{10^9}{10^6} = 10^{9-6} = 10^3$$

ABBREVIATIONS OF MEASURES AND WEIGHTS

The abbreviations of measures and weights which will be used in the forthcoming calculations are listed below.

cm. = centimeter
cc. = cubic centimeter
mm. = millimeter
cu. mm. = cubic millimeter
Gm. = gram
$\mu\mu$g or $\mu\gamma$ = micromicrogram

EQUIVALENTS OF MEASURES AND WEIGHTS

Centimeters deal with length. For example, your finger may be 7 centimeters in length.

Cubic centimeters, however, deal with volume. For example, a teaspoon of coffee may measure 5 cubic centimeters.

Millimeters deal with length. For example, your finger may be 70 millimeters in length.

Cubic millimeters, however, deal with volume. For example, a teaspoon of coffee may measure 5,000 cubic millimeters.

So much for an introduction to measures and weights.

Now, 1 centimeter equals 10 millimeters. Thus,

$$1 \text{ centimeter} = 10 \text{ millimeters}$$

The above equation deals with length. If we want it to deal with volume, we cube both sides of the equation. This is done as follows.

When we cube 1 centimeter, we get $1 \times 1 \times 1 = 1$ cubic centimeter. When we cube 10 millimeters, however, we get $10 \times 10 \times 10 = 1000$ cubic millimeters.

Therefore, 1 cubic centimeter equals 1000 cubic millimeters. Thus,

$$1 \text{ cubic centimeter} = 1000 \text{ cubic millimeters}$$

We can shorten the above equation by using abbreviations and mathematical shorthand. Thus,

$$1 \text{ cc.} = 10^3 \text{ cu. mm.}$$

A similar situation occurs when we change millimeters to microns. For example, consider the following:

One millimeter equals 1000 microns. Thus,

$$1 \text{ millimeter} = 1000 \text{ microns}$$

The above equation deals with length. If we want it to deal with volume, we cube both sides of the equation. This is done as follows.

When we cube 1 millimeter, we get $1 \times 1 \times 1 = 1$ cubic millimeter. When we cube 1000 microns, however, we get $1000 \times 1000 \times 1000 = 1,000,000,000$ cubic microns.

Therefore, 1 cubic millimeter equals 1,000,000,000 cubic microns. Thus,

$$1 \text{ cubic millimeter} = 1,000,000,000 \text{ cubic microns}$$

We can shorten the above equation by using abbreviations and mathematical shorthand. Thus,

$$1 \text{ cu. mm.} = 10^9 \text{ cu. microns}$$

One gram equals 1,000,000,000,000 micromicrograms. Thus,

$$1 \text{ gram} = 1,000,000,000,000 \text{ micromicrograms}$$

We can shorten the above equation by using abbreviations and mathematical shorthand. Thus,

$$1 \text{ Gm.} = 10^{12} \ \mu\mu g$$

We have just discussed the equivalents of measures and weights which will be used in the forthcoming calculations.

These equivalents of measures and weights are summarized in Table 24.

Table 24.—Equivalents of Measures and Weights

$$1 \text{ cm.} = 10 \text{ mm.}$$
$$1 \text{ cc.} = 10^3 \text{ cu. mm.}$$
$$1 \text{ mm.} = 10^3 \text{ microns}$$
$$1 \text{ cu. mm.} = 10^9 \text{ cu. microns}$$
$$1 \text{ Gm.} = 10^{12} \text{ micromicrograms}$$

ACCURACY OF LABORATORY EXAMINATIONS

Before turning to the calculations of the mean corpuscular values, we will briefly discuss the accuracy of the involved laboratory examinations.

To calculate the mean corpuscular values, it is necessary to have the patient's hemoglobin, red cell count, and hematocrit reading.

These examinations should be performed with the utmost accuracy.

If the red cell count is performed by the manual or microscopic method, the count should be made 3 times and the average of the 3 counts should be found and used in the calculations.

If it is at all possible, the red cell count should be made with an electronic cell counter because these instruments offer the utmost in accuracy.

CALCULATION OF THE MEAN CORPUSCULAR VOLUME

The mean corpuscular volume is the volume of the average erythrocyte. The mean corpuscular volume can be calculated by either the long method or the short method. The long method gives all the steps involved whereas the short method consolidates several steps. The procedures follow.

LONG METHOD

Given:

Patient's hematocrit reading   .   .   40%
Patient's red cell count .   .   .   .   5,000,000 cells per cu. mm. blood.

The above hematocrit reading may be written as .40, and the red cell count may be written as 5×10^6.

Problem:

Find the mean corpuscular volume.

Solution:

(1) Formula:

$$\text{Mean corpuscular volume} = \frac{\text{Cubic microns of cells in 1 cu. mm. of blood}}{\text{Number of cells in 1 cu. mm. of blood}}$$

(2) Finding the numerator:
From the table of measures and weights (page 362):

$$1 \text{ cu. mm.} = 10^9 \text{ cu. microns}$$

Therefore, 1 cubic millimeter of blood equals 10^9 cubic microns. What part of this 10^9 cubic microns is cells? The hematocrit reading of 40% tells us that 40% of this is cells. Therefore,

.40 $\times$ 10^9 is the number of cubic microns of cells in 1 cubic millimeter of blood. This is our numerator.

(3) Finding the denominator:
Since the patient's red cell count is given as 5,000,000 (5×10^6) cells per cu. mm., the denominator does not have to be found.

(4) Substituting in the formula of step (1):

$$\text{Mean corpuscular volume} = \frac{\text{Cubic microns of cells in 1 cu. mm. of blood}}{\text{Number of cells in 1 cu. mm. of blood}}$$

$$= \frac{.40 \times 10^9}{5 \times 10^6}$$

$$= \frac{.40 \times 10^{9-6}}{5}$$

$$= \frac{.40 \times 10^3}{5}$$

$$= \frac{.40 \times 1000}{5}$$

$$= \frac{400}{5}$$

$$= 80 \text{ cu. microns}$$

SHORT METHOD

Patient's hematocrit reading is 40% and RBC is 5,000,000.

$$\text{M.C.V.} = \frac{\text{Hematocrit} \times 10}{\text{RBC in millions}}$$

$$\text{M.C.V.} = \frac{40 \times 10}{5.0} = 80 \text{ cu. microns}$$

CALCULATION OF THE MEAN CORPUSCULAR HEMOGLOBIN

The mean corpuscular hemoglobin is the weight of hemoglobin in the average erythrocyte.

The mean corpuscular hemoglobin can be calculated by either the long method or the short method. The long method gives all the steps involved whereas the short method consolidates several steps. The procedures follow.

LONG METHOD

Given:

Patient's hemoglobin . . . 14 Gm. per 100 cc. blood
Patient's red cell count . . . 5,000,000 cells per cu. mm. blood.

The above hemoglobin may be written as $\dfrac{14\ \text{Gm.}}{100\ \text{cc.}}$

and the red cell count may be written as 5×10^6.

Problem:

Find the mean corpuscular hemoglobin

Solution:

(1) Formula:

$$\text{Mean corpuscular Hb.} = \frac{\text{Micromicrograms of Hb. in 1 cu. mm. of blood}}{\text{Number of cells in 1 cu. mm. of blood}}$$

(2) Finding the numerator:
The problem here is to convert the patient's 14 grams of hemoglobin per 100 cc. to micromicrograms per cu. mm. Thus, we want to

convert $\dfrac{14\ \text{Gm.}}{100\ \text{cc.}}$ to $\dfrac{\text{micromicrograms}}{\text{cu. mm.}}$. It is done as follows. From

the table of measures and weights (page 362) it is known that

$$1\ \text{Gm.} = 10^{12}\ \text{micromicrograms}$$
$$1\ \text{cc.} = 10^3\ \text{cu. mm.}$$

With this information, the patient's 14 Gm. of hemoglobin is converted to micromicrograms, and the 100 cc. of blood is converted to cu. mm. Thus,

$$\frac{14\ \text{Gm.}}{100\ \text{cc.}} \times \frac{10^{12}}{10^3} = \frac{14 \times 10^{12}\ \text{micromicrograms}}{100 \times 10^3\ \text{cu. mm.}}$$

By dividing the figures on the right hand side of the equal sign, we have the micromicrograms of Hb. in 1 cu. mm. of blood. Thus,

$$\frac{14 \times 10^{12}}{100 \times 10^3} = \frac{14 \times 10^{12}}{10^2 \times 10^3} = \frac{14 \times 10^{12}}{10^5} = 14 \times 10^{12-5}$$

$$= 14 \times 10^7 \text{ micromicrograms of Hb. in 1 cu. mm. of blood.}$$

This is our numerator.

(3) Finding the denominator:

Since the patient's red cell count is given as 5,000,000 (5×10^6) cells per cu. mm., the denominator does not have to be found.

(4) Substituting in the formula of step (1):

$$\text{Mean corpuscular Hb.} = \frac{\text{Micromicrograms of Hb. in 1 cu. mm. of blood}}{\text{Number of cells in 1 cu. mm. of blood}}$$

$$= \frac{14 \times 10^7}{5 \times 10^6}$$

$$= \frac{14 \times 10^{7-6}}{5}$$

$$= \frac{14 \times 10^1}{5}$$

$$= \frac{14 \times 10}{5}$$

$$= \frac{140}{5}$$

$$= 28 \text{ micromicrograms}$$

SHORT METHOD

Patient's hemoglobin is 14 grams and RBC is 5,000,000

$$\text{M.C.H.} = \frac{\text{Hb. in grams} \times 10}{\text{RBC in millions}}$$

$$\text{M.C.H.} = \frac{14 \times 10}{5.0}$$

$$= 28 \text{ micromicrograms}$$

CALCULATION OF THE MEAN CORPUSCULAR HEMOGLOBIN CONCENTRATION

The mean corpuscular hemoglobin concentration is the per cent of hemoglobin in the patient's packed red cell volume.

The term, mean corpuscular hemoglobin concentration, is a misnomer with respect to the formula.*

The mean corpuscular hemoglobin concentration can be calculated by either the long method or the short method. The long method gives all the steps involved whereas the short method consolidates several steps. The procedures follow.

LONG METHOD

Given:

Patient's hemoglobin . . . 14 Gm. per 100 cc. blood.
Patient's hematocrit reading . 40%

Problem:

Find the mean corpuscular hemoglobin concentration.

Solution:

(1) Formula:

$$\text{Mean corpuscular Hb. conc.} = \frac{\text{Gm. of Hb. in 100 cc. blood}}{\text{cc. of packed red cells in 100 cc. blood}} \times 100$$

(2) Finding the numerator:
Since the patient's hemoglobin is given as 14 Gm. per 100 cc. of blood, the numerator does not have to be found.

(3) Finding the denominator:
Since the hematocrit reading is the per cent of red cells in a given volume of blood, the cc. of packed red cells in 100 cc. of blood is found as follows.

Vol. of blood × Hematocrit reading = cc. of packed red cells in 100 cc. blood
100 cc.   × 40%   = 40 cc.

* From a mathematical point of view, whenever the word average or mean is found in a formula, the number of particles used to arrive at the average must be included in the denominator. This does not occur in the formula for the mean corpuscular hemoglobin concentration. Actually, what the formula does is to find the grams of hemoglobin per cubic centimeter of packed red cells. This is then multiplied by 100 and the "per cent" obtained.

26

(4) Substituting in the formula of step (1):

$$\text{Mean corpuscular Hb. conc.} = \frac{\text{Gm. of Hb. in 100 cc. blood}}{\text{cc. of packed red cells in 100 cc. blood}} \times 100$$

$$= \frac{14}{40} \times 100$$

$$= .35 \times 100$$

$$= 35\%$$

SHORT METHOD

Patient's Hb. is 14 grams and hematocrit reading is 40%.

$$\text{M.C.H.C.} = \frac{\text{Hb. in grams} \times 100}{\text{Hematocrit}}$$

$$\text{M.C.H.C.} = \frac{14 \times 100}{40}$$

$$= .35 \times 100$$

$$= 35\%$$

SUMMARY OF ABBREVIATIONS, NORMAL VALUES, AND SHORT METHODS

The student should memorize these abbreviations, normal values, and short methods for they will be useful on student examinations.

ABBREVIATIONS

mean corpuscular volume = M.C.V.
mean corpuscular hemoglobin = M.C.H.
mean corpuscular hemoglobin concentration = M.C.H.C.

NORMAL VALUES

M.C.V. = 80 to 90 cubic microns
M.C.H. = 27 to 32 micromicrograms ($\mu\mu$g)
M.C.H.C. = 33% to 38%

SHORT METHODS (EXAMPLES OF CALCULATIONS)

$$\text{Patient's values:} \quad \begin{aligned} \text{Hb.} &= 14 \text{ grams} \\ \text{RBC} &= 5.0 \text{ million} \\ \text{Hct.} &= 40\% \end{aligned}$$

$$\text{M.C.V.} = \frac{\text{Hct.} \times 10}{\text{RBC in millions}} = \frac{40 \times 10}{5.0} = 80 \text{ cu. microns}$$

$$\text{M.C.H.} = \frac{\text{Hb. in grams} \times 10}{\text{RBC in millions}} = \frac{14 \times 10}{5.0} = 28 \ \mu\mu\text{g}$$

$$\text{M.C.H.C.} = \frac{\text{Hb. in grams} \times 100}{\text{Hct.}} = \frac{14 \times 100}{40} = 35\%$$

Chapter 15

Red Cell Indexes

THE red cell indexes are often referred to as the red cell indices and some-times referred to as red cell sizing.

The discussion of the red cell indexes will cover the following:

Significance of the Red Cell Indexes
Difference Between Mean Corpuscular Values and Red Cell Indexes
Calculation of the Volume Index
Calculation of the Color Index
Calculation of the Saturation Index
Summary of Abbreviations, Normal Values, and Short Methods

The student review questions for the red cell indexes are numbered 188–191 and begin on page 746 of the Appendix.

SIGNIFICANCE OF THE RED CELL INDEXES

Hematologists have set up the following standard values:

Red cell count . . . .   5,000,000 per cu. mm.
Hemoglobin determination   . . .   14.5 grams per 100 cc.
Hematocrit reading. 42%

The red cell indexes are a comparison of the patient's values with the above standard values.

There are 3 red cell indexes: volume index, color index, and saturation index.

Let us consider the most commonly used red cell index—the color index. The color index is found with the following formula:

$$\text{Color index} = \frac{\dfrac{\text{Patient's hemoglobin}}{\text{Standard hemoglobin}}}{\dfrac{\text{Patient's red cell count}}{\text{Standard red cell count}}}$$

The numerator compares the patient's hemoglobin with the standard hemoglobin of 14.5 grams.

The denominator compares the patient's red cell count with the standard red cell count of 5,000,000.

After the above comparisons have been made, the result is expressed as a ratio. By dividing the ratio, we obtain the color index.

For example, suppose a patient had a red cell count of 5,000,000 and a hemoglobin determination of 14.5 grams. His color index would be found as follows:

$$\text{Color index} = \frac{\dfrac{\text{Patient's hemoglobin}}{\text{Standard hemoglobin}}}{\dfrac{\text{Patient's red cell count}}{\text{Standard red cell count}}}$$

$$= \frac{\dfrac{14.5}{14.5}}{\dfrac{5,000,000}{5,000,000}}$$

$$= \frac{1}{1}$$

$$= 1$$

This patient has a color index of 1. The normal values for the color index are 0.9 to 1.1. Consequently, this patient has a normal color index.

When a patient has a normal color index, his red cells contain the normal quota of hemoglobin.

Let's take another example. Suppose a patient had a red cell count of 4,500,000 and a hemoglobin determination of 7 grams. His color index would be found as follows:

$$\text{Color index} = \frac{\dfrac{\text{Patient's hemoglobin}}{\text{Standard hemoglobin}}}{\dfrac{\text{Patient's red cell count}}{\text{Standard red cell count}}}$$

$$= \frac{\dfrac{7.0}{14.5}}{\dfrac{4,500,000}{5,000,000}}$$

$$= \frac{.48}{.90}$$

$$= .53$$

$$= .5$$

This patient has a color index of 0.5. The normal values for the color index are 0.9 to 1.1. Consequently, this patient has a low color index.

When a patient has a low color index, his red cells do not contain the normal quota of hemoglobin.

A low color index, such as the one above, may be found in iron deficiency anemia.

Thus, the color index is a comparison of the patient's hemoglobin determination and red cell count with a given set of standard values.

The volume index and saturation index also compare the patient's values with the given set of standard values.

The volume index compares the patient's hematocrit reading and red cell count with the standard values.

Thus,

$$\text{Volume index} = \frac{\dfrac{\text{Patient's hematocrit reading}}{\text{Standard hematocrit reading}}}{\dfrac{\text{Patient's red cell count}}{\text{Standard red cell count}}}$$

The saturation index compares the patient's hemoglobin determination and hematocrit reading with the standard values.

Thus,

$$\text{Saturation index} = \frac{\dfrac{\text{Patient's hemoglobin determination}}{\text{Standard hemoglobin determination}}}{\dfrac{\text{Patient's hematocrit reading}}{\text{Standard hematocrit reading}}}$$

The normal values for the red cell indexes are given in Table 25.

Since the red cell indexes are concerned with the size and hemoglobin content of the red blood cells, they are useful in the diagnosis and treatment of the anemias.

The color index is usually calculated every time a red cell count and hemoglobin determination is performed. Thus, the color index is calcu-

Table 25.—Normal Values for the Red Cell Indexes

	Normal Values	*When Decreased*	*When Increased*
Volume Index	0.9 to 1.1	iron deficiency anemia	pernicious anemia
Color Index	0.9 to 1.1	iron deficiency anemia	pernicious anemia
Saturation Index	0.9 to 1.1	iron deficiency anemia	

lated about 2000 times a month by the average hospital laboratory and about 100 times a month by the average physician's office.

The volume index and saturation index, however, are rarely requested. They are only calculated about once a month by the average hospital laboratory and about once a year by the average physician's office.

The red cell indexes are usually abbreviated as follows:

volume index	V. I. or VI
color index	C. I. or CI
saturation index	S. I. or SI

DIFFERENCE BETWEEN MEAN CORPUSCULAR VALUES AND RED CELL INDEXES

Now let us turn to a subject which seems to confuse many students.

In the last chapter, we learned that the mean corpuscular values were concerned with the size and hemoglobin content of the red blood cells.

In this chapter, we learned that the red cell indexes are also concerned with the size and hemoglobin content of the red blood cells.

What is the difference between the mean corpuscular values and the red cell indexes?

To answer this question, let us first pursue the following analogy.

Suppose, for a moment, we go far afield: Let us talk about a baby.

Let us say that this baby is underweight. He weighs 15 pounds. He should weigh 30 pounds.

Now, we can talk about the *actual weight* of this baby. And, we can also talk about the *relative or comparative weight* of this baby.

If we talk about the actual weight, we might say: "The baby weighs 15 pounds. He should weigh about 30 pounds."

If we talk about the comparative weight, however, we might say: "The baby weighs one half the normal weight. Therefore, his weight index is $\frac{1}{2}$ or 0.5. His weight index should be about 1.0."

Now return to the mean corpuscular values and the red cell indexes.

Suppose we want some information about the hemoglobin in the patient's red cells.

One of the mean corpuscular values—the mean corpuscular hemoglobin —will give us information about the hemoglobin in the patient's red cells.

One of the red cell indexes—the color index—will also give us information about the hemoglobin in the patient's red cells.

The mean corpuscular hemoglobin might tell us: The hemoglobin in the red cell weighs 15 micromicrograms. It should weigh about 30 micromicrograms.

The color index might tell us: The hemoglobin in the red cell weighs one half the normal weight. Therefore, the color index is $\frac{1}{2}$ or 0.5. The color index should be about 1.0.

Now, both sources of information are telling us that the red cells are "underweight." But the mean corpuscular hemoglobin is giving us the *actual weight*. Whereas the color index is giving us the *comparative weight*.

Thus, the mean corpuscular hemoglobin presents an *actual value*. Whereas the color index presents a *comparative value*.

In a similar manner, the other mean corpuscular values—the mean corpuscular volume and the mean corpuscular hemoglobin concentration—also present *actual values*.

In a similar manner, the other red cell indexes—the volume index and the saturation index—also present *comparative values*.

By way of summary: The mean corpuscular values present actual values. The red cell indexes present comparative values.

The obvious question arises: Should we use the mean corpuscular values or should we use the red cell indexes?

Some physicians prefer the mean corpuscular values. These physicians are usually the research men. They want the "actual weight of the baby."

Other physicians, however, are content with the red cell indexes. They are satisfied with a "comparative weight of the baby."

And some physicians request neither the mean corpuscular values nor the red cell indexes.

These physicians simply say: "Forget about the actual weight and the comparative weight. Just take a look at the baby. After you've seen enough of them, you can tell if they're underweight."

These physicians, of course, are suggesting that you examine the actual red cells in the stained red cell examination.

The stained red cell examination, when properly performed, offers the most valuable information about the size and hemoglobin content of the red blood cells.

To obtain this information, proceed as follows: Study. Observe. And, "see enough babies."

CALCULATION OF THE VOLUME INDEX

The volume index can be calculated by either the long method or the short method. The long method gives all the steps involved whereas the short method consolidates several steps. The procedures follow.

LONG METHOD

Given:

	Patient	Standard
Hematocrit reading	38%	42%
Red cell count	4,500,000	5,000,000

Problem:

Find the volume index.

Solution:

(1) Formula:

$$\text{Volume index} = \frac{\dfrac{\text{Patient's hematocrit reading}}{\text{Standard hematocrit reading}}}{\dfrac{\text{Patient's red cell count}}{\text{Standard red cell count}}}$$

(2) Finding the numerator:

$$\frac{\text{Patient's hematocrit reading}}{\text{Standard hematocrit reading}} = \frac{.38}{.42} = .90$$

(3) Finding the denominator:

$$\frac{\text{Patient's red cell count}}{\text{Standard red cell count}} = \frac{4,500,000}{5,000,000} = .90$$

(4) Substituting in the formula of step (1):

$$\text{Volume index} = \frac{\dfrac{\text{Patient's hematocrit reading}}{\text{Standard hematocrit reading}}}{\dfrac{\text{Patient's red cell count}}{\text{Standard red cell count}}}$$

$$= \frac{.90}{.90}$$

$$= 1.0$$

SHORT METHOD

Patient's hematocrit reading is 38% and RBC is 4,500,000

$$V.I. = \frac{Hematocrit \times 0.118}{RBC \ in \ millions}$$

$$V.I. = \frac{38 \times 0.118}{4.5}$$

$$= 1.0$$

CALCULATION OF THE COLOR INDEX

The color index can be calculated by either the long method or the short method. The long method gives all the steps involved whereas the short method consolidates several steps. The procedures follow.

LONG METHOD

Given:

	Patient	Standard
Gm. of hemoglobin . . .	11.0	14.5
Red cell count	4,000,000	5,000,000

Problem:

Find the color index.

Solution:

(1) Formula:

$$\text{Color index} = \frac{\dfrac{\text{Patient's hemoglobin determination}}{\text{Standard hemoglobin determination}}}{\dfrac{\text{Patient's red cell count}}{\text{Standard red cell count}}}$$

(2) Finding the numerator:

$$\frac{\text{Patient's hemoglobin}}{\text{Standard hemoglobin}} = \frac{11.0}{14.5} = 0.76$$

(3) Finding the denominator:

$$\frac{\text{Patient's red cell count}}{\text{Standard red cell count}} = \frac{4,000,000}{5,000,000} = 0.80$$

(4) Substituting in the formula of step (1):

$$\text{Color index} = \frac{\dfrac{\text{Patient's hemoglobin determination}}{\text{Standard hemoglobin determination}}}{\dfrac{\text{Patient's red cell count}}{\text{Standard red cell count}}}$$

$$= \frac{0.76}{0.80}$$

$$= 0.95$$

By rounding off the 0.95, we obtain a color index of 1.0.

SHORT METHOD

Patient's hemoglobin is 76% (11 grams)* and RBC is 4,000,000.

$$\text{C.I.} = \frac{\text{Hb. in \%}}{\text{First 2 figures of RBC} \times 2}$$

$$\text{C.I.} = \frac{76}{40 \times 2}$$

$$= \frac{76}{80}$$

$$= 0.95$$

By rounding off the 0.95, we obtain a color index of 1.0.

Derivation of the Formula

$$\text{C.I.} = \frac{\text{Hb. in \%}}{\text{First 2 figures of RBC} \times 2}$$

The above formula for the short method was derived as indicated below. In the first equation below, you will note that we are using the "standard hemoglobin in per cent." The standard hemoglobin in per cent is 100%. This is equivalent to 14.5 grams.

From the original formula (page 377):

$$\text{C.I.} = \frac{\dfrac{\text{Patient's Hb. in \%}}{\text{Standard Hb. in \%}}}{\dfrac{\text{Patient's RBC}}{\text{Standard RBC}}}$$

Substituting 100 for the standard hemoglobin in per cent and 5,000,000 for the standard red cell count:

$$\text{C.I.} = \frac{\dfrac{\text{Patient's Hb. in \%}}{100}}{\dfrac{\text{Patient's RBC}}{5,000,000}}$$

* For table converting grams to per cent, see Table 8, page 189.

We can substitute ab for the first 2 figures of the patient's red cell count. Since the last 5 figures of the patient's red cell count will be zeros, we can make the following changes in the denominator:

$$\text{C.I.} = \frac{\dfrac{\text{Patient's Hb. in }\%}{100}}{\dfrac{\text{a,b00,000}}{5,000,000}}.$$

Cancelling the zeros:

$$\text{C.I.} = \frac{\dfrac{\text{Patient's Hb. in }\%}{100}}{\dfrac{\text{ab}}{50}}$$

Inverting and multiplying:

$$\text{C.I.} = \frac{\text{Patient's Hb. in }\%}{100} \times \frac{50}{\text{ab}}$$

Cancelling:

$$\text{C.I.} = \frac{\text{Patient's Hb. in }\%}{2} \times \frac{1}{\text{ab}}$$

Multiplying:

$$\text{C.I.} = \frac{\text{Patient's Hb. in }\%}{2\ \text{ab}}$$

Replacing ab with "First 2 figures of RBC":

$$\text{C.I.} = \frac{\text{Patient's Hb. in }\%}{2 \times \text{First 2 figures of RBC}}$$

Rearranging:

$$\text{C.I.} = \frac{\text{Hb. in }\%}{\text{First 2 figures of RBC} \times 2}$$

CALCULATION OF THE SATURATION INDEX

The saturation index can be calculated by either the long method or the short method. The long method gives all the steps involved whereas the short method consolidates several steps. The procedures follow.

LONG METHOD

Given:

	Patient	Standard
Gm. of hemoglobin . . .	12.0	14.5
Hematocrit reading . . .	36%	42%

Problem:

Find the saturation index.

Solution:

(1) Formula:

$$\text{Saturation index} = \frac{\dfrac{\text{Patient's hemoglobin determination}}{\text{Standard hemoglobin determination}}}{\dfrac{\text{Patient's hematocrit reading}}{\text{Standard hematocrit reading}}}$$

(2) Finding the numerator:

$$\frac{\text{Patient's hemoglobin}}{\text{Standard hemoglobin}} = \frac{12.0}{14.5} = 0.83$$

(3) Finding the denominator:

$$\frac{\text{Patient's hematocrit}}{\text{Standard hematocrit}} = \frac{36}{42} = 0.86$$

(4) Substituting in the formula of step (1):

$$\text{Saturation index} = \frac{\dfrac{\text{Patient's hemoglobin determination}}{\text{Standard hemoglobin determination}}}{\dfrac{\text{Patient's hematocrit reading}}{\text{Standard hematocrit reading}}}$$

$$= \frac{0.83}{0.86}$$

$$= 0.97$$

By rounding off the 0.97, we obtain a saturation index of 1.0.

SHORT METHOD

Patient's Hb. is 83% and hematocrit reading is 36%.

$$S.I. = \frac{Hb. \text{ in } \%}{Hematocrit \times 2.4}$$

$$S.I. = \frac{83}{36 \times 2.4}$$

$$= \frac{83}{86.4}$$

$$= 0.96$$

By rounding off the 0.96, we obtain a saturation index of 1.0.

SUMMARY OF ABBREVIATIONS, NORMAL VALUES, AND SHORT METHODS

ABBREVIATIONS

volume index   = V.I.
color index   = C.I.
saturation index = S.I.

NORMAL VALUES

V.I. = 0.9 to 1.1
C.I. = 0.9 to 1.1
S.I. = 0.9 to 1.1

SHORT METHODS

$$V.I. = \frac{Hematocrit \times 0.118}{RBC \text{ in millions}}$$

$$C.I. = \frac{Hb. \text{ in } \%}{\text{First 2 figures of RBC} \times 2}$$

$$S.I. = \frac{Hb. \text{ in } \%}{Hematocrit \times 2.4}$$

STUDENT NOTES

PART 4
Blood Coagulation Procedures

INTRODUCTION

Part 4 is made up of the following chapters:

The above blood coagulation procedures are used mainly in the diagnosis and treatment of the hemorrhagic diseases.

Chapter 16

Theory of Blood Coagulation

ONE of the simplest acts of nature, the clotting of blood, has not been explained by man. We compensate with big words and impressive theories. We use ten thousand well chosen words to say "we don't know."

Yet, somewhere in the wild forest of speculation flows the river of truth. Someday we will find this river. In the meantime, we must load our backs with a bundle of theory and push forward into the night.

An old theory and a new theory in the clotting of blood are presented below.

The student review questions for this chapter are numbered 192–205 and begin on page 746 of the Appendix.

OLD THEORY OF COAGULATION

According to the old theory, the following four substances are involved in coagulation:

1. thromboplastin   (throm-bo-plas′tin)
2. calcium   (kal′se-um)
3. prothrombin   (pro-throm′bin)
4. fibrinogen   (fi-brin′o-jen)

The first substance, thromboplastin, is found in tissue juices and platelet disintegration. The other three substances are present in the plasma portion of blood.

When you cut your finger and blood flows, thromboplastin is released from tissue juices and platelet disintegration.

This thromboplastin reacts with calcium and prothrombin to form thrombin. The thrombin reacts with fibrinogen to produce fibrin. The fibrin—a net-like substance—entangles the blood cells to form the clot.

Thus, we have the following reaction:

thromboplastin + calcium + prothrombin ⟶ thrombin
thrombin + fibrinogen ⟶ fibrin
fibrin + blood cells ⟶ blood clot

collected in heparin*, when necessary, will obviate the need for prophylactic calcium."

Factor V

"Factor V is the designation assigned to a substance previously known by many synonyms, the most common of which is "labile factor." This factor is derived from plasma globulin and is sometimes called an accelerator. This is because it speeds the conversion of prothrombin to thrombin in the presence of tissue thromboplastin. This conversion is relatively slow in the presence only of calcium (Factor IV) and thromboplastin (Factor III).

Because Factor V is consumed during the clotting of blood, it is not found in the serum. Although Factor V is related to prothrombin, its concentration in the blood is not reduced by a deficiency of vitamin K or by the action of coumarins, as mentioned above (Factor II). However, the amount of Factor V is reduced when the liver is damaged.

A clinical deficiency of Factor V causes a decrease in prothrombin activity, and congenital deficiency is called parahemophilia. Bleeding disorders may be controlled by transfusions of fresh whole blood, fresh citrated plasma, or fresh frozen plasma."

Factor VI

"Factor VI has not yet been assigned to any of the coagulation factors."

Factor VII

"Factor VII is stable to both heat and storage; hence, the many references to it as "stable factor." It has a high concentration in the serum, and stored serum is a practical source of it. Factor VII, like Factor V, is considered to be an accelerator in the conversion of prothrombin to thrombin. Therefore, severe deficiency will cause a decrease in prothrombin activity. However, Factor VII is not consumed during the clotting of blood and is, consequently, found in the serum following normal coagulation. Also, Factor VII is not essential for generation of thromboplastin activity (first stage of coagulation).

Congenital or neonatal deficiency of Factor VII occurs along with hypoprothrombinemia in hemorrhagic disease of the newborn. This is manifested by purpura and bleeding from the mucous membranes. An acquired deficiency may be caused by liver disease, deficiency of vitamin K, and by prothrombin depressants such as the coumarins. Administration of vitamin K_1 or its analogues is indicated in known cases of Factor VII deficiency but not in congenital deficiency. Excesses of Factor VII may

---

* Panheprin—heparin sodium, U.S.P., in various blood containers.

occur and have been associated reportedly with a high incidence of thrombo-embolism in the third trimester of pregnancy. Factor VII is replaced by administration of banked blood, banked or freeze-dried plasma, or stored serum."

Factor VIII

"Factor VIII is best described as "antihemophilic globulin," deficiency of which causes classic hemophilia A. This is the well-known hereditary disease in which a sex-linked characteristic is transmitted by females but in which hemorrhagic difficulties occur almost exclusively in males. In the classical form of the disease there is sufficient deficiency of the anti-hemophilic factor so that bleeding may occur spontaneously or after only minor trauma. It is now known, however, that milder degrees of the disease exist in which hemorrhage may follow only severe trauma or surgery such as tonsillectomy and adenoidectomy or dental extractions.

As an important precursor of thromboplastin, Factor VIII is essential in the first phase of clotting—the formation of intrinsic blood thromboplastin. Deficit of this factor causes reduction in the formation of thromboplastin as well as diminished conversion of prothrombin. As a result, clotting time is prolonged. Factor VIII seems to be almost completely utilized in the formation of a clot. A condition identical to human hemophilia A has been found in dogs, thus providing an opportunity for experimental study of this defect.*

Although the factor itself has not been obtained in a form at all pure, the fact has been established that its activity originates in the globulin fraction of normal plasma. Factor VIII is stable to heat, but unstable in storage. As much as 50 per cent may be lost when citrated blood is stored for 21 days or when fresh frozen plasma is stored for one month. However, platelet-free plasma which is rich in Factor VIII can be prepared and freeze-dried for stable storage. Activity, in this case, is preserved for as long as five years.

Fresh whole blood is a preferred replacement substance in the treatment of hemophilic bleeding episodes which result in significant lowering of the hemoglobin concentration. In instances where replacement of red cells is not required, fresh plasma or fresh frozen plasma is usually employed. The initial dose of plasma in the treatment of a hemophilic bleeding episode is usually 10 ml. per kilogram of body weight. The frequency of administration of plasma depends upon the type and degree of bleeding."

Factor IX

"Factor IX is another factor which is essential for the formation of intrinsic blood thromboplastin, but it influences the amount of thrombo-

* Graham, J. B., *et al.*:   Canine Hemophilia, J. Exper. Med., *90*, 97, August 1949.

plastin formed rather than the rate of its formation. Deficiency of this factor is inherited in the same way (as a sex-linked recessive trait) as deficiency of Factor VIII and is commonly called hemophilia B or Christmas disease after the surname of the first patient in whom this deficiency was characterized. With equal degrees of deficiency the same type of symptoms appear in hemophilia B as in hemophilia A.

Factor IX is found in normal plasma or serum associated with the globulins. It is unstable to heat but stable in storage. Consequently, defects of coagulation can be corrected by administration of fresh or stored blood, fresh or stored plasma, fresh or stored serum, and freeze-dried plasma or serum.

A point of interest — normal coagulation occurs when blood from a patient with hemophilia A is mixed with blood from a patient with hemophilia B; that is, the blood of either patient will correct the clotting defect in the other.

The presence of Factor IX in serum indicates that formation of a clot does not consume this factor. Deficiency of Factor IX occurs in hemorrhagic disease of the newborn and in liver disease. It is induced by administration of prothrombin depressants."

Factor X

"Factor X is the designation given to a substance frequently called Stuart-Prower factor, deficiency of which is believed to be inherited. Prothrombin depressants are thought to decrease this factor. Deficiency also occurs in hemorrhagic disease of the newborn, in liver disease, and in deficiency of vitamin K. The possible consequences of deficiency are nosebleeds, bleeding into a joint, or bleeding into the soft tissues. Plasma deficient in this factor shows defective generation of thromboplastin, impaired utilization of prothrombin, reduced prothrombin activity, and prolonged recalcified clotting time."

Factor XI

"Factor XI is also referred to as plasma thromboplastin antecedent or PTA. This is an important factor which plays a role in the formation of plasma thromboplastin. Deficiency of PTA is most commonly congenital in origin and produces the symptoms of mild hemophilia. This disease state, which is also called hemophilia C, differs from the other two types of hemophilia in that it is transmitted as a Mendelian dominant and, therefore, occurs in both males and females. PTA is not consumed during the process of clotting and, therefore, is found in serum as well as in plasma. The factor is stable to heat and storage. The coagulation disorder due to deficiency of this factor may be corrected by the administration of fresh or stored blood, plasma or serum."

Factor XII

"Factor XII is also referred to as the Hageman factor. The Hageman factor (named after the original patient) is a coagulation factor, the physiologic role of which is not yet completely understood. This factor is now known to be activated by contact with glass and to be important in the initiation of blood coagulation as it occurs outside the body. Inasmuch as patients with Hageman factor deficiency do not have hemorrhagic manifestations, the exact function of this factor in the maintenance of hemostasis is not yet completely understood."

Factor XIII

Factor XIII is also referred to as the fibrin stabilizing factor or FSF. This factor apparently strengthens the fibrin network, for it is essential for the formation of a stable fibrin clot.

MECHANISM OF COAGULATION

"As stated earlier, coagulation of the blood may be represented as occurring in three stages:

1. Formation of thromboplastic activity
2. Conversion of prothrombin to thrombin
3. Conversion of fibrinogen to fibrin

Isolation and description of coagulation by means of a simplified scheme is not intended to infer that it is a static process functioning independently of other bodily functions. On the contrary, the clotting of blood is a dynamic process acting in concert with other mechanisms to achieve and maintain hemostasis. For instance, Quick* emphasizes the role of contraction of blood vessels in hemostasis. He mentions that many of the agents affecting or taking part in coagulation are also utilized for other purposes.

Presented in Figure 144, page 393, is a simplified diagram of the steps involved in the formation of a blood clot. In this diagram, clotting is divided into three stages as outlined by Frost.† This graphic portrayal is purposely simplified to facilitate understanding of a very complex process.

The first phase of coagulation is the formation of thromboplastic activity. Initiation of the process of blood clotting is believed to begin with injury to the blood vessel which provides a contact surface and a site of accumulation of the platelets. The plasma factors involved in the formation of thromboplastin are Factor IV (calcium), Factor VIII (antihemophilic

* Quick, A. J.: Hemorrhagic Diseases, Lea & Febiger, Philadelphia, 1957, p. 14.
† Frost, J. W.: Coagulation Factors Relating to Obstetrics and Gynecology, J. M. Soc. New Jersey, 55, 596, November 1958.

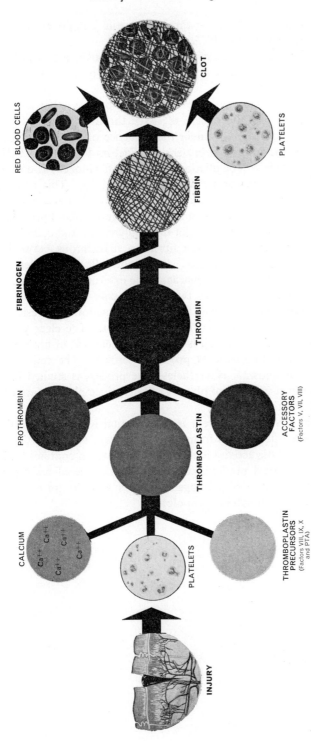

FIG. 144.—Schematic sequence of clot formation (courtesy of Abbott Laboratories).

globulin), Factor IX (plasma thromboplastin component), Factor X (Stuart-Prower factor), and PTA.

The second stage of coagulation involves the conversion of prothrombin to thrombin. In the actual coagulation of the blood the plasma thromboplastin, as mentioned before, is capable of converting prothrombin to thrombin directly. On the other hand, it is believed that an accessory mechanism exists with the release of tissue thromboplastin. Conversion of prothrombin to thrombin under the influence of this type of thromboplastin requires the additional presence of Factors V, VII, and VIII.

In the third stage of coagulation, Factor I (fibrinogen) is converted to fibrin by the thrombin formed in the second stage. This conversion is believed to be accelerated by calcium. Here thrombin acts enzymatically to break down the fibrinogen molecule into molecular fibrin and other substances. The molecules of fibrin then polymerize and combine end-to-end and side-to-side to form the fibrinous filamentous network or gel generally recognized as a fibrin clot. Red blood cells and platelets adhering to the fibrin clot give a clot its characteristic external appearance.

Normal coagulation involves two other events which occur after the actual formation of a clot. The first is clot retraction (syneresis) which is the consolidation or tightening of the fibrin clot. The clear yellow fluid expressed during this retraction is serum (*i.e.*, removal of fibrinogen from plasma by the clotting process produces serum). The reason for clot retraction is not known. Nevertheless, the process is studied in the test tube as an indirect measure of platelet activity, since platelets are necessary for normal retraction.

The second post-clotting event is the eventual lysis or dissolution of a fibrin clot, called fibrinolysis from the words fibrin and lysis. The source of normal fibrinolytic activity is the blood itself which contains an inactive enzyme usually called plasminogen. In the presence of activators from the tissues, the inactive plasminogen becomes plasmin, an active proteolytic enzyme which dissolves fibrin clots."

Chapter 17

Bleeding Time

The bleeding time is also referred to by the following terms: Bl. time, Bleeding t., skin bleeding time, capillary bleeding time, capillary contractility test, capillary retractability test, and blood vessel retractability test.

The bleeding time will be discussed under the following headings:

Significance of the Bleeding Time
Discussion of Procedures for the Bleeding Time
Duke Method for the Bleeding Time
Ivy Method for the Bleeding Time
Sources of Error in the Bleeding Time

The student review questions for the bleeding time are numbered 206–210 and begin on page 748 of the Appendix.

SIGNIFICANCE OF THE BLEEDING TIME

The bleeding time is the time required for a small cut to stop bleeding.

The bleeding time is usually performed by either the Duke method or the Ivy method.

The normal values for the Duke method are 1–3 minutes and the normal values for the Ivy method are 1–7 minutes.

The bleeding time is increased in those conditions listed in Table 27.

Table 27
Conditions Accompanied by an Abnormal Bleeding Time

scurvy	aplastic anemia
purpura hemorrhagica	multiple myeloma
symptomatic thrombocytopenic purpura	infectious mononucleosis
Glanzmann's disease	allergy
von Willebrand's disease	

What causes the bleeding time to increase in disease?
The bleeding time may increase in disease because of the following:

1. shortage of platelets
2. inadequate function of platelets
3. poor retractability of capillaries
4. deficiency of plasma factors

The bleeding time is mainly used in the diagnosis and treatment of the hemorrhagic diseases. These diseases deal with abnormal bleeding. They will be discussed in the section on diseases of the blood (page 641).

The bleeding time is also useful just before such operations as a tonsillectomy. In these cases, it may point to an abnormal bleeding process. This will warn the physician to take the proper surgical precautions.

The bleeding time is performed about 12 times a month by the average hospital laboratory and about 3 times a month by the average physician's office.

DISCUSSION OF PROCEDURES FOR THE BLEEDING TIME

The bleeding time may be performed by the following methods:

Duke Method
Ivy Method
Macfarlane Method
Adelson-Crosby Method

The Duke method is performed by using a sterile blood lancet to make a cut on either the finger or ear lobe, recording the time, touching a piece of filter paper to the cut every half minute until bleeding ceases, and recording the time.

The Ivy method is performed by wrapping a blood pressure cuff above the patient's elbow and inflating it to 40 millimeters pressure, using a sterile blood lancet to make a cut on the patient's forearm, recording the time, touching a piece of filter paper to the cut every half minute until bleeding ceases, and recording the time.

The Macfarlane method is performed by puncturing the ear lobe, recording the time, immersing the ear lobe in a 37° C. saline solution until bleeding ceases, and recording the time.

The Adelson-Crosby method is a rather complicated procedure and falls outside the realm of routine laboratory examinations.

The Ivy method is the preferred method of performing the bleeding time because the pressure on the blood vessels is standardized at 40 millimeters.

The normal values for the various methods of performing the bleeding time are generally considered to be:

Duke method   1–3 minutes
Ivy method   1–7 minutes
Macfarlane method   2–4 minutes

The normal values for the Duke method, however, may vary from laboratory to laboratory because this method has undergone various modifications.

At their very best, the methods of performing the bleeding time are considered rather crude and requests to repeat the test are frequently received.

The Duke method and the Ivy method are presented on the following pages.

DUKE METHOD FOR THE BLEEDING TIME

NECESSARY REAGENTS AND EQUIPMENT

1. Piece of filter paper
2. Watch with a second hand
3. Materials for a finger puncture: cotton balls or gauze pads, 70% alcohol, and sterile blood lancet.

Procedure

1. Observe the folded piece of filter paper in Figure 145.

   Note: At half-minute intervals, this filter paper had been touched to blood coming out of a finger puncture. Note that the blood spots on the filter paper get smaller and smaller. This indicates that the flow of blood is gradually stopping.

2. Obtain a piece of filter paper and a watch with a second hand.

3. Obtain the materials for a finger puncture: cotton balls or gauze pads, 70% alcohol, and a sterile blood lancet.

   Note: In place of the sterile blood lancet, some laboratories use an automatic spring lancet. This lancet has a blade which can be adjusted so it will cut to any desired depth. For this test, the blade is set so it will cut to a depth of 2 millimeters (about $\frac{1}{12}$ of an inch). This instrument is sterilized, of course, before it is used.

4. For this test, the blood must flow freely and naturally. Therefore, you do not massage or squeeze the finger.

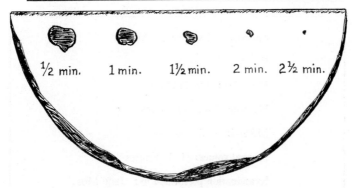

½ min.   1 min.   1½ min.   2 min.   2½ min.

Fig. 145.—Folded piece of filter paper showing the results of a normal bleeding time.

5. Moisten a piece of cotton with the 70% alcohol and thoroughly cleanse the ball of the patient's middle finger.

6. Allow about 1 minute to elapse so the finger will dry.

7. Using a sterile blood lancet, make a finger puncture deep enough to insure a free flow of blood.

8. Record the time.

9. Pick up your piece of filter paper and fold it in half.

10. Exactly $\frac{1}{2}$ minute after puncturing the finger, <u>lightly</u> touch the filter paper to the blood coming out of the puncture.

11. Repeat the above step every $\frac{1}{2}$ minute until blood ceases to flow.

12. Record the time at which blood ceased to flow.

    <u>Note:</u> Should the blood flow more than 15 minutes, proceed as follows: Discontinue the test, put a bandage on the wound, and report the test as "greater than 15 minutes."

13. The bleeding time is the time elapsed between the puncture of the finger and the cessation of bleeding (Fig. 145).

14. Determine the bleeding time from your recorded time data.

15. Moisten a piece of cotton with alcohol and cleanse the puncture on the patient's finger.

16. Make the report as illustrated in the sample report below.

17. Sample report:

Patient: Doe, Mr. John

Date: 7-7-72

Physician: Dr. Paul Aubry

Bleeding time: 3 minutes

Method: Duke method

Normal values: 1–3 minutes

Examination performed by: Jane Moss

IVY METHOD FOR THE BLEEDING TIME

NECESSARY REAGENTS AND EQUIPMENT

1. Piece of filter paper
2. Watch with a second hand
3. Blood pressure apparatus
4. Materials for a finger puncture: cotton balls or gauze pads, 70% alcohol, and a sterile blood lancet.

Procedure

1. Observe the folded piece of filter paper in Figure 145, page 397.

   Note: At half-minute intervals, this filter paper had been touched to blood coming out of a puncture. Note that the blood spots on the filter paper get smaller and smaller. This indicates the cessation of bleeding.

2. Obtain a piece of filter paper, a watch with a second hand, and a blood pressure kit.

3. Obtain the materials for a finger puncture: cotton balls or gauze pads, 70% alcohol, and a sterile blood lancet.

   Note: In place of the sterile lancet, some laboratories use an automatic spring lancet. This lancet has a blade which can be adjusted so it will cut to any desired depth. For this test, the blade is set so it will cut to a depth of 3 millimeters (about $\frac{1}{8}$ of an inch). This instrument is sterilized, of course, before it is used.

4. Wrap the blood pressure cuff just above the bend in the patient's elbow.

5. Inflate the blood pressure cuff to 40 millimeters pressure. (This standardizes the pressure.)

6. Moisten a piece of cotton with the 70% alcohol. Just below the bend in the elbow, cleanse the fleshy portion of the forearm. Then dry the area with a piece of dry cotton.

7. Pick up the sterile lancet. Choose an area free of veins. Make a rather deep puncture.

8. Record the time.

28

9. Pick up your piece of filter paper and fold it in half.

10. Exactly $\frac{1}{2}$ minute after puncturing the forearm, <u>lightly</u> touch the filter paper to the blood coming out of the puncture.

11. Repeat the above step every $\frac{1}{2}$ minute until blood ceases to flow.

12. Record the time at which blood ceased to flow.

    <u>Note</u>: Should the blood flow more than 15 minutes, proceed as follows: Discontinue the test, put a bandage on the wound, and report the test as "greater than 15 minutes."

13. The bleeding time is the time elapsed between the puncture of the forearm and the cessation of bleeding.

14. Determine the bleeding time from your recorded time data.

    <u>Note</u>: The accuracy of this test may be increased by performing 2 or 3 tests and taking the average. A different spot, of course, should be used for each puncture.

15. When the test is completed, moisten a piece of cotton with alcohol and cleanse the area. Then apply a "Band-aid" to the wound.

16. Make the report as indicated in the sample report below.

17. Sample report:

Patient: Mr. John Doe

Date: 7–7–72

Physician: Dr. John Jones

Bleeding time: 3 min.

Method: Ivy method

Normal values: 1–7 minutes

Technologist: Sandra Frisbie

SOURCES OF ERROR IN THE BLEEDING TIME

Mistakes in performing the bleeding time may cause the bleeding time to be decreased or increased.

These mistakes will decrease the bleeding time:

1. Failure to thoroughly cleanse the area to be punctured.
2. Choosing and puncturing a cold bloodless area.
3. Making only a superficial puncture.

These mistakes will increase the bleeding time:

1. Choosing and puncturing a red flushed area.
2. Making too deep a puncture.
3. Applying pressure to the punctured area.

Chapter 18

Coagulation Time

The coagulation time is also referred to as the coag. time, clotting time, and whole blood clotting time.

The coagulation time will be discussed under the following headings:

> Significance of the Coagulation Time
> Discussion of Procedures for the Coagulation Time
> Capillary Tube Method for the Coagulation Time
> Lee and White Method for the Coagulation Time
> Sources of Error in the Coagulation Time

The student review questions for the coagulation time are numbered 211–217 and begin on page 748 of the Appendix.

SIGNIFICANCE OF THE COAGULATION TIME

The coagulation time is the time required for blood to coagulate.

The normal values for the coagulation time vary with the method of determination.

The most commonly used methods and their normal values are:

Method	Normal Values
Capillary blood methods	
slide method	2–6 minutes
capillary tube method	2–6 minutes
Dale and Laidlaw method	1–3 minutes
Venous blood methods	
Lee and White method	5–15 minutes
Howell method	10–30 minutes
silicone tube method	20–60 minutes

Why do the capillary blood methods have shorter normal values than the venous blood methods?

You will recall that substances in tissue juices, essentially thromboplastin, assist blood coagulation.

In the capillary blood methods, the finger or ear lobe is punctured.

Tissue juices mix with the blood and assist in coagulation. Hence the coagulation time is relatively short.

In the venous blood methods, however, a needle goes through the skin and enters a vein. Tissue juices have little opportunity to mix with the blood and assist in coagulation. Hence the coagulation time is relatively long.

If the coagulation time is not properly reported, it can be very misleading. Suppose, for a moment, a coagulation time is reported as follows:

Name: Smith, Mr. John

Date: 7-7-72

Coagulation time: 30 minutes

Technologist: Judy Jones

Is this coagulation time normal or abnormal?

It could be either. If the Howell method was used to perform the test, it is *normal*. If the capillary tube method was used to perform the test, it is *decidedly abnormal*.

Consequently, in reporting the coagulation time, you should always include the method of determination and the normal values.

The coagulation time is increased in those conditions listed in Table 28.

In hemophilia, the coagulation time is greatly increased. In some cases, it may even exceed 100 minutes.

The coagulation time is mainly used in the diagnosis and treatment of the hemorrhagic diseases. These diseases deal with abnormal bleeding. They will be discussed in the section on diseases of the blood.

The coagulation time is also used just before such operations as a tonsillectomy. In these cases, it may point to an abnormal bleeding process. This will warn the physician to take the proper surgical precautions.

Table 28
Conditions Accompanied by an Increased Coagulation Time

hemophilia (Factor VIII deficiency)	Factor VII deficiency
hemorrhagic disease of the newborn	Factor IX deficiency (Christmas disease)
vitamin K deficiency	Factor XI deficiency (PTA deficiency)
heparin therapy	Factor XII deficiency (Hageman factor
Dicumarol therapy	deficiency)
fibrinogenopenia or afibrinogenemia	presence of circulating anticoagulants
melena neonatorum	anemia
Factor V deficiency (parahemophilia,	leukemia
Owen's disease)	pneumonia

The coagulation time is frequently requested.   It is performed about 100 times a month by the average hospital laboratory.   And it is run about 5 times a month by the average physician's office.

DISCUSSION OF PROCEDURES FOR THE COAGULATION TIME

The coagulation time may be performed by either capillary blood methods or venous blood methods.

The capillary blood methods are: (1) slide method, (2) capillary tube method, and (3) Dale and Laidlaw method.

The venous blood methods are: (1) Lee and White method, (2) Howell method, and (3) silicone tube method.

A synopsis of each method is given below.

The slide method is performed by puncturing the finger, recording the time, placing 3 drops of blood on a glass slide, drawing the point of a needle through the drops until fibrin threads appear, and recording the time.

The capillary tube method is performed by puncturing the finger, recording the time, filling a capillary tube with blood, breaking the capillary tube until a span of fibrin is seen, and recording the time.

The Dale and Laidlaw method is performed by puncturing the finger, recording the time, allowing the blood to flow into a capillary tube which contains a lead bead, immersing the capillary tube in 37° C. water, tilting the tube until the lead bead is held firmly by fibrin threads, and recording the time.

The Lee and White method is performed by obtaining a syringe, drawing blood from a vein and noting the time the blood enters the syringe, transferring the blood to 3 test tubes, tilting the tubes until coagulation takes place, and recording the time.

The Howell method is performed by coating a syringe with petrolatum, using this syringe to draw blood from a vein, recording the time the blood enters the syringe, transferring the blood to a test tube, tilting the tube until coagulation takes place, and recording the time.

The silicone tube method is performed by coating a syringe with silicone to decrease the contact of blood with glass (contact with glass promotes coagulation), drawing blood from a vein and noting the time the blood enters the siliconized syringe, transferring the blood to 2 siliconized test tubes, placing the tubes in a 37° C. water bath, tilting the tubes until coagulation takes place, and recording the time.

Of the above 6 methods for the coagulation time, the Lee and White method is the most widely used, being the method of choice in the majority of hospital laboratories.

The capillary tube method and the Lee and White method are given on the following pages.

CAPILLARY TUBE METHOD FOR THE COAGULATION TIME

NECESSARY REAGENTS AND EQUIPMENT

1. Watch with a second hand or a stop watch.
2. Materials for a finger puncture: cotton balls or gauze pads, 70% alcohol, and a sterile blood lancet.
3. Two *plain* capillary tubes. (A capillary tube is a glass tube about one half the length of a pencil and about as thick as the lead in a pencil. A capillary tube is illustrated in Fig. 146.) Make sure you have plain capillary tubes, that is, capillary tubes that are not coated with an anticoagulant.

Procedure

1. Obtain a watch with a second hand or a stop watch.
2. Obtain the materials for a finger puncture: cotton balls or gauze pads, 70% alcohol, and a sterile blood lancet.
3. Get 2 plain capillary tubes (Fig. 146, page 406).

   Note: Do not use capillary tubes coated with an anti-coagulant.
4. Observe the method of filling a capillary tube (Fig. 146).

   Note: Observe that one end of the capillary tube is placed in the drop of blood and the other end of the capillary tube is tilted downward so the blood will flow into the tube.
5. Moisten a piece of cotton with the 70% alcohol.
6. With the moistened cotton, cleanse the ball of the patient's middle finger.
7. Pick up a piece of dry cotton and thoroughly dry the ball of the finger.
8. Pick up the sterile blood lancet.
9. With your right hand, firmly grasp the sterile blood lancet.
10. With your left hand, firmly grasp the patient's middle finger.
11. Make a quick DEEP stab on the ball of the finger.

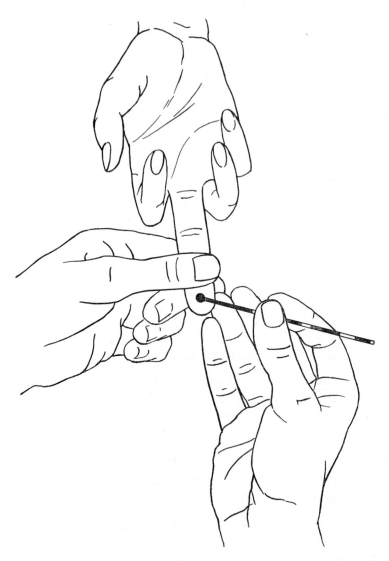

FIG. 146.—Method of filling a capillary tube. With his left hand, the technologist is holding the patient's finger. With his right hand, the technologist is holding one end of the capillary tube in the drop of blood and tilting the tube *downward* so blood will flow into the tube.

12. Gently massage the finger to produce blood.

13. Pick up a piece of dry cotton and wipe away the first drop of blood.

14. Pick up another piece of dry cotton and thoroughly dry the puncture area.

    Note: If the puncture area is not thoroughly dry, the blood will not form a rounded drop. It will run down the sides of the finger.

15. FIRMLY massage the finger to produce a LARGE rounded drop of blood.

16. When you have produced the large rounded drop of blood, record the time or start the stop watch.

17. Then pick up the capillary tube and hold it in your right hand.

18. Put one end of the capillary tube in the drop of blood and tilt the other end of the capillary tube downward (Fig. 146).

19. Allow the drop of blood to flow into the capillary tube.

20. Momentarily set the capillary tube on the table.

21. Quickly pick up a piece of dry cotton and thoroughly dry the puncture area.

22. FIRMLY massage the finger to produce another LARGE rounded drop of blood.

23. Quickly pick up the same capillary tube.

24. Put the same end of the capillary tube in the drop of blood and tilt the other end of the capillary tube downward.

25. Allow the drop of blood to flow into the capillary tube.

    Note: It does not make any difference if empty spaces are present in the column of blood in the capillary tube.

26. If the capillary tube is not filled with blood, repeat the above drying, massaging, and filling process.

27. When the capillary tube is filled with blood, place it on the table.

28. Pick up a piece of dry cotton and thoroughly dry the puncture area.

29. Then <u>FIRMLY</u> massage the finger to produce another <u>LARGE</u> rounded drop of blood.

   Note: If the finger puncture has dried up, of course, you will have to perform another finger puncture.

30. Pick up the second capillary tube and hold it in your right hand.

31. Put one end of the capillary tube in the drop of blood and tilt the other end of the capillary tube <u>downward.</u>

32. Allow the blood to flow into the capillary tube.

33. Momentarily set the capillary tube on the table.

34. Repeat the drying, massaging, and filling process until the capillary tube is at least half filled with blood.

35. When the two capillary tubes are filled with blood, allow 3 more minutes to elapse.

   Note: By allowing 3 minutes to elapse rather than 2 minutes, you will ensure the completion of the test if the coagulation time is prolonged or if you did not get enough blood.

36. When you have allowed the 3 minutes to elapse, pick up the first capillary tube.

37. Using both hands, hold the capillary tube as shown in Figure 147.

38. Now carefully break the capillary tube into two pieces, being careful not to pull the broken ends too far apart.

39. Look for a thread-like span of fibrin between the two broken ends (Fig. 148).

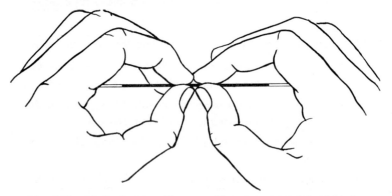

FIG. 147.—Method of breaking a capillary tube containing blood.

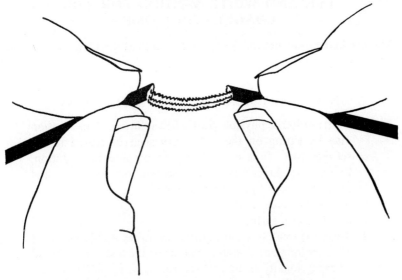

FIG. 148.—Span of fibrin between the two broken ends of a capillary tube containing blood.

40. If a span of fibrin is seen, record the time or stop the stop watch. Then proceed to step 42.

41. If a span of fibrin is not seen, continue breaking the capillary tube at half-minute intervals until the span of fibrin is seen. Then record the time or stop the stop watch.

42. The coagulation time is the time elapsed between the production of the large rounded drop of blood (step 16 above) and the appearance of the fibrin.

43. Determine the coagulation time from your time data.

44. Make the report as indicated in the sample report below.

45. Sample report:

> **Patient:** Doe, Mr. John
>
> **Date:** 7-7-72
>
> **Physician:** Dr. DeWitt Englund
>
> **Coagulation time:** 5 minutes
>
> **Method:** Capillary tube method
>
> **Normal values:** 2–6 minutes
>
> **Examination performed by:** Lee Walker

LEE AND WHITE METHOD FOR THE COAGULATION TIME

The Lee and White method is often referred to as the L and W method or the L–W coag. time.

NECESSARY REAGENTS AND EQUIPMENT

1. Bottle of sterile physiological saline solution. This solution may be sitting on the laboratory shelf or stored in the refrigerator. If it is necessary to prepare the solution, follow the directions in the section on solutions and reagents in the Appendix (page 698).
2. Sterile 20 gauge needle
3. Sterile 10 cc. syringe
4. Three (3) small test tubes; these test tubes should be about 3 inches long and $\frac{1}{3}$ inch in diameter; the test tubes should be exceptionally clean and well rinsed with distilled water; if possible, brand new test tubes should be used.
5. Wax marking pencil
6. Watch with a second hand
7. Tourniquet
8. 70% alcohol
9. Cotton balls or gauze pads

Procedure

1. Obtain a bottle of sterile physiological saline solution.

2. Get a sterile 20 gauge needle, sterile 10 cc. syringe, and 3 small test tubes (about 3 inches long and $\frac{1}{3}$ of an inch in diameter).

   Note: The above test tubes should be exceptionally clean and well rinsed with distilled water. If possible, use brand new test tubes. Dirty test tubes will hasten coagulation.

3. Thoroughly rinse the sterile 20 gauge needle and 10 cc. syringe with the sterile physiological saline solution. Also thoroughly rinse the 3 test tubes with the sterile physiological saline solution.

4. Label the test tubes #1, #2, and #3.

5. Obtain a watch with a second hand, a tourniquet, 70% alcohol, and some cotton balls or gauze pads

6. Take all of the above equipment to the patient.

7. Put the watch near the patient so you can observe the time.

8. Apply the tourniquet to the patient's arm and choose the best vein.

9. Make a "clean" venipuncture, attempting to enter the vein with a single direct thrust.

   Note: The purpose of the above technique is to minimize the amount of tissue juices withdrawn with the blood. Tissue juices mixed with blood will hasten coagulation.

10. Slowly withdraw blood, noting the time at which blood enters the syringe.

11. Continue withdrawing blood until you have about 5 cc. Then release the tourniquet. And withdraw the needle from the vein.

    Note: The blood should not be "foamy," that is, it should not contain air bubbles. Air bubbles in the blood may be caused by failure to have the needle completely in the vein or failure to have the needle firmly attached to the syringe. Air bubbles in the blood will hasten coagulation.

12. Remove the needle from the syringe.

13. Now gently transfer about 1 cc. of blood to each of the three test tubes.

    Note: Allow the blood to flow gently down the inside of each test tube. Excessive agitation will hasten coagulation.

14. There is a slight variation in the remainder of the procedure: Some laboratories put the test tubes in a test tube rack and continue the examination at room temperature. However, room temperature (about 20° C.) will retard coagulation. Other laboratories put the test tubes in a 37° C. water bath (or beaker containing water at 37° C.) and continue the examination at 37° C. The latter procedure is recommended.

15. Either put the 3 test tubes in a test tube rack at room temperature or put them in a 37° C. water bath.

16. Allow 4 minutes to elapse.

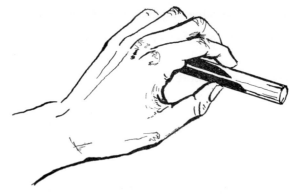

FIG. 149.—Completion of the coagulation time in the Lee and White method. Note that a blood clot has formed and therefore blood will not flow from the test tube.

17. Observe the completion of coagulation which is illustrated in Figure 149.

    Note: Coagulation is complete when the clot is so well formed that blood will not flow from the tube.

18. When the 4 minutes have elapsed, pick up tube #1.

19. At half-minute intervals, gently tilt the tube until a clot forms and blood will not flow from the tube (Fig. 149).

20. Now pick up tube #2.

21. At half-minute intervals, gently tilt the tube until a clot forms and blood will not flow from the tube.

22. Now pick up tube #3.

23. At half-minute intervals, gently tilt the tube until a clot forms and blood will not flow from the tube.

24. When the clot is so well formed that blood will not flow from tube #3, record the time.

25. The coagulation time is the time elapsed between the withdrawal of blood and the completion of coagulation in tube #3.

    Note: Three test tubes are used because each successive test tube is subjected to less tilting, therefore less agitation of the blood, and consequently a more accurate coagulation time.

26. Determine the coagulation time from your time data.

27. Make the report as indicated in the sample report below.

28. Sample report:

Patient: Mr. John Doe

Date: 7-7-72

Physician: Dr. John Jones

Coagulation time: 8 min.

Method: Lee and White

Normal values: 5–15 minutes

Technologist: Sandra Frisbie

SOURCES OF ERROR IN THE COAGULATION TIME

Coagulation will be hastened by the following:

1. Dirty test tubes.
2. Tissue juices mixed with blood. This may be caused by making several puncturing probes with the same needle or squeezing the finger.
3. Air bubbles in the blood. This may be caused by a faulty venipuncture. (Either failure to have the needle completely in the vein or having the needle loosely attached to the syringe.)
4. Excessive agitation of the blood. This may occur in transferring the blood from the syringe to the test tube. The blood should be allowed to flow gently down the inside of the test tube and not forcefully squirted into the test tube.

Coagulation will be retarded by the following:

1. Temperature below 35° C. (95° F.).
2. Temperature above 45° C. (113° F.).

Other factors affecting coagulation are:

1. Diameter of the test tube. The smaller the diameter, the more rapid the clot formation. Therefore, all test tubes should be the same diameter. (The blood clots faster in a test tube with a small diameter because the amount of foreign surface area [glass] to the amount of blood is increased.)

Chapter 19

Platelet Count

THE word platelet is an older and more popular name for a thrombocyte. Consequently, a platelet count may also be referred to as a thrombocyte count.

The platelet count will be considered under the following headings:

Platelets
Significance of the Platelet Count
Discussion of Procedures for the Platelet Count
Fonio Method for the Platelet Count
Rees and Ecker Method for the Platelet Count
Brecher-Cronkite Method for the Platelet Count
Sources of Error in the Platelet Count

The student review questions for the platelet count are numbered 218–233 and begin on page 749 of the Appendix.

PLATELETS

A platelet or thrombocyte goes through 4 stages of development:

Cell	Pronunciation
megakaryoblast	meg″ah-kar′e-o-blast
promegakaryocyte	pro-meg″ah-kar′e-o-sīt
megakaryocyte	meg″ah-kar′e-o-sīt
thrombocyte	throm′bo-sīt

The developing platelet lives in the bone marrow and the 4 stages of development are illustrated in Figure 150.

As shown in the illustration, the third stage of development is the mega-karyocyte. The outer edges of this cell break off and become thrombocytes. The thrombocytes accumulate in the bone marrow and are soon swept into the blood stream.

Technically speaking, of course, a platelet or thrombocyte is not a cell; it is a fragment of a cell.

Platelets come in various sizes and shapes. In diameter, they range between 2 and 4 microns. They are normally colorless, but with Wright's stain, they stain blue with pink granules.

414

Platelets literally stick together and they are frequently seen in groups of 3, 4, or 5.

A group of platelets is illustrated in the color plates which are opposite page 244 and page 526.

The platelets have 3 major functions:

1. They assist in the arrest of bleeding by sticking together and plugging holes in capillary walls.
2. They assist in coagulation by furnishing platelet factors and other substances.
3. They assist in clot retraction by "tying" fibrin threads into knots.

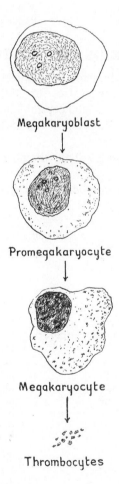

Megakaryoblast

Promegakaryocyte

Megakaryocyte

Thrombocytes

Fig. 150.—Development of platelets or thrombocytes.

29

The life span of a platelet was formerly thought to be 4 days. It is now, however, considered to be about 9 days.

As mentioned previously, the blood cells have recently undergone a change in terminology. The platelets now belong to the thrombocytic series of cells. The new name and old name for the cells in the thrombocytic series is given in Table 29.

Table 29.—New Name and Old Name for the Platelets

Thrombocytic Series of Cells

New Name for Cell	*Old Name for Cell*
Megakaryoblast	Megalokaryoblast
Promegakaryocyte	Promegalokaryocyte
Megakaryocyte	Megalokaryocyte
Thrombocyte	Platelet or thromboplastid

SIGNIFICANCE OF THE PLATELET COUNT

Although the normal values for the platelet count vary slightly from method to method, the normal values for clinical purposes are generally considered to be 150,000 to 400,000 per cubic millimeter of blood.

When the platelet count drops below the normal values, it is referred to as a thrombocytopenia.

When the platelet count rises above the normal values, it is referred to as a thrombocytosis.

A thrombocytopenia or thrombocytosis may be expected in those conditions listed in Table 30.

Table 30

Conditions Accompanied by Abnormal Platelet Counts

Low Platelet Count (thrombocytopenia)	High Platelet Count (thrombocytosis)
purpura hemorrhagica (idiopathic thrombocytopenic purpura)	after splenectomy
symptomatic thrombocytopenic purpura	polycythemia vera
aplastic anemia	acute posthemorrhagic anemia
pernicious anemia	myeloproliferative disorders
acute granulocytic leukemia	metastatic carcinoma
acute lymphocytic leukemia	chronic granulocytic leukemia
chronic lymphocytic leukemia	idiopathic thrombocythemia
monocytic leukemia	hemolytic anemia
plasmacytic leukemia	iron deficiency anemia
multiple myeloma	tuberculosis
Gaucher's disease	sickle cell anemia
diphtheria	after surgery *(immediatly after)*
typhoid fever	
acute rheumatic fever	

The platelet count may be below the normal values or above the normal values in certain normal conditions and activities. For example, the platelet count is below the normal values the first few days of life and also before menstruation. It is above the normal values at high altitudes and after severe exercise.

If the platelet count drops below 75,000 per cubic millimeter, a bleeding tendency is usually evident and the shortage of platelets affects several other coagulation tests.

For example, a low platelet count affects these tests as follows:

bleeding time	increases
clot retraction time	increases
prothrombin consumption time	decreases
capillary resistance test	positive

The platelet count is mainly used in the diagnosis and treatment of the hemorrhagic diseases.

A platelet count is also used in the treatment of leukemia. For example, a platelet count may be ordered during a course of x-ray therapy. If the platelet count is normal, it indicates that such treatment is producing a favorable effect.

The platelet count is frequently requested. It is performed about 100 times a month by the average hospital laboratory. And it is run about 5 times a month by the average physician's office.

DISCUSSION OF PROCEDURES FOR THE PLATELET COUNT

The platelet count may be performed by the following methods:

Indirect Methods
1. Fonio
2. Dameshek
3. Olef
4. Cramer and Bannerman

Direct Methods
1. Rees and Ecker
2. Brecher-Cronkite
3. Feissly and Ludin
4. Tocantins
5. Kristenson as modified by Lempert
6. Unopette
7. Automated Methods
    (1) Coulter Counter
    (2) Technicon Hemolab
    (3) Fisher Autocytometer
    (4) MK-4 Platelet Counter

What is the difference between the indirect methods and the direct methods?

In the indirect methods, the ratio of platelets to red cells is determined by a study of the blood smear. It is assumed that this ratio of platelets to red cells also exists in one cubic millimeter of blood. Therefore, the ratio is multiplied by the number of red cells in one cubic millimeter of blood.

The number of red cells in one cubic millimeter of blood, of course, is the red cell count.

To illustrate the calculation, consider the following: The blood smear shows 1 platelet to every 10 red cells. The red cell count is 5,000,000 cells per cubic millimeter.

Our ratio of platelets to red cells is therefore 1 to 10. This ratio times the red cell count gives us the platelet count:

$$\text{ratio} \times \text{red cell count} = \text{platelet count}$$
$$\tfrac{1}{10} \times 5,000,000 = 500,000$$

In the direct methods of performing the platelet count, the blood is diluted and the platelets are counted with either a microscope or an electronic instrument.

The indirect methods are less accurate, less widely used, and have slightly higher normal values than the direct methods.

We will present 1 indirect method and 2 direct methods. These methods are:

> Fonio Method
> Rees and Ecker Method
> Brecher-Cronkite Method

FONIO METHOD FOR THE PLATELET COUNT

NECESSARY REAGENTS AND EQUIPMENT

1. Finger tip blood or *fresh* anticoagulated blood
2. If finger tip blood is used, the following will be needed:
   a. materials for a finger puncture: several cotton balls or gauze pads, 70% alcohol, and a sterile blood lancet.
   b. bottle of 14% magnesium sulfate solution (This solution may be sitting on the laboratory shelf or stored in the refrigerator. If it is necessary to prepare the solution, follow the directions in the section on solutions and reagents in the Appendix, page 696.)
3. If fresh anticoagulated blood is used, the following will be needed:
   a. 2 wooden applicator sticks
4. Several glass slides
5. Red cell pipet
6. Red cell diluting fluid
7. Wright's stain
8. Counting chamber
9. Microscope

Procedure

1. Either <u>fresh</u> anticoagulated blood or finger tip blood may be used. If anticoagulated blood is used, it should not be over 1 hour old because the platelets disintegrate rapidly.

2. <u>If fresh anticoagulated blood is to be used,</u> obtain the following: the test tube of anticoagulated blood, a few glass slides, two wooden applicator sticks, a red cell pipet, and red cell diluting fluid. Mix the blood. Make a blood smear. Then proceed to step 9.

3. <u>If finger tip blood is to be used,</u> obtain the following: several cotton balls or gauze pads, 70% alcohol, a sterile blood lancet, several glass slides, and a bottle of 14% magnesium sulfate solution.

4. Moisten a piece of cotton with the 70% alcohol and cleanse the ball of the finger. Using a piece of <u>dry</u> cotton, thoroughly dry the finger.

5. Put a drop of the 14% magnesium sulfate solution on the ball of the finger and make a puncture through the solution.

   Note: This technique enables the blood to be diluted at once and helps to prevent clumping and also the disintegration of platelets.

6. Gently squeeze the finger so that the blood flows out of the puncture and mixes with the magnesium sulfate solution.

7. Touch a glass slide to the mixture and make a blood smear in the usual manner. Make another blood smear. The second smear, of course, will be held in reserve in case you make a mistake.

8. Dry the area with a piece of dry cotton and massage the finger to produce a rounded drop of blood.

9. Using the red cell pipet, dilute the blood for a red cell count by drawing blood to the 0.5 mark and red cell diluting fluid to the 101 mark.

10. Stain the blood smear with Wright's stain and buffer solution.

11. Thoroughly shake the red cell pipet for 3 minutes. Perform a red cell count. Make a record of your red cell count.

12. Put a drop of immersion oil on the thin portion of the stained blood smear. Then put the smear on the stage of the microscope. Using the oil immersion (95×) objective, bring the cells into view.

13. Make sure you are looking at the thin portion of the smear. The red cells in this area should not be overlapping, they should be spread out.

14. Observe the platelets which are illustrated in Plate 4, page 244 and Plate 15, page 526.

   Note: In Plate 4, there are 7 platelets. In Plate 15, there are 14 platelets. You will note that the platelets frequently come in groups of 2, 3, or 4.

15. Now it is necessary to count 1000 red cells (erythrocytes) and record the number of platelets seen during this count.

16. In order to narrow the microscopic field and thus make it easier to count the cells, some technologists put a piece of paper containing a "window" in the eyepiece of the microscope. Thus,

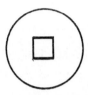

17. To make and insert this "window," proceed as follows: Remove the eyepiece from the microscope by simply lifting it up. Get a piece of paper and a scissors. Cut out a round piece of paper the same diameter as the eyepiece. Then cut the "window" in the piece of paper. Unscrew the top lens of the eyepiece. Put the round piece of paper containing the "window" on the shelf of the eyepiece. Screw the top lens back on the eyepiece. And return the eyepiece to the microscope.

18. Now count 1000 red cells (erythrocytes) and record the number of platelets seen during the count.

19. The platelet count equals the ratio of platelets to red cells times the red cell count.

20. For example, suppose you had the following data:

Red cell count = 5,000,000
Red cells counted on slide = 1,000
Platelets counted on slide = 50

21. Then the platelet count would be found as follows:

$$\text{Platelet count} = \frac{\text{Number of platelets counted on slide}}{\text{Number of red cells counted on slide}} \times \text{red cell count}$$

$$= \frac{50}{1000} \times 5,000,000$$

$$= \frac{1}{20} \times 5,000,000$$

$$= 250,000$$

22. Using your recorded data, make the calculations for your platelet count as indicated above.

23. Make the report as indicated in the sample report below.

24. Sample report:

Patient: Doe, Mr. John

Date: 7-7-72

Physician: Dr. James Dunn

Platelet Count: 350,000

Method: Fonio method

Normal values: 150,000 to 400,000 per cu. mm.

Examination performed by: Sandra Frisbie

REES AND ECKER METHOD FOR THE PLATELET COUNT

NECESSARY REAGENTS AND EQUIPMENT

1. Bottle of Rees and Ecker solution (This solution may be sitting in the refrigerator or on the laboratory shelf. If none is available, prepare the solution by following the directions on page 697 of the Appendix.)
2. Filter paper and funnel (Fig. 151, page 424)
3. Finger tip blood or *fresh* anticoagulated blood
4. Red cell pipet
5. Counting chamber
6. Microscope

Procedure

1. Obtain a bottle of Rees and Ecker solution and a clean small test tube.

2. Filter about 15 drops of the Rees and Ecker solution into the small test tube (the method of folding a filter paper is illustrated in Fig. 151, page 424).

   Note: This filtering process is absolutely necessary. It removes crystals and other debris which may be mistaken for platelets.

3. Either fresh anticoagulated blood or finger tip blood may be used. If anticoagulated blood is used, it must not be over 1 hour old because the platelets disintegrate rapidly.

4. If fresh anticoagulated blood is to be used, assemble the following: the anticoagulated blood, a red cell pipet, and the filtered Rees and Ecker solution. Mix the blood. Suck up blood to the 0.5 mark on the red cell pipet. Suck up the filtered Rees and Ecker solution to the 101 mark. Shake the pipet a few seconds. Then proceed to step 10.

5. If finger tip blood is to be used, obtain a red cell pipet and the filtered Rees and Ecker solution.

6. Assemble the materials for a finger puncture: several cotton balls or gauze pads, 70% alcohol, and a sterile blood lancet.

7. Make a rather deep finger puncture, wipe away the first drop, and make the blood flow out of the puncture.

8. As the blood flows out of the puncture, suck up blood to the 0.5 mark on the red cell pipet.

9. Then suck up the filtered Rees and Ecker solution to the 101 mark on the red cell pipet. Shake the pipet a few seconds.

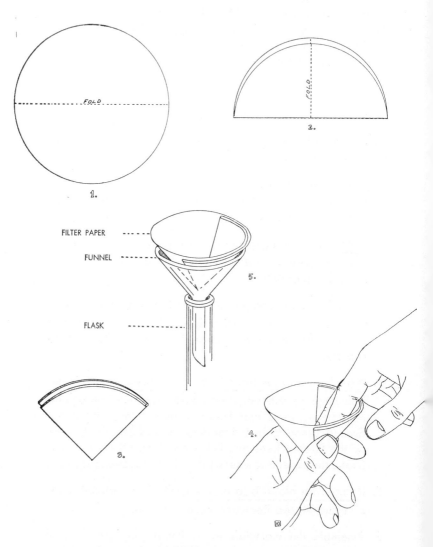

FILTER PAPER

FUNNEL

FLASK

FOLD

1.

2.

3.

4.

5.

FIG. 151.—Technique of folding a filter paper. (Seiverd, *Chemistry for Medical Technologists*, courtesy of C. V. Mosby Co.)

10. The remainder of the count should be completed within the next 30 minutes because the platelets disintegrate rapidly.

11. Thoroughly shake the pipet for 3 minutes.

12. Obtain a counting chamber which is used for the white cell count and red cell count.

13. Discard the first 4 drops from the pipet.

14. Charge either side of the counting chamber.

15. Put the counting chamber in a Petri dish. Moisten a piece of cotton with water and also put this in the Petri dish. Then cover the Petri dish. This decreases the evaporation.

16. Now let the preparation stand 5 minutes so the platelets can settle. Meanwhile, read the material below.

17. A platelet is a tiny glistening body about $\frac{1}{10}$ the size of a red cell. A heavy black circle has been drawn around a group of 3 platelets near the center of Figure 152.

    Note: The above illustration also contains 3 single platelets. Each single platelet is also surrounded by a heavy black circle. In the illustration, you would count and record 6 platelets.

18. After the 5 minutes have elapsed, remove the counting chamber from the Petri dish. Put the counting chamber on the stage of the microscope.

19. First bring the red cells into view with the $10 \times$ (16 mm.) objective. Then carefully switch to the $45 \times$ (4 mm.) objective.

20. Now lower the condenser to decrease the amount of light.

21. Using the fine adjustment, bring the cells into perfect focus.

22. The platelets are to be counted in the 5 "P" sections which are illustrated in Figure 153.

    Note: Each "P" section is the same as an "R" section which was used in the red cell count.

23. One "P" section, as you will see it through the $45 \times$ (4 mm.) objective, has been illustrated in Figure 152.

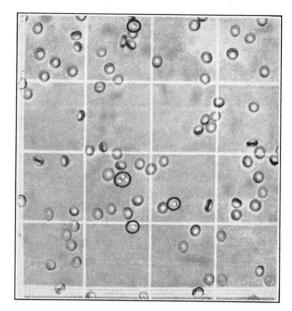

FIG. 152.—Platelets in one "P" section. A heavy black circle has been drawn around the platelets. Note the 3 platelets in a group near the center. Note the 3 single platelets. In the above illustration, you would count and record 6 platelets. The platelets were photographed through the 45× (4 mm.) objective of the microscope. (Courtesy of Mr. Cecil Gilliam.)

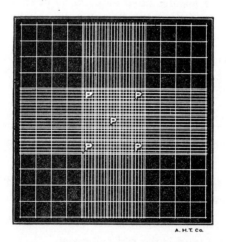

FIG. 153.—Sections of the counting chamber used in the platelet count. These 5 "P" sections are the same as the 5 "R" sections which were used for the red cell count.

24. Bring into view the "P" section in the upper left hand corner of the central ruled area (Fig. 153).

   Note: You can be sure you have the correct "P" section if the lines to the left and above the "P" section are not crossed or checkered.

25. Since the "P" section is the same as an "R" section, you will now have a microscopic field looking like Figure 152.

26. Slowly rotate the fine adjustment back and forth and look for tiny glistening objects that are about $\frac{1}{10}$ the size of red cells. These tiny glistening objects will become light and then dark as you rotate the fine adjustment back and forth. These tiny objects are platelets (Fig. 152).

   Note: Sometimes an object on the eyepiece of the microscope may resemble a platelet. To distinguish such objects from platelets, simply turn the eyepiece. If the object moves, it is on the eyepiece. Consequently, it is not a platelet.

27. If your platelet count is normal, you will see anywhere from 2 to 10 platelets in the entire "P" section.

28. When you search for platelets, you should: (1) Make sure your light is not too bright and (2) constantly rotate the fine adjustment back and forth.

29. Now count the platelets in this 1st "P" section and record the count.

30. Now move to the "P" section in the upper right hand corner of the heavily ruled area (Fig. 153).

   Note: This 2nd "P" section will be 4 large squares to the right. You can be sure you have the correct "P" section if the lines to the right and above the "P" section are not crossed or checkered.

31. Now count the platelets in this 2nd "P" section. Record the count.

32. Then count and record the platelets in the other 3 "P" sections which are illustrated in Figure 153.

33. When you have counted the platelets in the 5 "P" sections, add the 5 counts.

34. Thus, if your count is normal, you should have something like this:

Platelets in 1st "P" section = 4
Platelets in 2nd "P" section = 2
Platelets in 3rd "P" section = 6
Platelets in 4th "P" section = 10
Platelets in 5th "P" section = 8
            Total   30

35. If a total of 30 platelets were counted in the 5 "P" sections, the calculation is made as follows:

Total platelets   Dil. Cor.   Vol. cor.   Platelets
in 5 "P" sect. × factor × factor = in 1 cu. mm.
      30   ×   200   ×   50   = 300,000

36. The above dilution correction factor and volume correction factor are the same correction factors used in the red cell count and they have been derived in the same manner (page 170).

37. Using the above procedure, make the calculation for your platelet count.

Note: A short-cut method of making the calculation is to multiply your total count by 10,000 or "add 4 zeros." For example, if your total count was 30, you would "add 4 zeros" to 30 and get a count of 300,000.

38. Make the report as indicated in the sample report below.

39. Sample report:

> **Patient:** Doe, Mr. John
>
> **Date:** 7-7-72
>
> **Physician:** Dr. Paul Aubry
>
> **Platelet count:** 300,000
>
> **Method:** Rees and Ecker method
>
> **Normal values:** 150,000 to 400,000 per cu. mm.
>
> **Examination performed by:** Sandra Frisbie

40. Clean the pipet with the suction device used for cleaning the red and white cell pipets. If you wish to remove the blue stain, suck 70% alcohol into the pipet and allow to soak for a few hours.

BRECHER-CRONKITE METHOD FOR THE PLATELET COUNT

With an ordinary microscope, the platelets are identified on the basis of their size and shape. With a phase microscope, however, the platelets may be identified on the basis of their size, shape, and *structure*. This is made possible through a special arrangement of the optical system.

Consequently, with a phase microscope, the platelets may be easily identified and readily distinguished from debris, precipitated stain, and other foreign particles.

A phase microscope is used in the Brecher-Cronkite method of making a platelet count.

To make the platelet count by the Brecher-Cronkite method, you will need the special equipment listed below.

NECESSARY REAGENTS AND EQUIPMENT

1. Phase microscope equipped with a long working distance condenser, 43× annulus, 43× phase objective, and 10× oculars
2. Special counting chamber for phase microscope work
3. Special #1 coverslip to be used with the above counting chamber
4. Note: The above equipment may be obtained through your local medical supply house
5. Bottle of 1% ammonium oxalate solution. This solution is usually stored in the refrigerator. If it must be prepared, follow the directions in the section on solutions and reagents in the Appendix (page 695).

Procedure

1. Obtain the above equipment.
2. Obtain a bottle of 1% ammonium oxalate.
3. Filter about 2 cubic centimeters of the 1% ammonium oxalate solution into a clean medicine glass or a small test tube.
4. Either fresh anticoagulated blood or finger tip blood may be used. If anticoagulated blood is used, it should not be over 1 hour old because the platelets disintegrate rapidly.

   Note: In this test, the preferred anticoagulant is Sequestrene (EDTA) rather than ammonium and potassium oxalate. It is also preferable to use a siliconized syringe and siliconized serological test tube.

5. If fresh anticoagulated blood is to be used, proceed as follows: Obtain the anticoagulated blood and a red cell pipet. Mix the blood. Draw blood to the 0.5 mark in the red cell pipet. Draw the filtered 1% ammonium oxalate solution to the 101 mark. Shake the pipet for a few seconds. Then proceed to step 9.

6. If finger tip blood is to be used, proceed as follows: Obtain a red cell pipet and materials for a finger puncture: sterile lancet, 70% alcohol, and cotton balls or gauze pads.

7. Make a finger puncture and wipe away the first drop of blood.

8. Suck up blood to the 0.5 mark on the red cell pipet. Suck up the filtered 1% ammonium oxalate solution to the 101 mark. Shake the pipet for a few seconds.

9. Now shake the pipet thoroughly for 3 minutes. A mechanical shaker is preferred.

10. Discard the first 6 drops and charge the special counting chamber.

11. Put the counting chamber in a Petri dish. Moisten a piece of cotton with water and also put this in the Petri dish. Then cover the Petri dish. This decreases the evaporation.

12. Allow 15 minutes to elapse so the platelets can settle.

13. Then place the counting chamber on the stage of the phase microscope.

14. Using the 43× phase objective, bring the cells into view.

15. The platelets are round or oval bodies about $\frac{1}{10}$ the size of red cells (Fig. 154).

    Note: In the above illustration, some shadows of red cells may be seen in the background.

16. Now bring into view the "P" section in the upper left hand corner of the central ruled area (Fig. 153, page 426).

    Note: These 5 "P" sections in the above illustration are the same as the 5 "R" sections which are used in the red cell count.

17. Count the platelets in the "P" section.

18. Record the count.

19. Then count and record the platelets in the other 4 "P" sections which are illustrated in Figure 153, page 426.

20. Add the 5 counts.

21. If the 5 "P" sections had a total count of 30 platelets, the calculation is made as follows:

Total platelets   Dil. cor.   Vol. cor.   Platelets in
in 5 "P" sect. $\times$ factor $\times$ factor   = 1 cu. mm.

        30        $\times$ 200 $\times$ 50   = 300,000

22. The above dilution correction factor and volume correction factor are the same correction factors used in the red cell count and they have been derived in the same manner (page 170).

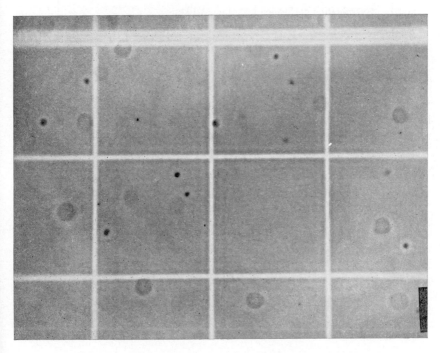

FIG. 154.—Platelets seen with the phase microscope. (Miale, J. B., *Laboratory Medicine—Hematology*, courtesy of C. V. Mosby Co.)

30

23. Using the above procedure, make the calculation for your platelet count.

Note: A short-cut method of making the calculation is to multiply your total count by 10,000 or "add 4 zeros." For example, 30 "plus 4 zeros" would make a count of 300,000.

24. Make the report as indicated in the sample report below.

25. Sample report:

Patient: Doe, Mr. John

Date: 7-7-72

Physician: Dr. Fred Meeker

Platelet count: 300,000

Method: Brecher-Cronkite method with phase microscope

Normal values: 150,000 to 400,000 per cu. mm.

Examination performed by: Lee Walker

SOURCES OF ERROR IN THE PLATELET COUNT

The platelet count is subject to an error of 10% to 20%. This error, however, is of little practical significance. Only wide deviations from the normal values are significant in diagnosis and therapy.

Errors in the platelet count may be caused by the following:

1. Squeezing the finger with heavy pressure to obtain the blood. (Heavy pressure may cause disintegration and agglutination of platelets, thus *decreasing* the count.)

2. Using dirty test tubes, pipets, or counting chamber. (Dirty glassware enables the platelets to stick to the dirt, thus *decreasing* the count.)

3. Using unfiltered diluting fluid. (Unfiltered diluting fluid contains debris and precipitated stain which may be mistaken for platelets, thus *increasing* the count.)

Chapter 20

Clot Retraction Time

The clot retraction time is also referred to as the clot-retraction time, clot retraction test, and measurement of clot retraction.

The clot retraction time will be discussed under the following headings:

>Significance of the Clot Retraction Time
>Discussion of Procedures for the Clot Retraction Time
>Single Tube Method for the Clot Retraction Time

The student review questions for the clot retraction time are numbered 234–238 and begin on page 751 of the Appendix.

SIGNIFICANCE OF THE CLOT RETRACTION TIME

The clot retraction time measures the ability of the blood clot to retract.

In normal blood, the clot reacts as follows: After 2 hours, there is partial retraction of the clot. After 24 hours, there is complete retraction of the clot (Fig. 155).

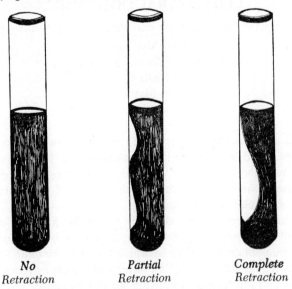

No
Retraction

Partial
Retraction

Complete
Retraction

FIG. 155.—Retraction of the blood clot.

433

When the platelet count is decreased, the clot retraction time is increased. Consequently, the platelets apparently play a major role in the retraction of the clot.

The clot retraction time is mainly used in the diagnosis of the hemorrhagic diseases. In purpura hemorrhagica, for example, the clot retraction time is greatly increased.   In a severe case, there is no retraction of the clot—even after 24 hours.

The clot retraction time is increased in those conditions listed in Table 31.

Table 31

Conditions Accompanied by an Increased Clot Retraction Time

thrombocytopenia
purpura hemorrhagica (idiopathic thrombocytopenic purpura)
Glanzmann's disease (hereditary hemorrhagic thrombasthenia)
aplastic anemia
acute leukemia
multiple myeloma
Hodgkin's disease
polycythemia

The clot retraction time is seldom requested. It is only performed about twice a month in the average hospital laboratory. And it is only run about once a year in the average physician's office.

DISCUSSION OF PROCEDURES FOR THE CLOT RETRACTION TIME

The clot retraction time may be performed by the following methods:

Single Tube Method
Macfarlane Serum Method
Tocantins Method
Budtz-Olsen Method
Stefanini-Dameshek Method

The single tube method is performed by withdrawing about 5 cubic centimeters of blood from the patient, transferring the blood to a test tube, placing the test tube in a 37° C. water bath, recording the degree of clot retraction after 2 hours, and recording the degree of clot retraction and appearance of the clot after 24 hours.

The Macfarlane serum method is performed by withdrawing 5 cubic centimeters of blood from the patient, transferring the blood to a graduated centrifuge tube containing a wire to which the clot can cling, placing the graduated centrifuge tube in a 37° C. water bath, allowing several hours to pass until the clot has formed, removing the clot by simply lifting the wire from the graduated centrifuge tube, reading the volume of serum in the graduated centrifuge tube, and calculating the percentage of serum as follows:

Calculation

$$\frac{\text{volume of serum obtained}}{\text{volume of blood used}} \times 100 = \text{per cent serum}$$

Example

$$\frac{3 \text{ cc.}}{5 \text{ cc.}} \times 100 = 60\% \text{ serum}$$

Normal Values

44% to 64% serum

The Tocantins, Budtz-Olsen, and Stefanini-Dameshek methods for the clot retraction time are not widely used and fall outside the realm of routine laboratory examinations.

The single tube method and Macfarlane serum method are widely used; however, these methods have undergone various modifications.

The single tube method for the clot retraction time is given on the following pages.

SINGLE TUBE METHOD FOR THE CLOT RETRACTION TIME

NECESSARY REAGENTS AND EQUIPMENT

1. One plain serological test tube (without anticoagulant)
2. Stopper for serological test tube
3. Materials for a venipuncture
4. 37° C. water bath or 37° C. incubator

Procedure

1. Obtain a plain serological test tube (without anticoagulant), a stopper for the serological test tube, and materials for a venipuncture: sterile 20 gauge needle, 10 cc. syringe, wax marking pencil, tourniquet, 70% alcohol, and cotton balls or gauze pads.

2. Write the patient's name on the test tube.

3. Make a venipuncture, withdraw about 5 cc. of blood, remove the needle from the syringe, and transfer the blood to the test tube.

4. Put the stopper in the mouth of the test tube.

5. Place the test tube in either a 37° C. water bath or a 37° C. incubator and allow 2 hours to elapse.

6. After 2 hours have elapsed, observe the clot.

7. Record your observation as <u>no retraction, partial retrac-tion,</u> or <u>complete retraction</u> (see Fig. 155, page 433).

    Note: Sometimes normal blood forms a clot in which the entire outer edges cling to the walls of the test tube. In such a clot, any retraction is not noticeable. Therefore, if the clot is sticking to the walls of the test tube, loosen it with a wooden applicator stick.

8. Put the test tube back in the 37° C. water bath or 37° C. incubator and allow 22 hours to elapse.

9. After the 22 hours have elapsed, make the following 2 examinations:

10. Examination #1: Observe the retraction of the clot. Record as <u>no retraction, partial retraction,</u> or <u>complete retraction</u> (see Fig. 155, page 433).

11. Examination #2: Observe the appearance of the clot. Record as firm or soft.

    Note: In normal blood, the clot is firm. In the presence of fibrinolysins or a deficiency of fibrinogen, the clot may be soft or partially dissolved.

12. Make your report as indicated in the sample report below.

13. Sample report:

Patient: Doe, Mr. John

Date: 7-7-72

Physician: Dr. James Mason

Clot retraction time:
        After 2 hours: partial retraction
        After 24 hours: complete retraction
        Appearance of clot: firm

Method: single tube method

Normal values: partial retraction after 2 hrs.
                  complete retraction after 24 hrs.
                  clot is firm

Examination performed by: Pat Eldridge

Chapter 21

Fibrinogen Deficiency Test

The fibrinogen deficiency test is also referred to by the following terms: plasma fibrinogen test, plasma fibrinogen titer, assay of fibrinogen, measurement of fibrinogen, test for afibrinogenemia, and test for hypofibrinogenemia.

The fibrinogen deficiency test will be discussed under the following headings:

Significance of the Fibrinogen Deficiency Test
Discussion of Procedures for the Fibrinogen Deficiency Test
Warner-Lambert Method for the Fibrinogen Deficiency Test
Fi-Test Method for the Fibrinogen Deficiency Test

The student review questions for the fibrinogen deficiency test are numbered 239–241 and begin on page 751 of the Appendix.

SIGNIFICANCE OF THE FIBRINOGEN DEFICIENCY TEST

Fibrinogen is a protein substance which is produced by the liver. It is used in the clotting of blood. During the clotting process, the fibrinogen is converted to fibrin.

The fibrinogen in the blood may be measured by the fibrinogen deficiency test.

The fibrinogen deficiency test has the normal values of 200 to 400 milligrams per 100 milliliters of plasma.

Values below normal may be expected in those conditions listed in Table 32.

Table 32

Conditions Accompanied by a Deficiency of Fibrinogen

congenital afibrinogenemia	presence of fibrinolysins
congenital hypofibrinogenemia	metastatic carcinoma
severe liver damage	acute granulocytic leukemia
during or following surgery	severe burns
severe hemorrhage	during intravascular clotting
complications during pregnancy	anaphylactic shock
abortion	scurvy

The fibrinogen deficiency test is mainly used in the diagnosis and treatment of the hemorrhagic diseases.

The fibrinogen deficiency test may also be useful during surgical hemorrhage or obstetrical bleeding. In such cases, a deficiency of fibrinogen may pinpoint an abnormality in the clotting mechanism and thereby enable corrective measures to be taken. Consequently, the fibrinogen deficiency test may sometimes be ordered as an emergency procedure.

The fibrinogen deficiency test is performed about 10 times a month by the average hospital laboratory and about 1 a month by the average physician's office.

DISCUSSION OF PROCEDURES FOR THE FIBRINOGEN DEFICIENCY TEST

The fibrinogen deficiency test may be performed by the following methods:

Screening Methods
1. Warner-Lambert method
2. Fi-Test method
3. Fibrindex method
4. Heat and Turbidity method

Quantitative Methods
1. Titration method
2. Colorimetric methods
3. Coagulation Analyzer method

The screening methods are rather simple methods which are generally performed by obtaining blood or plasma, adding a reagent, and inspecting the preparation for agglutination or clotting.

The quantitative methods are more involved procedures and they are usually performed in the chemistry department.

The screening methods make a rough estimation of fibrinogen whereas the quantitative methods make an exact determination of fibrinogen.

A rough estimation of fibrinogen, obtained from the screening methods, is sufficient for most clinical purposes.

We will present the following screening methods:

Warner-Lambert Method
Fi-Test Method

WARNER-LAMBERT METHOD FOR THE FIBRINOGEN DEFICIENCY TEST

This screening method for fibrinogen deficiency is performed by preparing plasma and adding physiological saline, adding this mixture to a solution of calcium and thromboplastin, observing the formation of a clot, and recording the time.

In this procedure, the calcium and thromboplastin are contained in the Simplastin reagent.

The procedure is given below.*

REAGENTS

Simplastin®
Pooled normal plasma or Diagnostic Plasma—
Warner-Chilcott

LIMITS OF THE TEST

1. Sufficient fibrinogen
2. Border line fibrinogen
3. Low fibrinogen

PERFORMING THE TEST

1. Draw a blood sample to obtain plasma following the procedure used to obtain plasma for a one-stage prothrombin assay.

2. Add 0.1 ml. plasma to 0.7 ml. 0.85 percent sodium chloride (physiological saline) and mix thoroughly.†

3. Blow 0.1 ml. of the diluted plasma into 0.2 ml. Simplastin which has been measured into a 10 × 75 mm. test tube.

4. Allow mixture to stand for 5 minutes at room temperature.

5. A the end of the 5 minute incubation period, observe clot formation by gently tilting tube to a horizontal position. Do not shake the tube or tilt repeatedly.

Note: The five-minute incubation period allows possible low prothrombin in the tested specimen to form sufficient thrombin to convert fibrinogen into fibrin. With prothrombin levels as low as 1 percent of normal, valid fibrinogen levels will be found.

* This procedure has been reproduced from the "Seminar on the Coagulation of Blood." It is presented through the courtesy of General Diagnostics Division, Warner-Lambert Pharmaceutical Company, Morris Plains, N. J.

† Because fibrinogen deficiencies in whole plasma do not become evident by clotting procedures until the fibrinogen level is 15 per cent of normal or less, this test is performed on plasma dilutions of 12.5 per cent.

INTERPRETATION

1. Solid or large sliding clot—sufficient fibrinogen.

2. Moderate sized sliding clot with some liquid—borderline fibrinogen.

3. Small clot to fibrin strands—low fibrinogen.

4. No visible sign of fibrin formation—very low fibrinogen. (To determine the size of the clot, compare the test to the control tubes.)

PLASMA CONTROL

Prepare the following dilutions of plasma in 0.85 percent sodium chloride (physiological saline):

Plasma	0.85 percent Sodium Chloride	
0.1 ml. plus	1.5 ml.	= sufficient fibrinogen
0.1 ml. plus	2.3 ml.	= borderline fibrinogen
0.1 ml. plus	3.1 ml.	= borderline fibrinogen
0.1 ml. plus	4.7 ml.	= low fibrinogen

1. Blow 0.1 ml. of each of the diluted plasma samples into 0.2 ml. amounts of Simplastin which have been measured into 10×75 mm. test tubes.

2. Allow the mixtures to stand for 5 minutes at room temperature.

3. At the end of the 5 minute incubation period, observe clot formation in the same manner as with the sample being tested. It is helpful to have the control sample running simultaneously with the patient's sample.

WARNING

It is essential in this test for the reagents to be absolutely free of fibrinolysin. If they are not, the clot will be partially or totally dissolved and erroneous results will be reported.

FI-TEST METHOD FOR THE FIBRINOGEN DEFICIENCY TEST*

Hyland FI-TEST® is a rapid slide screening test providing a simplified bedside or operating room procedure to screen for hypofibrinogenemia. The test utilizes 1 drop of heparinized whole blood obtained by finger prick and a reagent prepared from polystyrene latex. The reagent has been processed to give rapid and clear-cut reactions, distinguishing normal plasma fibrinogen levels from abnormally low levels (below 100 mg/100 ml). Sufficient materials are provided in each test package to perform 6 tests.

MATERIALS AND STORAGE

1. FI-TEST Latex Anti-Human Fibrinogen Reagent with dropper cap, 1 ml. Store between 2° C. and 8° C. Sodium azide, 0.1%, has been added as a preservative. Mix thoroughly before each use.
2. FI-TEST Glycine-Saline Buffer Diluent with dropper cap, six 3-ml vials. Store between 2° C. and 8° C.
3. FI-TEST Normal Control with dropper cap, 1 ml. Store between 2° C. and 8° C. Sodium azide, 0.1%, has been added as a preservative.
4. Six sterile, disposable blood lancets.
5. Six printed card slides.
6. Heparinized capillary pipets, one vial of 8.
7. One rubber bulb.
8. Toothpicks.

PERFORMANCE OF TEST

1. Bring test reagents to room temperature before use.

2. Using a capillary pipet, transfer 1 drop of heparinized whole blood specimen to one of the bottles of Glycine-Saline Buffer Diluent and mix by shaking.

3. Using the buffer dropper cap, place 1 drop of diluted blood specimen in a circle on one of the printed card slides

4. Using the Normal Control dropper cap, place 1 drop of Normal Control in the other oval on the same slide.

5. Mix Latex Anti-Human Fibrinogen Reagent thoroughly by shaking gently, and add 2 drops to each oval, using the dropper cap provided.

* Courtesy of Hyland, Division Travenol Laboratories, Inc., Los Angeles, Calif.

6. Mix reactants with separate toothpicks or wooden applicator sticks over an area approximately 20 × 25 mm. (most of the area within the oval).

7. Tilt card slowly from side to side for 15 to 20 seconds and observe for macroscopic agglutination.

INTERPRETATION

Agglutination in a degree comparable to that shown by the Normal Control: Normal plasma fibrinogen levels (250 to 400 mg/100 ml.) (See Note 1.)

No agglutination: Hypofibrinogenemia (plasma fibrinogen levels of 100 mg/100 ml or less).

NOTE

1. It has been reported that under unusual circumstances (e.g., fibrinolysis) the test may give falsely normal fibrinogen levels due to reaction with fibrinogen and/or fibrin breakdown products, rather than with clottable fibrinogen.[1,2]

References

1. Fletcher, A. P., Alkjaersig, N., Fisher, S., and Sherry, S.: The proteolysis of fibrinogen by plasmin: The identification of thrombin-clottable fibrinogen derivatives which polymerize abnormally. J. Lab. Clin. Med. **68**:780–802 (Nov.), 1966.
2. Bloom, A. L., and Campbell, N.: Defibrination syndrome with defective thrombin-fibrinogen reaction reversible by protamine. J. Clin. Pathol. **18**:786–789 (Nov.), 1965.

Chapter 22

Prothrombin Time

The prothrombin time is also referred to by the following terms: P T, pro time, prothrombin time test, P. T. test, and plasma prothrombin time.

The prothrombin time will be discussed under the following headings:

Significance of the Prothrombin Time
Discussion of Procedures for the Prothrombin Time
Exercises in Pipetting for the Beginner
Manual Method for Quick's One-Stage Prothrombin Time
Sources of Error in the Prothrombin Time

The student review questions for the prothrombin time are numbered 242–249 and begin on page 752 of the Appendix.

SIGNIFICANCE OF THE PROTHROMBIN TIME

Prothrombin is a protein substance which is produced by the liver. It is used in the clotting of blood. During the clotting process, the prothrombin is converted to thrombin.

What is the prothrombin time?

You will recall that the plasma of the blood contains many coagulation factors, among them being prothrombin, Factor V, Factor VII, and Factor X. The clotting ability of these combined plasma coagulation factors is referred to as the prothrombin time.

Thus, although the prothrombin time does not isolate and directly measure prothrombin, the test has become a suitable clinical means of determining the presence and functioning ability of prothrombin.

How is the prothrombin time performed?

The prothrombin time is performed by obtaining blood and preparing plasma. The plasma, of course, contains the prothrombin. The plasma is added to a mixture of calcium and thromboplastin. A clot forms. The time interval between the addition of the plasma and the appearance of the clot is called the prothrombin time.

In the above procedure, what is the purpose of the calcium?

The first step in the preparation of plasma is to add blood to an anti-coagulant. The anticoagulant removes calcium. Since calcium is one of the essential factors in coagulation, it must be restored to the system.

In the above procedure, what is the function of the thromboplastin?

The plasma contains prothrombin. In order for a clot to form, the prothrombin must be converted to thrombin. This conversion—prothrombin to thrombin—is assisted by thromboplastin.

The normal values for the prothrombin time are 11 to 16 seconds.

The prothrombin time is increased in those conditions listed in Table 33.

Table 33

Conditions Accompanied by an Increased Prothrombin Time

Dicumarol therapy	Factor VII deficiency
heparin therapy	Factor X deficiency
Panwarfin therapy	vitamin K deficiency
fibrinogen deficiency	hemorrhagic disease of the newborn
prothrombin deficiency	some liver diseases
Factor V deficiency	presence of circulating anticoagulants

The prothrombin time is often used in the diagnosis of disease. It finds even more extensive use, however, during the treatment of blood clots. A brief discussion follows.

When a patient has a blood clot, he receives a series of treatments with an anticoagulant such as Dicumarol or heparin. These anticoagulants delay coagulation. In so doing, they prevent the expansion of existing blood clots and hinder the formation of new blood clots.

Since the anticoagulant delays coagulation, it causes the prothrombin time to rise above the normal values of 11 to 16 seconds.

The prothrombin time, however, must be maintained within an "effective range." The effective range is usually considered to be 28 to 40 seconds.

What happens if the prothrombin time drops below the effective range of 28 to 40 seconds?

If the prothrombin time drops below 28 seconds, the treatment may be ineffective. For example, old clots may expand or new clots may form.

What happens if the prothrombin time rises above the effective range of 28 to 40 seconds?

If the prothrombin time rises above 40 seconds, the patient may hemorrhage. This could be serious—even fatal.

How is the prothrombin time maintained at the effective range of 28 to 40 seconds?

The prothrombin time is maintained at the effective range of 28 to 40 seconds by the following procedure:

1. A prothrombin time is run at frequent intervals. The usual practice is to run a prothrombin time each day.
2. After the prothrombin time is determined, the dosage of anticoagulant is adjusted:

3. If the prothrombin time is below 28 seconds, the dosage of anticoagulant is increased.
4. If the prothrombin time is above 40 seconds, the dosage of anticoagulant is decreased

Thus, the prothrombin time is a valuable test. It saves many lives. But it must be performed with extreme care and diligence.

In this test, perhaps more than any other, the health and welfare of a patient lies directly in the hands of a technologist.

The prothrombin time is frequently requested. It is performed about 600 times a month by the average hospital laboratory. And it is run about 10 times a month by the average physician's office.

DISCUSSION OF PROCEDURES FOR THE PROTHROMBIN TIME

The prothrombin time may be performed by either the one-stage procedure or the two-stage procedure.

The one-stage procedure is performed by withdrawing blood, centrifuging to obtain the plasma, adding plasma to a mixture of calcium and thromboplastin, recording the time, allowing the mixture to clot, and recording the time.

The two-stage procedure is performed by withdrawing blood and centrifuging to obtain the plasma; (stage 1) adding plasma to a solution of calcium and thromboplastin; (stage 2) removing samples of this mixture at various time intervals, adding the samples to a series of fibrinogen solutions, allowing the solutions to clot, and recording the time.

The one-stage procedure is simpler and more widely used than the two-stage procedure.

The one-stage procedure is usually performed as directed by Dr. A. J. Quick. This procedure is generally referred to as Quick's one-stage prothrombin time.

Quick's one-stage prothrombin time may be performed by the methods listed below.

MANUAL METHODS
1. Tilt tube method
2. Wire loop method

AUTOMATED METHODS
1. Fibrometer method
2. Hemolab method
3. Clotex method
4. Emdeco method
5. Electra 500 method
6. Hemochron method
7. Thrombitron method

The manual method for Quick's one-stage prothrombin time is given on the following pages.

To perform the manual method, however, the student must be able to pipet.

If the student is already familiar with pipetting, he can skip the following exercises in pipetting and go directly to the procedure (page 453).

If the student has not learned to pipet, he should first perform the following exercises in pipetting and then turn to the procedure.

EXERCISES IN PIPETTING FOR THE BEGINNER

These exercises should be performed by students who have not learned to pipet. The exercises will take about 30 minutes.

In pipetting, volume may be referred to in two ways. One way is to use the term cc. This stands for cubic centimeter. The other way is to use the term ml. This stands for milliliter.

For all practical purposes, one cubic centimeter equals one milliliter. Thus, one textbook may direct you to add 5 cc. of a reagent and another textbook may direct you to add 5 ml. of the reagent. In either case, you would be adding the same quantity of the reagent.

A note of precaution for beginners: *Never use the same pipet to measure two different reagents.* For example, never use a pipet to measure 5 milliliters of an acid and then use the same pipet to measure 5 milliliters of a base.

NECESSARY EQUIPMENT

1. A 5 milliliter serological pipet (Fig. 156)
2. A 1 milliliter serological pipet graduated in hundreds (Fig. 156)
3. A 2 milliliter volumetric pipet (Fig. 156)
4. A 400 milliliter beaker (Fig. 157)
5. Either a 50 milliliter or 100 milliliter graduate (Fig. 157)
6. An 0.1 milliliter micro pipet (Fig. 156)
7. 5 serological test tubes (Fig. 47, page 84)

Procedure

1. Obtain a 5 milliliter serological pipet, a 1 milliliter serological pipet graduated in hundreds, and a 2 milliliter volumetric pipet (Fig. 156).

2. Obtain a 400 milliliter beaker and either a 50 milliliter or 100 milliliter graduate (Fig. 157).

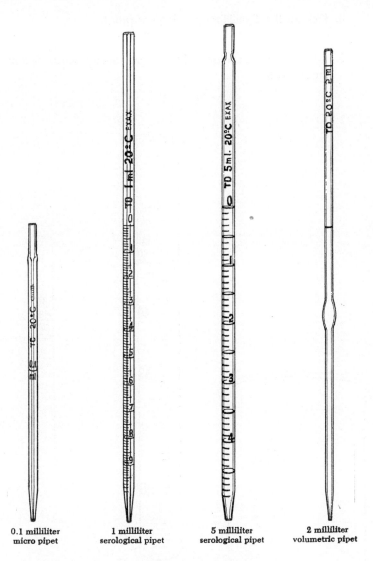

0.1 milliliter   1 milliliter   5 milliliter   2 milliliter
micro pipet   serological pipet   serological pipet   volumetric pipet

Fig. 156.—Pipets used in hematology.

3. Add water to the beaker until it is about half full.

4. Pick up the 5 milliliter serological pipet.

5. Observe the technique of pipetting which is illustrated in Figure 158.

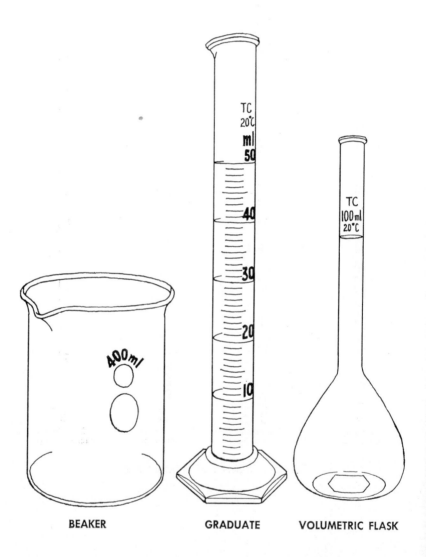

Fig. 157.—Beaker, graduate, and volumetric flask.

6. Using your 5 milliliter pipet, suck up water until it is a little bit above the "0" mark. Quickly put the index finger of your right hand over the opening in the top of the pipet. This holds the water in the pipet.

Note: If your index finger is wet, it is difficult to control the flow of fluid. Therefore, try to keep your index finger dry.

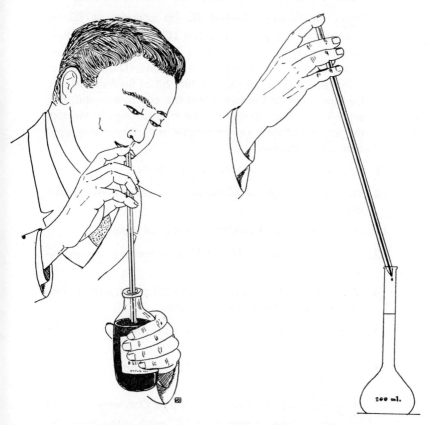

FIG. 158.—Technique of pipetting with a serological pipet. (Seiverd, *Chemistry for Medical Technologists*, courtesy of C. V. Mosby Co.)

1. Suck up fluid until it is a little above the "O" mark.
2. Quickly put your index finger over the top of the pipet.
3. By controlling the flow with your index finger, allow the fluid to drain to the "O" mark.
4. When the fluid reaches the "O" mark, press down firmly with your index finger. This holds the fluid on the "O" mark.
5. Then transfer the pipet to a container.
6. And allow the fluid to drain to the desired mark.

7. Controlling the flow with your index finger, allow the water to drain to the "0" mark. When the water reaches the "0" mark, press down with your index finger to hold the water on the "0" mark.

8. Now transfer the pipet to the graduate. Hold the tip of the pipet against the inside wall of the graduate. Then release the pressure on your index finger and allow the water to run down the inside wall of the graduate.

   Note: Pipets are labelled TC (to contain) or TD (to deliver). If a pipet is labelled TC, the tiny bit of fluid remaining in the tip should be blown out of the pipet into the container. If a pipet is labelled TD and has 1 or 2 frosted rings at the top, the tiny bit of fluid should also be blown out of the pipet into the container. But, if a pipet is labelled TD and has no frosted rings at the top, the tiny bit of fluid should remain in the tip of the pipet and be discarded.

9. Repeat the above process 4 more times.

10. You should now have 25 milliliters of water in the graduate.

11. Now pick up the 1 milliliter serological pipet.

12. In a similar manner, add 1 milliliter of water to the graduate.

13. Using the same 1 milliliter serological pipet, add 4 more milliliters of water to the graduate.

14. You should now have 30 milliliters of water in the graduate.

15. Using the 5 milliliter serological pipet, add 2 milliliters of water to the graduate.

   Note: This may be done in two ways: One way is to suck up water a little bit above the "0" mark, allow the water to drain to the "0" mark, transfer the pipet to the graduate, and allow the water to drain to the "2" mark. The other way is to suck up water a little bit above the "3" mark, allow the water to drain to the "3" mark, transfer the pipet to the graduate, and allow the entire contents to drain out of the pipet.

16. Using the 5 milliliter serological pipet, add 3 milliliters of water to the graduate.

17. You should now have 35 milliliters of water in the graduate.

18. Pick up the 2 milliliter volumetric pipet. Observe the mark or circle just above the bulb of the pipet. This mark or circle is the 2 milliliter mark.

19. Now suck up water until it is just a little bit above the 2 milliliter mark, allow the water to drain to the 2 milliliter mark, and then press down with your index finger to hold the water on the 2 milliliter mark.

20. Put the tip of the pipet against the inside wall of the graduate and allow the water to drain out of the pipet.

21. Using the same 2 milliliter volumetric pipet, add 2 more milliliters of water to the graduate.

22. Now again pick up the 1 milliliter serological pipet.

23. Using the 1 milliliter serological pipet, add 0.5 milliliter of water to the graduate.

    Note: You can do this two ways: One way is to suck up water to the "0" mark, transfer the pipet to the graduate, and let the water drain to the ".5" mark. The other way is to suck up water to the ".5" mark, transfer the pipet to the graduate, and let the entire contents drain out of the pipet.

24. Now add 0.1 milliliter of water to the graduate.

    Note: The best way to do this is to suck up water to the "0" mark, transfer the pipet to the graduate, and allow the water to drain to the ".1" mark.

25. Now add 0.4 milliliter of water to the graduate.

    Note: The best way to do this is to suck up water to the "0" mark, transfer the pipet to the graduate, and allow the water to drain to the ".4" mark.

26. You should now have 40 milliliters of water in the graduate.

27. Discard the water in the graduate

28. Now get 4 serological test tubes.

29. Pick up the 1 millilter serological pipe .

30. Now proceed as follows:

31. Suck up water to the "0" mark on the 1 milliliter serological pipet.

32. Transfer the tip of the pipet to the bottom of a serological test tube. Allow the water to drain to the ".2" mark.

33. Now transfer the tip of the pipet to the bottom of another serological test tube. Allow the water to drain to the ".4" mark.

34. Now transfer the tip of the pipet to the bottom of another serological test tube. Allow the water to drain to the ".6" mark.

35. Now transfer the tip of the pipet to the bottom of another serological test tube. Allow the water to drain to the ".8" mark.

36. Discard the 0.2 milliliter of water remaining in the pipet.

37. You should now, of course, have 0.2 milliliter of water in each serological test tube.

38. Obtain an 0.1 milliliter micro pipet (Fig. 156, page 447).

39. The 0.1 milliliter micro pipet holds only 0.1 milliliter. This pipet is calibrated TC (to contain). In other words, the entire contents of this pipet must always be blown out. The 0.1 milliliter micro pipet is used in the determination of the prothrombin time.

40. Get another serological test tube.

41. Using the 0.1 milliliter micro pipet, suck up water to the "0.1" mark.

42. Transfer the tip of the pipet almost to the bottom of the serological test tube.

43. Now forcibly blow out the contents into the serological test tube.

44. Using the same pipet and test tube, repeat the above procedure 4 more times. Thus, you should have 0.5 milliliter of water in the serological test tube.

45. Using the same equipment, repeat this entire exercise 3 more times, beginning on page 446.

46. Note: You should never use the same pipet to transfer two different reagents.

MANUAL METHOD FOR QUICK'S ONE-STAGE PROTHROMBIN TIME

NECESSARY REAGENTS AND EQUIPMENT

For the convenience of the instructor and the future reference of the student, the necessary reagents and equipment for the prothrombin time are listed below.

The first 6 items listed below are used in the preparation of plasma.

These first 6 items will not be necessary if the instructor obtains the plasma and allows the students to start with Step 2 (see note for instructor on page 454).

Items to Prepare Plasma

1. 0.1 M (molar) sodium oxalate solution. This is a 1.34% solution of sodium oxalate. Directions for preparing this solution may be found in the Appendix on page 698.
2. One 10 cc. or 15 cc. graduated centrifuge tube. This is optional. You may use a serological test tube in place of this.
3. One 5 milliliter serological pipet. This is not necessary if you use a graduated centrifuge tube to prepare the plasma.
4. Materials for a venipuncture: sterile 20 gauge needle, 10 cc. syringe, tourniquet, 70% alcohol, cotton balls or gauze pads, and wax marking pencil.
5. Centrifuge.
6. One 2 milliliter volumetric pipet. This is not necessary if you use a medicine dropper to transfer the plasma.

Items to Perform Test

1. Normal plasma to be used as the control. Normal plasma is known and sold under various trade names. Among the more commonly used brands are the following: Diagnostic Plasma, Normal Plasma Control, Solu-Trol, and Standardized Normal Plasma.
2. Thromboplastin reagent. The thromboplastin reagent is known and sold under various trade names. Among the more commonly used brands are the following: Simplastin, Calsoplastin, Solu-Plastin, Activated Thromboplastin (Dade).
3. Two 1 milliliter serological pipets graduated in hundreds.
4. Four 0.1 milliliter micro pipets.
5. Wax marking pencil.

6. 10 serological test tubes. In place of these test tubes, you may use Kahn tubes (small tubes about 3 inches in length).
7. One 37° C. water bath. If this is not available, you can improvise by getting a 400 milliliter beaker, adding water until it is about one third full, putting a thermometer in the beaker, and heating the water to 37° C. During the test, the temperature should not rise above 39° C. nor drop below 35° C.
8. Large clock with a second hand or a stop watch.
9. #22 nichrome wire loop. This is not necessary if the tilt tube method is used to determine the end-point.

PROCEDURE

The procedure for the prothrombin time is broken down into 5 steps:

Step 1: Preparing the Patient's Plasma
Step 2: Preparing the Control Plasma
Step 3: Preparing the Thromboplastin Reagent
Step 4: Performing the Test
Step 5: Reporting the Test

The above 5 steps are considered in detail on the following pages.

Note to Instructor

In schools having a large enrollment, it is suggested that the instructor prepare the patient's plasma and start the students on Step 2: Preparing the Control Plasma.

Instead of actually preparing the patient's plasma, however, the instructor may purchase some control plasma (Diagnostic Plasma, Solu-Trol, or any other brand name). This, of course, is normal plasma. It may be used in place of the patient's plasma.

The instructor may also dilute this control plasma with physiological saline and use such preparations as "unknowns." For example, 0.2 milliliter of normal plasma plus 0.8 milliliter of physiological saline will make an "unknown" plasma having a prothrombin time of approximately 30 seconds.

The instructor may issue the "unknowns" to students and thereby check the accuracy of their technique.

STEP 1: PREPARING THE PATIENT'S PLASMA

1. Obtain a bottle of 0.1 M (molar) sodium oxalate. This bottle may also be labelled 1.34% sodium oxalate.

   Note: This solution is usually sitting on the laboratory shelf or in the refrigerator. The solution should be clear; it should not contain any precipitate. If it must be prepared, follow the directions on page 698 of the Appendix.

2. Get a 15 cc. graduated centrifuge tube or a serological test tube.

   Note: The 15 cc. graduated centrifuge tube is usually used. However, these tubes sometimes break during the process of centrifuging the blood.

3. If you are using a 15 cc. graduated centrifuge tube, you will not have to put a 5 cc. mark on the tube because it is already graduated in cubic centimeters. Therefore, skip the next step and proceed to step 5 below.

4. If you are using a serological test tube, put a 5 cc. mark on the test tube as follows: Get another serological test tube of equal size. Using a 5 milliliter serological pipet, add exactly 5 milliliters of water to this 2nd test tube. Get a wax marking pencil. Hold the 2 serological test tubes together and brace their bottoms on the table. Observe the 5 cc. level of water in the 2nd test tube. Now put a mark on the 1st test tube indicating the 5 cc. level. This 5 cc. level, of course, will be indicated by the 5 cc. level of water in the 2nd test tube.

5. Get a 1 milliliter serological pipet.

6. Add exactly 0.5 milliliter (not 0.1 milliliter!) of 0.1 M sodium oxalate to your 15 cc. graduated centrifuge tube or serological test tube.

7. Obtain the materials for a venipuncture: sterile 20 gauge needle, 10 cc. syringe, tourniquet, 70% alcohol, cotton balls or gauze pads, and wax marking pencil.

8. Write the patient's name on the test tube containing the 0.5 milliliter of 0.1 M sodium oxalate.

9. Make a venipuncture and withdraw a little more than 5 cc. of blood.

10. Remove the needle from the syringe.

11. Put the neck of the syringe in the test tube containing the 0.5 milliliter of sodium oxalate.

12. Add blood to the test tube until you reach the 5 cc. level.

   Note: This measurement must be exact. The test tube must contain 0.5 milliliter of the sodium oxalate and 4.5 cc. of blood. Some technologists prefer to measure the 4.5 cc. of blood by putting several cotton balls or gauze pads over the neck of the syringe, holding the syringe with the tip pointing upward, and forcing blood out until they reach the 4.5 cc. level on the syringe.

13. To prevent the blood from clotting, quickly proceed with the following:

14. Put a stopper in the mouth of the test tube. Do not shake the test tube. But mix the blood and sodium oxalate by completely inverting the test tube 8 to 10 times.

15. Within the next 30 minutes, centrifuge the blood at 2000 RPM (revolutions per minute) for 10 minutes.

16. When the blood has centrifuged for 10 minutes, remove the test tube from the centrifuge.

17. Obtain the plasma by either one of the following methods:
   Method 1:
   Using a clean dry medicine dropper, suction up the plasma and transfer about 1 milliliter to a serological test tube. The plasma should not contain any red cells. If it does, it must be centrifuged for 5 minutes at 2000 RPM. Then it must be poured into another serological test tube.
   Method 2:
   Get a 2 milliliter volumetric pipet. Observe the technique of removing the plasma which is illustrated in Figure 159.   Note that the index finger of the left hand is braced on both the pipet and the lip of the test tube. This prevents the pipet from slipping into the red cells. In the manner illustrated in Figure 159, suck up about 1 milliliter of the plasma. Transfer the plasma to a serological test tube. The plasma should not contain any red cells. If it does, it must be centrifuged for 5 minutes at 2000 RPM.   Then it must be poured into another serological test tube.

18. After you have transferred the plasma to a serological test tube, label the test tube Patient's Plasma.

19. If you are going to perform the test within the next few minutes, put the test tube containing the patient's plasma in a 37° C. water bath.

    Note: If a water bath is not available, you can improvise by getting a 400 milliliter beaker, adding water until it is about one third full, putting a thermometer in the water, and heating the water to 37° C. During the test, the water should not rise above 39° C. nor drop below 35° C.

20. If you are not going to perform the test within the next few minutes, the plasma may be stored in the refrigerator (4° C.) for a maximum of 4 hours. Upon removal from the refrigerator, it should be mixed by inverting the test tube 10 to 12 times and then put in the 37° C. water bath for 5 minutes.

21. Now proceed to Step 2: Preparing the Control Plasma.

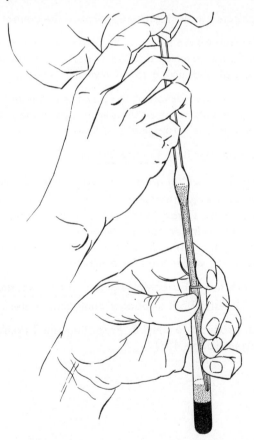

Fig. 159.—Method of removing plasma from oxalated blood.

STEP 2:   PREPARING THE CONTROL PLASMA

Since this is a very sensitive test, a control must be run to test the activity of the reagents.   The control is a sample of normal plasma.   It is referred to as *Control Plasma*.

The control plasma is known and sold under various trade names. Among the more commonly used brands are the following:

1. Diagnostic Plasma
2. Normal Plasma Control
3. Solu-Trol
4. Standardized Normal Plasma

The control plasma is stored in the refrigerator.

1. Obtain one of the above brands of control plasma and the literature which accompanies the control plasma.

2. As directed in the literature, prepare the control plasma.

3. Note: The above step usually consists of simply adding a specified amount of distilled water to the powder in a small vial and mixing to dissolve the powder.

4. After you have dissolved the powder in the vial with the specified amount of distilled water, pour the contents of the vial into a serological test tube.

5. Label the test tube Control Plasma.

   Note: This control plasma keeps about 2 days (see accompanying literature).   When it is not being used, it should be stored in the refrigerator.   Upon removal from the refrigerator, it should be mixed by gently inverting the test tube 10 times.   Then it should be put in a 37° C. water bath for 5 minutes.

6. Put the test tube containing the Control Plasma in the 37° C. water bath or beaker containing water at 37° C.

7. Then proceed to Step 3: Preparing the Thromboplastin Reagent (page 459).

STEP 3:   PREPARING THE THROMBOPLASTIN REAGENT

The thromboplastin reagent is known and sold under various trade names.   Among the more commonly used brands are the following:

1. Simplastin
2. Calsoplastin
3. Solu-Plastin
4. Activated Thromboplastin (Dade)

The first 2 thromboplastin reagents listed above also contain the required amount of calcium.   The last 2, however, issue the thromboplastin and calcium in separate containers.

The thromboplastin reagent is stored in the refrigerator.

1. Obtain one of the above brands of thromboplastin reagent and the literature which accompanies the reagent.

2. As directed in the literature, prepare the thromboplastin reagent.

3. Note: The above step consists of either (1) adding a specified amount of distilled water to a powder in a small vial or (2) mixing two liquid reagents.

4. After you have prepared the thromboplastin reagent as directed in the literature which accompanies the reagent, pour the thromboplastin reagent into a serological test tube.

5. Label the test tube Thromboplastin Reagent.

   Note: This thromboplastin reagent keeps 1 day.   When it is not being used, it should be stored in the refrigerator. Upon removal from the refrigerator, it should be gently mixed by inverting the test tube 10 times.   Then it should be put in the 37° C. water bath for 5 minutes.

6. Put the test tube containing the Thromboplastin Reagent in either a water bath at 37° C. or a 400 milliliter beaker containing water at 37° C.

7. Then proceed to Step 4: Performing the Test (page 460).

STEP 4:   PERFORMING THE TEST

Your water bath should now contain 3 test tubes: *Patient's Plasma*, *Control Plasma*, and *Thromboplastin Reagent*.   These 3 items, of course, were prepared in steps 1, 2, and 3.

1. Get 4 <u>clean, dry</u> serological test tubes.

2. Label one test tube <u>Control</u>.   Label one test tube <u>Patient #1</u>. Label one test tube <u>Patient #2</u>.   Label one test tube <u>Patient #3</u>.

3. Put the 4 test tubes in the 37° C. water bath or beaker containing water at 37° C.

4. Get a 1 milliliter serological pipet which is graduated in hundreds.   This pipet has 100 markings.   Ten marks represent 0.1 milliliter.   Twenty marks represent 0.2 milliliter.   Forty marks represent 0.4 milliliter.   By way of analogy: each mark represents a penny, the total 100 marks representing one dollar.

   <u>Note</u>: If the student has not learned to pipet, he should first perform the pipetting exercises given on page 446.

5. Suck up the <u>Thromboplastin Reagent</u> to the "0" mark on the 1 milliliter serological pipet.

6. Add <u>exactly</u> 0.2 milliliter of the <u>Thromboplastin Reagent</u> to the <u>bottom</u> of the test tube labelled <u>Control</u>.

   <u>Note</u>: You do not let the <u>Thromboplastin Reagent</u> drain down the side of the test tube because it may not all reach the bottom of the test tube.

7. Now add <u>exactly</u> 0.2 milliliter of the <u>Thromboplastin Reagent</u> to the <u>bottom</u> of the test tube labelled <u>Patient #1</u>.

8. Now add <u>exactly</u> 0.2 milliliter of the <u>Thromboplastin Reagent</u> to the <u>bottom</u> of the test tube labelled <u>Patient #2</u>.

9. Now add <u>exactly</u> 0.2 milliliter of the <u>Thromboplastin Reagent</u> to the <u>bottom</u> of the test tube labelled <u>Patient #3</u>.

10. You should have 0.2 milliliter of <u>Thromboplastin Reagent</u> left in the 1 milliliter serological pipet.   Return this to your test tube labelled <u>Thromboplastin Reagent</u>.

11. In the following steps, some technologists use a stop watch to record the time. Other technologists simply use a large clock with a second hand and note the time. For example, they start each test when the second hand is on 12. Then it is a simple matter to note the time in seconds. This naturally leaves both hands free to conduct the test.

12. In the following steps, some technologists use the tilt tube method of determining the end-point. Other technologists use the wire loop method of determining the end-point.

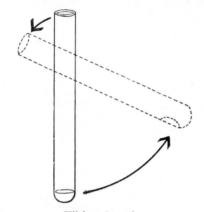

Tilting the tube

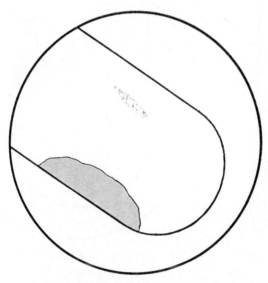

Jelly-like clot in bottom of test tube

Fig. 160.—End-point of the prothrombin time using the tilt tube method.

13. The end-point with the tilt tube method is illustrated in Figure 160.

14. The end-point with the wire loop method is illustrated in Figure 161.

15. Get an 0.1 milliliter <u>micro pipet.</u> This micro pipet is a small pipet which holds only 0.1 milliliter.

16. Suck up the <u>Control Plasma</u> to the 0.1 mark.

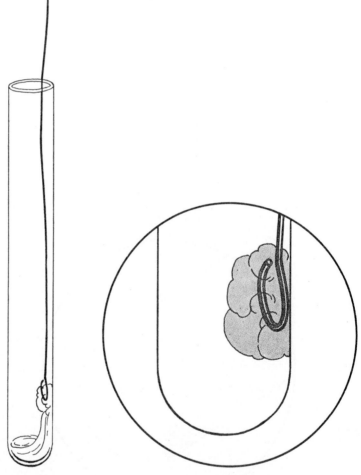

WIRE LOOP
scooping up mixture
in bottom of test tube.

JELLY-LIKE CLOT
sticking to wire loop

FIG. 161.—End-point of the prothrombin time using the wire loop method.

17. Put the tip of the pipet <u>almost</u> to the bottom of the test tube labelled <u>Control</u>.

18. Now forcibly blow out the contents and immediately note the time or start the stop watch.

19. Quickly pick up the test tube. Mix as follows: Hold the top of the tube in your left hand. Tap the bottom of the tube 3 times with your right hand.

20. If you are using the tilt tube method of determining the end-point, quickly proceed with the following: At about one second intervals, repeatedly tilt the test tube from a vertical to an almost horizontal position until a jelly-like clot appears (Fig. 160).

21. If you are using the wire loop method of determining the end-point, quickly proceed with the following: Pick up the wire loop. Put the loop <u>into</u> the mixture in the bottom of the test tube. Now continuously scoop through the mixture, averaging about 2 scoops a second, until a jelly-like clot appears (Fig. 161).

22. The instant the clot appears, note the time or stop the stop watch.

23. The prothrombin time is the time elapsed between the addition of the plasma and the appearance of the clot.

24. From your time data, determine the prothrombin time for your <u>Control Plasma</u>.

25. Write down the prothrombin time for your <u>Control Plasma</u>.

26. The <u>Control Plasma</u> should have a prothrombin time of 13, 14, 15, or 16 seconds. If the <u>Control Plasma</u> does not have a prothrombin time of 13, 14, 15, or 16 seconds, something is wrong with your reagents, equipment, or technique.

27. If your <u>Control Plasma</u> does not have a prothrombin time of 13, 14, 15, or 16 seconds, <u>do not continue the test until you have worked out the mistakes in your procedure.</u>

28. <u>Note</u>: The most common mistakes are the following:

    (1) Mistakes in pipetting: Using the wrong amounts of thromboplastin reagent or plasma during the test. Using the wrong amounts of sodium oxalate or blood during the preparation of the patient's plasma.

    (2) Wet or unclean glassware: Using wet pipets or dirty test tubes.

    (3) Faulty reagents: Using old or <u>improperly prepared reagents</u>.

    (4) Not following the directions <u>exactly</u> as outlined.

29. When your <u>Control Plasma</u> falls within the normal limits of 13–16 seconds, continue as follows:

30. Get another 0.1 milliliter <u>micro pipet</u>.

31. Suck up <u>exactly</u> 0.1 milliliter of the <u>Patient's Plasma</u>.

32. Put the tip of the pipet <u>almost</u> to the bottom of the test tube labelled <u>Patient #1</u>.

33. Now forcibly blow out the contents and immediately note the time or start the stop watch.

34. Quickly pick up the test tube. Mix as follows: Hold the top of the test tube with your left hand. Tap the bottom of the test tube 3 times with your right hand.

35. If you are using the tilt tube method of determining the end-point, quickly proceed with the following: At about one second intervals, repeatedly tilt the test tube from a vertical to an almost horizontal position until a jelly-like clot appears (Fig. 160).

36. If you are using the wire loop method of determining the end-point, quickly proceed with the following: Pick up the wire loop. Put the loop <u>into</u> the mixture in the bottom of the test tube. Now continuously scoop through the mixture, averaging about 2 scoops a second, until a jelly-like clot appears (Fig. 161).

37. The instant the clot appears, note the time or stop the stop watch.

38. The prothrombin time is the time elapsed between the addition of the plasma and the appearance of the clot.

39. From your time data, determine the prothrombin time for your Patient #1 test tube.

40. Write down the prothrombin time for your Patient #1 test tube.

41. Now get another 0.1 milliliter micro pipet. Suck up exactly 0.1 milliliter of the patient's plasma. Put the tip of the pipet almost to the bottom of the test tube labelled Patient #2. Forcibly blow out the contents and immediately note the time or start the stop watch.

42. Quickly pick up the test tube. Mix as follows: Hold the top of the test tube with your left hand. Tap the bottom of the test tube 3 times with your right hand.

43. If you are using the tilt tube method of determining the end-point, quickly proceed with the following: At about one second intervals, repeatedly tilt the test tube from a vertical to an almost horizontal position until a jelly-like clot appears (Fig. 160).

44. If you are using the wire loop method of determining the end-point, quickly proceed with the following: Pick up the wire loop. Put the loop into the mixture in the bottom of the test tube. Now continuously scoop through the mixture, averaging about 2 scoops a second, until a jelly-like clot appears (Fig. 161).

45. The instant the clot appears, note the time or stop the stop watch.

46. The prothrombin time is the time elapsed between the addition of the plasma and the appearance of the clot.

47. Using your time data, determine the prothrombin time for your Patient #2 test tube.

48. Write down the prothrombin time for your Patient #2 test tube.

49. Now get another 0.1 milliliter micro pipet. Suck up exactly 0.1 milliliter of the patient's plasma. Put the tip of the pipet almost to the bottom of the test tube labelled Patient #3. Forcibly blow out the contents and immediately note the time or start the stop watch.

50. Quickly pick up the test tube. Mix as follows: Hold the top of the test tube with your left hand. Tap the bottom of the test tube 3 times with your right hand.

51. If you are using the tilt tube method of determining the end-point, quickly proceed with the following: At about one second intervals, repeatedly tilt the test tube from a vertical to an almost horizontal position until a jelly-like clot appears (Fig. 160).

52. If you are using the wire loop method of determining the end-point, quickly proceed with the following: Pick up the wire loop. Put the loop into the mixture in the bottom of the test tube. Now continuously scoop through the mixture, averaging about 2 scoops a second, until a jelly-like clot appears (Fig. 161).

53. The instant the clot appears, note the time or stop the stop watch.

54. The prothrombin time is the time elapsed between the addition of the plasma and the appearance of the clot.

55. Using your time data, determine the prothrombin time for your Patient #3 test tube.

56. Write down the prothrombin time for your Patient #3 test tube.

57. You should now have the following data:

    Control test tube   _____ seconds
    Patient #1 test tube _____ seconds
    Patient #2 test tube _____ seconds
    Patient #3 test tube _____ seconds

58. Now proceed to Step 5: Reporting the Test (page 467).

STEP 5:   REPORTING THE TEST

1. Find the average of the patient's 3 prothrombin times. Then use this average as your patient's prothrombin time.

2. Example:

   Patient #1 test tube = 16 seconds
   Patient #2 test tube = 15 seconds
   Patient #3 test tube = 14 seconds

                                       45

                           15   average
                        3) 45

3. Therefore, the above patient's prothrombin time is 15 seconds.

4. If your average prothrombin time comes out with a fraction, disregard the fraction. For example, if your average is 15.3 seconds, use 15 seconds.

5. If any 2 prothrombin times with the Patient's Plasma differ by more than 2 seconds, something is wrong with your reagents, equipment, or technique. For example, you should not have a prothrombin time of 20 seconds with the Patient #1 test tube and a prothrombin time of 15 seconds with the Patient #2 test tube.

6. In reporting the prothrombin time, some laboratories report the Control's Time and the Patient's Time. Other laboratories report the Control's Time, Patient's Time, and also the Prothrombin Activity.

   Note: The prothrombin activity may be found by either referring to the literature which comes with your thromboplastin reagent or by following the directions given below.

7. Find the prothrombin activity by either referring to the literature which comes with your thromboplastin reagent or by following the directions given below (page 468).

8. Then make your report as indicated in the sample report below.

9. Sample report:

Patient: Doe, Mr. John

Date: 7-7-72

Physician: Dr. Thomas Goodman

Prothrombin time:

    Control   15 seconds

    Patient   30 seconds

    Prothrombin activity   20%

Method: Quick's one-stage method

Examination performed by: Lee Walker

How to Find the Prothrombin Activity

The prothrombin activity is a comparison of the patient's prothrombin time to normal prothrombin time. It is found as indicated below.

You must have the following data:

Prothrombin time for your Control

Prothrombin time for the Patient

Now find the column in Figure 162 which represents your control's time. If your control's time is 14 seconds, the column on the left is used. If your control's time is 15 seconds, the column in the middle is used. And if your control's time is 16 seconds, the column on the right is used.

Refer to the correct column for your particular control, get the patient's prothrombin time, and read off the prothrombin activity

Example: Suppose the control's time is 15 seconds. We would then use the 15 second control column. This is the middle column in Figure 162.

Now suppose the patient's prothrombin time is 17 seconds. By referring to this middle column, we find that a patient's prothrombin time of 17 seconds gives a prothrombin activity of 72 per cent.

For the data appearing in Figure 162, we are indebted to a paper written by Dr. Milton R. Bronstein which appeared in the journal of the Medical Society of New Jersey, Vol. 49, December 1952.

14-second Control Column		15-second Control Column		16-second Control Column	
Patient's Pro-thrombin Time	Pro-throm-bin Activity	Patient's Pro-thrombin Time	Pro-throm-bin Activity	Patient's Pro-thrombin Time	Pro-throm-bin Activity
14 sec.	100%	15 sec.	100%	16 sec.	100%
15 sec.	86%	16 sec.	86%	17 sec.	86%
16 sec.	72%	17 sec. →	72%	18 sec.	75%
17 sec.	60%	18 sec.	61%	19 sec.	63%
18 sec.	49%	19 sec.	50%	20 sec.	50%
19 sec.	44%	20 sec.	45%	21 sec.	46%
20 sec.	40%	21 sec.	41%	22 sec.	39%
21 sec.	35%	22 sec.	35%	23 sec.	36%
22 sec.	28%	23 sec.	34%	24 sec.	34%
23 sec.	27%	24 sec.	30%	25 sec.	29%
24 sec.	25%	25 sec.	27%	26 sec.	25%
25 sec.	23%	26 sec.	24%	27 sec.	24%
26 sec.	21%	27 sec.	23%	28 sec.	24%
27 sec.	20%	28 sec.	22%	29 sec.	23%
28 sec.	19%	29 sec.	21%	30 sec.	21%
29 sec.	18%	30 sec.	20%	31 sec.	20%
30 sec.	17%	31 sec.	19%	32 sec.	19%
31 sec.	16%	32 sec.	18%	33 sec.	18%
32 sec.	16%	33 sec.	17%	34 sec.	16%
33 sec.	15%	34 sec.	16%	35 sec.	16%
34 sec.	14%	35 sec.	16%	36 sec.	15%
35 sec.	13%	36 sec.	15%	37 sec.	15%
36 sec.	12.5%	37 sec.	14%	38 sec.	14%
more than 36 sec.	less than 12.5%	38 sec.	13%	39 sec.	13%
		39 sec.	13%	40 sec.	13%
		40 sec.	12.5%	41 sec.	12.5%
		more than 40 sec.	less than 12.5%	more than 41 sec.	less than 12.5%

Fig. 162.—Finding the prothrombin activity. Example: Suppose the control's time is 15 seconds. We would then use the 15 second control column. This is the middle column. Now suppose the patient's prothrombin time is 17 seconds. By referring to this middle column, we find that a patient's prothrombin time of 17 seconds gives a prothrombin activity of 72 per cent.

SOURCES OF ERROR IN THE PROTHROMBIN TIME

Errors in performing the prothrombin time are frequently made by the beginner.

The 10 most common errors are caused by the following:

1. Using incorrect anticoagulant in preparing the patient's plasma. The correct anticoagulant is 0.1 M (1.34%) sodium oxalate.

2. Using incorrect amount of anticoagulant in preparing the patient's plasma. The correct amount is 0.5 ml.

3. Using old or contaminated anticoagulant in preparing the patient's plasma. The anticoagulant should be clear and free of any precipitate.

4. Using incorrect amount of the patient's blood in preparing the patient's plasma. The correct amount of blood is *exactly* 4.5 ml.

5. Using patient's plasma which is old or hemolyzed. The plasma should be prepared within 30 minutes after the withdrawal of blood. The plasma should be used immediately or stored for no longer than 4 hours in the refrigerator at 4° C.

6. Using old or outdated control plasma or thromboplastin reagent. The directions accompanying these items should be strictly followed.

7. Using dirty or wet test tubes in performing the test.

8. Using dirty or wet pipets in performing the test.

9. Making mistakes in pipetting, that is, adding the wrong quantities of thromboplastin reagent, control plasma, or patient's plasma.

10. *Failing to follow directions EXACTLY as given* for (1) preparing the patient's plasma, (2) preparing the control plasma, (3) preparing the thromboplastin reagent, or (4) performing the test.

Chapter 23

Partial Thromboplastin Time

The partial thromboplastin time is often abbreviated PTT and it is sometimes referred to as the partial thromboplastin time test.

The discussion will cover the partial thromboplastin time and the activated partial thromboplastin time.*

The student review questions for this chapter are numbered 250–252 and begin on page 753 of the Appendix.

PARTIAL THROMBOPLASTIN TIME

PRINCIPLE

The partial thromboplastin time is nothing more than a simple clotting time with one less variable. Platelet variability is controlled with a phospholipid reagent providing maximum activity. The test measures those plasma factors involved in the generation of plasma thromboplastin. Platelet function and factor VII are not measured.

REAGENTS

a. partial thromboplastin reagent (THROMBOFAX)
b. 0.02 M calcium chloride reagent
c. normal plasma (ORTHO Plasma Coagulation Control)

METHOD

1. Incubate in a 37° C water bath for 5 minutes before use, sufficient THROMBOFAX reagent for the number of tests to be performed; sufficient calcium chloride reagent for the number of tests to be performed; do not incubate plasma.

2. Add to a 12 × 75 mm test tube 0.1 ml of the plasma to be tested and 0.1 ml prewarmed THROMBOFAX reagent.

* This discussion has been reprinted from the recent publication "Coagulation Procedures." It is presented through the courtesy of Ortho Diagnostics, Raritan, New Jersey.

3. Place the tube in a 37°C water bath for 30 seconds.

4. While holding the tube in the water bath, blow 0.1 ml of the prewarmed calcium chloride reagent into the plasma-THROMBOFAX mixture. Start a stop watch simultaneously with the addition of the calcium chloride reagent.

5. Shake the tube briefly to mix contents. Replace tube into test tube rack and do not disturb during the 60 seconds incubation.

6. Following the incubation period remove the tube from the water bath, gently tilt back and forth until fibrin strands appear. Stop the watch the instant the first appearance of fibrin is noted. A solid clot follows.

7. Record the number of seconds on the stop watch.

8. A control should be run using the procedure outlined in steps 1–6 above. This control may be ORTHO Plasma Coagulation Control or freshly drawn normal plasma.

RESULTS

1. Normal THROMBOFAX time = 100 seconds or less.
2. Abnormal THROMBOFAX time = Greater than 100 seconds.

In some instances, plasma samples will be clotted when the tube is removed from the water bath at 60 seconds. The THROMBOFAX time should be reported as "less than 60 seconds." The laboratory performing the procedure should establish their own range of normal values.

References

Langdell, R. D., Wagner, R. H., and Brinkhous, K. M., 1953: Effect of Antihemophilic Factor on One-Stage Clotting Tests. J. Lab. Clin. Med. 47:637.

Rodman, N. F., Barrow, E. M., and Graham, J. B., 1958: Diagnosis and Control of the Hemophloid States with the Partial Thromboplastin (PTT) Test. Amer. J. Clin. Pathol. 29:525.

ACTIVATED PARTIAL THROMBOPLASTIN TIME

PRINCIPLE

The variable of plasma contact may be controlled by exposing the plasma to a specified amount of an activator for a standard amount of time. The contact will shorten the number of seconds required for normal plasma to clot and narrow the limits of the normal range.

REAGENTS

a. partial thromboplastin reagent (THROMBOFAX)
b. 0.02 M calcium chloride reagent
c. Celite reagent—Ortho Research Foundation 5043-A
d. normal plasma (ORTHO Plasma Coagulation Control)

METHOD

1. Immediately before use prepare a 1:1 ratio of the plasma to be tested and Celite reagent. The quantity should be sufficient for duplicate testing, use a 12 × 75 mm test tube.

2. Agitate the plasma-Celite mixture on a mechanical mixer for 15 seconds or by hand for 30 seconds to activate the plasma.

3. Pipette 0.1 ml of THROMBOFAX into a test tube (12 × 75 mm) in a 37° C water bath. Add 0.2 ml of the plasma-Celite mixture, mix and incubate 5 to 6 minutes.

4. While holding the tube in the water bath blow 0.1 ml of the prewarmed calcium chloride reagent into the plasma-Celite mixture. Start a stop watch simultaneously with the addition of the calcium chloride reagent. Shake the tube briefly to mix the contents.

5. Replace the tube into the water bath and do not disturb during the 30 seconds incubation.

6. Following the incubation period, remove the tube from the water bath, gently tilt back and forth until fibrin strands appear. Stop the watch the instant the first appearance of fibrin is noted. A solid clot follows.

7. Record the number of seconds on the stop watch.

8. A control should be run using the procedure outlined in steps 1–7 above. This control may be ORTHO Plasma Coagulation Control or freshly drawn normal plasma.

RESULTS

Normal plasmas will clot in approximately 40 seconds. The laboratory performing the procedure should establish its own range of normal values.

References

Modified technique of Struver, G., and Bittner, D. L., Department of Pathology, Saint Mary Hospital, San Francisco, California.

Chapter 24

Supplemental Coagulation Procedures

In this chapter, we will discuss 7 coagulation procedures and very briefly mention 17 additional coagulation procedures.

The material will be presented in the following order:

Prothrombin Consumption Time
Plasma Thrombin Time
Plasma Recalcification Time
Capillary Resistance Test
Fibrinolysin Test
Euglobulin Clot Lysis Time
Factor VIII Assay
Additional Coagulation Procedures

The student review questions for this chapter are numbered 253–276 and begin on page 753 of the Appendix.

Let us now discuss the 7 coagulation procedures listed above.

The majority of these 7 coagulation procedures are simple procedures which are performed in a manner similar to Quick's one-stage prothrombin time.

Thus, you will find that you are obtaining blood, preparing plasma or serum, mixing it with a reagent or reagents, recording the time, observing the formation of a clot, and recording the time.

The frequency of performing these 7 coagulation procedures differs from laboratory to laboratory and locality to locality.

For example, the plasma recalcification time may be run 2,000 times a year by one laboratory and not even run once a year by another laboratory.

In presenting these 7 coagulation procedures, we have drawn heavily upon recent publications in the field.

(Some of these publications may be obtained free of charge by simply writing to the company which produces and distributes the reagent.)

PROTHROMBIN CONSUMPTION TIME*

The prothrombin consumption time is also referred to as the prothrombin consumption test and the serum prothrombin time.

* This discussion has been reprinted from the recent publication "Blood Coagulation." It is presented through the courtesy of General Diagnostics Division, Warner-Lambert Pharmaceutical Company, Morris Plains, N. J.

INTRODUCTION

Abnormal results of the prothrombin consumption time indicate a deficiency in the production of plasma thromboplastin. The procedure below is a modification of the procedure by Sussman, Cohen and Gittler. Because Simplastin-A contains fibrinogen, its use eliminates the need for two reagents, simplifying both the preparation of reagents and the test procedure.

REAGENTS

Simplastin-A—The complete prothrombin consumption reagent.
Verify Normal—As the test system control.

PROCEDURE

1. Allow blood to clot in a test tube at room temperature. After clotting, place in a 37° C water bath for 2 hours. Centrifuge at 1700 rpm for 10 minutes and carefully separate the serum. (Serum may be stored at 5° C for a maximum of 2 hours before using in the test.)

2. Simplastin-A contains optimum amounts of Factor V, fibrinogen, calcium and sodium chloride. To reconstitute, add 4.0 ml. distilled water.

3. Place the serum to be tested in a water bath at 37° C for 5 minutes.

4. Pipet 0.2 ml. Simplastin-A suspension into a test tube. Place in a water bath at 37° C for 5 minutes.

5. With a micropipet transfer 0.1 ml. of the serum into the tube containing the Simplastin-A suspension.

6. Blow out pipet quickly and start timer simultaneously, preferably by a foot treadle.

7. Immediately insert a small No. 22 nichrome wire loop stirrer into the tube. Move loop across bottom of tube in sweeping motions about two times per second. (The "tilt tube" method may be used if preferred.)

8. The clot is formed in a fine web. When it appears, stop watch and record time.

9. Be sure recapped vial of Simplastin-A is immediately replaced in refrigerator.

REPORTING RESULTS OF
PROTHROMBIN CONSUMPTION TIME

Normal serum prothrombin times may vary from laboratory to laboratory and should be established for each laboratory. In general, however, with Simplastin-A, prothrombin consumption times of over 20 seconds are normal. Times of 18 to 20 seconds are usually considered normal; interpretation depends on further testing. Times of less than 18 seconds are abnormal.

PLASMA THROMBIN TIME*

The plasma thrombin time is also referred to as the plasma thrombin clotting time, thrombin time, and thrombin test.

PRINCIPLE

Plasma is clotted by thrombin. The plasma thrombin clotting time is dependent on (*a*) the strength of the thrombin, (*b*) the concentration of fibrinogen in the plasma, (*c*) the presence of any antithrombin substances such as heparin, (*d*) temperature.

EQUIPMENT AND REAGENTS

1. Water bath, 37° C.
2. Timer.
3. Test tubes, 13 × 100 mm.
4. Thrombin (5,000 NIH units).
5. Saline, 0.85%.
6. Normal plasma.
7. Unknown plasma.

PROCEDURE

1. *Dilution of thrombin.* Dilute the dried material with saline so that 0.1 ml. of thrombin clots 0.1 ml. of normal plasma in 12–15 sec. The units of thrombin may vary from bottle to bottle; however, when a bottle is reconstituted with 10 ml. of saline, the concentration approximates 500 U. per milliliter. A 1:1,000 dilution of this stock solution will have a final concentration of approximately 0.5 U. per milliliter, 0.1 ml. of which will clot 0.1 ml. of plasma in the standard time.

* This discussion has been reprinted from "Laboratory Methods in Blood Coagulation." It is presented through the courtesy of the author, James W. Eichelberger Jr., and the publisher, Hoeber Medical Division of Harper & Row.

2. To a clean test tube containing 0.1 ml. of normal plasma add 0.1 ml. of standard thrombin. Start the timer immediately upon the addition of the thrombin and time the formation of the clot.

3. Repeat Step 2 using the unknown plasma.

NORMAL VALUES

The normal values are 12–15 seconds.

RESULTS

1. The thrombin time of the unknown plasma is prolonged when there is an appreciable amount of heparin or heparin-like substance in the plasma. The test is sometimes abnormal in liver disease, and occasionally the plasma of the newborn has a prolonged thrombin time.
2. A normal thrombin time may be observed in patients known to be undergoing heparin therapy. Presumably this is due to a low concentration of heparin in the patient's plasma which may be detectable when a lower concentration of thrombin is used.

PLASMA RECALCIFICATION TIME*

The plasma recalcification time is also referred to as the plasma clotting time, recalcification time test, calcium clotting time, and calcium clotting time test.

INTRODUCTION

Plasma, if recalcified, will usually clot within 1–2 minutes. Since tissue juices are absent in this test system, clotting will depend on intrinsic prothrombinase formation. As platelets are required for the formation of intrinsic prothrombinase, it is of utmost importance to regulate the separation of plasma which will standardize the number of platelets.

The recalcification time is prolonged in Classical Hemophilia, Christmas Disease, Factor X deficiency, Factor V deficiency, Factor VII deficiency, prothrombin and fibrinogen deficiencies, and in the presence of a circulating anticoagulant.

* This discussion has been reprinted from the recent publication "FibroSystem Manual of Methods for the Coagulation Laboratory." It is presented through the courtesy of BioQuest, Division of Becton, Dickinson and Company, P. O. Box 175, Cockeysville, Maryland   21030.

EQUIPMENT REQUIRED

Stop watch
VACUTAINER tubes or sterile syringes and needles
Test tubes
Pipettes

REAGENTS REQUIRED

FIBROTROL normal plasma control
Sodium oxalate 0.1 M
Calcium chloride 0.025 M

PREPARATION OF PLASMA SPECIMENS

1. Withdraw 4.5 ml. venous blood into a Vacutainer tube containing sodium oxalate or obtain 4.5 ml. of blood by venipuncture and immediately mix with 0.5 ml. of sodium oxalate solution.
2. Within 30 minutes, centrifuge the oxalated blood at 50g for five minutes. Transfer plasma to a clean dry test tube and refrigerate until test is performed.

PROCEDURE

1. Place 0.025 M calcium chloride solution into a small test tube and place in a 37° C. water bath.

2. Add 0.2 ml. of patient's plasma to a 12 × 75 mm test tube and place in a 37° C. water bath for 2–3 minutes.

3. Forcibly blow 0.2 ml. of 0.025 M calcium chloride into the tube containing the plasma, start timer and accurately measure the time required for clot formation. Formation of the clot can be observed by gently tilting the tube back and forth from a horizontal position or by drawing a loop of No. 20 Nichrome wire through the mixture.

   Note: The end point is defined as the first formation of fibrin threads.

REPORTING RESULTS

The recalcification time is reported in seconds. Normal range is 90–120 seconds.

Reference

Miale, J. B.: *Laboratory Medicine—Hematology*, 2nd edition, 1962, The
C. V. Mosby Company, St. Louis.

CAPILLARY RESISTANCE TEST

The capillary resistance test is also referred to as the capillary fragility
test, tourniquet test, cuff test, Rumpel-Leede test, R-L test, and Rumpel-
Leede phenomenon.

The discussion will cover the significance of the capillary resistance test,
the methods of performing the capillary resistance test, and the Rumpel-
Leede method for the capillary resistance test.

SIGNIFICANCE OF THE CAPILLARY RESISTANCE TEST

The capillary resistance test measures the ability of the capillaries to
resist pressure.

In health, the capillaries in the arm will resist a pressure of 100 millimeters.

In purpura hemorrhagica, however, the capillaries in the arm will break
or rupture after a pressure of 100 millimeters. Tiny spots will then appear.
These spots are hemorrhages or petechiae (Fig. 163, page 480).

The capillary resistance test is positive in those conditions listed in
Table 34.

Table 34

Conditions Accompanied by a Positive Capillary Resistance Test

purpura hemorrhagica (idiopathic thrombo-cytopenic purpura)	chronic nephritis
	measles
purpura simplex	influenza
scurvy	scarlet fever
hypofibrinogenemia	achylia gastrica
vitamin K deficiency	
aplastic anemia	

METHODS OF PERFORMING
THE CAPILLARY RESISTANCE TEST

The capillary resistance test may be performed by either the tourniquet
methods or the suction cup method.

The tourniquet methods are: Rumpel-Leede method, Hess method,
Quick method, Weil method, and Bell method.

The suction cup method is usually the Elliott method.

33

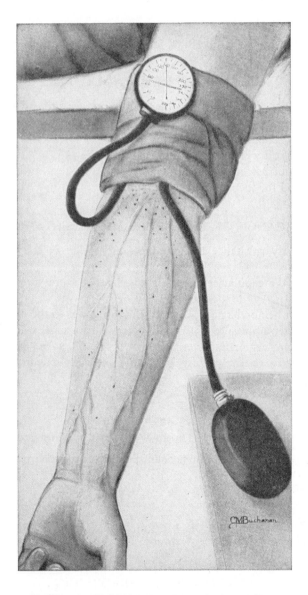

FIG. 163.—A positive capillary resistance test. Note the tiny spots on the arm. These tiny spots are hemorrhages. They are referred to as petechiae. (From Kracke, Roy R., "Diseases of the Blood," 2nd edition, courtesy of J. B. Lippincott Co.)

In many hospitals, the capillary resistance test is not performed by a technologist; it is performed by an intern or resident physician.

The Rumpel-Leede method for performing the capillary resistance test is given below.

RUMPEL-LEEDE METHOD FOR THE CAPILLARY RESISTANCE TEST

Necessary Reagents and Equipment

1. Pen or wax marking pencil
2. Blood pressure apparatus

Procedure

1. Obtain a pen or wax marking pencil and a blood pressure apparatus.

2. Using the pen or wax marking pencil, mark any tiny hemorrhages or petechiae that are already present on the patient's arm (Fig. 163).

   Note: The above petechiae, of course, will be disregarded in the count.

3. Just above the bend in the elbow, wrap the cuff of the blood pressure apparatus.

4. Inflate the blood pressure apparatus to 100 millimeters pressure.

5. Maintain the 100 millimeters pressure for 5 minutes.

6. Release the pressure and allow 15 minutes to elapse.

7. Observe the petechiae which are illustrated in Figure 163, page 480.

   Note: In making your count, you should disregard any petechiae within one half inch of the blood pressure cuff. These petechiae may be due to a pinching of the skin by the blood pressure cuff.

8. After the 15 minutes have elapsed, proceed as follows: Disregarding any petechiae within one half inch of the blood pressure cuff, count the number of fresh petechiae produced.

9. If less than 10 fresh petechiae are present, report the test as negative.

10. If 10 to 20 fresh petechiae are present, report the test as doubtful.

11. If more than 20 fresh petechiae are present, report the test as positive.

12. A sample report is given below.

13. Sample report:

Patient: Mr. John Doe

Date: 7-7-72

Capillary resistance test:

   Positive; 35 petechiae produced by
   100 millimeters pressure

Method: Rumpel-Leede

Normal and abnormal values:
           Negative: less than 10 petechiae produced by
           100 millimeters pressure.
           Doubtful: 10 to 20 petechiae produced by 100
           millimeters pressure.
           Positive: more than 20 petechiae produced by
           100 millimeters pressure.

Technologist: Carol Moffatt

FIBRINOLYSIN TEST*

INTRODUCTION

Circulating in the blood along with factors of the clotting mechanism is a fibrinolytic substance—fibrinolysin—capable of dissolving clots.

In the normal blood this action is taking place continually, setting up a balance against the clotting mechanism. In cases where there is an excess of this substance, its action can be demonstrated by several simple laboratory tests.

An abnormal amount of fibrinolysin speeds up the lysis (destruction) of the fibrin clot. The patient sample should be compared to a normal control for a period of 24 hours. Although any difference in the dissolving action between the patient sample and the normal control is clinically significant,

* This discussion has been reprinted from the recent publication "Blood Coagulation." It is presented through the courtesy of General Diagnostics Division, Warner-Lambert Pharmaceutical Company, Morris Plains, N. J.

a difference evident within the first hour indicates a very high titer of fibrinolysin. For more specific testing the following method may be used:

EQUIPMENT

Centrifuge
Graduated centrifuge tubes
Sterile syringes
13 × 75 mm. test tubes
Water bath with thermometer
Ice bath

REAGENTS

Fibrinogen Warner-Chilcott
Verify Normal (Diagnostic Plasma)
Thrombin (Parke, Davis Bovine Thrombin has been found to be satisfactory for this test.)
Sodium oxalate or citrate 0.1 M (use the anticoagulant you use for your prothrombin-time test.)

PROCEDURE

1. Reconstitute 2 vials of Fibrinogen Warner-Chilcott as directed on the package insert.

2. Draw 9.0 ml. of blood from the patient and mix with 1.0 ml. of the anticoagulant. Collect just before running the test and keep the specimen chilled in a crushed ice bath.

3. Reconstitute Diagnostic Plasma as directed for use as the normal plasma.

4. Spin the patient's sample down and separate the plasma. Place both the patient's sample and the reconstituted Diagnostic Plasma in the ice bath.

5. Into four 13 × 75 mm. test tubes that have been numbered and placed in the 37° C water bath add:
   Tube 1: 0.5 ml. Verify Normal (Diagnostic Plasma) and 0.5 ml. patient's plasma.
   Tube 2: 1.0 ml. Verify Normal (Diagnostic Plasma) (this will be a control).
   Tube 3: 0.5 ml. fibrinogen solution and 0.5 ml. patient's plasma.
   Tube 4: 1.0 ml. fibrinogen solution (this will be a control).

6. To each of the four tubes add 0.1 ml. (containing about 10 units) of the thrombin solution.

RESULTS

1. Fibrin clots should form within a few seconds after the thrombin has been added to the tubes.
2. Tubes 2 and 4 are the control tubes.
3. Lysis in Tube 2 will be slow compared to lysis in Tube 1 when the patient's plasma contains increased fibrinolysin.
4. In the normal individual, lysis in Tube 3 is faster than in Tube 1, since fibrinogen contains no antifibrinolysin. There should be no lysis in Tube 4.
5. The patient's tubes are compared against the controls and are recorded as plus or minus. This is a highly subjective test that indicates a probable yes or no answer. There is no quantitative means of reporting.

EUGLOBULIN CLOT LYSIS TIME*

SIGNIFICANCE

"Euglobulin clot lysis measures over-all fibrinolysis, but is especially sensitive to increased quantities of the activator of plasminogen. It is particularly useful in patients whose blood is incoagulable due to the administration of heparin for cardiac surgery procedures, since the euglobulin fraction of plasma is separated from inhibitors and then clotted with thrombin. Also, the procedure can be completed in a relatively short period of time."

REAGENTS

1. Sodium citrate solution, 3.8%.
2. Buffered saline solution. Dilute 1 part sodium barbital acetate buffer (pH 7.42) with 4 parts normal saline solution. Tris buffered saline solution may be used.
3. Thrombin solution. To 1000 units of bovine topical thrombin, add 5 ml. 50% glycerol in normal saline solution (200 u/ml.). Store in the freezer until ready to use.
4. Carbon dioxide stream from a tank of medical carbon dioxide.

PROCEDURE

1. Collect blood with 3.8% sodium citrate solution (4 ml blood to 1 ml citrate). Store in ice bath for no longer than 30 minutes.

* This discussion has been reprinted from "Laboratory Evaluation of Hemostasis." Courtesy of the author, Dr. Marjorie S. Sirridge, and the publisher Lea & Febiger.

2. Centrifuge 5 minutes at 3000 rpm.

3. Place 1 ml plasma in a 50 ml Erlenmeyer flask containing 15 ml distilled water.

4. Blow a stream of CO_2 over the surface of the mixture for 4 minutes while rotating the flask manually or with a mechanical stirrer. A globulin precipitate forms quickly.

5. Centrifuge the contents of the flask in a centrifuge tube for 5 minutes and discard the supernatant, wiping the walls of the tube dry with a cotton applicator.

6. Re-dissolve the euglobulin precipitate in 1 ml buffered saline solution and place two 0.3 ml aliquots in each of 2 tubes.

7. Clot these aliquots with 0.01 ml thrombin.

8. Incubate the tubes at 37° C and observe for clot dissolution. The end point is complete dissolution of the clot.

NORMAL VALUES

Values below 120 minutes indicate increased fibrinolytic activity, more precisely activator activity.

References

von Kaulla, K. N., and Schultz, R. L.: Methods for the Evaluation of Human Fibrinolysis. Studies with Two Combined Techniques. Amer. J. Clin. Path., 29:104, 1958.

von Kaulla, K. N.: *Chemistry of Thrombolysis, Human Fibrinolytic Enzymes.* Springfield, Ill., Charles C Thomas, 1963.

FACTOR VIII ASSAY*

PRINCIPLE

The prolonged partial thromboplastin time of a hemophilic plasma is shortened by the addition of normal plasma. The degree of correction is proportional to the amount of factor VIII in the normal (or unknown) plasma.

* This discussion has been reprinted from "Laboratory Methods in Blood Coagulation." Courtesy of the author, James W. Eichelberger, Jr., and the publisher, Hoeber Medical Division of Harper & Row.

EQUIPMENT AND REAGENTS

1. Water bath, 37° C.
2. Ice bath
3. Test tubes, plain glass and silicone-coated, 10 × 100 mm. and 15 × 120 mm.
4. Calcium chloride, 0.025 M.
5. Sodium citrate, 0.1 M.
6. Barbital-saline buffer, pH 7.4
7. Cephalin, 3%
8. Kaolin, 2%
9. Normal control plasma
10. Patient's plasma
11. Factor VIII-deficient plasma (stored in silicone-coated tubes at −20° C.).

PROCEDURE

1. Withdraw 9 ml. of the patient's blood in a silicone-coated syringe and add to a silicone-coated tube containing 1.0 ml. of sodium citrate. Collect blood from the normal control in the same manner. The samples should be centrifuged immediately and the plasmas transferred to silicone-coated tubes and placed in the ice bath.

2. Thaw the factor VIII-deficient substrate plasma at 37° C. and place in the ice bath until ready for use.

3. Prepare a 1:35 dilution of the cephalin by adding 0.1 ml. of the stock to 3.4 ml. of saline.

4. Prepare a 1:1 suspension of the cephalin and kaolin by mixing 2.0 ml. of each. The cephalin-kaolin reagent should always be mixed well before pipetting.

5. Prepare the dilution curve prior to the assay of the unknown plasma. It is preferable to have at least six fresh normal plasmas which are pooled and assayed each time a new batch of substrate plasma is prepared. Otherwise, a single plasma may be used to prepare the daily dilution curve. Always dilute the normal plasmas in silicone-coated tubes and keep on ice until ready for use. Using barbital-saline buffer, serially dilute the plasmas 1:5, 1:10, 1:20, 1:40, 1:80, 1:160, and 1:320. The dilutions represent 100, 50, 25, 12.5, 6.25, 3.1, and 1.5% factor VIII activity.

6. In a plain glass test tube add:

   a. 0.1 ml. of factor VIII-deficient plasma substrate,
   b. 0.1 ml. of cephalin-kaolin reagent,
   c. 0.1 ml. of 1:5 diluted normal plasma.

Incubate in the water bath for 2 min. with occasional mixing.

Add 0.1 ml. of calcium chloride. The tube should be kept in the water bath, mixed gently every 15–20 sec., and observed after 50 sec. The normal plasma should clot in 60–80 sec.

7. Repeat Step 6 for each of the normal plasma dilutions. Duplicate determinations should agree within 3–5 sec. The results, plotted on log-log paper, should give an approximately straight line.

8. Dilute the patient's plasma 1:5 and 1:10 (additional dilutions are optional) and assay in a similar manner. Read the clotting times on the assay curve to determine the percentage of factor VIII activity.

Results

Example of a Factor VIII Assay in a Normal Person and a Hemophiliac

Clotting time (sec.)	Plasma Dilution						
	1:5	1:10	1:20	1:40	1:80	1:160	1:320
Normal	65	74	85.5	93.2	101	105	113
Patient	92.8	103	107	115	121		

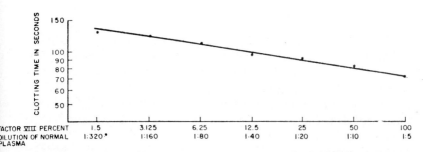

Factor VIII activity dilution curve plotted on log-log paper. The 1:5 dilution represents 100% factor VIII activity. Curve is typical of dilution curves obtained for plasma factor assays.

ADDITIONAL COAGULATION PROCEDURES

In this section, 17 coagulation procedures will be alphabetically listed and briefly discussed.

With an occasional exception, these 17 coagulation procedures are not even run once a year by the average hospital laboratory. However, this rough estimate may be subject to some glaring exceptions. For example, Owren's thrombotest and the thromboplastin generation test are very popular tests in some areas of the United States.

Aspirin Tolerance Test

The aspirin tolerance test is performed by running a bleeding time on the patient, giving the patient a dose of aspirin, and running another bleeding time.

The second bleeding time is two or three times the normal values in von Willebrand's disease and platelet dysfunction.

Circulating Anticoagulant Examination

A circulating anticoagulant is an anticoagulant which circulates in the blood, hinders the normal clotting of blood, and causes a hemorrhagic syndrome.

The circulating anticoagulant examination is performed by (Step 1) adding the patient's blood to normal blood and determining the clotting time of the mixture, (Step 2) determining the clotting time of normal blood, and (Step 3) comparing the clotting time of the mixture with the clotting time of normal blood.

If the mixture clots slower than normal blood, a circulating anticoagulant is assumed to be present in the patient's blood.

A circulating anticoagulant may be introduced into the blood during various types of therapy, such as heparin therapy, and it may be present in the blood in hemophilia and leukemia.

Contact Activation Test

The contact of plasma with glass activates clotting.

The degree of activation may be measured by the contact activation test.

The test is performed by exposing the plasma to kaolin or celite and determining the clotting time.

Defective activation may be found in either factor XI deficiency or factor XII deficiency.

Factor V Assay

Factor V assay is performed in a manner similar to the prothrombin time.
Factor V deficiency is found in parahemophilia.

Factor VII Assay

Factor VII assay is also performed in a manner similar to the prothrombin time.

Factor VII deficiency causes abnormal bleeding.

Factor VII deficiency may be seen as an inherited condition, in vitamin K deficiency, during coumarin therapy, and in liver disease.

Factor XI Assay

Factor XI assay is another relatively simple clotting procedure.

Factor XI deficiency is an inherited condition, confined mainly to Jews, and characterized by mild episodes of bleeding.

Factor XIII Deficiency Test

The factor XIII deficiency test is also referred to as the fibrin stabilizing factor test and the FSF test.

The factor XIII deficiency test is based on the following principle:

(1) A plasma clot formed from normal blood will not dissolve in a 5 M solution of urea.

(2) A plasma clot formed from blood deficient in factor XIII will dissolve in a 5 M solution of urea.

Factor XIII deficiency is the most recently discovered clotting defect, it may be inherited or acquired, and it is characterized by abnormal bleeding.

Hicks-Pitney Test

The Hicks-Pitney test is a modification of the thromboplastin generation test.

The Hicks-Pitney test may be used as a screening procedure to detect any deficiencies in the generation of intrinsic thromboplastin.

The Hicks-Pitney test has the following normal values: 7–12 second clotting time after a generation time of 5 minutes or less.

Values above normal are indicative of a defect in coagulation; this defect may be pinpointed by running the more involved thromboplastin generation test.

Plasma Antithrombin Test

The plasma antithrombin test is also referred to as the plasma antithrombin detection test and the thrombin titration.

The plasma antithrombin test may be used to detect the presence of heparin or a heparin-like substance in the patient's plasma.

The plasma antithrombin test is performed by titrating the patient's plasma with thrombin solutions of decreasing concentrations.

Platelet Adhesiveness Estimation

The platelet adhesiveness estimation may be performed by the Hellem method, Salzman method, or Borchgrevink method.

In the method of Hellem, a platelet count is made on a sample of the patient's blood, another sample of the patient's blood is filtered to expose the platelets to a foreign surface, a platelet count is then run on the filtered sample of blood, and the difference in the two platelet counts is considered an indication of platelet adhesiveness.

Platelet adhesiveness is usually reduced in von Willebrand's disease.

Platelet Antibody Test

The platelet antibody test is also referred to as the platelet antibody detection test and the platelet-agglutination test.

The platelet antibody test is usually performed by obtaining the patient's whole blood, allowing the blood to clot at 37° C. and then putting it in the refrigerator at 4° C. for 12–24 hours, centrifuging to obtain the serum, inactivating the serum at 56° C. for 30 minutes, adsorbing the serum with barium sulfate, adding the inactivated and adsorbed serum to a suspension of platelets, and inspecting the preparation for agglutination with the naked eye or the low power (10×) objective of the microscope.

The platelet antibody test may be useful in cases of thrombocytopenia induced by drugs or chemical agents.

Platelet Antiglobulin Consumption Test

The platelet antiglobulin consumption test is performed by (Step 1) exposing Coombs' anti-human globulin serum to platelets, centrifuging and removing the serum, making serial dilutions of the serum, adding anti-D sensitized cells to the serial dilutions, inspecting the preparations for clumping, and recording the highest titer showing clumping; (Step 2) repeating the test using Coombs' anti-human globulin serum which has *not* been exposed to platelets and recording the highest titer showing clumping; and (Step 3) comparing the two highest titers.

If the highest titer of Step 1 and the highest titer of Step 2 differ by 3 tubes or more, the test is considered positive.

The exact significance of a positive platelet antiglobulin consumption test has not been firmly established.

However, the test has been found to be positive in many cases of purpura hemorrhagica (idiopathic thrombocytopenic purpura).

Platelet Factor 3 Assay

The platelet factor 3 assay may be used to determine the thromboplastin generating ability of a patient's platelets.

This test is rather involved and it is usually performed by either the method of Husom or the method of Bonnin and Cheney.

Prothrombin and Proconvertin Test

The prothrombin and proconvertin test is also referred to as the prothrombin and proconvertin time and the P and P test.

The prothrombin and proconvertin test is similar to the one-stage prothrombin time, the main difference being that the plasma is diluted in order to make the test more sensitive.

The prothrombin and proconvertin test is used in the control of anticoagulant therapy. The test is reported in per cent activity. And the therapeutic range is generally considered to be 10%–25% activity.

Stypven Time

Russell's viper is the name of a snake in Asia. The venom from this snake is sold under the trade mark of Stypven. Hence, Stypven is Russell's viper venom.

Stypven reacts in a test tube in a manner similar to intrinsic thromboplastin.

If Stypven is substituted for thromboplastin in Quick's one-stage prothrombin time, the test is referred to as the Stypven time.

The Stypven time has the same normal values as the prothrombin time, that is, 11–16 seconds.

The Stypven time reveals normal values in a factor VII deficiency and elevated values in a factor X deficiency.

Consequently, the Stypven time may be used to distinguish between a factor VII deficiency and a factor X deficiency.

Thromboplastin Generation Test

The thromboplastin generation test is also referred to as TGT.

The thromboplastin generation test is designed to pinpoint deficiencies in the production of thromboplastin. It is a long involved tedious procedure. And it is usually performed by a technologist specializing in blood coagulation procedures.

Thrombotest

The thrombotest is sometimes referred to as Owren's thrombotest or Thrombotest Owren.

The thrombotest is performed in a manner similar to the one-stage prothrombin time.

The thrombotest is used in the control of anticoagulant therapy. It is reported in per cent activity, the normal range being 70%–130% activity. The therapeutic range is generally considered to be 10%–20% activity.

STUDENT NOTES

PART 5

Miscellaneous Tests

INTRODUCTION

Part 5, Miscellaneous Tests, is made up of the following:

If a test in the chapter entitled Tests Rarely Requested gains any degree of popularity, it will be moved up to the chapter entitled Tests Seldom Requested.

By a similar token, if a test in the chapter entitled Tests Seldom Requested increases in usefulness, it will be moved up to occupy a single chapter.

And, if a test now being presented in a single chapter of this text decreases in widespread use, it will be dropped back to either Tests Seldom Requested or Tests Rarely Requested.

In this way, the tests which are required to meet the curriculum requirements of the hematology department may be kept in their proper perspective.

Some additional tests, that are not performed in the hematology department but which are useful in diagnosing blood diseases, will be mentioned in the dictionary in the Appendix.

Chapter 25

Eosinophil Count

The eosinophil count is also referred to as the direct eosinophil count, total eosinophil count, absolute eosinophil count, and circulating eosinophile count.

The discussion will cover the significance of the eosinophil count and the procedure for the eosinophil count.

The student review questions for the eosinophil count are numbered 277–283 and begin on page 755 of the Appendix.

SIGNIFICANCE OF THE EOSINOPHIL COUNT

In the differential white cell count, we determined the percentage of eosinophils in a random sample of 100 white cells. Although this information is useful, it is sometimes necessary to make a more accurate determination, that is, to determine the number of eosinophils per cubic millimeter of blood. The number of eosinophils per cubic millimeter of blood is determined by making an eosinophil count.

The normal values for the eosinophil count are 50 to 400 eosinophils per cubic millimeter of blood.

When the eosinophil count drops below the normal values, the condition is known as eosinopenia (e-o-sin-o-pe′ne-ah).

When the eosinophil count rises above the normal values, the condition is known as eosinophilia (e″o-sin-o-fil′e-ah).

An eosinopenia or eosinophilia may be found in those conditions listed in Table 35.

The eosinophil count is performed about 6 times a month by the average hospital laboratory and about 2 times a year by the average physician's office.

PROCEDURE FOR THE EOSINOPHIL COUNT

The procedure for the eosinophil count consists of diluting the blood with an eosinophil diluting fluid, charging a counting chamber, counting the eosinophils with a microscope, and making a calculation.

The necessary reagents and equipment are listed below and the procedure follows.

494

Table 35

Conditions Accompanied by Abnormal Eosinophil Counts

Eosinopenia (low eosinophil count)	*Eosinophilia* (high eosinophil count)
hyperadrenalism (Cushing's disease)	allergies
administration of ACTH	skin diseases
after major surgery	parasitic infestations
severe infections	chronic granulocytic leukemia
eclampsia	scarlet fever
shock	Hodgkin's disease
	tuberculosis
	brucellosis
	copper poisoning
	digitalis administration
	insulin administration
	after splenectomy

NECESSARY REAGENTS AND EQUIPMENT

1. One of the following eosinophil diluting fluids:

   (*a*) *Phloxine Diluting Fluid*
   To prepare: Pour 50 ml. of propylene glycol into a bottle. Add 40 ml. of distilled water. Add 10 ml. of a 1% water solution of phloxine. Add 1 ml. of a 10% water solution of sodium carbonate. Mix. Filter. Store at room temperature. Keeps 1 month.

   (*b*) *Pilot's Solution*
   To prepare: Pour 50 ml. of propylene glycol into a container. Add 40 ml. of distilled water. Add 10 ml. of a 1% water solution of phloxine. Add 1 ml. of a 10% water solution of sodium carbonate. Add 100 units of heparin. Mix. Filter. Store at room temperature. Keeps 1 month.

   (Function of ingredients: The heparin keeps the cells from clumping; the sodium carbonate lyses all white cells except eosinophils; the phloxine stains the eosinophils red; and the propylene glycol renders the red cells invisible.)

   (*c*) Other diluting fluids which may be used are: Tannen's diluting fluid, Randolph's diluting fluid, Manner's diluting fluid, Dunger's diluting fluid, and Discombe's diluting fluid. For preparation, see the section on solutions and reagents in the Appendix.

2. Finger tip blood or fresh anticoagulated blood. If fresh anticoagulated blood is used, it must be used within 4 hours after it is withdrawn.
3. White cell pipet
4. Microscope
5. Any one of the following 3 counting chambers may be used:

34

(*a*) Improved Neubauer ruling counting chamber. This counting chamber is the counting chamber generally used for the white cell count and red cell count. It has 2 sections. Each section has an area of 9 square millimeters and a depth of 0.1 millimeter. Therefore, the volume of 1 section is $9 \times .1 = .9$ cubic millimeter. The volume of the 2 sections is $2 \times .9 = 1.8$ cubic millimeters. (See Fig. 164, page 498.)

(*b*) Fuchs-Rosenthal counting chamber. This is a special counting chamber offering greater volume than the above counting chamber. It has 2 sections. Each section has an area of 16 square millimeters and a depth of 0.2 millimeter. Therefore, the volume of 1 section is $16 \times .2 = 3.2$ cubic millimeters. The volume of the 2 sections is $2 \times 3.2 = 6.4$ cubic millimeters.

(*c*) Speirs-Levy counting chamber. This counting chamber has 4 sections. Each section has an area of 10 square millimeters and a depth of 0.2 millimeter. Therefore, the volume of 1 section is $10 \times .2 = 2.0$ cubic millimeters. The volume of the 4 sections is $4 \times 2 = 8$ cubic millimeters.

Procedure

1. Obtain a bottle of eosinophil diluting fluid.

   Note: Any one of the above eosinophil diluting fluids may be used.

2. Obtain a white cell pipet and rubber sucking tube.

3. Either finger tip blood or fresh anticoagulated blood may be used.

4. If finger tip blood is to be used, obtain the materials for a finger puncture: cotton balls or gauze pads, 70% alcohol, and a sterile blood lancet. Make a finger puncture. Wipe away the first drop of blood. Massage the finger to produce a rounded drop of blood. Then proceed to step 6 below.

5. If fresh anticoagulated blood is to be used, mix the blood by completely inverting the test tube 10 to 12 times.

   Note: The anticoagulated blood must not be over 4 hours old.

6. Using the white cell pipet, suck up blood to the 1.0 mark.

7. Then suck up the eosinophil diluting fluid to the 11.0 mark. (This is a 1 in 10 dilution.)

8. Allow the pipet to sit for 15 minutes.

   Note: This gives the eosinophils an opportunity to accept the stain.

9. Shake the pipet for 2 to 3 minutes.

10. Discard the first 4 drops.

11. Now charge all sections of the counting chamber.

    Note:
    (1) If you are using the Improved Neubauer ruling counting chamber, charge the side usually used for the white cell count and also the side usually used for the red cell count.
    (2) If you are using the Fuchs-Rosenthal counting chamber, charge the 2 sections.
    (3) If you are using the Speirs-Levy counting chamber, charge the 4 sections.

12. Place the counting chamber on the stage of a microscope.

13. Using the $10 \times$ (16 mm.) objective, bring the cells into view.

    Note: It makes no difference which section of the counting chamber is used to start the count.

14. Scan several fields and note that the eosinophils are pink or red in color.

15. The eosinophils are to be counted in all sections of your counting chamber.

    Note: If you are using the Improved Neubauer ruling counting chamber, the ruled area of one section is illustrated in Figure 164, page 498.

16. Therefore, using the $10 \times$ (16 mm.) objective, count the eosinophils in all sections of your counting chamber.

17. Make a record of your total count.

18. A sample calculation for each particular counting chamber is given below.

19. Pick out the sample calculation for your particular counting chamber and make your calculation accordingly.

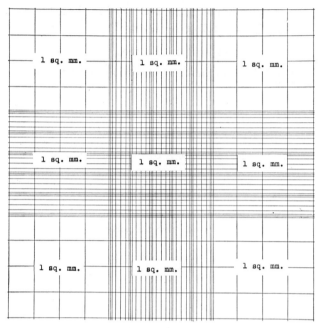

Fig. 164.—Improved Neubauer ruling. Ruled area to be counted in the eosinoph count and spinal cell count. The ruled area is 9 square millimeters. The countin chamber is 0.1 millimeter deep. Therefore, the volume is 9 × .1 = .9 cubic mil meter. The volume of 2 similar sections is 2 × .9 = 1.8 cubic millimeters. (Illus tration courtesy of Bausch & Lomb Co.)

20. Calculation with the Improved Neubauer ruling counting chamber:

Let us say your total count was 40. Then your eosinophil count would be:

Eosinophil count =

| Total number of eosinophils counted | × | dilution correction factor | × | volume correction factor |

$$= 40 \times 10 \times \frac{1}{1.8}$$

$$= \frac{400}{1.8}$$

$$= 222 \text{ per cubic millimeter}$$

Thus, you multiply your total count by 10 and divide by 1.8

21. Calculation with the Fuchs-Rosenthal counting chamber:
Let us say your total count was 142. Then your eosinophil count would be:

Eosinophil count =

total number of eosinophils counted	×	dilution correction factor	×	volume correction factor
= 142	×	10	×	$\dfrac{1}{6.4}$

$$= \frac{1420}{6.4}$$

= 222 per cubic millimeter

Thus, you multiply your total count by 10 and divide by 6.4.

22. Calculation with the Speirs-Levy counting chamber:
Let us say your total count was 178. Then your eosinophil count would be:

Eosinophil count =

total number of eosinophils counted	×	dilution correction factor	×	volume correction factor
= 178	×	10	×	$\dfrac{1}{8}$

$$= \frac{1780}{8}$$

= 222 per cubic millimeter

Thus, you multiply your total count by 10 and divide by 8.

23. After you have made your calculation, make out your report as indicated in the sample report below.

24. Sample report:

Patient: Doe, Mr. John

Date: 7-7-72

Physician: Dr. Paul Rodgers

Eosinophil count: 222 eosinophils per cu. mm.

Normal values: 50 to 400 per cu. mm.

Examination performed by: Betty Snow

Chapter 26

Spinal Cell Count

THE spinal cell count is sometimes referred to as the cerebrospinal flu
cell count, CSF cell count, cytological examination of cerebrospinal flui
or the enumeration of cellular elements in cerebrospinal fluid.

The discussion will cover the significance of the spinal cell count and tl
procedure for the spinal cell count.

The student review questions for the spinal cell count are number
284–286 and begin on page 756 of the Appendix.

SIGNIFICANCE OF THE SPINAL CELL COUNT

The cells found in spinal fluid are usually white cells. Sometime
however, red cells produced by the puncture itself may be seen.

The normal values for the spinal cell count are 0 to 10 white cells p
cubic millimeter.

The spinal cell count rises above the normal values in meningitis, encep
alitis, poliomyelitis, and latent syphilis. In the above diseases, the wh
cell count may vary from 20 to 1000 cells per cubic millimeter.

The white cells found in spinal fluid are lymphocytes and neutrophi
segmented cells.

If the white cell count is within the normal values of 0 to 10, the ty
of white cells present is of no diagnostic significance.

If the white cell count is above the normal values of 0 to 10, howev
the type of white cells present may be of diagnostic significance.

For example, the lymphocytes are increased in anterior poliomyel
whereas the neutrophilic segmented cells are increased in influen
meningitis.

The lymphocytes usually outnumber the neutrophilic segmented cells
the following diseases:

> anterior poliomyelitis
> tuberculosis meningitis
> epidemic encephalitis
> latent syphilis

500

The neutrophilic segmented cells outnumber the lymphocytes in the following diseases:

influenzal meningitis

pneumococcus meningitis

pyogenic meningitis

epidemic meningitis

The type of white cells present, of course, is determined by making a differential white cell count of the spinal fluid.

Spinal fluid often contains contagious material. Therefore, take particular precautions in handling the specimens.

The spinal cell count is performed about 35 times a month by the average hospital laboratory and about once a year by the average physician's office.

PROCEDURE FOR THE SPINAL CELL COUNT

The spinal cell count consists of a total white cell count and, if necessary, a differential white cell count.

The total white cell count is performed by charging a counting chamber, counting the white cells with a microscope, and making a calculation.

If the total white cell count is within the normal values of 0 to 10, it is unnecessary to make a differential white cell count. If the total white cell count is elevated, however, a differential white cell count should be performed.

The differential white cell count is performed by making a smear, staining the cells, placing the slide on the stage of the microscope, and tabulating the different types of white cells.

The necessary reagents and equipment for the total white cell count and differential white cell count are listed below. The procedures follow.

NECESSARY REAGENTS AND EQUIPMENT

1. Precaution: Handle the spinal fluid with care! It may contain contagious material!
2. Fresh spinal fluid. Since the cells disintegrate rapidly, the cells should be counted within 1 hour after the spinal fluid is withdrawn.
3. 3 small test tubes
4. 2 medicine droppers
5. 10% acetic acid
6. Counting chamber
7. Microscope
8. Centrifuge
9. 3 glass slides
10. Either of the following stains:
    (a) 1% methyl alcohol solution of methylene blue
    (b) Wright's stain and buffer solution

PROCEDURE FOR THE TOTAL WHITE CELL COUNT

1. Precaution: Handle the spinal fluid with care! It may contain contagious material!

2. Mix the spinal fluid by completely inverting the test tube 10 to 12 times.

   Note: If the spinal fluid is pink or grossly bloody, make a record of this observation and include it in your report.

3. Using a medicine dropper, transfer 9 drops of the spinal fluid to a small test tube.

4. To this small test tube containing the 9 drops of spinal fluid, add 1 drop of 10% acetic acid.

   Note: The above 9 in 10 dilution is usually made in a white cell pipet. However, the procedure described above is much safer for the beginner since it eliminates the possibility of sucking any spinal fluid into his mouth. The purpose of the dilution is to hemolyze any red cells which may be present.

5. Mix as follows: Hold the top of the test tube with your left hand. Gently tap the bottom of the test tube with your right hand.

6. Allow 5 minutes to elapse.

7. Mix again.

8. Obtain a counting chamber and coverglass which is normally used for the white cell count and red cell count.

9. Using a medicine dropper, suction up a few drops of this spinal fluid containing the 1 drop of 10% acetic acid.

10. Using the medicine dropper, carefully charge either side of the counting chamber.

11. Place the counting chamber on the stage of a microscope.

12. Bring the cells into view with the $10\times$ (16 mm.) objective of the microscope.

    Note: The nucleus in the neutrophilic segmented cells will be bright and clear. The nucleus in the lymphocytes will appear round. The red cells will either be absent or appear as "shadows."

13. Turn to Figure 164, page 498.

14. The white cells are to be counted in the nine 1 square millimeter sections illustrated in Figure 164.

15. Count the white cells in the nine 1 square millimeter sections.

16. Record the total number of white cells counted in the nine 1 square millimeter sections.

    Note: For all practical purposes, the total number of white cells counted may be used as your spinal cell count. However, two minor correction factors are necessary to make the count more "scientific." Therefore, continue with the following steps.

17. To avoid contagion, first proceed as follows:

18. Place the counting chamber and coverglass in a beaker of 70% alcohol and allow to soak for about 4 hours.

19. Place the test tube containing the 9 drops of spinal fluid and 1 drop of 10% acetic acid in the beaker of 70% alcohol. Allow to soak for about 4 hours.

20. Now, to make your calculation, you must multiply your total number of white cells by 2 correction factors.

21. First, since you diluted 9 drops of spinal fluid with 1 drop of 10% acetic acid, you must multiply your total count by $\frac{10}{9}$.

22. Second, by counting the white cells in the nine 1 square millimeter sections, you have counted the white cells in 0.9 cubic millimeter. The report, however, is to be given as the number of white cells in 1.0 cubic millimeter. Therefore, you must multiply your total count by $\frac{1.0}{0.9}$ $\left(\text{or } \frac{10}{9}\right)$.

23. Now calculate the number of white cells in 1 cubic millimeter by multiplying your total count by the correction factors $\frac{10}{9}$ and $\frac{10}{9}$.

24. Example:

    The total count was 9. Multiplying this 9 by $\frac{10}{9}$ and $\frac{10}{9}$, we have $9 \times \frac{10}{9} \times \frac{10}{9} = 11$ white cells per cu. mm.

25. If the number of white cells per cubic millimeter falls within the normal range of 0 to 10, there is no point in making a differential white cell count. In such cases, make out your report as indicated in the sample report below.

26. Sample report:

```
┌─────────────────────────────────────────────────────────────┐
│                                                              │
│     Patient:     Doe, Mr. John                               │
│                                                              │
│     Date:        7–7–72                                      │
│                                                              │
│     Physician:  Dr. James Jennings                           │
│                                                              │
│     Spinal cell count:  6 white cells per cu. mm.            │
│                                                              │
│     Normal values:    0 to 10 white cells per cu. mm.        │
│                                                              │
│     Examination performed by:  Betty Snow                    │
│                                                              │
└─────────────────────────────────────────────────────────────┘
```

27. If the number of white cells per cubic millimeter is above the normal range of 0 to 10, proceed to make a differential white cell count as directed below.

PROCEDURE FOR THE DIFFERENTIAL WHITE CELL COUNT

1. Carefully pour 1 or 2 milliliters of fresh <u>unaltered</u> spinal fluid into a small test tube.

2. Centrifuge at high speed for 10 minutes.

3. Pour off and discard the supernatant fluid.

4. The test tube will now contain the cells and about 1 drop of spinal fluid.

5. Mix the contents of the test tube as follows: Hold the top of the test tube with your left hand. Gently tap the bottom of the test tube with your right hand.

6. Pour some of the above mixture onto a glass slide and make a smear in the usual manner.

7. Allow the smear to thoroughly dry.

   <u>Note</u>: The drying process will take about 20 minutes. <u>Very gentle</u> heat may be applied. Excessive heat will distort the white cells.

8. Either of the following stains may be used:

(1) 1% methyl alcohol solution of methylene blue

(2) Wright's stain and buffer solution

The methylene blue stain is preferred. This stain is applied to the smear for about 12 minutes and then <u>very gently</u> drained off by slightly tilting the slide. If the draining off process is not gentle, the smear may be flushed off the slide.

9. Now stain the smear with either 1% methyl alcohol solution of methylene blue or Wright's stain and buffer solution.

10. Allow the smear to thoroughly dry. (It takes at least 10 minutes.)

11. Put a drop of immersion oil on the smear and put the smear on the stage of the microscope.

12. Using the oil immersion (95×) objective of the microscope, record the number of lymphocytes and neutrophilic segmented cells seen while counting 100 white cells.

13. Record the percentages found.

14. Example:

    40 lymphocytes and 60 neutrophilic segmented cells were recorded while counting 100 white cells. Therefore, there are 40% lymphocytes and 60% neutrophilic segmented cells.

15. Make the report as indicated in the sample report below.

16. Sample report:

Patient: Doe, Mr. John

Date: 7-7-72

Physician: Dr. James Johnson

Spinal cell count:

Total white cell count = 112 white cells per cu. mm.

Normal values = 0 to 10 white cells per cu. mm.

Differential white cell count:

Lymphocytes	40%
Neutrophilic segmented cells	60%

Examination performed by: Betty Snow

Chapter 27

L. E. Cell Examination

L. E. stands for lupus erythematosus (lu'pus er-ith-e'mah-to'sus).

The L. E. cell examination is also referred to as the LE cell test, Lupus Erythematosus test, L. E. preparation, and LE prep.

The L. E. cell examination will be discussed under the following headings:

> Introduction to the L. E. Cell Examination
> Discussion of Procedures for Preparing the Smear
> Blood Clot Method of Preparing the Smear
> Examination of the Smear for L. E. Cells

The student review questions for the L. E. cell examination are numbered 287–293 and begin on page 756 of the Appendix.

INTRODUCTION TO THE L. E. CELL EXAMINATION

Systemic lupus erythematosus is also referred to as S. L. E. and disseminated lupus erythematosus.

Systemic lupus erythematosus is a disease affecting the connective tissues of the body. It is associated with skin eruptions on the face, neck, and extremities. The cause of this disease is unknown. And it occurs most frequently in women of child bearing age.

The plasma of the blood frequently contains an L. E. factor. This L. E. factor is a gamma globulin which acts as an antibody. It acts upon a white cell and causes a chemical change in the nucleus.

The nucleus then assumes the shape of a round body. This round body is ingested by a neutrophilic segmented cell. The combination of neutrophilic segmented cell and ingested round body is called an L. E. cell.

Three L. E. cells are shown above the numbers 3, 4, and 5 in Plate 14.

In this illustration, also make the following two observations:

(1) The nucleus of the neutrophilic segmented cell acts like a pair of pincers and surrounds or engulfs the round body. Thus, the neutrophilic segmented cell becomes the "cannibal" and the round body becomes the "meal."

(2) Cell number 6 consists of a round body which is being attacked by four neutrophilic segmented cells. Eventually, one of these neutrophilic segmented cells will win the meal.

506

PLATE 14

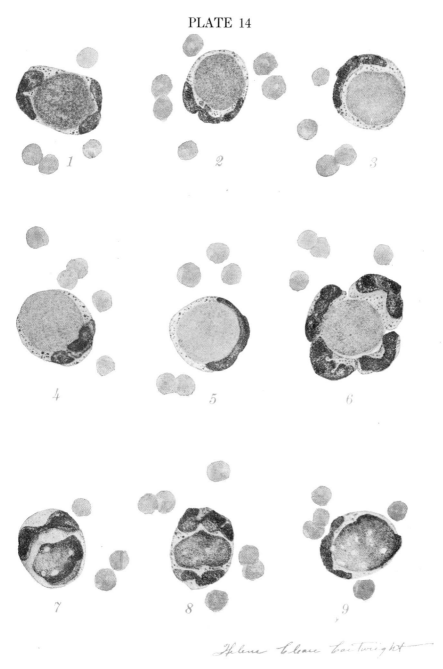

"L.E." Cells and "Tart" Cells (Nucleophagocytosis). Cells 1 to 6 are from the blood of a patient with disseminated lupus erythematosus. Cells 1, 2 and 3 show the characteristic progressive loss of nuclear detail and staining quality which take place in affected nuclei. Cell 1 by itself could not be identified as an L.E. cell. Cells 3, 4 and 5, however, are typical, fully developed L.E. cells and show the complete loss of nuclear detail. No. 6 is a small "rosette." As yet the nuclear mass has not been engulfed by any one of the phagocytes.

Nucleophagocytosis (cells 7, 8 and 9) must be distinguished from the L.E. phenomenon. Note that the engulfed material in 7, 8 and 9 retains some of its original chromatin pattern. The nuclear chromatin stains more darkly than in fully developed L.E. cells and is condensed about the edges. Vacuolization is also present. (Wintrobe, *Clinical Hematology*, 6th edition.)

What is the difference between an L. E. cell and a tart cell?

A cell known as a tart cell may be present in the blood of patients who are sensitive to various drugs. The tart cell also contains ingested material. It is also illustrated in Plate 14 (cells 7, 8, and 9).

Since the L. E. cell and tart cell both contain ingested material, they look somewhat alike. The distinguishing characteristics of the L. E. cell and tart cell will now be considered.

In an L. E. cell, the ingested body is round, smooth, and evenly stained. Note cells 3, 4, and 5 in Plate 14.

In a tart cell, the ingested body is irregular, coarse, and unevenly stained. Note cells 7, 8, and 9 in Plate 14.

The L. E. cell examination is performed about 25 times a month by the average hospital laboratory and about once a month by the average physician's office.

DISCUSSION OF PROCEDURES FOR PREPARING THE SMEAR

The various methods of preparing the smear for the L. E. cell examination have the following principle.

The L. E. factor in the patient's serum or plasma is allowed to react with white cells, the reaction produces a crop of L. E. cells, and the L. E. cells are then harvested.

The smear for the L. E. cell examination may be prepared by the following methods:

> Blood Clot Method
> Rotary or Defibrinated Method
> Slide Method
> Capillary Tube Method

The blood clot method of Zimmer and Hargraves is performed as follows: The blood is withdrawn, allowed to clot, and incubated.

Using two wooden applicator sticks, the clot is then thoroughly mashed up in its own serum.

The mixture is centrifuged.

The top layer of cells containing the white cells is transferred to a Wintrobe tube and centrifuged again.

The buffy coat or top layer of white cells is then removed and used to make the smear.

The blood clot method of Magath and Winkle is performed in the above manner except that the "mashing up" process is performed by forcing the clotted blood through a wire sieve or strainer.

The rotary or defibrinated method of Zinkham and Conley is performed as follows:

The blood is withdrawn, placed in a flask containing heparin and glass beads, and allowed to incubate at room temperature for 90 minutes.

The flask is then rotated for 30 minutes, the blood is transferred to a Wintrobe tube, and the Wintrobe tube is centrifuged.

The buffy coat or top layer of white cells is then removed and used to make the smear.

The slide method of Snapper and Nathan is performed as follows:

A drop of either of the following is placed on a glass slide.

(1) normal blood

(2) concentrated white cells from a normal hematocrit reading

This preparation is incubated, washed, and allowed to dry.

One drop of the patient's finger tip blood is then added to the above preparation.

The specimen is incubated.

The incubation allows the L. E. factor in the patient's blood to act upon the white cells of the normal blood.

The specimen is then dried and serves as the smear.

The capillary tube method of Mudick is performed as follows:

Either finger tip blood or anticoagulated blood from the patient is drawn into a capillary tube.

The capillary tube is then centrifuged.

A wire stylet is inserted into the capillary tube and the buffy coat and plasma are thoroughly mixed.

The preparation is incubated and centrifuged again.

The buffy coat or top layer of white cells is obtained and used to make the smear.

All the above methods of preparing the smear for the L. E. cell examination are currently in use.

The blood clot method of preparing the smear is given below.

BLOOD CLOT METHOD OF PREPARING THE SMEAR

NECESSARY REAGENTS AND EQUIPMENT

1. Materials for a venipuncture: sterile 20 gauge needle, 10 cc. syringe, cotton balls or gauze pads, 70% alcohol, tourniquet, and wax marking pencil
2. 2 serological test tubes
3. 2 wooden applicator sticks or #40 wire sieve or tea strainer
4. 2 Wintrobe tubes
5. Wintrobe pipet
6. Centrifuge
7. 3 glass slides
8. Wright's stain and buffer solution

Procedure

1. Assemble the materials for a venipuncture: sterile 20 gauge needle, 10 cc. syringe, cotton balls or gauze pads, 70% alcohol, tourniquet, and wax marking pencil.

2. Obtain a serological test tube.

3. Make a venipuncture, withdraw about 8 cc. of blood, and transfer the blood to the test tube.

4. Either allow the blood to stand at room temperature for 2 hours or place the blood in a 37° C. incubator for 30 minutes.

5. Then thoroughly mash up the blood clot by either method a or method b below:

6. Method a:

   Using 2 wooden applicator sticks, forcefully and deliberately poke through the blood clot 15 to 20 times.

7. Method b:

   Force the blood clot and serum through a #40 wire sieve. (Some technologists use an ordinary tea strainer.)

8. Allow the mashed up blood to remain at room temperature for 1 hour.

9. Then pour all the fluid portion, that is, the bloody serum, into another test tube.

10. Place the test tube containing the bloody serum in the centrifuge.

11. Centrifuge at 2000 RPM for 20 minutes.

12. Using a Wintrobe pipet, remove and discard the serum above the cells.

13. Using the Wintrobe pipet, remove about 1 cc. of the top layer of cells.

14. Now transfer these cells to a Wintrobe tube.

15. Centrifuge the Wintrobe tube at 2000 RPM for 20 minutes.

16. Using the Wintrobe pipet, remove and discard any serum which is above the grayish white layer of cells (buffy coat).

17. Using the Wintrobe pipet, carefully transfer the grayish white layer of cells to a glass slide.

18. Make several blood smears in the usual manner.

19. Allow the smears to dry.

20. Stain the smears with Wright's stain and buffer solution.

21. Allow the smears to dry.

22. Then turn to the examination of the smear for L. E. cells which is given below.

EXAMINATION OF THE SMEAR FOR L. E. CELLS

1. Put a drop of immersion oil on one of the stained smears.

2. Place the smear on the stage of the microscope and bring the cells into view with the oil immersion (95×) objective of the microscope.

3. Observe the L. E. cells which are illustrated in Plate 14, page 506.

   Note: Cells 3, 4, and 5 are typical L. E. cells. Observe that the central area is round, smooth, and evenly stained. Cells 7, 8, and 9 are tart cells. Observe that the central area is irregular, coarse, and unevenly stained. The tart cells should neither be counted nor reported.

4. At least 2 typical L. E. cells should be seen before the examination can be considered positive.

5. Now inspect 1000 white cells and record the number of L. E. cells seen.

6. If your inspection revealed 2 or more typical L. E. cells, report the examination as positive.

7. If your inspection revealed less than 2 typical L. E. cells, report the examination as negative.

8. Make out your report as indicated in the sample report below.

9. Sample report:

Patient: Doe, Mr. John

Date: 7-7-72

Physician: Dr. DeWitt Englund

L. E. cell examination: positive

Examination performed by: Norma Greene

Chapter 28

Fetal Hemoglobin Determination

Fetal hemoglobin is often referred to as F hemoglobin, hemoglobin F, Hb F, HbF, and Hb-F.

The fetal hemoglobin determination will be discussed under the following headings:

Significance of the Fetal Hemoglobin Determination
Discussion of Procedures for the Fetal Hemoglobin Determination
Alkali Denaturation Method for the Fetal Hemoglobin Determination

The student review questions for the fetal hemoglobin determination are numbered 294–299 and begin on page 757 of the Appendix.

SIGNIFICANCE OF THE FETAL HEMOGLOBIN DETERMINATION

Fetal hemoglobin is a normal hemoglobin which is manufactured in the red cells of the fetus and infant.

At birth, 50%–90% of the hemoglobin is fetal hemoglobin.

Under normal conditions, the manufacture of fetal hemoglobin is replaced by the manufacture of adult hemoglobin during the first year of life.

In an anemia known as thalassemia, however, an inherited abnormality occurs in the manufacture of hemoglobin. The effect of this abnormality is to allow the continued production of fetal hemoglobin and hinder the manufacture of adult hemoglobin. The end result is a decrease in the quantity and quality of erythrocytes.

The continued production of fetal hemoglobin may occur on a minor scale or a major scale. If it occurs on a minor scale, the anemia is referred to as thalassemia minor. If it occurs on a major scale, the anemia is referred to as thalassemia major.

Thus, the fetal hemoglobin determination may be useful in the diagnosis of thalassemia.

The fetal hemoglobin determination has the following normal values:

0% – 4%   .   .   before the age of 2 years
0% – 2%   .   .   after the age of 2 years

35

511

The fetal hemoglobin determination reveals values of 5%–10% in thalassemia minor and values of 40%–90% in thalassemia major.

The fetal hemoglobin determination may also show values above normal in aplastic anemia, hereditary spherocytic anemia, sickle cell anemia, hemoglobin H disease, and erythremic myelosis.

The fetal hemoglobin determination is performed about once a month by the average hospital laboratory and about once a year by the average physician's office.

DISCUSSION OF PROCEDURES FOR THE FETAL HEMOGLOBIN DETERMINATION

The fetal hemoglobin determination may be performed by the following methods:

> alkali denaturation method
> blood slide methods
> electrophoretic methods

The alkali denaturation method is based on the following principle:

With the exception of fetal hemoglobin, all hemoglobins are easily modified or denatured by an alkali.

The alkali denaturation method of Singer, Chernoff, and Singer is performed as follows:

A hemoglobin solution or hemolysate is prepared from the patient's blood.

A sample of the hemoglobin solution is taken. The hemoglobin concentration is determined. This hemoglobin concentration represents the total hemoglobin, that is, all types of hemoglobin which may be present.

A second sample of the hemoglobin solution is then taken. The alkali, potassium hydroxide, is added. This denatures all hemoglobins *except* fetal hemoglobin. The denatured material is removed. The remaining hemoglobin is fetal hemoglobin. The hemoglobin concentration is determined. And the value obtained represents fetal hemoglobin.

The fetal hemoglobin is expressed as a percentage of the total hemoglobin.

Thus,

$$\text{Per cent fetal Hb} = \frac{\text{Hb in 2nd sample (fetal Hb)}}{\text{Hb in 1st sample (total Hb)}} \times 100$$

The alkali denaturation method for the fetal hemoglobin determination is given below.

ALKALI DENATURATION METHOD FOR THE FETAL HEMOGLOBIN DETERMINATION

The discussion will cover (1) the necessary reagents and equipment, (2) the preparation of the patient's hemoglobin solution, and (3) the procedure.

NECESSARY REAGENTS AND EQUIPMENT

1. 5 ml. of the patient's anticoagulated blood
2. physiological (0.85%) saline solution
3. distilled water
4. toluene
5. N/12 potassium hydroxide (pH 12.7). This is the alkali solution. It may be obtained from your local medical supply house. The solution should be stored in a plastic bottle at 4° C.
6. acidified 50% saturated solution of ammonium sulfate. Preparation: To 100 ml. of a saturated solution of ammonium sulfate, add 100 ml. of distilled water and 0.5 ml. of concentrated (10 N) hydrochloric acid. Mix.
7. centrifuge
8. spectrophotometer
9. stopwatch or timer
10. #44 Whatman filter paper and funnel
11. water bath maintained at 20° C.

PREPARATION OF THE PATIENT'S HEMOGLOBIN SOLUTION

1. Obtain 5 ml. of the patient's anticoagulated blood.

2. Pour the blood into a <u>graduated</u> centrifuge tube.

3. Centrifuge the blood.

4. Remove the blood from the centrifuge and discard the plasma.

5. Wash the red cells 3 times as follows: Add 10 ml. of physiological saline, mix, centrifuge, and discard the physiological saline.

6. After the last centrifuging and discarding of the physiological saline, centrifuge the red cells once more to make sure they are well packed.

7. Then note and record the volume of <u>packed</u> red cells.

8. For each 1 ml. of packed red cells, add 1.4 ml. of distilled water and 0.4 ml. of toluene.

   Note: A simple way to perform this step is to take a Wintrobe pipet and remove and discard the packed red cells above the 1 ml. mark, thus leaving exactly 1 ml. of packed red cells. Then simply add 1.4 ml. of distilled water and 0.4 ml. of toluene.

9. Shake vigorously for 5 minutes.

10. Centrifuge at 3000 RPM for 15 minutes.

11. Using a cotton swab, remove and discard the top layer of toluene.

12. Insert a pipet below the plug of stromal material and remove the hemoglobin solution.

13. Filter the hemoglobin solution through a #44 Whatman filter paper.

    Note: The filtered solution should not be cloudy. If it is cloudy: take two pieces of filter paper, make a double filter, and re-filter.

14. Pour the filtered solution into a test tube and label Patient's Hemoglobin Solution.

15. This hemoglobin solution has a hemoglobin concentration of about 10 grams per 100 ml.

16. If this hemoglobin solution is kept in a tightly capped bottle and stored in the refrigerator at 4° C., it will keep about 1 year.

PROCEDURE

1. Add 0.02 ml. of the above patient's hemoglobin solution to 5 ml. of distilled water. Mix. (This is a dilution of 0.02 in 5.02).

2. Using distilled water as the blank, set the spectrophotometer at 540 mμ.

3. Now insert the diluted hemoglobin solution in the spectrophotometer.

4. Read and make a record of the optical density (O. D.).

5. Remove the diluted hemoglobin solution from the spectrophotometer and discard it.

6. Pipet 1.6 ml. of the N/12 potassium hydroxide into a small test tube.

7. Place the test tube in the 20° C. water bath.

8. Allow about 8 minutes to pass so that the solution becomes adjusted to the 20° C. temperature.

   Note: It is essential that the temperature be maintained between 19° C. and 21° C.

9. After the 8 minutes have elapsed, proceed with the following steps which must be performed in quick succession:

10. To the test tube of potassium hydroxide in the water bath, add 0.1 ml. of the patient's hemoglobin solution and immediately start the stopwatch or timer.

11. Quickly remove the test tube from the water bath, mix the contents by holding the top of the test tube with your left hand and tapping the bottom of the test tube with your right hand, and then quickly return the test tube to the water bath.

12. Exactly 60 seconds after adding the patient's hemoglobin solution, proceed with the following:

13. Add 3.4 ml. of the acidified 50% saturated solution of ammonium sulfate.

   Note: This stops the reaction and precipitates the denatured hemoglobin.

14. Mix by inverting the test tube about 6 times.

15. Now filter the solution through a #44 Whatman filter paper.

   Note: The solution may be colored but it should be perfectly clear. If it is not clear, take two #44 Whatman filter papers, make a double filter, and re-filter the solution.

16. Pour the clear filtered solution into a test tube.

17. Using distilled water as the blank, again set the spectrophotometer at 540 mμ.

18. Then insert your clear filtered solution into the spectro-photometer.

19. Read and <u>make a record</u> of the optical density (O.D.).

20. With the two O. D. (optical density) readings from the spectrophotometer, a calculation is now made using the formula:

Per cent fetal Hb =

$$\frac{\text{O. D. fetal Hb (2nd reading)}}{\text{O. D. total Hb (1st reading)}} \times 0.203 \times 100$$

21. Explanation of factor 0.203: The dilution of the 1st sample of the patient's hemoglobin solution was

$$\frac{5.02}{0.02} = 251$$

The dilution of the 2nd sample of the patient's hemoglobin solution was

$$\frac{5.1}{0.1} = 51$$

Therefore, the dilution correction factor is

$$\frac{51}{251} = 0.203$$

22. A sample calculation is given below:
    1st O. D. reading was 20
    2nd O. D. reading was 40

Per cent fetal Hb =

$$\frac{\text{O. D. fetal Hb (2nd reading)}}{\text{O. D. total Hb (1st reading)}} \times 0.203 \times 100$$

$$= \frac{40}{20} \times 0.203 \times 100$$

$$= 2 \times 0.203 \times 100$$

$$= 0.203 \times 200$$

$$= 40.6$$

$$= 41$$

23. Using your two recorded O. D. (optical density) readings from the spectrophotometer, make your calculation in the above manner.

24. Then make out your report as shown in the sample report below.

25. Sample report:

Patient: Doe, Mr. John

Date: 7-7-72

Physician: Dr. James Mason

Fetal hemoglobin determination: 41%

Method: Alkali denaturation method

Normal values: 0%–2%

Examination performed by: Betty Snow

Chapter 29

Hemoglobin Electrophoretic Separations

The act of electrically separating the components of hemoglobin is referred to as hemoglobin electrophoretic separations.

Hemoglobin electrophoretic separations are also referred to as the abnormal hemoglobin examination and hemoglobin electrophoresis.

We will consider the significance of hemoglobin electrophoretic separations and present a brief discussion of the procedures for hemoglobin electrophoretic separations.

The student review questions for hemoglobin electrophoretic separations are numbered 300–309 and begin on page 757 of the Appendix.

SIGNIFICANCE OF HEMOGLOBIN ELECTROPHORETIC SEPARATIONS

We have 3 normal hemoglobin molecules:

hemoglobin A (Hb A)
hemoglobin A_2 (Hb A_2)
hemoglobin F (Hb F)

Hemoglobin A is the major normal adult hemoglobin molecule. This molecule has 2 alpha chains and 2 beta chains. Each chain is linked to a heme group.

Hemoglobin A_2 is a minor normal adult hemoglobin molecule, being present in normal blood to the extent of 1.5%–3.5%. This molecule has 2 alpha chains and 2 delta chains. Each chain is linked to a heme group.

Hemoglobin F is the normal fetal hemoglobin molecule. During the first two years of life, this hemoglobin is present in the blood to the extent of 0%–4%. The molecule has 2 alpha chains and 2 gamma chains. Each chain is linked to a heme group.

The 3 normal hemoglobin molecules—Hb A, Hb A_2, and Hb F—are illustrated in Figure 165.

As stated above, hemoglobin F is a normal hemoglobin. However, sometimes large quantities of hemoglobin F are found in the blood of children and young adults. This condition is unnatural and it can lead to a severe anemia.

518

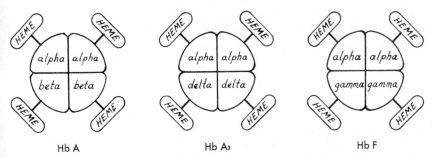

Hb A   Hb A₂   Hb F

Fig. 165.—The three normal hemoglobin molecules.

Now let us leave the normal hemoglobins and turn to the abnormal hemoglobins.

The term "abnormal hemoglobins" is generally reserved for those hemoglobins which are found in the so-called hemoglobin diseases or hemoglobinopathies.

These abnormal hemoglobins differ from the normal hemoglobins in molecular structure.

To date, we have found about 100 abnormal hemoglobins.

Among the more commonly encountered abnormal hemoglobins are the following: Hb S, Hb C, Hb D, Hb E, and Hb H.

All the abnormal hemoglobins are genetically transmitted.

Let us briefly consider the transmission and effects of an abnormal hemoglobin, using hemoglobin S as an example.

If a person inherits a gene for normal hemoglobin A from one parent and a gene for abnormal hemoglobin S from the other parent, his hemoglobin pattern is said to be heterozygous.

If a person inherits a gene for abnormal hemoglobin S from both parents, his hemoglobin pattern is said to be homozygous.

The person with the heterozygous hemoglobin pattern may have sickle cell trait; whereas the person with the homozygous hemoglobin pattern may have sickle cell anemia.

Persons with sickle cell trait may transmit the disease but they are usually not affected with an anemia or any physical symptoms of the disease.

Persons with sickle cell anemia, however, have a severe anemia with all the physical symptoms and they usually die before they reach 21.

In sickle cell trait, the blood reveals about 65% Hb A and about 35% Hb S; in sickle cell anemia, however, the blood reveals about 90% Hb S.

Thus, the percentage of hemoglobin S in the blood may be a vital indicator, pointing to the very life or death of the patient.

What does the blood reveal in thalassemia?

In thalassemia minor, the blood reveals about 8% Hb F; in thalassemia major, however, the blood reveals about 65% Hb F.

In thalassemia minor, the patient usually lives; in thalassemia major, the patient usually dies.

Thus, we see that the percentage of normal and abnormal hemoglobin in the blood is a vital indicator.

We may determine the percentage of normal and abnormal hemoglobin by performing hemoglobin electrophoretic separations.

Hemoglobin electrophoretic separations are performed about once a month by the average hospital laboratory and about once a year by the average physician's office.

DISCUSSION OF PROCEDURES FOR HEMOGLOBIN ELECTROPHORETIC SEPARATIONS

The word electrophoresis comes from two Greek words. The first portion denotes electricity and the second portion means bearing. Thus, electrophoresis means bearing electricity.

Electrophoresis may be defined as the movement of charged particles on various media under the influence of an electric current.

The particles are placed on "race tracks" or media such as paper, starch, or gel. An electric current is applied. The particles move at speeds governed by their weight and electric charge.

The particles under our immediate consideration are hemoglobins A, A_2, F, S, C, D, E, and H.

Some of these hemoglobins are slow and others are fast.

By running the patient's blood against known hemoglobins, we can identify the different hemoglobins.

The relative speeds of the various hemoglobins on filter paper using 0.05 M barbital buffer solution at a pH of 8.6 are illustrated in Figure 166.

You will note that some of the normal and abnormal hemoglobins run dead heats, that is, they migrate at the same speed.

For example, Hb H and Hb I migrate at the same speed; Hb S and Hb D migrate at the same speed; and Hb F and Hb G migrate at the same speed.

How do we separate these hemoglobins?

Such hemoglobins can usually be separated by altering the conditions of the race.

For example, we can change the race track or media. We can change the solution in which the hemoglobin is suspended. And we can change the pH of the solution.

Thus, Hb H and Hb I may be separated by using filter paper media, a phosphate buffer solution, and a pH of 6.5.

Hb S and Hb D may be separated by using a phosphate buffer solution in which they have different solubilities.

Hb F and Hb G may be differentiated by running the alkali denaturation test which we learned in the preceding chapter.

Hemoglobin electrophoretic separations may be carried out with the following media: filter paper, starch block, agar gel, acrylamide gel, and cellulose acetate.

Since hemoglobin electrophoretic separations are usually run in the chemistry department, we will not present a step-by-step procedure.

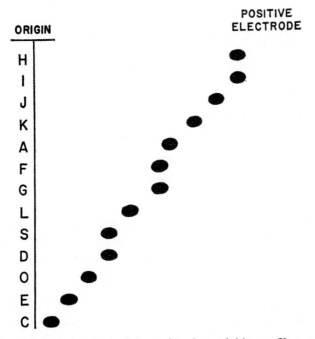

FIG. 166.—Relative migrations of the various hemoglobins on filter paper using 0.05 M barbital buffer solution at a pH of 8.6. (Reproduced from the revised edition of "A Syllabus of Laboratory Examinations in Clinical Diagnosis" by Page and Culver, published by Harvard University Press.)

Chapter 30

Bone Marrow Smears

BONE marrow smears will be discussed under the following headings:

Significance of Bone Marrow Smears
Preparation and Staining of Bone Marrow Smears
Study of Cells Seen in Bone Marrow Smears
Examination of Bone Marrow Smears

The student review questions for bone marrow smears are numbered 310–317 and begin on page 758 of the Appendix.

SIGNIFICANCE OF BONE MARROW SMEARS

The red cells, white cells, and platelets are manufactured in the bone marrow. If the manufacturing process is abnormal, it may indicate disease The manufacturing process may be studied by obtaining a smear of the bone marrow and evaluating the cells.

The normal values for bone marrow smears are given in Table 36.

What is the M:E ratio?

The M:E stands for myeloid-erythroid. Thus, the M:E ratio is the myeloid-erythroid ratio. It is the ratio of white cells to nucleated red cells.

For example, if a bone marrow smear shows 80% white cells and 20% nucleated red cells, the M:E ratio is 4:1.

The M:E ratio is often referred to as the WBC:Nucleated RBC ratio.

The average M:E ratio is 4:1, with a normal range of 6:1 to 2:1.

An increased M:E ratio (7:1 or more) may be found in infections, granulocytic leukemia, leukemoid reactions, and a decrease in the number of nucleated red cells.

A decreased M:E ratio (1:1 or less) may be encountered in either a decrease in the production of white cells or an increase in the production of red cells.

Bone marrow smears are of particular interest to the physician in the following diseases: aplastic anemia, pernicious anemia, leukemia, purpura hemorrhagica, agranulocytosis, and multiple myeloma.

Table 36

Normal Values for Bone Marrow Smears

Cell	Normal Values in Per Cent
WHITE CELLS	
Myeloblasts	0 to 5
Progranulocytes	2 to 8
Neutrophilic myelocytes	4 to 16
Neutrophilic metamyelocytes	5 to 20
Neutrophilic band cells	10 to 35
Neutrophilic segmented cells	7 to 30
Eosinophilic cells	1 to 4
Basophilic cells	0 to 1
Lymphocytes	5 to 15
Monocytes	0 to 5
Plasmacytes	0 to 1
Red Cells	
Rubriblasts	0 to 1
Prorubricytes	1 to 4
Rubricytes	3 to 10
Metarubricytes	4 to 25
(total nucleated red cells)	(8 to 30)
PLATELETS	
Megakaryocytes	0 to 3
M:E ratio	4:1

The more significant bone marrow abnormalities in some of the diseases which we will study are summarized in Table 37.

Bone marrow smears are obtained and evaluated about 10 times a month by the average hospital laboratory and about once a year by the average physician's office.

PREPARATION AND STAINING OF BONE MARROW SMEARS

The physician furnishes the equipment for the bone marrow puncture. The technologist furnishes about 10 "extra clean" glass slides and materials for a finger puncture.

Table 37

The More Significant Bone Marrow Abnormalities in Various Diseases

Disease	Abnormality	Normal Values
aplastic anemia	hypoplastic (defective and incomplete development of cells)	normoplastic
iron deficiency anemia	hyperplastic (overactive); increase in nucleated red cells (30%—60%)	normoplastic 8% — 30%
pernicious anemia	increase in nucleated red cells (30%—50%); presence of "pernicious anemia type" nucleated red cells	8% — 30%
hereditary spherocytic anemia	increase in nucleated red cells (30%—60%)	8% — 30%
sickle cell anemia	increase in nucleated red cells (40%—70%)	8% — 30%
thalassemia major	increase in nucleated red cells (30%—60%)	8% — 30%
acute granulocytic leukemia	increase in myeloblasts (15%—50%)	0% — 5%
chronic granulocytic leukemia	increase in myeloblasts (5%—15%)	0% — 5%
acute lymphocytic leukemia	increase in lymphoblasts (15%—75%)	0%
chronic lymphocytic leukemia	increase in lymphocytes (30%—90%)	5% — 15%
monocytic leukemia	increase in monocytes (20%—60%)	0% — 5%
plasmacytic leukemia	increase in plasmacytes (15%—75%)	0% — 1%
purpura hemorrhagica (idiopathic thrombocytopenic purpura)	number of megakaryocytes is normal or increased; platelet formation is decreased	0% — 3%
polycythemia vera	hyperplastic; percentage of white cells, red cells, and platelets is normal	normoplastic
agranulocytosis	granulocytes are decreased during height of disease but increased during recovery; percentage of nucleated red cells is normal; percentage of megakaryocytes is normal	8% — 30% 0% — 3%
infectious mononucleosis	increase in lymphocytes (15%—35%)	5% — 15%
multiple myeloma	10%—90% myeloma cells	0%
Hodgkin's disease	presence of Sternberg-Reed cells	0
Gaucher's disease	presence of Gaucher's cells	0

The physician prepares the patient, makes a puncture of the bone (usually the sternum), and withdraws about 0.3 cubic centimeter of bone marrow. This is passed to the technologist who should proceed as follows:

1. Place a small amount of bone marrow on a glass slide.

2. Make a bone marrow smear in the same manner that you would make a blood smear.

   Note: The smear may appear uneven and "lumpy" due to the presence of fatty material and bone marrow fragments.

3. Make about 5 more bone marrow smears.

4. Make a finger puncture on the patient.

5. Make two blood smears for a differential white cell count.

6. Write the patient's name and date on both the bone marrow smears and blood smears.

   Note: The blood smears are taken for the purpose of correlating the findings in the bone marrow with the findings in the blood.

7. Allow the bone marrow smears and the blood smears to dry. (It takes about 20 minutes for bone marrow smears to dry.)

8. Then stain both the bone marrow smears and blood smears with Wright's stain and buffer solution.

   Note: Bone marrow smears are thicker than ordinary blood smears. Therefore, they should be stained a few minutes longer than ordinary blood smears. Some technologists even double the staining time. For example, they leave the Wright's stain on for 2 minutes rather than the usual 1 minute; they leave the mixture of Wright's stain and buffer solution on for 16 minutes rather than the usual 8 minutes.

9. After staining the bone marrow smears and blood smears, allow them to dry. (It requires about 10 minutes.)

10. Make the study of bone marrow cells which is given below.

STUDY OF CELLS SEEN IN BONE MARROW SMEARS

A bone marrow smear contains practically the whole spectrum of blood cells and it therefore offers the student an excellent opportunity to study the different types of blood cells.

Since the student is already familiar with neutrophilic segmented cells and neutrophilic band cells, we have not included these cells in our forthcoming illustration.

The student should study the bone marrow cells by making the comparisons given in items 1–13 below.

1. In the lower right hand corner of Plate 15, note the difference between the monocyte and the neutrophilic metamyelocyte.

2. In the upper portion of Plate 15, note the difference between the rubricyte and the two lymphocytes.

3. On the right side of the plate, note the difference in the three myelocytes: eosinophilic myelocyte, neutrophilic myelocyte, and basophilic myelocyte.

4. On the right side of the plate, note the difference between the neutrophilic myelocyte and the neutrophilic metamyelocyte.

5. In the upper right side of the plate, note the difference between the lymphocyte and the metarubricyte.

6. In the lower portion of the plate, note the difference between the progranulocyte without granules and the progranulocyte with granules.

7. On the left side of the plate, note the difference between the prorubricyte and the lymphocyte just below it.

8. On the left side of the plate, note the difference between the monocyte and the lymphocyte.

9. On the extreme left side of the plate, note the very slight difference in the three "blast" cells: the rubriblast, lymphoblast, and myeloblast. The difference in these three "blast" cells is somewhat like the difference in three newborn babies.

10. On the right side of the plate, note the platelets being released from the megakaryocyte.

11. On the left side of the plate, note the difference in the prorubricyte, plasmacyte, and lymphocyte.

PLATE 15   CELLS OF THE BON

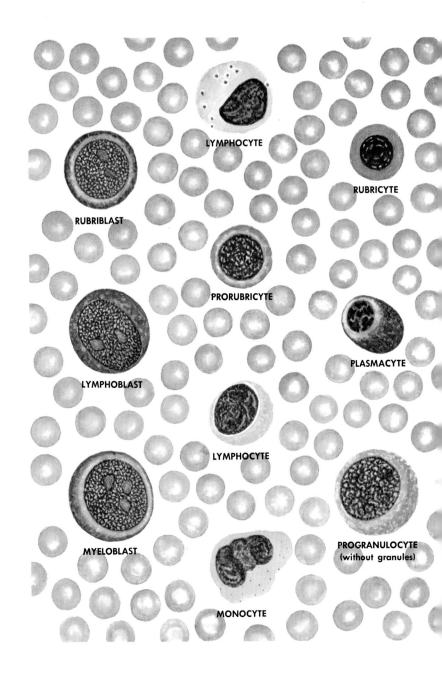

LYMPHOCYTE

RUBRICYTE

RUBRIBLAST

PRORUBRICYTE

PLASMACYTE

LYMPHOBLAST

LYMPHOCYTE

MYELOBLAST

PROGRANULOCYTE
(without granules)

MONOCYTE

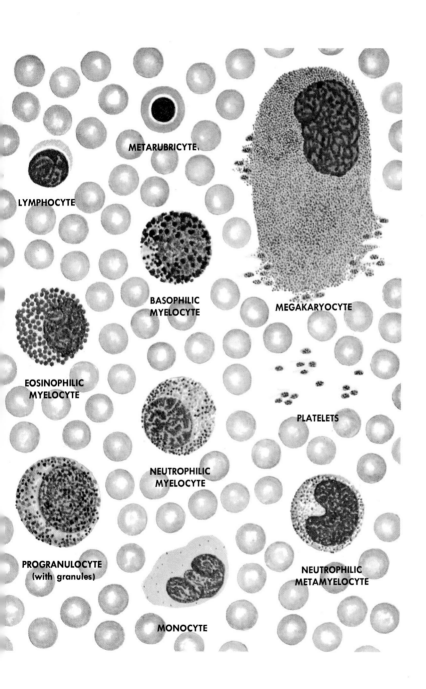

METARUBRICYTE

LYMPHOCYTE

BASOPHILIC
MYELOCYTE

MEGAKARYOCYTE

EOSINOPHILIC
MYELOCYTE

PLATELETS

NEUTROPHILIC
MYELOCYTE

PROGRANULOCYTE
(with granules)

NEUTROPHILIC
METAMYELOCYTE

MONOCYTE

12. In the lower portion of the plate, going from left to right, note the difference in the young cells of the neutrophilic series: myeloblast, progranulocyte (without granules), progranulocyte (with granules), neutrophilic myelocyte, and neutrophilic metamyelocyte.

13. In the upper portion of the plate, going from left to right, note the difference in the young cells of the erythrocytic series: rubriblast, prorubricyte, rubricyte, and metarubricyte.

14. After you have made this study of bone marrow cells, turn to the examination of bone marrow smears which is given below.

EXAMINATION OF BONE MARROW SMEARS

1. After studying the cells of the bone marrow as directed above, proceed with the following.

2. Some instructors require the student to classify and tabulate each nucleated red cell.

3. Other instructors require the student to simply tabulate each nucleated red cell without classifying it as a rubriblast, prorubricyte, rubricyte, or metarubricyte.

4. The latter procedure is recommended for beginners.

5. Therefore, unless you are otherwise instructed, simply tabulate all nucleated red cells without classifying them. Thus, if you see 1 rubriblast, 2 prorubricytes, and 1 rubricyte, mark down 4 nucleated red cells.

6. Obtain a piece of paper and write down the names of the blood cells as shown in the sample work-sheet for a bone marrow examination (Fig. 167, page 528).

7. Place a drop of immersion oil on the thin area of a bone marrow smear.

8. Put the bone marrow smear on the stage of the microscope and bring the cells into view with the oil immersion (95$\times$) objective of the microscope.

9. Move the smear until you find a spot where the cells are fairly well distributed.

Note: You should never count the cells in an area where the cells are clumped or bunched together because the distribution will not be even and consequently the sample will not be representative.

Cells	Tabulation	Totals
myeloblasts	///	3
progranulocytes	~~////~~	5
neutrophilic myelocytes . .	~~////~~ ~~////~~	10
neutrophilic metamyelocytes .	~~////~~ ~~////~~ //	12
neutrophilic band cells . .	~~////~~ ~~////~~ ~~////~~ /	16
neutrophilic segmented cells .	~~////~~ ~~////~~ ~~////~~ ~~////~~ ///	23
eosinophilic cells	/	1
basophilic cells		
lymphocytes	~~////~~ ////	9
monocytes	/	1
plasmacytes.		————
		80
nucleated red cells . . .	~~////~~ ~~////~~ ~~////~~ ~~////~~	20
megakaryocytes		
unidentified cells	//	
M:E ratio	4:1	

FIG. 167.—Sample work-sheet for a bone marrow examination.

10. When you find an area where the cells are fairly well distributed, identify and record the cells in this microscopic field.

11. Then move the smear to another microscopic field where the cells are fairly well distributed.

12. Identify and record the cells in this microscopic field.

13. Continue the above process until you have identified and recorded 100 cells.

14. Note: If you wish to increase the accuracy of your report, identify and record another 100 cells. Then take the average for each cell. For example, if you found 2 myeloblasts in your first 100 cells and 4 myeloblasts in your second 100 cells, the average would be 3 myeloblasts.

15. When you have completed your examination, ask your instructor or pathologist to check the values you obtained.

16. Give the bone marrow smears and also the blood smears to the pathologist or physician for evaluation and diagnosis.

17. Note: If possible, save one of the bone marrow smears for future study and reference.

Chapter 31

Additional Staining Procedures

THIS chapter considers the following additional staining procedures:

Siderocyte Stain
Heinz Body Stain
Peroxidase Stain
Alkaline Phosphatase Stain
Giemsa Stain
Feulgen Stain
Miscellaneous Stains

The siderocyte stain and Heinz body stain are for red cells.

The peroxidase stain and alkaline phosphatase stain are for white cells.

These four stains are run several times a year by the average hospital laboratory.

The remaining stains vary in importance.

The student review questions for additional staining procedures are numbered 318–335 and begin on page 759 of the Appendix.

SIDEROCYTE STAIN

The siderocyte stain is also referred to as the Prussian blue stain and Prussian blue reaction.

The discussion will cover the significance of the siderocyte stain and the procedure for the siderocyte stain.

SIGNIFICANCE OF THE SIDEROCYTE STAIN

Sideros is Greek for iron.

A siderocyte is an erythrocyte containing free iron; a sideroblast is a nucleated red cell containing free iron.

The free iron can not be identified on an ordinary blood smear stained with Wright's stain and a special stain must be used.

When stained with a Prussian blue reagent, the free iron appears as tiny blue or blue-green granules.

Siderocytes have been illustrated in Plate 11, page 278.

In health, 0%–1% of the erythrocytes are siderocytes.

In some conditions, 1%–30% of the erythrocytes may be siderocytes.

Among these conditions are thalassemia major, lead poisoning, and following splenectomy.

A rise in the percentage of siderocytes usually indicates an abnormality in the synthesis of hemoglobin.

PROCEDURE FOR THE SIDEROCYTE STAIN

Necessary Reagents

1. absolute methyl alcohol
2. 2% potassium ferrocyanide solution.
   To prepare: Place 2 grams of potassium ferrocyanide in a brown bottle. Add 100 ml. of distilled water. Mix. *Keeps only 1 month.*
3. 2% (about 0.2 N) hydrochloric acid solution
4. either one of the following counterstains may be used:
   a. 0.1% aqueous solution of eosin
   b. 0.1% aqueous solution of safranin
5. preparation of solutions given in Appendix, page 696–697

Procedure

1. Using either finger tip blood or anticoagulated blood, make a blood smear in the usual manner.

2. Allow the smear to dry.

3. Fix the cells by placing the smear in the absolute methyl alcohol for 10 minutes.

4. Remove the smear and allow it to dry.

5. Make a freshly prepared Prussian blue reagent as follows:
   Pour 50 ml. of the 2% potassium ferrocyanide solution into a flask.
   Add 50 ml. of the 2% (about 0.2 N) hydrochloric acid. Mix.

6. Place the smear on a staining rack, in a staining dish, or in a 100 ml. beaker.

7. Completely cover the smear with the freshly prepared Prussian blue reagent.

8. Allow to stain for 15 minutes.

9. Then wash the smear in a gentle stream of distilled water for about 5 minutes.

10. Using either the 0.1% aqueous solution of eosin or the 0.1% aqueous solution of safranin, counterstain the smear for 1 minute.

11. Then wash the smear with distilled water and allow to dry.

12. Place a drop of immersion oil on the <u>thin area</u> of the smear.

13. Using the oil immersion (95×) objective of the microscope, bring the cells into view.

14. Find an area where the red cells are spread out and evenly distributed.

15. The siderocytes will be the red cells containing blue or blue-green granules. See Plate 11, page 278.

16. Now the problem is to count 1000 red cells (erythrocytes and siderocytes) and record the number of siderocytes seen.

17. Therefore, count 1000 red cells, making a record every time you see a siderocyte.

18. The per cent siderocytes is found as follows:

Per cent siderocytes

$$= \frac{\text{number of siderocytes recorded}}{\text{1000 red cells (erythrocytes plus siderocytes)}} \times 100$$

19. Sample calculation

Let us say you recorded 50 siderocytes while counting the 1000 red cells.

Then,

Per cent siderocytes

$$= \frac{\text{number of siderocytes recorded}}{\text{1000 red cells (erythrocytes plus siderocytes)}} \times 100$$

$$= \frac{50}{1000} \times 100$$

$$= \frac{5000}{1000}$$

$$= 5\%$$

20. Make your calculation as shown above.

21. Report the per cent siderocytes.

22. Normal values: 0%–1%

23. 1%–30% siderocytes may be seen in thalassemia major, lead poisoning, and after removal of the spleen.

HEINZ BODY STAIN

The discussion will cover the significance of the Heinz body stain and the procedure for the Heinz body stain.

SIGNIFICANCE OF THE HEINZ BODY STAIN

A Heinz body is a small particle which may be present in an erythrocyte. It is believed that this small particle is precipitated hemoglobin. And its presence indicates some injury to the erythrocyte.

Heinz bodies are not normally present in erythrocytes.

5%–75% of the erythrocytes may contain Heinz bodies in:

(1) hemolytic anemia caused by drug poisoning
(2) after removal of the spleen (splenectomy)

Among the many drugs responsible for the presence of Heinz bodies are phenylhydrazine, primaquine, and nitrobenzene. These drugs have an oxidizing activity. This oxidizing activity apparently interferes with the normal functioning of hemoglobin in some individuals.

The procedure for the Heinz body stain follows.

PROCEDURE FOR THE HEINZ BODY STAIN

Heinz bodies may be observed as round refractile bodies on wet unstained preparations of blood.

Heinz bodies can not be identified on blood smears stained with Wright's stain. Hence, a special stain must be used. The special stains most frequently employed are either a methyl violet solution or a brilliant cresyl blue solution.

With a methyl violet solution, the Heinz bodies appear as deep purple particles.

The procedure using a methyl violet solution is given below.

Necessary Reagent

0.5% physiological saline solution of methyl violet. To prepare: Add 0.5 gram of methyl violet to 100 ml. of physiological saline solution. Shake thoroughly for a few minutes. Filter into a clean bottle.

Procedure

1. Place 3 drops of the above methyl violet solution in a small test tube.

2. Add 3 drops of either finger tip blood or fresh anti-coagulated blood to the 3 drops of methyl violet solution.

3. Mix and allow to stand for 15 minutes.

4. Mix again and make a blood smear in the usual manner.

5. Allow the smear to dry.

6. Place a drop of immersion oil on the <u>thin area</u> of the smear.

7. Bring the cells into view with the oil immersion (95×) objective of the microscope.

8. Find an area where the red cells are spread out and evenly distributed.

9. With this methyl violet solution, the Heinz bodies appear as deep purple particles. The particles may vary in size from barely visible dots to spheres occupying almost half the space in the erythrocyte. The particles usually lie near the edge of the cell. Several particles may be present in a single erythrocyte.

10. Now the problem is to count 1000 red cells (normal erythrocytes and erythrocytes containing Heinz bodies) and make a record every time you see an erythrocyte containing a Heinz body.

11. Therefore, count 1000 red cells, making a record every time you see an erythrocyte containing a Heinz body.

12. The per cent erythrocytes containing Heinz bodies is found as follows:

Per cent erythrocytes containing Heinz bodies

$$= \frac{\text{number of erythrocytes containing Heinz bodies recorded}}{\text{1000 red cells (normal erythrocytes plus erythrocytes containing Heinz bodies)}} \times 100$$

13. Sample calculation

Let us say you recorded 50 erythrocytes containing Heinz bodies while counting the 1000 red cells.

Then,

Per cent erythrocytes containing Heinz bodies

$$= \frac{\text{number of erythrocytes containing Heinz bodies recorded}}{\text{1000 red cells (normal erythrocytes plus erythrocytes containing Heinz bodies)}} \times 100$$

$$= \frac{50}{1000} \times 100$$

$$= \frac{5000}{1000}$$

$$= 5\%$$

14. Make your calculation as shown above.

15. Report the per cent erythrocytes containing Heinz bodies.

16. Normal values: none

17. 5%–75% of the erythrocytes may contain Heinz bodies in hemolytic anemia caused by drug poisoning and after removal of the spleen.

PEROXIDASE STAIN

The peroxidase stain is often referred to as the peroxidase reaction and it is sometimes referred to as the oxydase stain or oxydase reaction.

The discussion will cover the significance of the peroxidase stain and the procedure for the peroxidase stain.

SIGNIFICANCE OF THE PEROXIDASE STAIN

The treatment of leukemia may vary with the form of leukemia.

The form of leukemia is usually identified by finding the white cell series which predominates. For example, if the granulocytic series predominates, the leukemia is granulocytic leukemia; if the lymphocytic series predominates, the leukemia is lymphocytic leukemia.

The predominating white cell series, however, may be difficult to establish, especially if a distinction must be made between the young cells of the
granulocytic series and the young cells of the lymphocytic series.

The predominating white cell series can generally be established by performing a peroxidase stain.

The peroxidase stain functions as follows:

The cytoplasm of some blood cells contains the enzyme peroxidase
whereas the cytoplasm of other blood cells does not contain the enzyme
peroxidase.

If the enzyme peroxidase is present in the cytoplasm, it will liberate the
oxygen in a hydrogen peroxide solution.

The liberated oxygen will react with benzidine.

This reaction will then produce colored granules in the cytoplasm.

If colored granules are present in the cytoplasm, the cell is said to be
peroxidase positive; if colored granules are not present in the cytoplasm,
the cell is said to be peroxidase negative.

The peroxidase positive cells are:

progranulocytes	eosinophils
neutrophilic myelocytes	basophils (?)
neutrophilic metamyelocytes	most monocytes
neutrophilic band cells	
neutrophilic segmented cells	

The peroxidase negative cells are:

myeloblasts	lymphoblasts	plasmablasts	monoblasts
	prolymphocytes	proplasmacytes	promonocytes
	lymphocytes	plasmacytes	some monocytes
rubriblasts			
prorubricytes			
rubricytes			
metarubricytes			

Thus, we may conclude:

(1) With the exception of the myeloblast, which is peroxidase negative,
all cells of the granulocytic series are peroxidase positive.
(2) All cells of the lymphocytic series and plasmacytic series are peroxidase negative.
(3) The cells of the monocytic series may be peroxidase positive or
peroxidase negative.
(4) Nucleated red cells are peroxidase negative.

Some peroxidase positive neutrophils are illustrated in Figure 168.

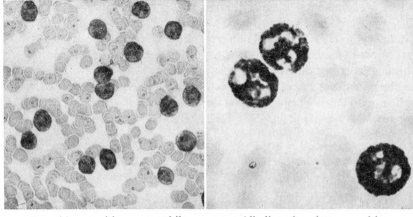

Peroxidase positive neutrophils   Alkaline phosphatase positive
                                                    neutrophils

FIG. 168.—Peroxidase positive neutrophils and alkaline phosphatase positive neutrophils. (Reproduced from the 7th edition of "Bray's Clinical Laboratory Methods" revised by Bauer, Ackermann, and Toro and published by the C. V. Mosby Co.)

The color of the granules varies with the method of staining. For example, the granules may be bluish green, blue, purple, or brown. Also, if granulation is present, the degree of granulation may be light, medium, or heavy.

How can the peroxidase stain be useful in diagnosis?

The peroxidase stain can be useful in distinguishing between acute granulocytic leukemia and acute lymphocytic leukemia.

In acute granulocytic leukemia, 5%–25% of the white cells are peroxidase positive; in acute lymphocytic leukemia, 95%–100% of the white cells are peroxidase negative.

Why are *only* 5%–25% of the white cells peroxidase positive in acute granulocytic leukemia?

Acute granulocytic leukemia is accompanied by a differential white cell count showing 15%–50% myeloblasts.

Myeloblasts are peroxidase negative but they *belong to the granulocytic series.*

With the possible exception of an occasional monocyte, the 5%–25% peroxidase positive cells also *belong to the granulocytic series.*

Thus, 20%–75% of the white cells *belong to the granulocytic series.*

Therefore, the chances are good that the granulocytic series is the predominating white cell series.

If the granulocytic series is the predominating white cell series, the leukemia is acute granulocytic leukemia rather than acute lymphocytic leukemia.

The procedure for the peroxidase stain follows.

PROCEDURE FOR THE PEROXIDASE STAIN

The peroxidase stain may be performed by the following methods:

> Sato and Sekiya method
> Goodpasture's method
> Kaplow's method
> Graham-Knoll method
> Jacoby's method
> Washburn's method modified
>   by Osgood and Ashworth
> Hattori's method

All of the above methods are in current use and have their respective advocates.

The time honored method of Sato and Sekiya is given below.

Necessary Solutions

1. 0.5% aqueous solution of copper sulfate. To prepare: Add 0.5 gram of anhydrous copper sulfate to 100 ml. of distilled water. Mix.
2. Saturated benzidine solution. To prepare: Add 0.5 gram of reagent grade benzidine to 400 ml. of distilled water. Shake vigorously for a few minutes. Store in a brown bottle.
3. 3% hydrogen peroxide solution. This solution should be newly purchased and not old or deteriorated. It should be kept in a tightly capped brown bottle and stored in the refrigerator.
4. 1% aqueous solution of safranin. To prepare: Add 1 gram of safranin to 100 ml. of distilled water. Mix.

Procedure

1. Prepare a benzidine-hydrogen peroxide reagent as follows:
   Filter 100 ml. of the saturated benzidine solution into a flask.
   Add exactly 2 drops of the 3% hydrogen peroxide solution. Mix.

2. Make a blood smear from either finger tip blood or fresh anticoagulated blood.

3. Allow the blood smear to dry and then place it on a staining rack.

4. Cover the blood smear with the 0.5% aqueous solution of copper sulfate.

5. Allow to stand for 1 minute.

6. Pour off the 0.5% aqueous solution of copper sulfate and do not wash.

7. Cover the blood smear with the freshly prepared benzidine-hydrogen peroxide reagent.

8. Allow to stand for 8 minutes.

9. Wash with distiiled water.

10. Allow the blood smear to dry. (Takes about 10 minutes.)

11. Cover the blood smear with the 1% aqueous solution of safranin.

12. Allow to stand for 2 minutes.

13. Wash with distilled water.

14. Allow the blood smear to dry. (Takes a few minutes.)

15. Meanwhile, read the following description of peroxidase positive cells and peroxidase negative cells.

16. The erythrocytes in this smear will appear as shadow forms.

17. The peroxidase positive cells will have granules. The granules will be bluish-green to bluish-black in color. The degree of granulation may be light, medium, or heavy.

18. Some peroxidase positive cells with heavy granulation are illustrated in Figure 168, page 536.

19. The peroxidase negative cells will not have granules. The majority of peroxidase negative cells will be colored red.

20. Now place a drop of immersion oil on the thin area of your stained blood smear.

21. Bring the cells into view with the oil immersion (95×) objective of the microscope.

22. Inspect 100 white cells and record the number of peroxidase positive cells and the number of peroxidase negative cells.

   Note: Any nucleated red cells which may be present will be peroxidase negative. Simply skip these nucleated red cells.

23. Determine the per cent peroxidase positive cells and the per cent peroxidase negative cells.

24. Sample calculation
   If your inspection of 100 white cells revealed 20 peroxidase positive cells and 80 peroxidase negative, you would have 20% peroxidase positive cells and 80% peroxidase negative cells.

25. Report the per cent peroxidase positive cells and the per cent peroxidase negative cells.

26. In acute granulocytic leukemia, 5%–25% of the white cells are peroxidase positive; in acute lymphocytic leukemia, 95%–100% of the white cells are peroxidase negative.

ALKALINE PHOSPHATASE STAIN

The alkaline phosphatase stain is also referred to as the alkaline phosphatase score, alkaline phosphatase test, alkaline phosphatase activity of neutrophils, leukocyte alkaline phosphatase test, LAP test, and alkaline phosphatase cytochemical test.

The discussion will cover the significance of the alkaline phosphatase stain and the procedure for the alkaline phosphatase stain.

SIGNIFICANCE OF THE ALKALINE PHOSPHATASE STAIN

An enzyme, alkaline phosphatase, is present in neutrophilic segmented cells, neutrophilic band cells, and neutrophilic metamyelocytes.

The amount of alkaline phosphatase which is present may be roughly estimated by performing an alkaline phosphatase stain.

The normal values for the alkaline phosphatase stain are 13 to 100.

Values below normal may be found in chronic granulocytic leukemia, acute granulocytic leukemia, paroxysmal nocturnal hemoglobinuria, infectious mononucleosis, and hereditary hypophosphatasia.

Values above normal may be found in neutrophilic leukemoid reactions, polycythemia vera, and pregnancy.

What is a neutrophilic leukemoid reaction?

A neutrophilic leukemoid reaction is any reaction producing a blood picture resembling granulocytic leukemia.

A neutrophilic leukemoid reaction may be seen in mercury poisoning, Hodgkin's disease, myeloid metaplasia, meningitis, the presence of tumors, and many other conditions.

The alkaline phosphatase stain is primarily used to distinguish between chronic granulocytic leukemia and neutrophilic leukemoid reactions.

For example, the following bloods may reveal the following alkaline phosphatase scores:

blood in chronic granulocytic leukemia	blood in health	blood in neutrophilic leukemoid reactions
0 – 13	13 – 100	100 – 400

The method of scoring is given in the following procedure.

PROCEDURE FOR THE ALKALINE PHOSPHATASE STAIN

It is a good policy to run a high positive control and a low negative control with this test.

A high positive control may be prepared by making a blood smear from the blood of a woman in the 6th–9th month of pregnancy.

A low negative control may be prepared by making a blood smear from normal blood, fixing the smear with the fixative solution (listed below), and then boiling the smear for 2 minutes. (Carol Sievers)

The above high positive control smear and low negative control smear may be stained and inspected along with the patient's smear.

Since this test is largely based on a person's ability to judge color, it is suggested that the student run the following:

(1) a high positive control smear
(2) a low negative control smear
(3) a normal blood smear (containing 55%–80% neutrophils)

The student should obtain an alkaline phosphatase score of 100–400 on the high positive control smear, a score of 0–13 on the low negative control smear, and a score of 30–80 on the normal blood smear (normal values are 13–100).

If the student obtains the above values, his "scoring eye" is in fairly good shape.

The alkaline phosphatase stain is usually performed by the method of Kaplow.

The necessary solutions and reagents are listed below and the procedure follows.

Necessary Solutions and Reagents

1. Fixative solution.

   Add 40 ml. of formalin (36%–39% formaldehyde) to 360 ml. of absolute methanol (absolute methyl alcohol). Mix. When not in use, keep this solution in a tightly capped bottle and store in the *freezing unit* of a refrigerator. Keeps indefinitely.

2. Stock 0.2 M propanediol solution.

   Dissolve 10.5 grams of 2-amino-2-methyl-1, 3-propanediol (reagent may be purchased from Eastman Kodak Co., Rochester, N. Y.) in 500 ml. of distilled water. Mix. Store in the refrigerator. Keeps indefinitely.

3. Working 0.05 M propanediol buffer (pH 9.75).

   To 125 ml. of stock 0.2 M propanediol solution, add 25 ml. of 0.1 N hydrochloric acid. Mix. Dilute to 500 ml. with distilled water. Mix. Store in refrigerator. Keeps indefinitely. *Before using, allow to come to room temperature.*

4. Sodium alpha naphthyl acid phosphate.

   This reagent may be purchased from Dajac Laboratories, Leominster, Mass.

5. Fast blue RR.

   This reagent is a commercial preparation of the diazonium salt of 4-benzoyl-2,5 methoxyaniline. It may be purchased from either the General Dyestuff Corporation, Boston, Mass. or Borden Chemical Company, Philadelphia, Penna.

6. Counterstain.

   Mayer's hematoxylin stain. This stain may be prepared as follows: To 500 ml. of distilled water, add 1 gram of hematoxylin (color index no. 75290). Mix. Heat just to boiling and add another 500 ml. of distilled water. Mix. Add 0.2 gram of reagent grade sodium iodate. Mix. Add 50 grams of aluminum potassium sulfate (12 H_2O). Mix. Pour into a large flask or bottle and shake for about 1 minute. Filter. Store in a brown bottle at room temperature. Keeps indefinitely.

Procedure

1. Remove the working 0.05 M propanediol buffer (pH 9.75) from the refrigerator and allow it to come to room temperature. (Takes about 45 minutes)

2. Using either finger tip blood or fresh oxalated or heparinized blood, make a patient's blood smear.

   Note: Do not use blood containing the anticoagulant EDTA.

3. Remove the fixative solution from the freezing unit of the refrigerator and pour about 100 ml. into a 100 ml. beaker.

4. Bring this fixative solution to a temperature of about 5° C.

5. Then dip the patient's blood smear in the fixative solution for 30 seconds.

   Note: If you are also running a positive control smear, a negative control smear, or a normal control smear, also dip these smears in the fixative solution for 30 seconds. Then continue to treat these smears exactly as directed for the patient's smear.

6. Now wash the blood smears in gentle running tap water for about 10 seconds.

7. Make a freshly prepared substrate mixture as follows: First make sure the working 0.05 M propanediol buffer (pH 9.75) has adjusted to room temperature. Then pour 70 ml. of the working 0.05 M propanediol buffer (pH 9.75) into a flask. Add 70 mg. of the sodium alpha naphthyl acid phosphate. Mix. Add 70 mg. of the fast blue RR (diazonium salt of 4-benzoyl-2,5 methoxyaniline). Shake for about 15 seconds. This mixture has a pH of 9.5 to 9.6.

8. If you are using a staining rack to stain the smears, filter this freshly prepared substrate mixture directly onto the smears.

9. If you are using a Coplin staining jar to stain the smears, filter this freshly prepared substrate mixture directly into the Coplin staining jar containing the smears.

10. Allow the substrate mixture to remain in contact with the smears for 10 minutes at room temperature.

11. Then wash the smears in gently running tap water for about 10 seconds.

12. Counterstain the smears with the Mayer's hematoxylin stain for 4 minutes.

13. Then again wash the smears in gently running tap water for about 10 seconds.

14. Allow the smears to dry.

15. Note: If you are running a positive control smear and a negative control smear, find the alkaline phosphatase score on these smears <u>before</u> you inspect the patient's smear.

16. Note: The positive control smear should have a score between 100 and 400. The negative control smear should have a score between 0 and 13.

17. Now treat <u>each</u> of the smears you are running in the following manner:

18. Place a drop of immersion oil on the <u>thin area</u> of the smear and bring the cells into view with the oil immersion (95×) objective of the microscope.

19. Alkaline phosphatase positive neutrophils are illustrated in Figure 168, page 536.

20. Now the problem is to grade a total of 100 cells. The cells to be graded are the neutrophilic segmented cells, neutrophilic band cells, and neutrophilic metamyelocytes. All the other cells in the smear are neither counted nor graded.

21. The grading is done as follows:

    0   cytoplasm is colorless

    1+   cytoplasm is pale brown and has no granular precipitate

    2+   cytoplasm is brown with a small amount of granular precipitate

    3+   cytoplasm is brownish black with a moderate amount of granular precipitate

    4+   cytoplasm is black with a large amount of granular precipitate

22. The recording is done as shown in the sample recording sheet (Fig. 169, page 544).

23. Grading and recording the cells as directed above, grade and record 100 consecutive neutrophilic segmented cells, neutrophilic band cells, and neutrophilic metamyelocytes.

24. After you have graded and recorded 100 cells, make your calculation as directed below.

37

Cell	Number Recorded					Totals
"0" cells	ЖЖ	ЖЖ	ЖЖ	ЖЖ	ЖЖ	
	ЖЖ	ЖЖ	ЖЖ	ЖЖ	ЖЖ	
	ЖЖ	ЖЖ	ЖЖ	ЖЖ		
						70
"1+" cells	ЖЖ	ЖЖ	ЖЖ	ЖЖ		20
"2+" cells	ЖЖ	ЖЖ				10
"3+" cells						
"4+" cells						

FIG. 169.—Sample recording sheet for the alkaline phosphatase stain. In the above recording sheet, the technologist saw and recorded 70 "0" cells, 20 "1+" cells, 10 "2+" cells, no "3+" cells, and no "4+" cells.

25. Multiply the quantity of each cell times the value for each cell. For example, if you saw and recorded 70 of the "0" cells, you would multiply 70 $\times$ 0, getting a score of 0. If you saw and recorded 10 of the "2+" cells, you would multiply 10 $\times$ 2, getting a score of 20. A sample calculation is given below.

26. Sample calculation

cell	quantity (number seen)	value	score
"0" cell	70	0	0
"1+" cell	20	1	20
"2+" cell	10	2	20
"3+" cell	0	3	0
"4+" cell	0	4	0
Alkaline phosphatase score			40

27. After you have made your calculations, report your alkaline phosphatase score.

   Note: If you ran a positive control smear and a negative control smear, also include these scores in your report.

28. The normal values for an alkaline phosphatase score are 13–100.

29. Values of 0–13 may be seen in chronic granulocytic leukemia.

30. Values of 100–400 may be seen in neutrophilic leukemoid reactions.

GIEMSA STAIN

The Giemsa stain is widely used for staining blood smears and malaria smears.

This stain is a complicated mixture of dyes: azure, eosin, and methylene blue.

The preparation of the Giemsa stock solution is given below and the procedure for the Giemsa stain follows.

PREPARATION OF GIEMSA STOCK SOLUTION

Add 5 grams of powdered Giemsa stain to 330 ml. of reagent grade glycerol. Mix. Place in a 60° C. oven for 2 hours. Allow to cool. Mix. With constant stirring, slowly add 330 ml. of acetone-free absolute methyl alcohol. Transfer to a bottle. Shake for a few minutes. Label the bottle *Giemsa Stock Solution*. Filter before use.

PROCEDURE FOR THE GIEMSA STAIN

Necessary Reagents

1. Acetone-free absolute methyl alcohol.
2. Giemsa stock solution. For preparation, see directions above.
3. pH 6.8 buffer solution. For preparation, see buffer solution, under Wright's stain and buffer solution, page 699.

Procedure

1. Fix the blood smear by putting it in the acetone-free absolute methyl alcohol for 2 minutes.

2. Make a fresh batch of Giemsa working solution as follows:

   (1) Filter the Giemsa stock solution until you have 10 ml.
   (2) Add this 10 ml. of filtered Giemsa stock solution to 90 ml. of the pH 6.8 buffer solution.
   (3) Mix.

3. Use either Method A or Method B below.

4. Method A

Place the smear on a staining rack. With the fresh batch of Giemsa working solution, fully cover the smear so that the solution is almost brimming over. Allow to stain for 20 minutes. Then flush the excess stain off with distilled water.

5. Method B

Put the smear in a staining jar or 100 ml. beaker. Completely cover the smear with the fresh batch of Giemsa working solution. Allow to stain for 20 minutes. Remove and wash with distilled water.

6. Allow the smear to dry.

FEULGEN STAIN

The Feulgen stain is also referred to as the Feulgen reaction.
The Feulgen stain is specific for deoxyribonucleic acid (DNA).
This stain will clearly define the nucleoli in the nucleus of immature cells.
Hence the stain makes it easier to identify and count immature cells.
The Feulgen stain calls for the use of several stains and reagents, the procedure is rather involved, and it is usually run in the histology or tissue department.

MISCELLANEOUS STAINS

The miscellaneous stains will be alphabetically listed and briefly discussed.

Basophilic Aggregation Stain

The basophilic aggregation stain has been used to demonstrate the basophilic stippling of erythrocytes seen in lead poisoning.

Deoxyribonucleic Acid (DNA) Stain

See Feulgen stain above.

Inclusion Body Stain

The inclusion body stain may be useful in identifying the particles seen in erythrocytes in hemoglobin H disease and hemoglobin Zurich disease.

Jenner's Stain

Jenner's stain is also known as the May-Grünwald stain.
This stain is a forerunner of Wright's stain.
It is used to stain blood smears.

Manson Stain

The Manson stain is sometimes referred to as Manson's methylene blue stain.
This stain has been used to demonstrate the basophilic stippling of erythrocytes seen in lead poisoning.

May-Grünwald Stain

The May-Grünwald stain is also known as Jenner's stain.
This stain is similar to Wright's stain.
It is used to stain blood smears.

May-Grünwald-Giemsa Stain

As the name implies, the May-Grünwald-Giemsa stain is a mixture of the May-Grünwald stain and Giemsa stain.
This stain is similar to Wright's stain.
It is used to stain blood smears.

Pappenheim's Stain

Pappenheim's stain is used to identify basophilic granules and nuclear fragments in erythrocytes.

Periodic Acid-Schiff Stain

The periodic acid-Schiff stain is also referred to as the P. A. S. stain, Periodic-Acid-Schiff reaction, PAS reaction, and PAS reaction for glycogen.
This stain is useful in identifying and classifying immature cells of the blood and bone marrow.
It may be useful in differentiating erythremic myelosis from sideroblastic anemia.
The procedure for the stain is rather involved and it is usually run in the histology or tissue department.

Ribonucleic Acid (RNA) Stain

See Unna-Pappenheim stain below.

Romanowsky's Stain

A polychrome stain is a stain of many colors.

Romanowsky's stain is sometimes referred to as the original polychrome stain.

Romanowsky's stain is the forerunner of Wright's stain, Giemsa stain, Jenner's stain, May-Grünwald stain, May-Grünwald-Giemsa stain, and Wright-Giemsa stain.

Basically, all the above stains are alcoholic solutions of two dyes—eosin and methylene blue.

Sudan Black B Stain

The sudan black B stain may be used in the same capacity as the peroxidase stain, that is, it may be used in establishing the identity of the predominating white cell series.

The sudan black B stain acts upon any lipid or fatty material which may be present in a cell.

Cells of the granulocytic series that contain granules generally take the stain and are said to be sudanophilic.

Cells of the lymphocytic series do not take the stain and are said to be sudanophobic.

Supravital Stain

A supravital stain is used to stain and inspect living cells which have been removed from the body.

This stain enables the white cells to remain alive and mobile. It does not stain the nucleus or cytoplasm. But it stains significant structures, mainly the mitochondria, in the cytoplasm.

In myeloblasts, the mitochondria are small, numerous in number, and scattered throughout the cytoplasm.

In lymphoblasts, the mitochondria are large, relatively few in number, and usually grouped around the nucleus.

Hence the supravital stain may be useful in distinguishing between myeloblasts and lymphoblasts.

Unna-Pappenheim Stain

The Unna-Pappenheim stain will reveal the presence of ribonucleic acid (RNA).

Ribonucleic acid is present in the cytoplasm of plasmacytes.

Hence this stain may be used to identify plasmacytes.

Vital Stain

A vital stain is also referred to as an intravital stain.

A vital stain is the "staining of a tissue by a dye which is introduced into a living organism and which, by virtue of elective attraction to certain tissues, will stain these tissues." (From Dorland's Medical Dictionary.)

Wright-Giemsa Stain

As the name implies, the Wright-Giemsa stain is a combination of Wright's stain and Giemsa stain.

Chapter 32

Tests Seldom Requested

THIS chapter considers 7 tests which may be run several times a year by the hematology department in the average hospital laboratory.

The discussion will cover the following:

> Ham Test
> Donath-Landsteiner Test
> Glucose-6-phosphate Dehydrogenase Deficiency Test
> Sia Test
> Thorn Eosinophil Test
> Nasal or Sputum Smear for Eosinophil Estimation
> Buffy Coat Preparations

The student review questions for this chapter are numbered 336–348 and begin on page 761 of the Appendix.

HAM TEST

The Ham test is also referred to as Ham's test for paroxysmal nocturnal hemoglobinuria, Ham's test for P. N. H., Ham's acidified serum test, acid-serum test, acid-serum hemolysis test, acid hemolysis test, and acid hemolysin test.

The Ham test involves mixing the patient's red cells with acidified serum and inspecting the mixture for hemolysis.

This test is reported as positive or negative; the test is positive in paroxysmal nocturnal hemoglobinuria.

The method of performing the test has undergone various modifications and refinements.

The necessary reagents and equipment are listed below and a procedure for the test follows.

NECESSARY REAGENTS AND EQUIPMENT

1. Materials for a venipuncture
2. Small flask
3. Ten glass beads
4. Physiological (0.85%) saline solution

5. 0.2 N hydrochloric acid solution.

6. Fresh normal compatible serum.
   (About 1.5 ml. of fresh serum from a normal person with the same blood group as the patient.)

7. Centrifuge

8. 37° C. incubator or 37° C water bath

Procedure

1. Place the 10 glass beads in the small flask.

2. Withdraw 10 ml. of blood from the patient and transfer it to the flask.

3. Immediately start to gently swirl the flask and continue swirling the flask until you can no longer hear the beads hitting the wall of the flask.

4. Pour this defibrinated blood into a test tube.

5. Centrifuge the defibrinated blood.

6. Discard the serum.

7. Wash the cells 3 times as follows:
   Add 5 ml. of the physiological (0.85%) saline solution, mix, centrifuge, and discard the physiological (0.85%) saline solution above the cells.

8. Then make a 50% suspension of cells in the physiological (0.85%) saline solution.

   Note: For every 1 ml. of packed red cells, add 1 ml. of physiological (0.85%) saline solution.

9. Pour the 50% suspension of cells into a test tube and label 50% Suspension of Patient's Cells.

10. Pipet 0.5 ml. of the fresh normal compatible serum into a small test tube. Label the test tube Test.

11. Pipet 0.5 ml. of the fresh normal compatible serum into another small test tube. Label this test tube Control.

12. Add 0.05 ml. of the 0.2 N hydrochloric acid to the test tube labelled Test. Mix.

    Note: Do not add any of the hydrochloric acid to the test tube labelled Control.

13. Add 1 drop of the <u>50% Suspension of Patient's Cells</u> to each test tube.

14. Tap the bottom of each test tube to mix the contents.

15. Incubate both test tubes at 37° C. for 1 hour.

16. Then centrifuge both test tubes at 1000 RPM for 2 minutes.

17. Remove the test tubes from the centrifuge and inspect the fluid portion of each test tube.

18. If the fluid portion of both test tubes is colorless, the test is negative.

19. If the fluid portion of the <u>Control</u> is colorless and the fluid portion of the <u>Test</u> is pink, the test is positive.

20. Note: A false positive test may occur in hereditary spherocytic anemia. If this is suspected by the physician, the test should be repeated, using acidified serum previously inactivated at 56° C. for 30 minutes. Since P. N. H. red cells require complement for hemolysis, the modified test will be negative in P. N. H. but will remain positive in hereditary spherocytic anemia. (Miale)

21. Report the test as positive or negative.

    Note: If the test is positive, make a notation in your report regarding the possibility of a false positive test due to hereditary spherocytic anemia.

22. Further control test:
    A further control may be run by selecting a student or other normal person in place of the patient and performing the test exactly as outlined above. At the conclusion of the test, the fluid portion of the test tube labelled <u>Test</u> and the fluid portion of the test tube labelled <u>Control</u> should be colorless indicating the absence of hemolysis.

DONATH-LANDSTEINER TEST

The Donath-Landsteiner test is also referred to as the Donath-Landsteiner reaction, Donath-Landsteiner hemolysin test, D-L hemolysin test, D-L antibody test, Donath-Landsteiner test for cold-warm hemoylsins, Donath-Landsteiner test for paroxysmal cold hemoglobinuria, and Donath-Landsteiner test for P. C. H.

The Donath-Landsteiner test may be performed by a simple screening procedure or by the more involved titration procedure.

The screening procedure is performed by obtaining the patient's blood, chilling it to a low temperature, warming it to body temperature, and then inspecting the serum for hemolysis.

The Donath-Landsteiner test is positive in paroxysmal cold hemoglobinuria.

The screening procedure is given below.

NECESSARY REAGENTS AND EQUIPMENT

1. Materials for a venipuncture
2. Two plain test tubes (no anticoagulant)
3. Crushed ice water bath (about 4° C.)
4. 37° C. incubator or 37° C. water bath

Procedure

1. Warm the syringe and two plain test tubes to body temperature (37° C.) by holding them tightly in your fists for a few minutes.

2. Withdraw 10 ml. of blood from the patient and transfer 5 ml. to each test tube.

3. Label one test tube Control.

4. Put this test tube labelled Control in the 37° C. incubator or 37° C. water bath.

5. Label the other test tube Test.

6. Place this test tube labelled Test in the crushed ice water bath (about 4° C.) for 30 minutes.

7. At the end of the 30 minutes, remove the test tube from the crushed ice water bath and put it in the 37° C. incubator or 37° C. water bath.

8. Allow 90 minutes to elapse.

9. When the 90 minutes have elapsed, remove the test tubes and inspect the serum in each test tube.

10. If the serum in both test tubes is free of hemolysis (shows no pink tinge), report the test as negative.

11. If the serum in the test tube labelled Test shows hemolysis (a pink tinge) and the serum in the test tube labelled Control is free of hemolysis (no pink tinge), report the test as positive.

GLUCOSE-6-PHOSPHATE DEHYDROGENASE DEFICIENCY TEST

The glucose-6-phosphate dehydrogenase deficiency test is also referred to as the G6PD deficiency test, G-6-PD deficiency test, G6PD test, and G-6-PD test.

Glucose-6-phosphate dehydrogenase is an enzyme which is present in normal red cells.

This enzyme is involved in a series of reactions that protect the red cell from injury by oxidant drugs.

If the enzyme is deficient and an oxidant drug is present, however, the red cells are subject to hemolysis and a hemolytic anemia may follow.

A deficiency of the enzyme is an inherited characteristic. The deficiency is found in about 10% of the Negro population. And it is also quite common among Caucasians and Orientals.

Among the many oxidant drugs that may be responsible for this condition are sulfanilamide, antipyrine, phenacetin, acetanilide, and the antimalarial drug primaquine.

Thus, the glucose-6-phosphate dehydrogenase deficiency test is useful in diagnosing hemolytic anemia caused by oxidant drugs.

Several methods are currently available for performing the test.

The fluorescence spot test or screening test for G-6-PD deficiency is given below.

NECESSARY REAGENTS AND EQUIPMENT

1. Reaction mixture. The ingredients of this reaction mixture are listed below. A stable form of this reaction mixture may be purchased from Hyland Laboratories, 4501 Colorado Blvd., Los Angeles, Calif., 90039.

   a. Glucose-6-phosphate (0.01 M) . . . . 0.1 ml.
   b. TPN (0.0075 M) . . . . 0.1 ml.
   c. Saponin (1%) . . . . 0.2 ml.
   d. Potassium phosphate buffer, pH 7.4 (0.25 M). 0.3 ml.
   e. Distilled water . . . . 0.3 ml.

2. A long wavelength (465 mμ) source of ultra violet (UV) light
3. Materials for a venipuncture
4. Control A few milliliters of normal anticoagulated blood prepared with the anticoagulant EDTA or heparin

Procedure

1. Using either heparin or EDTA as the anticoagulant, withdraw about 5 cc. of blood from the patient and prepare anticoagulated blood.

2. Obtain 2 small test tubes. Label one <u>Patient.</u> Label the other <u>Control.</u>

3. Place 0.2 ml. of the above reaction mixture in each test tube.

4. To the test tube labelled <u>Patient,</u> add 0.02 ml. of the patient's anticoagulated blood.

5. To the test tube labelled <u>Control,</u> add 0.02 ml. of the Control's anticoagulated blood.

6. Gently tap the bottom of each test tube to mix the contents.

7. Allow the 2 test tubes to stand for 5 minutes.

8. Then obtain a No. 1 Whatman filter paper.

9. Again gently tap the bottom of each test tube to mix the contents.

10. Take the test tube labelled <u>Patient,</u> remove 1 drop, and place it on the filter paper.

11. Label the spot <u>P.</u>

12. Take the test tube labelled <u>Control,</u> remove 1 drop, and place it on the filter paper about 2 inches to the right of the patient's drop.

13. Label the spot <u>C.</u>

14. Allow the 2 spots to <u>thoroughly</u> dry. (Takes about 10 minutes)

15. Making sure the spots are thoroughly dry, examine the spots under the ultra violet light.

16. The spot labelled <u>C</u> (Control) should fluoresce brightly, indicating that the G-6-PD activity is normal.

17. If the spot labelled <u>P</u> (Patient) fluoresces brightly, the patient's G-6-PD activity is normal.

18. If the spot labelled <u>P</u> (Patient) does not fluoresce, the patient's G-6-PD activity is deficient.

19. Report your results. An example follows.

20. Example

Screening Test for G-6-PD Deficiency

Patient: G-6-PD is normal

Control: G-6-PD is normal

SIA TEST

The Sia test is also referred to as the Sia test for macroglobulins, macroglobulinemia test, and euglobulin test.

The Sia test is positive in about 1 out of every 4 cases of Waldenström's macroglobulinemia.

Procedure

1. Withdraw about 5 cc. of blood from the patient and prepare serum.

2. Obtain a 100 ml. graduate and fill it to the very top with distilled water.

3. Using a medicine dropper, allow 1 large drop of serum to fall into the water. (Hold the medicine dropper almost horizontal.)

4. If no turbidity or precipitate appears within 1 minute, report the test as negative.

5. If a heavy coarse precipitate appears and gradually falls to the bottom of the graduate, report the test as positive.

6. If a light fine precipitate appears and remains in suspension, report the test as doubtful.

THORN EOSINOPHIL TEST

The Thorn eosinophil test is also referred to as the Thorn ACTH test, ACTH stimulation test, and eosinophil depression test.

The Thorn eosinophil test is sometimes performed in conjunction with the Thorn uric acid excretion test and these two tests should not be confused.

The Thorn eosinophil test is a test for adrenal cortical function.

The test is performed as follows:

The technologist makes a finger puncture on the patient and performs an eosinophil count (number per cubic millimeter).

The physician gives the patient an injection of ACTH (adrenocorticotropic hormone).

Four hours after the injection of ACTH, the technologist performs another eosinophil count on the patient.

If the adrenal cortical function is normal, the eosinophil count will act as follows:

The eosinophil count before the injection will be about twice the value of the eosinophil count after the injection. For example, the eosinophil count before the injection may be 200. The eosinophil count after the injection may be 100.

If the adrenal cortical function is decreased, the eosinophil count will act as follows:

The eosinophil count before the injection will be approximately the same as the eosinophil count after the injection. For example, the eosinophil count before the injection may be 200. The eosinophil count after the injection may be 195.

When the adrenal cortical function is decreased, it indicates hypoadrenalism (Addison's disease).

NASAL OR SPUTUM SMEAR FOR
EOSINOPHIL ESTIMATION

An eosinophil estimation of a nasal smear or sputum smear may occasionally be requested.

A nasal smear showing 20%–30% eosinophils may be seen in allergies.

A sputum smear showing a high percentage of eosinophils may be seen in asthmatic bronchitis.

Procedure

1. Allow the nasal smear or sputum smear to thoroughly dry.

   Note: Do not use heat to hasten drying.

2. Stain the smear with a diluted Wright's stain in the following manner:

3. Distribute 35 drops of Wright's stain evenly over the smear. Immediately distribute 35 drops of buffer solution evenly over the Wright's stain. Mix thoroughly by blowing on the solutions.

4. Allow to stain for 10 minutes.

   Note: With this smear, you do not flush the excess stain off the slide because you may flush the smear off the slide.

5. At the end of the 10 minute staining time, gently tilt the slide and allow the excess stain to drain off the smear.

6. Then gently wash the smear with a small amount of distilled water.

7. Allow the smear to thoroughly dry. (Takes about 15 minutes) Do not blot the smear to hasten drying.

8. Place a drop of immersion oil on the smear.

9. Using the oil immersion (95×) objective of the microscope, bring the cells into view.

10. The eosinophils will be the cells with the coarse pink or red granules in the cytoplasm.

11. Skip all the broad flat epithelial cells.

12. If the smear is a nasal smear:

    (a) Count and tabulate 200 consecutive eosinophils and neutrophils.
    (b) Report the percentage of eosinophils and the percentage of neutrophils.
    (c) Example
        50 eosinophils and 150 neutrophils were seen. Therefore, the nasal smear shows 25% eosinophils and 75% neutrophils.

13. If the smear is a sputum smear:

    (a) Count and tabulate 200 consecutive eosinophils and monocytes.
    (b) Report the percentage of eosinophils and the percentage of monocytes.
    (c) Example
        40 eosinophils and 160 monocytes were seen. Therefore, the sputum smear shows 20% eosinophils and 80% monocytes.

BUFFY COAT PREPARATIONS

When anticoagulated blood is centrifuged for about 30 minutes, the white cells gradually rise and form a thin grayish-white layer above the red cells.

This thin grayish-white layer of white cells is known as a buffy coat; it is also referred to as the white cell cream or leukocytic cream.

If the buffy coat is used to prepare a blood smear, the preparation is called a buffy coat preparation.

Thus, a buffy coat preparation is simply a blood smear made from a concentrated specimen of white cells.

A buffy coat preparation is useful in facilitating the search for immature white cells seen in aleukemic leukemia, a phase of leukemia in which the immature white cells are few in number.

Procedure

1. Obtain 6 cc. of fresh Sequestrenized (EDTA) blood.

2. Mix the blood.

   Note: After the blood is withdrawn and mixed, it should not be allowed to stand. The buffy coat should be obtained immediately.

3. To obtain the buffy coat, use either Method A or Method B below.

4. Method A

   Fill 2 Wintrobe tubes with the blood. Centrifuge the Wintrobe tubes at 3000 RPM for 15 minutes. Remove and discard the plasma. Remove the buffy coat and prepare several smears in the usual manner.

5. Method B

   Centrifuge the blood in the test tube at 3000 RPM for 45 minutes. Remove 0.5 ml. of the plasma and transfer it to a small test tube. Remove and discard the remaining plasma. Remove all the buffy coat. (Some red cells and plasma may be included.) Transfer the buffy coat to the small test tube containing the 0.5 ml. of plasma. Very gently invert the small test tube about 10 times. (Do not shake!) Prepare several smears in the usual manner.

6. Stain the blood smears with Wright's stain and buffer solution.

7. Refer the blood smears to the physician or pathologist for evaluation.

8. Note: It requires considerable experience to evaluate buffy coat preparations.

9. If the blood smear is from a patient with leukemia, try to save a blood smear for future reference in studying immature white cells.

Chapter 33

Tests Rarely Requested

THIS chapter will briefly discuss 32 tests which are performed about once a year in the average hematology department.

Some additional tests, which are not performed in the hematology department but are useful in diagnosing blood diseases, will be mentioned in the dictionary in the Appendix.

The discussion will cover the following:

Autohemolysis Test
Basophil Count
Benzidine Test
Blood Specific Gravity Determination
Blood Viscosity Determination
Carboxyhemoglobin (Carbon Monoxide
    Hemoglobin) Determination
Crosby's Test
Ehrlich's Finger Test
Evans Blue Test
Ferrohemoglobin Solubility Test
Glutathione Reductase Deficiency Test
Haptoglobin Determination
Hemolytic Index
Katayama's Test
Mean Corpuscular Thickness
Methemalbumin Examination
Methemoglobin Determination
Myoglobin Determination
Plasma Hemoglobin Determination
Polyvinylpyrrolidone Test
Pyroglobulin Test
Pyruvic Kinase Deficiency Test
Red Cell Diameter Examination
Red Cell Mechanical Fragility Test
Rosenbach's Test for P. C. H.
Sanford's Method for P. C. H.
Schlesinger's Test for Urobilin
Sedimentation Index

Sulfhemoglobin Examination
Teichmann's Test for Blood
Trypsin Test
Wet Blood Film Examination

The student review questions for this chapter are numbered 349–359 and begin on page 762 of the Appendix.

Autohemolysis Test

Autohemolysis is the rupture or hemolysis of a person's red cells by his own plasma or serum.

The autohemolysis test may be performed by either a screening test or a quantitative test.

The normal values for the screening test are little or no hemolysis.

The normal values for the quantitative test are: lysis at 48 hours is 0.40%–4.50% without glucose and lysis at 48 hours is 0.03%–0.40% with glucose.

Values above normal may be found in hereditary spherocytic anemia, paroxysmal nocturnal hemoglobinuria, acquired autoimmune hemolytic anemia, and hemolytic anemia caused by drugs or chemicals.

Basophil Count

The basophil count is also referred to as the absolute basophil count.

The basophil count may be performed by Cooper's toluidine blue method.

The normal values are 10–100 basophils per cubic millimeter of blood.

Values above normal may be found in granulocytic leukemia and basophilic leukemia.

Benzidine Test

This is a test for the presence of blood.

To 5 cc. of a saturated solution of benzidine in glacial acetic acid, add 5 cc. of a fresh solution of 3% hydrogen peroxide. Mix.

To the above reagent, add 1 cc. of the specimen (the unknown). Mix.

If the mixture turns blue, it indicates the presence of blood.

Blood Specific Gravity Determination

The specific gravity of blood is the weight of a given volume of blood compared to the weight of an equal volume of distilled water (at 4° C.).

The specific gravity of blood may be determined in the same manner as the specific gravity method for determining hemoglobin (page 179).

The normal values for the specific gravity of blood are 1.048–1.066.

Values below normal may be found in anemia; values above normal may be found in polycythemia vera.

Blood Viscosity Determination

The viscosity or "thickness" of blood may be measured with a viscosimeter.

The normal values for the blood viscosity determination are 4.8–5.2 times the viscosity of distilled water.

Values below normal may be found in anemia; values above normal may be found in polycythemia vera

Carboxyhemoglobin (Carbon Monoxide Hemoglobin) Determination

The carboxyhemoglobin determination may be performed by a chemical method and a spectroscopic examination.

The normal values (symptom-free values) for the carboxyhemoglobin determination are generally considered to be 0% to 10%.

Values of 40% to 80% may be found in carbon monoxide poisoning.

The pigment carboxyhemoglobin, which is found in carbon monoxide poisoning, gives blood a brilliant cherry red color.

Crosby's Test

Crosby's test is also referred to as the thrombin test of Crosby for P. N. H. (paroxysmal nocturnal hemoglobinuria).

Crosby's test is reported as *negative* if no hemolysis occurs and *positive* if hemolysis occurs.

Crosby's test is positive in paroxysmal nocturnal hemoglobinuria.

Ehrlich's Finger Test

Ehrlich's finger test is performed by tightly binding the patient's finger with a rubber band, immersing the finger in ice water and then in warm (40° C.) water, making a finger puncture to obtain blood, centrifuging the blood, and inspecting the serum for hemolysis.

If the serum is pink, hemolysis is present and the test is positive.

Ehrlich's finger test is positive in paroxysmal cold hemoglobinuria (P. C. H.).

Evans Blue Test

The Evans blue test may be used to determine the total plasma volume.

A measured quantity of the dye, Evans blue, is injected into the patient.

The resulting dilution of the dye by the plasma is determined. The greater the dilution of the dye, the greater the volume of plasma.

When the total plasma volume has been determined, the total red cell volume and total blood volume can be found.

The total red cell volume and total blood volume are increased in polycythemia vera.

Ferrohemoglobin Solubility Test

The ferrohemoglobin solubility test is a colorimetric procedure which may be used to differentiate between hemoglobin S and hemoglobin D.

The test is based on the principle that hemoglobin S has a low solubility in a phosphate buffer solution whereas hemoglobin D has a high solubility in a phosphate buffer solution.

Glutathione Reductase Deficiency Test

Glutathione reductase is an enzyme which is found in erythrocytes.

A deficiency of this enzyme in erythrocytes is believed to increase the susceptibility of erythrocytes to oxidant drugs.

The increased susceptibility of erythrocytes to oxidant drugs may lead to increased hemolysis of erythrocytes and a resulting hemolytic anemia.

The glutathione reductase deficiency test is a simple screening procedure which examines a treated specimen of blood for fluorescence under the rays of an ultra violet light.

Haptoglobin Determination

Haptoglobin is a glycoprotein which is present in the plasma. It binds free hemoglobin. And it may aid in conveying the free hemoglobin to the spleen.

The normal values for the binding capacity of haptoglobin are generally considered to be 40–190 milligrams of free hemoglobin per 100 milliliters of serum.

Values above normal may be found in inflammatory conditions and values below normal may be seen in hemolytic anemia and severe liver disease.

The haptoglobin determination, which may be performed by electrophoretic methods, is also referred to as the serum haptoglobin determination and the haptoglobin-binding capacity.

Hemolytic Index

An increase in the destruction of erythrocytes may be revealed by calculating the hemolytic index.

The formula is:

$$\text{Hemolytic index} = \frac{\begin{array}{c}\text{mg. of daily fecal urobilinogen}\\\text{(average of 4 days)}\end{array} \times 100}{\begin{array}{c}\text{grams of hemoglobin per 100 ml.}\\\text{of blood}\end{array} \times \dfrac{\text{total blood volume}}{100}}$$

The normal values are 11 to 21.

Values below normal may be found in iron deficiency anemia and values above normal may be found in hemolytic anemia.

Katayama's Test

This is a simple test for carbon monoxide poisoning.

To 5 drops of blood, add 10 cc. of water, 5 drops of fresh orange-colored ammonium sulfide (the gas dissolved in water), and a few drops of 10% acetic acid. Mix.

With normal blood, the mixture turns a greenish-gray or greenish-brown color.

With blood containing carbon monoxide, the mixture turns a rose-red color; the deeper the rose-red color, the greater the concentration of carbon monoxide.

Mean Corpuscular Thickness

The mean corpuscular thickness of erythrocytes may be determined with the following formula:

$$\text{M. C. T.} = \frac{\text{mean corpuscular volume}}{\pi\left(\dfrac{\text{mean diameter}}{2}\right)^2}$$

The mean corpuscular thickness of erythrocytes is 2.0 microns, with a normal range of 1.8–2.2 microns.

Methemalbumin Examination

Methemalbumin is a compound formed by the union of albumin and heme.

Methemalbumin may be present in the plasma in some cases of hemolytic anemia.

The methemalbumin examination is often referred to as Schumm's test.

The examination is performed by obtaining plasma and examining it with a spectroscope for characteristic absorption bands.

Methemoglobin Determination

Methemoglobin is a compound formed by the oxidation of hemoglobin. Normally, about 0.01% to 0.30% of the total hemoglobin is methemoglobin.

Increased amounts of methemoglobin may be found in toxic conditions caused by oxidizing drugs.

The methemoglobin determination is performed by obtaining plasma and examining it with a spectroscope for characteristic absorption bands.

Myoglobin Determination

Myoglobin is a globin found in muscle.

Myoglobin may be present in the urine after any rapid destruction of skeletal muscle.

The myoglobin determination may be performed by a chemical procedure and also by an electrophoretic procedure.

Plasma Hemoglobin Determination

The plasma hemoglobin determination is also referred to as the free hemoglobin determination and the serum hemoglobin determination.

The normal values for the plasma hemoglobin determination are 2 to 3 milligrams per 100 milliliters of serum.

Values above normal may occur in some cases of hemolytic anemia and in any condition associated with the sudden and extensive destruction of erythrocytes.

The plasma hemoglobin determination is usually performed in the chemistry department.

Polyvinylpyrrolidone Test

The polyvinylpyrrolidone test is sometimes referred to as the PVP test.

This is a test for incomplete antibodies.

The PVP test is usually performed in the blood bank department.

Pyroglobulin Test

Pyroglobulin is a globulin which is not normally present in serum. If present, it will precipitate when serum is heated to 56° C. And it will not redissolve upon boiling or cooling.

Pyroglobulin may be found in the serum in some cases of multiple myeloma and lymphosarcoma; it may also be present in some patients for whom no diagnosis can be established.

The pyroglobulin test is usually performed in the chemistry department.

Pyruvic Kinase Deficiency Test

Pyruvic kinase (PK) is an enzyme which is present in erythrocytes.

If this enzyme is deficient, increased hemolysis may occur and a hemolytic anemia may follow.

The pyruvic kinase deficiency test may be performed by a simple screening procedure and also by a more involved enzyme assay procedure.

The screening procedure consists of examining a treated specimen of blood for fluorescence under the rays of an ultra violet light.

Red Cell Diameter Examination

The red cell diameter examination is also referred to as the red cell diameter, mean corpuscular diameter, MCD, erythrocyte mean corpuscular diameter, Price-Jones count, and Price-Jones curve.

Among the more commonly known methods of performing the red cell diameter examination are the Price-Jones method, Haden-Hausser method, Nicholson method, and the Watson image shearing eyepiece (WISE) method.

The normal range for the diameter of red cells—the erythrocytes—is 7.0 to 8.0 microns.

Values below the normal range may be found in iron deficiency anemia and values above the normal range may be found in pernicious anemia.

Red Cell Mechanical Fragility Test

The red cell mechanical fragility test is performed by obtaining blood, adding glass or quartz beads, rotating the blood and beads in a flask for 60 minutes, and determining the extent of hemolysis.

The normal values are 2%–5% hemolysis.

Values above normal may be found in sickle cell anemia, thalassemia major, and acquired autoimmune hemolytic anemia.

Rosenbach's Test for P. C. H.

Rosenbach's test is useful in diagnosing paroxysmal cold hemoglobinuria (P. C. H.).

If cold hemolysins are present in the patient's blood, immersion of the hands or feet in ice water for 10 to 20 minutes will be followed by symptoms of paroxysmal cold hemoglobinuria.

Paroxysmal cold hemoglobinuria is discussed in the section on blood diseases (page 615).

Sanford's Method for P. C. H.

To the patient's red cells and serum, guinea pig complement and physiological (0.85%) saline are added. The mixture is placed in the refrigerator for 30 minutes and then incubated at 37° C. for 2 hours. If hemolysis is present, the test is positive for paroxysmal cold hemoglobinuria (P. C. H.).

Schlesinger's Test for Urobilin

In some cases of hemolytic anemia, the urine may contain abnormal amounts of a colorless compound, urobilinogen.

If the urine remains in a bottle or other container for a short time, the following reaction occurs.

The colorless compound, urobilinogen, is oxidized to a brown pigment, urobilin.

Schlesinger's test for urobilin is performed as follows:

Obtain 10 cc. of urine, add 2 cc. of 10% calcium chloride, mix, and filter. This removes any bile.

To the filtered solution, add a few drops of Lugol's iodine solution and mix. This oxidizes urobilinogen to urobilin.

Add 10 cc. of a saturated alcoholic solution of zinc acetate, mix, and filter. This solution reacts with urobilin to produce a green fluorescence.

Allow the filtered solution to stand about 1 hour.

If possible, perform the following inspection in the sunlight.

Hold the test tube containing the solution against a dark background. Using a hand lens, concentrate the light on the solution. Note the color of the solution.

If a greenish fluorescence is observed, the test is positive for urobilin.

Sedimentation Index

According to Dorland's Medical Dictionary, the sedimentation index is "the logarithm of the number of millimeters of sedimentation of erythrocytes that would have occurred in 100 minutes at the maximum rate of sedimentation observed at 10 minute intervals over a 2–2$\frac{1}{2}$ hour period."

Sulfhemoglobin Examination

Sulfhemoglobin is an abnormal hemoglobin pigment.

The presence of sulfhemoglobin in the blood may be caused by oxidant drugs.

A simple screening test may be performed by shaking anticoagulated blood vigorously for about 15 minutes.

If the blood turns a mauve-lavender color, it indicates the presence of sulfhemoglobin.

Teichmann's Test for Blood

Place 1 drop of the suspected liquid (or solid) on a glass slide. Add a crystal of sodium chloride and a drop of glacial acetic acid. Mix thoroughly with an applicator stick, spreading the preparation so that it covers the area of a nickel.

Gently heat over a flame for a few minutes and then allow about 30 minutes to elapse.

Inspect the preparation with the naked eye or the low power ($10\times$ or 16 mm.) objective of the microscope.

If rhombic shaped ( ) crystals of hemin are observed, the presence of blood is indicated.

If you wish to run a positive control, proceed as follows:

Put 1 drop of blood in about 5 drops of water. Mix. Allow about 10 minutes to elapse. Mix again. Using this preparation as the suspected liquid, repeat the above test and observe the rhombic shaped crystals of hemin.

Trypsin Test

Trypsin is an enzyme secreted by the pancreas.

Two so-called trypsin tests are currently in use: (1) a test for trypsin in feces or duodenal fluid and (2) a trypsin test for incomplete antibodies.

The test for trypsin in feces or duodenal fluid may be useful in diagnosing diseases of the pancreas. With the method of Gross, a tryptic activity below 2.5 is considered *abnormal*. This test is usually run in the chemistry department.

The trypsin test for incomplete antibodies may be useful in some cases of hemolytic anemia. This test is usually run in the blood bank department.

Wet Blood Film Examination

A *small* drop (about the size of a pinhead) of fresh blood is placed on a glass slide. The edges of a coverglass are rimmed with petroleum jelly. The coverglass is placed over the drop of blood and pressed down so that the blood cells are spread out. (For technique, see pages 342, 343.)

The preparation is examined first with the $10\times$ (16 mm.) objective of the microscope, next with the $45\times$ (4 mm.) objective, and finally with the oil immersion ($95\times$) objective.

The following basic observations are made: red cells, white cells, platelets, and blood dust.

PART 6
Blood Diseases

INTRODUCTION

THIS section will deal with 28 blood diseases which the medical technologist usually encounters and 17 blood diseases and anomalies which he rarely encounters.

The more commonly encountered diseases will be discussed with respect to (1) basic clinical information, (2) factors affecting laboratory examinations, and (3) results of laboratory examinations.

The basic clinical information will present a bird's-eye view of the etiology, symptoms, diagnosis, treatment, and prognosis.

The factors affecting laboratory examinations will be concerned with such questions as the following:

Why is the hemoglobin low in iron deficiency anemia? What causes the white cell count to be high in chronic granulocytic leukemia? What is the reason for the increased coagulation time in hemophilia?

The results of the laboratory examinations will be concerned with contrasting the values in health with the values in the particular disease.

For example, in health, the white cell count is 5,000 to 10,000 per cubic millimeter; but in chronic granulocytic leukemia, the white cell count may be 100,000 to 800,000 per cubic millimeter.

The blood diseases will be organized and presented as follows:

Chapter 34 The Anemias
Chapter 35 The Leukemias
Chapter 36 Hemorrhagic Diseases
Chapter 37 Miscellaneous Blood Diseases

We will adhere to the terminology for blood diseases which is recommended in the third edition of *Current Medical Terminology*, edited by Dr. Burgess L. Gordon, and published by the American Medical Association.

Chapter 34

The Anemias

Anemia is pronounced ah-ne' me-ah. The word comes from the Greek. It means lack of blood.

Anemia is a condition which is characterized by a low red cell count, a low hemoglobin, or a combination of the two.

The anemias will be discussed under the following headings:

> Introduction to the Anemias
> Aplastic and Deficiency Anemias
> Hemolytic Anemias
> Posthemorrhagic Anemias

The student review questions for the anemias are numbered 360–430 and begin on page 763 of the Appendix.

INTRODUCTION TO THE ANEMIAS

The introductory material deals with the life of the red cell and classifications of the anemias.

LIFE OF THE RED CELL

The discussion will cover the birth, work, and death of the red cell.

Birth of the Red Cell

The production of erythrocytes is referred to as erythropoiesis.

When the body needs erythrocytes, a hormone called erythropoietin is summoned. This hormone stimulates a primitive cell in the bone marrow. This primitive cell becomes an infant red cell—a rubriblast.

The rubriblast begins to grow. It has a nucleus and multiplies by division. The cells which are produced in turn grow and multiply by division.

After going through these stages of development, the cell is ready to manufacture hemoglobin.

The manufacture of hemoglobin requires many materials. Among the essential materials are iron, protoporphyrin, amino acids, ribonucleic acid, and enzymes. Some of these materials are made by the cell and some are received from the bone marrow.

When the manufacture of hemoglobin is well under way, the cell extrudes the nucleus and becomes a reticulocyte.

The reticulocyte completes the manufacture of hemoglobin, makes preparations to leave the bone marrow, and becomes an erythrocyte.

Thus, the erythrocyte, complete with hemoglobin, stands poised on the threshold of the bone marrow, ready to enter the blood stream.

The above stages in the development of the erythrocyte require about 6 days and, by the process of division and multiplication, 1 rubriblast gives rise to 16 erythrocytes.

What controls the production of erythrocytes?

The production of erythrocytes is controlled by the oxygen supply to the tissues. When the oxygen supply to the tissues decreases, the production of erythrocytes increases. For example, at high altitudes, the oxygen supply decreases and the production of erythrocytes increases.

Each day, about 200 billion fresh young erythrocytes are born. And each day, about 200 billion tired old erythrocytes die. Thus, a normal balance exists between erythrocyte production and erythrocyte destruction.

Work of the Red Cell

If the daily production of 200 billion erythrocytes were packed in a graduate, they would occupy about 20 milliliters. This volume is less than the volume of a small glass of tomato juice. If these same erythrocytes were laid side by side in a row, however, they would extend about 1000 miles!

Thus, the amount of surface area obtained from these tiny particles falls in the realm of fantasy. This extensive surface area makes them ideally equipped to perform their function in life. And, this function is the diffusion and exchange of gases.

When the erythrocyte enters the blood stream, it is fully equipped with hemoglobin and ready to perform its function in life.

One erythrocyte contains 200 to 300 million molecules of hemoglobin. Each molecule of hemoglobin contains iron. This iron is the key factor in the hemoglobin molecule, for it enables the hemoglobin to form a temporary union with oxygen.

The erythrocyte is swept along by the blood stream and enters the lungs. In the lungs, the oxygen pressure is high. The hemoglobin therefore forms a temporary union with the oxygen.

Thus,

$$\text{hemoglobin plus oxygen} \longrightarrow \text{oxygenated hemoglobin (oxyhemoglobin)}$$

The erythrocyte is then swept along by the blood stream and enters a tissue.

In the tissue, the oxygen pressure is low. The hemoglobin therefore gives up the oxygen.

Thus,

hemoglobin minus oxygen $\longrightarrow$ reduced hemoglobin

When the oxygen is released, the erythrocyte receives carbon dioxide. This gas is mostly carried in the form of bicarbonate.

Then the erythrocyte, again swept along by the blood stream, leaves the tissue and returns to the lungs.

In the lungs, the erythrocyte releases the carbon dioxide. It then forms the temporary union with oxygen. And thus the cycle is complete.

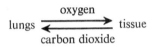

This shuttle service between lungs and tissues is necessary to sustain life; and the erythrocyte works endlessly to perform its vital mission. After 120 days and nights of faithful service, the old erythrocyte is literally worn out. Aged, depleted, and fragmented, it is now resigned to the drama of its dying days.

Death of the Red Cell

The erythrocyte usually goes home to the bone marrow to die.

The dying erythrocyte's journey to the bone marrow is the height of efficiency, for it enables the bone marrow to re-use the iron in the cell and thus forego having this mineral transported from afar.

The grimy task of dismantling the dying erythrocyte falls to a scavenger or phagocyte; a phagocyte is simply a white cell which has turned cannibal.

Attracted by the smell of death, the phagocyte hunkers over and devours rhe erythrocyte.

After the phagocyte has digested the erythrocyte, the iron from the erythrocyte is recovered.

The iron is then transported by transferrin and soon enters another infant red cell.

Thus, the iron literally bridges the gap between life and death; in effect, it receives immortality from the dying erythrocyte.

This final act completes the cycle in our saga of the red cell.

CLASSIFICATIONS OF THE ANEMIAS

The anemias have two basic classifications: morphological and etiological. The morphological classification deals with the size and hemoglobin concentration of the erythrocytes. The etiological classification is concerned with the cause of the anemia. A brief discussion of each classification follows.

Morphological Classification

In this discussion, we will assume that the student has learned a few definitions about red cells from chapters 8 and 14.

We will first discuss the size of the erythrocytes, then the hemoglobin concentration of the erythrocytes, and finally combine the size and hemoglobin concentration to form the morphological classification.

The erythrocytes may be grouped according to size: small, normal, or large. Thus, erythrocytes may be microcytic, normocytic, or macrocytic.

The size of the erythrocytes is found by calculating the mean corpuscular volume (MCV).

The mean corpuscular volume has a normal range of 80 to 90 cubic microns. If the erythrocytes are within this range, they are normocytic. If the erythrocytes are below this range, they are microcytic. If the erythrocytes are above this range, they are macrocytic.

The erythrocytes may *also* be grouped according to hemoglobin concentration: normal or decreased. Thus, the erythrocytes may be normochromic or hypochromic.

The hemoglobin concentration of the erythrocytes is found by calculating the mean corpuscular hemoglobin concentration (MCHC).

The mean corpuscular hemoglobin concentration has a normal range of 33% to 38%. If the erythrocytes are within this range, they are normochromic. If the erythrocytes are below this range, they are hypochromic.

Now, suppose we combine the size and hemoglobin concentration to describe the erythrocytes and the corresponding anemia. A few examples follow.

If the erythrocytes are small and deficient in hemoglobin, they are microcytic hypochromic erythrocytes. These microcytic hypochromic erythrocytes morphologically classify the anemia as a microcytic hypochromic anemia.

If the erythrocytes are large and normal in hemoglobin, they are macrocytic normochromic erythrocytes. These macrocytic normochromic erythrocytes morphologically classify the anemia as a macrocytic normochromic anemia.

The erythrocytes seen in the above two examples are shown in Figure 170.

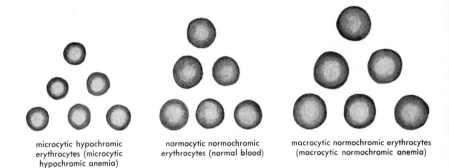

microcytic hypochromic   normocytic normochromic   macrocytic normochromic erythrocytes
erythrocytes (microcytic   erythrocytes (normal blood)   (macrocytic normochromic anemia)
hypochromic anemia)

FIG. 170.—Two examples of erythrocytes seen in the morphological classification
of the anemias. (Stain: Wright's; Magnification: 1500×.)

It is apparent that various combinations of size and hemoglobin concentration are theoretically possible. For example, erythrocytes which are normal in size could be either normal in hemoglobin or deficient in hemoglobin.

However, only three combinations of size and hemoglobin concentration are commonly found. These three combinations are:

> microcytic hypochromic erythrocytes
> macrocytic normochromic erythrocytes
> normocytic normochromic erythrocytes

The above three combinations of size and hemoglobin concentration make up the morphological classification of the anemias which we have summarized in Table 38.

Table 38

Morphological Classification of the Anemias

Erythrocytes	Size of Erythrocytes (MCV)	Hemoglobin Concentration of Erythrocytes (MCHC)	Anemia	Example
microcytic hypochromic	below normal	below normal	microcytic hypochromic	iron deficiency anemia
macrocytic normochromic	above normal	normal	macrocytic normochromic	pernicious anemia
normocytic normochromic	normal	normal	normocytic normochromic	aplastic anemia

In Table 38, iron deficiency anemia is given as an example of a microcytic hypochromic anemia.

We may, of course, have several microcytic hypochromic anemias in addition to iron deficiency anemia.

We may also have several macrocytic normochromic anemias in addition to pernicious anemia.

In Table 38, note the following about the normocytic normochromic classification.

The erythrocytes are normal in size and normal in hemoglobin concentration, but an anemia is present. Why? This anemia, the so-called normocytic normochromic anemia, is not caused by an abnormal size or hemoglobin concentration of the erythrocytes. It is due to a *decrease in the number of erythrocytes.*

Etiological Classification

The etiological classification deals with "causes" and, when a classification deals with "causes," it may be misleading and cumbersome.

For example, yesterday sickle cell anemia was "caused" by sickle cells. Today it is "caused" by inheriting certain genes. Tomorrow it may be "caused" by a man marrying the wrong woman.

It seems absurd for the student of medical technology to be called upon to wrestle with classifications of blood diseases. It would seem far better to spend the allotted time increasing the speed and accuracy of performing laboratory examinations. However, since it is necessary to present some etiological classification, a simple basic one will be considered.

Anemia may be caused by a decrease in red cell production, increase in red cell destruction, or loss of red cells. A few examples follow.

If the red cell factories in the bone marrow do not receive the proper raw materials, the production of red cells is decreased, and anemia results. If the red cell factories go on strike, the production of red cells goes down, and anemia follows.

Should the red cells leave the bone marrow, enter the blood stream, and then rupture because of faulty manufacture or attack by antibodies, increased red cell destruction occurs, and anemia results.

Finally, extensive bleeding from an injury or lesion will cause loss of red cells and anemia follows.

Thus, we may classify the anemias under 3 general headings:

1. anemias due to decreased red cell production
2. anemias due to increased red cell destruction
3. anemias due to loss of red cells

The anemias due to decreased red cell production fall into a group called the aplastic and deficiency anemias.

The anemias due to increased red cell destruction fall into a group called the hemolytic anemias.

The anemias due to loss of red cells fall into a group called the posthemorrhagic anemias.

Thus, we have 3 broad groups of anemias:

> aplastic and deficiency anemias
> hemolytic anemias
> posthemorrhagic anemias

The aplastic and deficiency anemias which we will consider are: aplastic anemia, iron deficiency anemia, and pernicious anemia.

The hemolytic anemias which we will consider are: hereditary spherocytic anemia, sickle cell anemia, thalassemia major, paroxysmal nocturnal hemoglobinuria, paroxysmal cold hemoglobinuria, acquired autoimmune hemolytic anemia, and erythroblastosis fetalis.

The posthemorrhagic anemias which we will consider are: acute posthemorrhagic anemia and chronic posthemorrhagic anemia.

The basic etiological classification which has just been presented is summarized in Table 39.

Table 39.—Etiological Classification of the Anemias

Cause	Group	Specific Anemia
Anemias Due to Decreased Red Cell Production	Aplastic and Deficiency Anemias	aplastic anemia iron deficiency anemia pernicious anemia
Anemias Due to Increased Red Cell Destruction	Hemolytic Anemias	hereditary spherocytic anemia sickle cell anemia thalassemia major paroxysmal nocturnal hemoglobinuria paroxysmal cold hemoglobinuria acquired autoimmune hemolytic anemia erythroblastosis fetalis
Anemias Due to Loss of Red Cells	Posthemorrhagic Anemias	acute posthemorrhagic anemia chronic posthemorrhagic anemia

We will now discuss the 12 specific anemias under the 3 group headings:

> Aplastic and Deficiency Anemias
> Hemolytic Anemias
> Posthemorrhagic Anemias

APLASTIC AND DEFICIENCY ANEMIAS

This section considers the anemias resulting from a decrease in the production of red cells.

The anemias which will be discussed are aplastic anemia, iron deficiency anemia, and pernicious anemia.

APLASTIC ANEMIA

Aplastic means failure to develop. In this instance, it refers to the bone marrow's failure to develop.

Aplastic anemia is often referred to by the following synonyms: primary refractory anemia, aregeneratory anemia, hypoplastic anemia, and panmyelophthis.

Aplastic anemia will be discussed under the following headings: basic clinical information, factors affecting laboratory examinations, results of laboratory examinations, and miscellaneous information.

Basic Clinical Information

Aplastic anemia is a severe disease of the blood which is characterized by failure of the bone marrow to produce the normal number of red cells, white cells, and platelets.

Aplastic anemia is usually caused by the action of drugs, chemicals, or radiation on the bone marrow.

Among the many drugs which may cause aplastic anemia are sulfonamides, salvarsan, and streptomycin.

Among the many chemicals which may cause aplastic anemia are arsenic, benzene, and insecticides.

If aplastic anemia is caused by radiation, the radiation may be from radium, x-rays, or atomic explosions.

Sometimes the cause of aplastic anemia cannot be determined and it is then referred to as idiopathic aplastic anemia.

Aplastic anemia appears to be on the increase. It may affect anyone: man, woman, or child.

The typical patient complains about headaches, weakness, fatigue, and difficulty in breathing. Thus, the symptoms are meager.

The doctor observes that the patient is pale, has fever and a high pulse rate, there is bleeding into the skin and from the mucous membranes, and the mouth contains ulcers.

The diagnosis will be made from the results of the physical examination and laboratory examinations.

The routine laboratory examinations usually include a white cell count, red cell count, hemoglobin, color index, differential white cell count, stained red cell examination, platelet count, and reticulocyte count.

Additional laboratory examinations may include a hematocrit reading, bleeding time, clot retraction time, capillary resistance test, serum iron, and bone marrow examination.

If the patient has aplastic anemia, the treatment will be aimed at (1) removing the cause, (2) controlling bleeding and infection, (3) supplying blood by means of transfusions, and (4) stimulating the bone marrow to produce blood cells.

The outlook or prognosis for a patient with aplastic anemia varies. The patient may (1) recover, (2) die within six months or (3) live for as long as eighteen years.

Now let us consider the manner in which this disease affects the laboratory examinations.

Factors Affecting Laboratory Examinations

In aplastic anemia, the bone marrow fails to produce the normal number of red cells, white cells, and platelets.

Thus, aplastic anemia is characterized by a pancytopenia, that is, a poverty or decrease of all blood cells.

Because the production of blood cells is decreased, the following tests are below normal: red cell count, white cell count, hemoglobin determination, hematocrit reading, and platelet count.

The reticulocyte count is usually decreased.

Since the red cells that are produced are normal in size and color, the color index is normal.

Because the bone marrow is not producing granulocytes, the differential white cell count shows a decrease in granulocytes and an increase in lymphocytes (which are formed in the lymphatic system rather than in the bone marrow).

Since the platelet count is low, those tests affected by a shortage of platelets are altered. Thus, the bleeding time is increased, the clot retraction time is increased, and the capillary resistance test is positive.

Because the production of red cells is decreased, the iron which is normally used in their manufacture goes unused. This iron soon builds up in the blood stream. And, the test for serum iron shows increased values.

Since the manufacture of red cells, white cells, and platelets is almost at a standstill, the bone marrow examination reveals few developing cells. Thus, the bone marrow is said to be hypoplastic.

The results of the laboratory examinations in aplastic anemia are summarized in Table 40.

Table 40
Results of Laboratory Examinations in Aplastic Anemia

Laboratory Examinations	Results	Values in this Disease	Values in Health
White cell count	Decreased	1,000 to 3,000 per cu. mm.	5,000 to 10,000 per cu. mm.
Red cell count	Decreased	0.5 to 2.5 million per cu. mm.	4.0 to 6.0 million per cu. mm.
Hemoglobin determination	Decreased	1 to 7 grams per 100 cc.	12 to 18 grams per 100 cc.
Color index	Normal	0.9 to 1.1	0.9 to 1.1
Differential white cell count	Decrease in granulocytes	0% to 20%	55% to 81%
	Increase in lymphocytes	50% to 90%	20% to 35%
Stained red cell examination (RBC morphology)	Normal	Red cells are normal in size and color	Red cells are normal in size and color
Platelet count (thrombocyte count)	Decreased	5,000 to 50,000 per cu. mm.	150,000 to 400,000 per cu. mm.
Reticulocyte count	Usually decreased	0% to 0.5%	1% to 2%
Hematocrit reading	Decreased	8% to 24%	37% to 54%
Bleeding time	Increased	3 to 8 min. (Duke method)	1 to 3 min. (Duke method)
Clot retraction time	Increased	Poor retraction after 2 hours and after 24 hours	Partial retraction after 2 hours and complete retraction in 24 hours
Capillary resistance test	Positive	20 to 40 petechiae produced by 100 millimeters pressure	0 to 10 petechiae produced by 100 millimeters pressure
Serum iron	Increased	200 to 2,000 micrograms per 100 ml.	70 to 180 micrograms per 100 ml.
Bone marrow examination	Hypoplastic	Decreased production of blood cells	Normal production of blood cells

Miscellaneous Information

In aplastic anemia, the red cells are normal in size and therefore the anemia is normocytic. The red cells are normal in color and thus the anemia is normochromic. Consequently, aplastic anemia is morphologically classified as a normocytic normochromic anemia.

IRON DEFICIENCY ANEMIA

Iron deficiency anemia is also referred to as hypochromic microcytic anemia, chronic hypochromic anemia, idiopathic hypochromic anemia, and chlorosis.

The discussion will cover basic clinical information, factors affecting laboratory examinations, results of laboratory examinations. and miscellaneous information.

Basic Clinical Information

Iron deficiency anemia is a disease of the blood which is characterized by a defective development of red cells resulting in the production of small pale erythrocytes.

Iron deficiency anemia may be caused by (1) deficiency of iron in the diet, (2) poor absorption or utilization of iron, or (3) chronic loss of blood.

This anemia is usually confined to women.

The typical patient complains about headaches, weakness, nervousness, difficulty in breathing, menstrual irregularities, abdominal pains, and numbness in the arms and legs.

The doctor observes that the patient is pale, has brittle fingernails, and her hair and skin appear dry and "dead." He may find fissures at the corners of her mouth and he may also find an enlarged heart, spleen, and liver.

The diagnosis will be made from the results of the physical examination and laboratory examinations.

The routine laboratory examinations usually include a red cell count, hemoglobin determination, color index, stained red cell examination, and hematocrit reading.

Additional laboratory examinations may include a volume index, red cell diameter, mean corpuscular hemoglobin, mean corpuscular volume, mean corpuscular hemoglobin concentration, serum iron, total iron-binding capacity, and bone marrow examination.

If the patient does have iron deficiency anemia, treatment will be aimed at restoring iron to the system by means of injection or oral medication.

The outlook is favorable, most patients recover in 2 or 3 weeks.

Now let us consider the manner in which this disease affects the laboratory examinations.

Factors Affecting Laboratory Examinations

As the name implies, iron deficiency anemia is caused by iron deficiency.

Iron is a vital material in the manufacture of hemoglobin. When iron is deficient, the production of hemoglobin is deficient. The deficient production of hemoglobin is observed in the red cells of the blood smear. These red cells are small and pale as illustrated in Figure 171, page 583.

The stained red cell examination therefore shows small red cells (microcytosis). These red cells are paler than normal (hypochromia).

The stained red cell examination also usually shows variation in the size of the cells (anisocytosis) and variation in the shape of the cells (poikilocytosis).

Since the red cells are deficient in hemoglobin, the hemoglobin determination drops below the normal values.

In iron deficiency anemia, the hemoglobin determination is markedly decreased but the red cell count is only slightly decreased.

For example, the hemoglobin determination might be decreased 60% but the red cell count may only be decreased 20%.

Thus, we might have a hemoglobin of 6 grams (40%) and a red cell count of 4,000,000.

This would give us the following color index:

$$\text{Color index} = \frac{\text{Hemoglobin in percent}}{\text{First 2 figures of RBC} \times 2}$$

$$= \frac{40}{40 \times 2}$$

$$= \frac{40}{80} = 0.5$$

Thus, in iron deficiency anemia, the color index is below the normal range of 0.9 to 1.1. This, of course, is due to the deficiency of hemoglobin within the red cell.

Since the red cells are deficient in hemoglobin, the weight of hemoglobin in the average red cell is below normal. Thus, the mean corpuscular hemoglobin (MCH) is decreased.

Because the red cells are smaller than normal, the following tests are decreased: red cell diameter, volume index, and mean corpuscular volume (MCV).

Since the red cells are not filled with hemoglobin, the concentration of hemoglobin in the average red cell is below normal. Thus, the mean corpuscular hemoglobin concentration (MCHC) is decreased.

Because the hemoglobin and red cell count are decreased, the hematocrit reading is decreased.

Since the iron in the system is decreased, the serum iron is decreased; and the total iron-binding capacity (TIBC) is increased.

The bone marrow examination shows that the bone marrow is (1) hyperplastic, that is, overactive and (2) shows an increase in nucleated red cells.

The results of the laboratory examinations in iron deficiency anemia are summarized in Table 41.

Table 41

Results of Laboratory Examinations in Iron Deficiency Anemia

Laboratory Examinations	Results	Values in this Disease	Values in Health
Red cell count	Decreased	3 to 5 million per cu. mm.	4 to 6 million per cu. mm.
Hemoglobin determination	Decreased	4 to 10 grams per 100 cc.	12 to 18 grams per 100 cc.
Color index	Decreased	0.4 to 0.8	0.9 to 1.1
Stained red cell examination (RBC morphology)	Microcytosis	present	absent
	Hypochromia	present	absent
	Anisocytosis	present	absent
	Poikilocytosis	present	absent
Hematocrit reading	Decreased	10% to 25%	37% to 54%
Mean corpuscular hemoglobin (MCH)	Decreased	5 to 25 micro-micrograms	27 to 32 micro-micrograms
Red cell diameter	Decreased	6 to 7 microns	7 to 8 microns
Volume index	Decreased	0.4 to 0.8	0.9 to 1.1
Mean corpuscular volume (MCV)	Decreased	60 to 80 cubic microns	80 to 90 cubic microns
Mean corpuscular hemoglobin concentration (MCHC)	Decreased	20% to 30%	33% to 38%
Serum iron	Decreased	10 to 30 micro-grams per 100 ml.	70 to 180 micro-grams per 100 ml.
Total iron-binding capacity (TIBC)	Increased	360 to 450 micro-grams per 100 ml.	300 to 360 micro-grams per 100 ml.
Bone marrow examination	Hyperplastic. Increase in nucleated red cells.	30% to 60%	8% to 30%

Miscellaneous Information

The miscellaneous information is concerned with pyridoxine deficiency anemia and classifications of iron deficiency anemia.

Iron deficiency anemia may be confused with a microcytic hypochromic anemia caused by a deficiency of pyridoxine (vitamin B_6). These two anemias may be distinguished by a test for serum iron. In iron deficiency anemia, the serum iron is decreased; whereas in pyridoxine deficiency anemia, the serum iron is increased.

In iron deficiency anemia, the red cells are small and therefore the anemia is microcytic. The red cells, lacking hemoglobin, are pale and thus the anemia is hypochromic. Consequently, iron deficiency anemia is morphologically classified as a microcytic hypochromic anemia.

Since iron deficiency anemia is caused by a deficiency of iron, it is etiologically classified as a deficiency anemia.

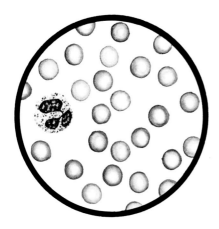 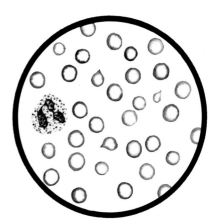

Blood Smear in Health

Note:

1. The red cells are normal in size.
2. The red cells are normal in color.

Blood Smear in Iron Deficiency Anemia

Note:

1. The red cells are smaller than the red cells in health.
2. The red cells are paler than the red cells in health.
3. The red cells show a slight variation in size.
4. The red cells show a slight variation in shape.

FIG. 171.—Blood smear in health compared with blood smear in iron deficiency anemia. (Stain: Wright's; Magnification: 1000×)

PERNICIOUS ANEMIA

Pernicious anemia may be referred to by the following terms: Addison's anemia, Biermer's anemia, primary anemia, the initials P. A. (for pernicious anemia), and megaloblastic anemia due to vitamin B_{12} deficiency.

The discussion will cover basic clinical information, the red cell in pernicious anemia, factors affecting laboratory examinations, results of laboratory examinations, and miscellaneous information.

Basic Clinical Information

Pernicious anemia is a disease of the blood which is characterized by a defective development of the red cells resulting in the production of greatly enlarged erythrocytes.

Pernicious anemia is caused by failure of the stomach to secrete an intrinsic factor. Lack of this intrinsic factor prevents absorption of vitaman B_{12} into the blood stream. Absence of vitamin B_{12} in the blood stream and bone marrow results in the abnormal development of red cells.

The typical patient complains about being weak, having a sore tongue, numbness or tingling in the arms and legs, shortness of breath, loss of appetite, loss of weight, diarrhea, pain in the chest, and the usual addition: "I've been feeling this way a long, long time."

The doctor observes that the patient is pale, has lemon colored skin, a smooth glazed tongue, a high pulse rate, impaired coordination, decreased vibratory sense, and a systolic murmur.

The diagnosis will be made from the results of the physical examination and laboratory examinations.

The routine laboratory examinations usually include a white cell count, red cell count, hemoglobin, color index, differential white cell count, stained red cell examination, platelet count, gastric analysis, and Schilling test.

Additional laboratory examinations may include a red cell diameter, volume index, mean corpuscular volume, mean corpuscular hemoglobin, mean corpuscular hemoglobin concentration, erythrocyte survival time, reticulocyte count, serum bilirubin, urine urobilinogen, bone marrow examination, and serum vitamin B_{12} examination.

If the patient does have pernicious anemia, treatment will be aimed at restoring vitamin B_{12} to the system.

After 3 weeks treatment, the symptoms usually subside.

Now let us consider the red cell in pernicious anemia.

The Red Cell in Pernicious Anemia

As previously mentioned, the development of a red cell takes place in the bone marrow. This development has one objective. This objective is to fill the cell with hemoglobin.

During the process, the cell acts somewhat like an organism. The nucleus acts as the "brain" directing the manufacture of hemoglobin. The cytoplasm acts as the "body" being filled with hemoglobin.

Now, if the cell has the necessary raw materials, (1) the nucleus develops *normally* and (2) the cytoplasm develops *normally*. The result is the production of a normal erythrocyte.

But, if the cell lacks vitamin B_{12}, (1) the nucleus develops *abnormally* and (2) the cytoplasm develops *normally*. The result is the production of a malformed erythrocyte.

This malformed erythrocyte is called a macrocyte. It looks like this:

malformed erythrocyte   normal erythrocyte
(macrocyte)

As you can see, the macrocyte is a giant of an erythrocyte. It is a virtual Frankenstein among normal erythrocytes. But this Frankenstein of an erythrocyte is internally defective.

When the macrocyte leaves the bone marrow and enters the blood stream, it performs duties similar to a normal erythrocyte. Thus, it trudges back and forth between lungs and tissues, first carrying oxygen and then carbon dioxide. But, because it is internally defective, it breaks down at an early age.

The average macrocyte lives only $\frac{1}{3}$ the lifetime of a normal erythrocyte. Because of this short life, it fails to complete the work load of a normal erythrocyte.

By way of summary:

In pernicious anemia, the bone marrow, lacking vitamin B_{12}, produces fewer erythrocytes. The erythrocytes it does produce are unusually large and well filled with hemoglobin. But these erythrocytes are internally defective, breaking down at an early age.

Now let us consider some terminology regarding the developing red cell in pernicious anemia.

The developing red cell in health and in pernicious anemia is illustrated in Figure 172.

| Development of Red Cell in Health | Development of Red Cell in Pernicious Anemia |
| (erythrocytic series) | (megaloblastic series) |

rubriblast   "pernicious anemia type" rubriblast

prorubricyte   "pernicious anemia type" prorubricyte

rubricyte   "pernicious anemia type" rubricyte

metarubricyte   "pernicious anemia type" metarubricyte

reticulocyte   reticulocyte

erythrocyte   macrocyte

FIG. 172.—Development of the red cell in health and in pernicious anemia. (Magnification: 1500×.)

You will note that the first 4 cells in the developing red cell contain a nucleus. You will recall that these cells are therefore called nucleated red cells.

The nucleated red cells in pernicious anemia may be distinguished from the nucleated red cells in health on the following basis.

(1) The nucleated red cells in pernicious anemia are slightly larger than the nucleated red cells in health.

(2) The nucleated red cells in pernicious anemia have a nucleus which is loosely knit, whereas the nucleated red cells in health have a nucleus which is closely knit.

The nucleated red cells seen in pernicious anemia were formerly known as the nucleated red cells of the *megaloblastic series.*

The new name and old name for the nucleated red cells seen in pernicious anemia are given in Table 42.

Table 42

New Name and Old Name for Nucleated Red Cells Seen in Pernicious Anemia

New Name	*Old Name*
"pernicious anemia type" rubriblast	promegaloblast
"pernicious anemia type" prorubricyte	basophilic megaloblast
"pernicious anemia type" rubricyte	polychromatophilic megaloblast
"pernicious anemia type" metarubricyte	orthochromatic megaloblast

Now let us consider the manner in which the decreased red cell production and malformed erythrocytes affect the laboratory examinations in pernicious anemia.

Factors Affecting Laboratory Examinations

In the stained red cell examination, some normal erythrocytes are present, but the majority of erythrocytes are large erythrocytes called macrocytes. The macrocytes are well filled with hemoglobin. A blood smear showing the macrocytes of pernicious anemia is illustrated in Figure 173, page 588.

Since the bone marrow is plagued by the deficiency of vitamin B_{12}, the production of red cells is decreased. Thus, the red cell count falls from a normal range of 4–6 million to 1–3 million per cubic millimeter.

The hemoglobin is also decreased, but not so much as the red cell count. For example, the hemoglobin may be decreased 50% but the red cell count may be decreased 60%. This is due to the presence of the large red cells well filled with hemoglobin. They have the effect of "buoying up" the hemoglobin values.

Since the erythrocytes are large and well filled with hemoglobin, the color index *increases.* It usually goes from a normal range of 0.9–1.1 to 1.1–1.6.

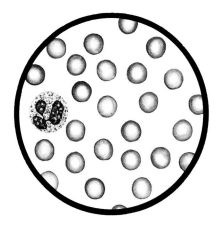 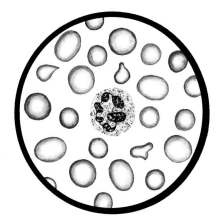

Blood Smear in Health

Note:

1. The normal size of the erythrocytes.

2. The normal shape of the erythrocytes.

Blood Smear in Pernicious Anemia

Note:

1. The large erythrocytes (macrocytes); compare these large erythrocytes with the normal erythrocytes in the illustration on the left.

2. The variation in the size of the erythrocytes (anisocytosis).

3. The variation in the shape of the erythrocytes (poikilocytosis).

4. The hypersegmented neutrophil in the center.

FIG. 173.—Blood smear in health compared with blood smear in pernicious anemia. (Stain: Wright's; Magnification: 1000×)

Thus, with a hemoglobin of 7.5 grams (52%) and a red cell count of 2,000,000, we would have the following color index:

$$\text{Color index} = \frac{\text{Hemoglobin in percent}}{\text{First 2 figures of RBC} \times 2}$$

$$= \frac{52}{20 \times 2}$$

$$= \frac{52}{40}$$

$$= 1.3$$

Because a high color index is rarely encountered and because it is often confusing to students, let us take a moment to discuss the color index in pernicious anemia.

You understand, of course, that the color index is simply an expression of the relationship between *weight* and *number*, that is, the *weight* of hemoglobin to the *number* of red cells.

Now, let us pursue the following analogy.

Suppose you had 10 babies weighing 10 pounds each. The relationship between *weight* and *number* would be:

$$\frac{\text{weight}}{\text{number}} \quad \frac{10}{10} = 1.0$$

Now suppose you had 10 babies and they weighed 13 pounds each. The relationship between *weight* and *number* would be:

$$\frac{\text{weight}}{\text{number}} \quad \frac{13}{10} = 1.3$$

In pernicious anemia, the cells (babies) are large and contain more hemoglobin, thus giving a high color index.

In pernicious anemia, the *number* of red cells is also decreased, and this adds to the increase in the color index.

For example, suppose you only had 8 babies and they weighed 13 pounds each. The relationship between *weight* and *number* would be:

$$\frac{\text{weight}}{\text{number}} \quad \frac{13}{8} = 1.6$$

The most significant finding for the medical technologist is a blood smear showing a decided increase in large erythrocytes (macrocytosis), a variation in the size of the erythrocytes (anisocytosis), a variation in the shape of the erythrocytes (poikilocytosis), and hypersegmented neutrophils (Fig. 173).

Since the macrocytes are unusually large, the following tests show increased values: red cell diameter, volume index, and mean corpuscular volume.

Because the macrocytes are unusually large and well filled with hemoglobin, the weight of hemoglobin in the average red cell is also increased. Thus, the mean corpuscular hemoglobin (MCH) shows increased values.

Since the macrocytes are filled with hemoglobin, the concentration of hemoglobin in the average red cell is normal. Thus, the mean corpuscular hemoglobin concentration (MCHC) is normal.

Because the erythrocytes are internally defective, they break down at an early age. Thus, the erythrocyte survival time is decreased.

The decreased production of red cells causes a decrease in the reticulocyte count; the increased destruction of red cells causes an increase in the serum bilirubin and also in the urine urobilinogen.

The bone marrow examination reveals an increase in nucleated red cells, the nucleated red cells being of the "megaloblastic series."

The white cell count and platelet count are below normal, probably also caused by the vitamin deficiency.

The gastric analysis reveals the absence of free hydrochloric acid (achlorhydria) even after stimulation with histamine.

Since the stomach fails to secrete an intrinsic factor, the Schilling test is positive.

Because the body lacks vitamin B_{12}, the serum vitamin B_{12} is decreased. (This test may be determined chemically or by measuring the growth response of certain bacteria.)

The results of the laboratory examinations in pernicious anemia are summarized in Table 43.

The classifications of pernicious anemia and some related macrocytic anemias will be discussed on page 592.

Table 43

Results of Laboratory Examinations in Pernicious Anemia

Laboratory Examinations	Results	Values in this Disease	Values in Health
White cell count	Decreased	2,000 to 4,000 per cu. mm.	5,000 to 10,000 per cu. mm.
Red cell count	Decreased	1 to 3 million per cu. mm.	4 to 6 million per cu. mm.
Hemoglobin determination	Decreased	4 to 12 grams per 100 cc.	12 to 18 grams per 100 cc.
Color index	Increased	1.1 to 1.6	0.9 to 1.1

Table 43.—(*Continued*)

Laboratory Examinations	Results	Values in this Disease	Values in Health
Differential white cell count	Decrease in granulocytes	10% to 40%	55% to 81%
	Presence of hypersegmented neutrophils	2% to 8%	0%
Stained red cell examination (RBC morphology)	Macrocytosis	present	absent
	Anisocytosis	present	absent
	Poikilocytosis	present	absent
	Polychromato-philia	present	absent
	Nucleated red cells	0 to 5 per 100 white cells	0 per 100 white cells
Platelet count	Decreased	50,000 to 150,000 per cu. mm.	150,000 to 400,000 per cu. mm.
Gastric analysis	Achlorhydria	0 degrees of free hydrochloric acid	20 to 70 degrees of free hydrochloric acid
Schilling test	Positive	will not absorb vitamin B_{12}	will absorb vitamin B_{12}
Red cell diameter	Increased	8.0 to 9.0 microns	7.0 to 8.0 microns
Volume index	Increased	1.1 to 1.6	0.9 to 1.1
Mean corpuscular volume (MCV)	Increased	95 to 150 cubic microns	80 to 90 cubic microns
Mean corpuscular hemoglobin (MCH)	Increased	33 to 53 micromicrograms	27 to 32 micromicrograms
Mean corpuscular hemoglobin concentration (MCHC)	Normal	33% to 38%	33% to 38%
Erythrocyte survival time	Decreased	10 to 30 days half-life (Ashby)	55 to 65 days half-life (Ashby)
Reticulocyte count	Decreased	0%	1% to 2%
Serum bilirubin	Increased	0.8 to 2.0 mg/100 ml.	0.2 to 0.8 mg/100 ml.
Urine urobilinogen	Increased	2 to 4 Ehrlich units in 24 hrs.	1 to 2 Ehrlich units in 24 hrs.
Bone marrow examination	Increase in nucleated red cells.	30% to 50%	8% to 30%
	"P.A. Type" nucleated red cells.	present	absent
Serum vitamin B_{12}	Decreased	varies with method	varies with method

Miscellaneous Information

The miscellaneous information will cover the classifications of pernicious anemia and list the anemias which are related to pernicious anemia.

Because the red cell development is abnormal and results in the production of greatly enlarged erythrocytes or macrocytes, pernicious anemia is classified morphologically as a macrocytic anemia.

And, since the red cells are normal in color, it is further morphologically classified as a macrocytic normochromic anemia.

Since pernicious anemia is caused by the absence or deficiency of a vital material in red cell development, it is classified etiologically as a deficiency anemia.

Due to the bone marrow's production of large nucleated red cells called "megaloblasts," pernicious anemia is also referred to as a megaloblastic anemia.

Thus, pernicious anemia has the following classifications:

      macrocytic anemia
      macrocytic normochromic anemia
      deficiency anemia
      megaloblastic anemia

Pernicious anemia is a typical example of the macrocytic anemias.

Among other macrocytic anemias are the following: tropical sprue, idiopathic steatorrhea, tropical macrocytic anemia, macrocytic anemia of pregnancy, macrocytic anemia of hypothyroidism, macrocytic anemia in lesions of the stomach, macrocytic anemia caused by *Diphyllobothrium latum* (fish tapeworm) infestation, macrocytic anemia caused by drugs such as Dilantin, Mysoline, 5-fluorouracil, or 6-mercaptopurine, and refractory megaloblastic and "achrestic" anemias.

HEMOLYTIC ANEMIAS

This section considers seven anemias resulting from an increase in the destruction of red cells.

The material covers the following:

      General Discussion of the Hemolytic Anemias
      Hereditary Spherocytic Anemia
      Sickle Cell Anemia
      Thalassemia Major
      Paroxysmal Nocturnal Hemoglobinuria
      Paroxysmal Cold Hemoglobinuria
      Acquired Autoimmune Hemolytic Anemia
      Erythroblastosis Fetalis

GENERAL DISCUSSION OF THE HEMOLYTIC ANEMIAS

The discussion will cover the rupture of the red cell, the results of hemolysis, and the classification of the hemolytic anemias.

Rupture of the Red Cell

In the hemolytic anemias, the erythrocyte breaks down or hemolyzes at an early age. The breakdown may occur in the liver, spleen, blood stream, or bone marrow. The location of the breakdown depends upon such factors as the cause of the breakdown and the rate of the breakdown.

When the erythrocyte breaks down, it liberates hemoglobin. The hemoglobin decomposes into iron, globin, and bilirubin. The iron and globin are saved by the body and used again.

The bilirubin, a red pigment, is absorbed by a fluid, bile. After absorption by the bile, the bilirubin may be used again or excreted as urobilinogen in the urine or feces.

The basic steps in the decomposition of hemoglobin are illustrated in Figure 174.

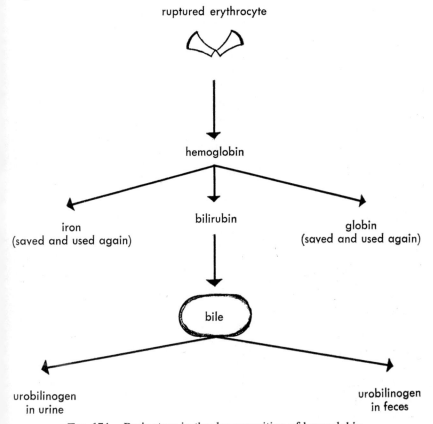

FIG. 174.—Basic steps in the decomposition of hemoglobin.

When 1 milliliter of erythrocytes breaks down, it liberates 10 milligrams of bilirubin and 1 milligram of iron. Consequently, a rising tide of bilirubin and iron is often observed in the hemolytic anemias.

Results of Hemolysis

An increased breakdown or hemolysis of red cells is the one common finding in all hemolytic anemias.

The increased breakdown of the red cells (1) alters the blood, urine, and feces, and (2) stimulates the bone marrow to produce more red cells.

First, let us consider the alterations in the blood, urine, and feces.

These alterations in blood, urine, and feces are largely dependent upon the rate of red cell breakdown.

The rate of red cell breakdown may be slow or rapid.

If the rate of red cell breakdown is slow, the laboratory findings are as follows.

The blood shows an increase in bilirubin. The urine and feces usually show an increase in urobilinogen.

If the rate of red cell breakdown is rapid and a large amount of blood is destroyed, the laboratory findings are as follows.

The blood shows a decrease in the red cell count, an increase in plasma hemoglobin, and the presence of methemalbumin. The latter substance, methemalbumin, is formed by the union of heme and albumin.

The urine shows casts, albumin, hemosiderin, hemoglobin, and methemoglobin. The latter substance, methemoglobin, is an oxidation product of hemoglobin.

The feces show an increase in urobilinogen.

Now let us consider the manner in which the increased hemolysis affects the bone marrow.

The increased breakdown of the red cells stimulates the bone marrow to produce more red cells.

The overactivity of the bone marrow is reflected by an increase in the reticulocyte count, platelet count, white cell count, and a blood smear showing anisocytosis, poikilocytosis, polychromatophilia, basophilic stippling, and nucleated red cells.

The laboratory signs of increased red cell destruction and production are summarized in Table 44.

Classification of the Hemolytic Anemias

The hemolytic anemias may be broken down into two broad groups: the intracorpuscular hemolytic anemias and the extracorpuscular hemolytic anemias.

Table 44

Signs of Increased Red Cell Destruction and Production

Signs of Increased Red Cell Destruction

Blood
1. decrease in red cell count
2. increase in bilirubin
3. increase in plasma hemoglobin
4. presence of methemalbumin

Urine
1. casts
2. albumin
3. hemosiderin
4. hemoglobin
5. methemoglobin
6. urobilinogen usually increased

Feces
1. urobilinogen increased

Signs of Increased Red Cell Production

Blood
1. increase in reticulocyte count, platelet count, and white cell count
2. blood smear shows anisocytosis, poikilocytosis, polychromatophilia, basophilic stippling, and nucleated red cells

The intracorpuscular hemolytic anemias are usually inherited whereas the extracorpuscular hemolytic anemias are usually acquired.

The intracorpuscular hemolytic anemias are due to a defect in the erythrocytes.

Thus, when erythrocytes from a patient with an intracorpuscular hemolytic anemia are transfused into a normal person, the transfused erythrocytes have a *decreased* life span. On the other hand, when normal erythrocytes are transfused into a patient with an intracorpuscular hemolytic anemia, the normal erythrocytes have a normal life span.

These erythrocyte survival tests indicate that the fault is in the erythrocytes and not in the plasma.

The intracorpuscular hemolytic anemias which we will consider are hereditary spherocytic anemia, sickle cell anemia, thalassemia major, and paroxysmal nocturnal hemoglobinuria.

The extracorpuscular hemolytic anemias are caused by a factor outside the erythrocytes.

Thus, when normal erythrocytes are transfused into a patient with an extracorpuscular hemolytic anemia, the normal erythrocytes have a

40

decreased life span. On the other hand, when erythrocytes from a patient with an extracorpuscular hemolytic anemia are transfused into a normal person, the transfused erythrocytes have a normal life span.

These erythrocyte survival tests indicate that the fault is in the plasma and not in the erythrocytes.

The extracorpuscular hemolytic anemias which we will discuss are paroxysmal cold hemoglobinuria, acquired autoimmune hemolytic anemia, and erythroblastosis fetalis.

The classification of the hemolytic anemias is given in Table 45.

Table 45.—Classification of the Hemolytic Anemias

Group	Specific Anemia
Intracorpuscular Hemolytic Anemias	hereditary spherocytic anemia
	sickle cell anemia
	thalassemia major
	paroxysmal nocturnal hemoglobinuria
Extracorpuscular Hemolytic Anemias	paroxysmal cold hemoglobinuria
	acquired autoimmune hemolytic anemia
	erythroblastosis fetalis

Each of the seven hemolytic anemias mentioned above will now be discussed in detail.

HEREDITARY SPHEROCYTIC ANEMIA

Hereditary spherocytic anemia is often referred to by the following synonyms: congenital hemolytic anemia, congenital hemolytic icterus, congenital hemolytic jaundice, spherocytic jaundice, acholuric jaundice, and hereditary spherocytosis.

The discussion will cover basic clinical information, factors affecting laboratory examinations, results of laboratory examinations, and miscellaneous information.

Basic Clinical Information

Hereditary spherocytic anemia is an inherited hemolytic anemia which is characterized by the production of sphere shaped erythrocytes having an increased osmotic fragility and decreased life span.

The disease may affect man, woman, or child.

The typical patient complains about being weak, having abdominal pains, and loss of appetite. Thus, the symptoms are meager.

The doctor observes that the patient has a fever and an enlarged spleen; he may also find jaundice, gallstones, an enlarged liver, and ulcers on the legs.

The diagnosis will be made from the results of the physical examination and laboratory examinations, with the results of the laboratory examinations being extremely significant to the physician.

The routine laboratory examinations usually include a white cell count, red cell count, hemoglobin determination, differential white cell count, stained red cell examination, hematocrit reading, reticulocyte count, red cell osmotic fragility test, serum bilirubin, and direct Coombs' test.

Additional laboratory examinations may include an icteric index, red cell diameter, erythrocyte survival time, serum iron, urine urobilinogen, and bone marrow examination.

Hereditary spherocytic anemia is not fatal and the outlook for the patient is usually favorable.

The disease may be mild or severe. If it is mild, few problems arise. If it is severe, however, it may be desirable to remove the spleen. When the spleen is removed, complete recovery generally follows.

The removal of the spleen is believed to be beneficial because the spleen apparently acts as a trap which catches and destroys the sphere shaped erythrocytes. Hence, when the trap is removed, the erythrocytes are no longer destroyed.

Now let us consider the manner in which hereditary spherocytic anemia affects the laboratory examinations.

Factors Affecting Laboratory Examinations

In this anemia, we see the following drama and conflict within the body.

The bone marrow, acting under the direction of the mendelian laws of heredity, produces malformed erythrocytes.

And the spleen, acting as judge, jury, and executioner, pulls these malformed erythrocytes out of the circulation, destroys them, and tosses their remains back into the blood stream.

Such is the drama and the conflict in hereditary spherocytic anemia.

The anemia is characterized by good periods and bad periods. During the good periods or remissions, the patient is apparently in good health. But during the bad periods or relapses, he may become jaundiced or show other signs of anemia.

The blood picture during remissions is usually normal. The blood picture during relapses changes drastically. These changes are discussed below.

Fatigue, infection, or exposure to cold may trigger a sudden increase in the breakdown of erythrocytes.

The increased breakdown of erythrocytes causes the red cell count and hemoglobin determination to drop below normal.

Since the red cell count and hemoglobin determination drop below normal, the hematocrit reading drops below normal.

The bone marrow endeavors to compensate for the increased breakdown of erythrocytes and sends immature red cells into the blood stream. Consequently, the reticulocyte count goes up and nucleated red cells appear in the blood smear.

About one-third of the erythrocytes coming into the blood stream are malformed erythrocytes—the spherocytes.

The spherocytes are sphere shaped and consequently they are thicker than normal biconcave erythrocytes.

What do these thick cells look like on a blood smear?

In a blood smear, the spherocytes are lying flat and viewed from above (like a coin lying on a table).

Since the spherocytes are thicker than normal erythrocytes, the central portion appears darkly stained.

The appearance of normal erythrocytes and spherocytes in the blood smear is illustrated in Figure 175.

Normal Erythrocytes	Spherocytes
Note the pale area in the center of the cells. This is due to their normal biconcave shape.	Note that the central portion is darkly stained and not pale as in the normal erythrocyte. This is due to the abnormal sphere shape of the cell.

FIG. 175.—Appearance of normal erythrocytes and spherocytes in the blood smear. (Stain: Wright's; Magnification: 2000×.)

Suppose we stand the spherocyte on end (like a coin). Now suppose we view it from the side (like looking at the edge of the coin).

We see that the spherocyte has a smaller diameter than a normal erythrocyte. The difference in diameter between the two cells is somewhat like the difference in diameter between a nickel and a quarter.

The diameter of a spherocyte and a normal erythrocyte is illustrated in Figure 176.

Since the spherocyte has a smaller diameter than a normal erythrocyte, decreased values are found in tests which measure the red cell diameter.

The spherocyte, however, compensates for the decrease in diameter by being fatter in the middle.

Thus, the spherocyte is the roly-poly among red cells. It is short and fat. And this structure enables it to maintain a volume and hemoglobin content which is practically normal.

Since the spherocyte is practically normal in volume and hemoglobin content, the red cell indexes and mean corpuscular values are usually normal.

Thus, the volume index, color index, and saturation index are usually normal.

And the mean corpuscular volume, mean corpuscular hemoglobin, and mean corpuscular hemoglobin concentration are usually normal.

Now, suppose water *simultaneously* enters the spherocyte and normal erythrocyte illustrated in Figure 176.

Which cell will be the first to rupture?

Since the spherocyte is almost round, it is already nearer the breaking point; therefore, it will be the first to rupture.

Hence, the spherocyte is said to have a greater osmotic fragility than a normal erythrocyte.

Consequently, in hereditary spherocytic anemia, the red cell osmotic fragility test shows increased values.

Because the spherocytes only live about 14 days (against a normal life expectancy of 120 days), the erythrocyte survival time shows decreased values.

Since the dying spherocytes leave behind their iron and bilirubin, these elements are increased in the blood and urobilinogen is increased in the urine.

The excess bilirubin in the blood causes the icteric index to rise.

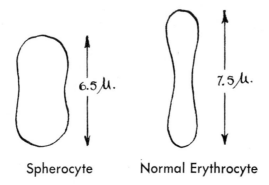

Spherocyte   Normal Erythrocyte

Note:

1. The spherocyte has a diameter of 6.5 microns where-
    as the normal erythrocyte has a diameter of 7.5
    microns.

2. The spherocyte is puffed up or "fatter" than a normal
    erythrocyte.

Fig. 176.—Spherocyte and normal erythrocyte viewed from the side.

Because the breakdown of red cells is due to malformation of the cells and is not caused by antibodies in the blood, the direct Coombs' (antiglobulin) test is negative.

Since the bone marrow is endeavoring to produce more red cells, a bone marrow examination reveals an increase in nucleated red cells.

The increased activity of the bone marrow causes the white cell count to rise and the differential white cell count to show immature white cells.

In the stained red cell examination, about $\frac{1}{3}$ of the red cells are spherocytes and the other $\frac{2}{3}$ are normal erythrocytes.

Some erythrocytes are larger than usual and may, in fact, be reticulocytes (lacking their special stain).

These large erythrocytes, which are probably reticulocytes, usually show some degree of polychromatophilia.

The stained red cell examination thus shows spherocytosis and anisocytosis. It also shows a few nucleated red cells.

Blood smears showing the spherocytes and reticulocytes of hereditary spherocytic anemia are illustrated in Figure 177.

The results of the laboratory examinations in hereditary spherocytic anemia during a relapse are summarized in Table 46, page 602.

Miscellaneous Information

Since hereditary spherocytic anemia is caused by an increase in the hemolysis of red cells, it is etiologically classified as a hemolytic anemia.

In mild cases, the anemia is usually normocytic but occasionally may be microcytic.

In severe cases, the anemia may appear to be slightly macrocytic. This is due to the greatly increased number of reticulocytes (10% to 50%). The reticulocytes are larger than erythrocytes and, without their special stain, appear in the blood smear as large erythrocytes. Consequently, the increased number of reticulocytes makes the anemia appear to be macrocytic.

Because of the above discrepancies in the size of the red cells, hereditary spherocytic anemia does not fall into any definite morphological classification.

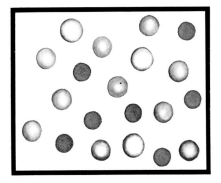 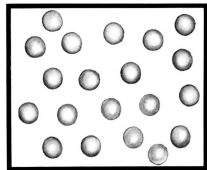

Blood Smear in Hereditary Spherocytic Anemia Showing Spherocytes

Note that about one third of the erythrocytes are small and darkly stained. These cells are spherocytes. (Blood smear was stained with Wright's stain.)

Blood Smear in Health Showing Normal Erythrocytes

Note that the erythrocytes are normal in size and color. (Blood smear was stained with Wright's stain.)

The granular net-like mass in the reticulocyte can not be seen when the cell is stained only with Wright's stain. And the cell is then looked upon as a large erythrocyte. A special stain, however, brings out the granular net-like mass. The cell then reveals its identity as a reticulocyte.

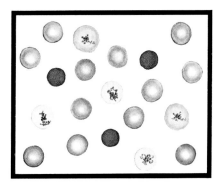

Blood Smear in Hereditary Spherocytic Anemia Showing Reticulocytes

Note the granular net-like mass in some of the larger cells. These cells are reticulocytes. (This blood smear was first stained with a special stain to bring out the reticulum in the reticulocyte and then counter-stained with Wright's stain.)

FIG. 177.—Spherocytes and reticulocytes in hereditary spherocytic anemia. (Magnification 1000×)

Table 46

Results of Laboratory Examinations in
Hereditary Spherocytic Anemia During a Relapse

Laboratory Examinations	Results	Values in this Disease	Values in Health
White cell count	Increased	10,000 to 30,000 per cu. mm.	5,000 to 10,000 per cu. mm.
Red cell count	Decreased	1.5 to 4.0 million per cu. mm.	4.0 to 6.0 million per cu. mm.
Hemoglobin determination	Decreased	4 to 10 grams per 100 cc.	12 to 18 grams per 100 cc.
Differential white cell count	Myelocytes Metamyelocytes	0% to 2% 6% to 12%	0% 0%
Stained red cell examination (RBC morphology)	Spherocytosis Anisocytosis Nucleated red cells	present present 0 to 10 per 100 white cells	absent absent 0 per 100 white cells
Hematocrit reading	Decreased	12% to 30%	37% to 54%
Reticulocyte count	Increased	10% to 50%	1% to 2%
Red cell osmotic fragility test	Increased	hemol. begins .50% hemol. ends .40%	hemol. begins .44% hemol. ends .34%
Serum bilirubin	Increased	0.8 to 5.0 mg. per 100 ml.	0.2 to 0.8 mg. per 100 ml.
Direct Coombs' test	Negative	negative	negative
Icteric index	Increased	15 to 30 units	4 to 6 units
Red cell diameter	Decreased	6.0 to 7.0 microns	7.0 to 8.0 microns
Erythrocyte survival time	Decreased	average survival 14 days	55 to 65 days half-life (Ashby method)
Serum iron	Increased	180 to 225 micrograms per 100 ml.	70 to 180 micrograms per 100 ml.
Urine urobilinogen	Increased	2 to 6 Ehrlich units in 24 hrs.	1 to 2 Ehrlich units in 24 hrs.
Bone marrow examination	Increase in nucleated red cells	30% to 60%	8% to 30%

SICKLE CELL ANEMIA

Sickle cell anemia is often referred to by the following synonyms: homozygous hemoglobin S disease, drepanocytic anemia, menisocytosis, sicklemia, and Herrick's syndrome.

The discussion will cover basic clinical information, factors affecting laboratory examinations, results of laboratory examinations, and miscellaneous information.

Basic Clinical Information

Let us consider the hemoglobin in sickle cell anemia and sickle cell trait.

Hemoglobin A is normal hemoglobin; hemoglobin S is an abnormal hemoglobin. These two hemoglobins differ in molecular structure. This difference in molecular structure is responsible for sickle cell anemia and sickle cell trait.

Sickle cell anemia is caused by inheriting a gene for hemoglobin S from both parents. Such a person has genes SS and is said to be homozygous. His red cells contain hemoglobin S.

Sickle cell trait is caused by inheriting a gene for hemoglobin A from one parent and a gene for hemoglobin S from the other parent. Such a person has genes AS and is said to be heterozygous. His red cells contain a mixture of hemoglobin A and hemoglobin S.

Persons with sickle cell anemia have a severe anemia with all the physical symptoms and they usually die before they reach the age of 21.

Persons with sickle cell trait may transmit the disease but they are usually not affected with an anemia or any physical symptoms of the disease.

In most instances, persons with sickle cell trait can look forward to a normal life.

Sickle cell anemia and sickle cell trait are usually confined to Negroes or persons of Negro ancestry. Sickle cell anemia affects about 1% of all Negroes and sickle cell trait is found in about 10% of all Negroes. The disease and the trait may affect either male or female.

The patient in sickle cell anemia is usually a Negro child or young adult.

A typical patient complains about having pains in the stomach, arms, legs, and joints. He may also complain about being tired, tense, and nervous.

The doctor notes that the patient is a Negro and observes that he has a short trunk, long thin arms and legs, a tower-shaped head, a rotund stomach, ulcers on the lower part of the legs, an enlarged liver, and an enlarged heart with systolic murmur.

The diagnosis will be made from the results of the physical examination and laboratory examinations.

The routine laboratory examinations usually include a white cell count, red cell count, hemoglobin determination, differential white cell count, stained red cell examination, hematocrit reading, reticulocyte count, sickle cell examination, red cell osmotic fragility test, and abnormal hemoglobin examination.

Additional laboratory examinations may include a urine analysis, urine urobilinogen, sedimentation rate, serum bilirubin, platelet count, erythrocyte survival time, red cell mechanical fragility test, and bone marrow examination.

If the patient does have sickle cell anemia, he is usually cautioned against travelling to mountainous regions and also cautioned against travelling in non-pressurized planes.

Such precautions are necessary because the sickling tendency is increased when the oxygen content of the air is decreased.

Sickle cell anemia does not have any satisfactory treatment.

Now let us consider the manner in which this disease affects the laboratory examinations.

Factors Affecting Laboratory Examinations

In sickle cell anemia, the bone marrow is producing a decreased number of erythrocytes. These erythrocytes are malformed and subject to sickling and premature hemolysis.

The decreased production of erythrocytes results in a decrease in the red cell count, hemoglobin determination, and hematocrit reading.

When oxygen is scarce, the malformed erythrocytes tend to buckle or assume a sickle shape. These sickled erythrocytes are illustrated in Fig. 178.

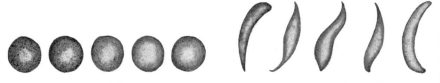

Normal Erythrocytes   Sickled Erythrocytes

Fig. 178.—Normal erythrocytes and sickled erythrocytes
(stained with Wright's stain and magnified 1500×).

Sickled erythrocytes are also referred to as sickle cells, sickled red cells, sickle-shaped erythrocytes, drepanocytes, and menisocytes.

An environment of lowered oxygen content is encountered in the small capillaries. Here the erythrocytes buckle or sickle. The sickle cells, because of their long thin shape, get stuck. This slows up the flow of blood somewhat like an auto accident slows up the flow of traffic. Then the sickle cells—stuck, stranded, and fragile—begin to rupture.

Table 47

Results of Laboratory Examinations in Sickle Cell Anemia

Laboratory Examinations	Results	Values in this Disease	Values in Health
White cell count	Increased	10,000 to 30,000 per cu. mm.	5,000 to 10,000 per cu. mm.
Red ceil count	Decreased	1 to 4 million per cu. mm.	4 to 6 million per cu. mm.
Hemoglobin determination	Decreased	3 to 12 grams per 100 cc.	12 to 18 grams per 100 cc.
Differential white cell count	Myelocytes	1% to 5%	0%
	Metamyelocytes	5% to 10%	0%
Stained red cell examination	Sickle cells	present	absent
	Anisocytosis	present	absent
	Poikilocytosis	present	absent
	Polychromatophilia	present	absent
	Target cells	present	absent
	Basophilic stippling	present	absent
	Nucleated red cells	2 to 30 per 100 white cells	0 per 100 white cells
Hematocrit reading	Decreased	10% to 30%	37% to 54%
Reticulocyte count	Increased	10% to 40%	1% to 2%
Sickle cell exam	Positive	Positive	
Red cell osmotic fragility test	Decreased	hemol. begins .38% hemol. ends .30%	hemol. begins .44% hemol. ends .34%
Abnormal hemoglobin exam (Hemoglobin electrophoresis)	Positive	Hb-S and Hb-F	Hb-A
Urine analysis	Albumin	positive	negative
	Casts	present	absent
Urine urobilinogen	Increased	2 to 4 Ehrlich units in 24 hrs.	1 to 2 Ehrlich units in 24 hrs.
Sedimentation rate	Decreased	varies with method	varies with method
Serum bilirubin	Increased	1.0 to 3.0 mg. per 100 ml.	0.2 to 0.8 mg. per 100 ml.
Platelet count	Increased	400,000 to 500,000 per cu. mm.	150,000 to 400,000 per cu. mm.
Erythrocyte survival time	Decreased	1 to 19 days half-life (Cr^{51} method)	28 to 38 days half-life (Cr^{51} method)
Red cell mechanical fragility test	Increased	5% to 25% hemolysis	2% to 5% hemolysis
Bone marrow examination	Increase in nucleated red cells	40% to 70%	8% to 30%

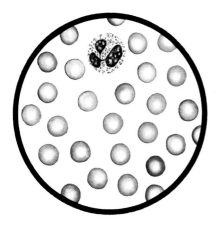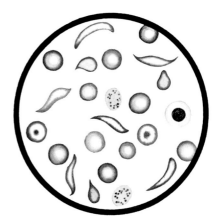

Blood Smear in Health	**Blood Smear in Sickle Cell Anemia**
<u>Note:</u>	<u>Note:</u>
1. The normal size of the red cells.	1. The 6 sickle cells.
2. The normal shape of the red cells.	2. Anisocytosis (variation in size of red cells).
	3. Poikilocytosis (variation in shape of red cells).
	4. Polychromatophilia (gray color of some red cells).
	5. Target cells (red cells with a dot in the center).
	6. Basophilic stippling (coarse granulation in some red cells).
	7. The nucleated red cell at 3 o'clock.

FIG. 179.—Blood smear in health compared with blood smear in sickle cell anemia. (Stain: Wright's; Magnification: 1000×)

Miscellaneous Information for Sickle Cell Anemia

The miscellaneous information will first touch lightly on abnormal hemoglobins and then summarize the classifications for sickle cell anemia. Normal adult hemoglobin is called hemoglobin A. Normal fetal hemoglobin is called hemoglobin F. The latter hemoglobin, hemoglobin F, is usually present in only small quantities after the first year of life.

The suffix -*pathy* means disease; thus, a hemoglobinopathy is a hemoglobin disease.

Sickle cell anemia, caused by an abnormal hemoglobin molecule, is the most common hemoglobinopathy.

In sickle cell anemia, the erythrocytes contain 75% or more of hemoglobin S. In sickle cell trait, the erythrocytes contain only 25% to 45% of hemoglobin S. Thus, the amount of hemoglobin S which is present seems to be a factor in the severity of the condition.

Other abnormal hemoglobin molecules, such as hemoglobin C and hemoglobin D, cause other hemoglobin diseases. Among these diseases are hemoglobin C disease, hemoglobin D disease, sickle cell— hemoglobin C disease, and sickle cell— hemoglobin D disease.

These diseases are rare and a detailed discussion is unnecessary for the average medical technologist. However, some relevant information regarding these hemoglobin diseases or hemoglobinopathies is given in Table 48.

Table 48.—Some Hemoglobin Diseases (Hemoglobinopathies)

Disease or Trait	Genes Responsible	Hemoglobins Detected	Sickling Activity	Severity of Anemia
Sickle cell anemia	SS	S + F	present	+ + +
Sickle cell trait	AS	A + S	present	±
Hb C disease	CC	C + (F)	absent	±
Hb D disease	DD	D + (F)	absent	—
Sickle cell—Hb C disease	SC	S + C + (F)	present	— to + + +
Sickle cell—Hb D disease	SD	S + D	present	+ + +

Since sickle cell anemia is associated with the hemolysis of red cells, it is classified as a hemolytic anemia. Because the defect is in the red cells, it is further classified as an intracorpuscular hemolytic anemia. Since sickle cell anemia is inherited and not acquired, it is also classified as an inherited hemolytic anemia.

The mean corpuscular volume is within the normal range of 80 to 90 cubic microns; thus, the anemia is normocytic. The mean corpuscular hemoglobin concentration is within the normal range of 33% to 38%;

thus, the anemia is normochromic. Consequently, sickle cell anemia is morphologically classified as a normocytic normochromic anemia.

Because sickle cell anemia is caused by an abnormal hemoglobin molecule, it is also classified as a hemoglobinopathy.

THALASSEMIA MAJOR

The word, thalassemia, comes from two Greek words. The *thalass* portion means sea and the *emia* portion means blood. Thus, thalassemia means sea blood.

The word came into being because the disease, sea blood or thalassemia, was first discovered in persons living near the Mediterranean sea.

The disease, thalassemia major, is often referred to by the following synonyms: Cooley's anemia, Mediterranean anemia, homozygous thalassemia, target cell anemia, hereditary leptocytosis, and erythroblastic anemia.

The discussion of thalassemia major will cover basic clinical information, factors affecting laboratory examinations, results of laboratory examinations, and miscellaneous information.

Basic Clinical Information

Thalassemia is an inherited disease.

If a child inherits the thalassemia gene from both parents, he is said to be homozygous. He then has the severe form of the disease. This is known as *thalassemia major.*

If a child inherits the thalassemia gene from one parent and a normal gene from the other parent, he is said to be heterozygous. He then has the mild form of the disease. This is known as *thalassemia minor.*

Thalassemia major will now be discussed; thalassemia minor will be considered under miscellaneous information.

In thalassemia major, an abnormality occurs in the synthesis of hemoglobin within the red cells. Even after the first year of life, the red cells continue to produce fetal hemoglobin in place of adult hemoglobin. The end result is the manufacture of poorly constructed erythrocytes having blotches of hemoglobin randomly distributed throughout the cell. This defect in cell structure is accompanied by a defect in the utilization of iron.

Thalassemia major may affect either sex and it occurs most frequently in the children of Italians, Greeks, Syrians, and Armenians.

The typical patient is a child who complains about being weak, tired, and stomach-sick; he may also complain about difficulty in breathing and a pounding heart.

The doctor observes that the child is of Italian, Greek, Syrian, or Armenian extraction.

The doctor also observes that the child has prominent facial bones, slanting eyes, and yellow skin.

The above combination of facial features has been described as a "Mongolian" face.

The doctor further observes that the child's head appears too large for his body and that his liver and spleen are enlarged.

If the patient does have thalassemia major, very little can be done in the way of treatment.

The majority of patients die in childhood.

The diagnosis will be made from the results of the physical examination and laboratory examinations.

The routine laboratory examinations usually include a white cell count, red cell count, hemoglobin determination, differential white cell count, stained red cell examination, hematocrit reading, reticulocyte count, red cell osmotic fragility test, icteric index, serum bilirubin, fetal hemoglobin determination, and abnormal hemoglobin examination.

Additional laboratory examinations may include a mean corpuscular volume, mean corpuscular hemoglobin, mean corpuscular hemoglobin concentration, red cell mechanical fragility test, erythrocyte survival time, plasma hemoglobin determination, urine urobilinogen, fecal urobilinogen, bone marrow examination, siderocyte count, and serum iron.

Now let us consider the manner in which this disease affects the laboratory examinations.

Factors Affecting Laboratory Examinations

In thalassemia major, we find an inherited fault in the manufacture of erythrocytes. Thus, we see the bone marrow producing (1) a decreased number of erythrocytes and (2) malformed erythrocytes.

The decreased number of erythrocytes causes the following tests to drop below normal: red cell count, hemoglobin determination, and hematocrit reading.

The malformed erythrocytes which are produced contain blotches of hemoglobin in various parts of the cell and assume many varied shapes.

Thus, the stained red cell examination shows target cells, ovalocytes, hypochromia, anisocytosis, poikilocytosis, polychromatophilia, basophilic stippling, Cabot rings, and Howell-Jolly bodies. It also shows nucleated red cells.

A blood smear in thalassemia major is illustrated in Plate 16, page 614.

The target cells are a common occurrence in this disease; these cells are also referred to as Mexican hat cells and leptocytes (thin cells).

Because the volume occupied by the average red cell is decreased, the mean corpuscular volume is below normal.

Since the weight of hemoglobin in the average red cell is decreased, the mean corpuscular hemoglobin is below normal.

Because the concentration of hemoglobin in the average red cell is decreased, the mean corpuscular hemoglobin concentration is below normal.

The malformed erythrocytes are subject to mechanical fracture and thus the red cell mechanical fragility test shows increased values.

The life span of the malformed erythrocytes is decreased and the erythrocyte survival time is therefore below normal.

The debris from the early death of the red cells causes a rise in the icteric index, serum bilirubin, plasma hemoglobin, urine urobilinogen, and fecal urobilinogen.

The bone marrow endeavors to compensate for the loss of red cells and becomes overactive or hyperplastic. Thus, the bone marrow examination shows an increase in nucleated red cells.

The overactive bone marrow causes the reticulocyte count to rise and, as previously indicated, nucleated red cells to appear in the blood smear.

As a by-product of this overactivity in the bone marrow, the white cell count goes up and the differential white cell count reveals immature white cells.

The target cells in this disease are longer and thinner than normal erythrocytes (see Fig. 180).

Because of their shape, water entering the target cells causes them to rupture at a slower rate than normal erythrocytes. Thus, decreased values are found in the red cell osmotic fragility test.

The fetal hemoglobin determination reveals that 40%–90% of the hemoglobin is fetal hemoglobin.

The abnormal hemoglobin examination reveals large quantities of hemoglobin F and small quantities of hemoglobin A_2.

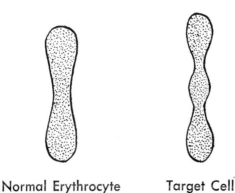

Normal Erythrocyte   Target Cell

FIG. 180.—Normal erythrocyte and target cell. (The cells are standing on end, like a coin; and viewed from the side, like looking at the edge of the coin.)

Because of the faulty utilization of iron in the synthesis of hemoglobin, some erythrocytes contain free iron, and the siderocyte count is increased.

Due to the increased breakdown of red cells and the decreased usage of iron, the iron content of the blood rises. Consequently, the test for serum iron shows increased values.

The results of the laboratory examinations in thalassemia major will be summarized in Table 50 and the cells of the blood smear will be illustrated in the accompanying Plate 16 (page 614).

Miscellaneous Information

The miscellaneous information will first consider the classifications of thalassemia major and then discuss thalassemia minor.

In thalassemia major, the mean corpuscular volume is below normal and thus the anemia is microcytic. The mean corpuscular hemoglobin concentration is below normal and thus the anemia is hypochromic. Consequently, thalassemia major is morphologically classified as a microcytic hypochromic anemia.

Because the red cells are subject to hemolysis, the anemia is classified as a hemolytic anemia.

Since the factor for the hemolysis is inside the red cell and not outside the red cell, the anemia is further classified as an intracorpuscular hemolytic anemia.

As the disease is inherited and not acquired, it is also classified as a congenital hemolytic anemia.

Since thalassemia major is caused by an inherited defect in the manufacture of hemoglobin, it is classified as a hemoglobin disease or hemoglobinopathy.

This anemia is also referred to as the microcytic hypochromic anemia that is not deficient in iron.

Thus, thalassemia major may be classified as a:

1. microcytic hypochromic anemia
2. hemolytic anemia
3. intracorpuscular hemolytic anemia
4. congenital hemolytic anemia
5. hemoglobinopathy
6. microcytic hypochromic anemia
   not deficient in iron

As previously stated, thalassemia major is considered the severe form of the disease and thalassemia minor is considered the mild form of the disease.

Now let us consider thalassemia minor.

Thalassemia minor is also referred to as Cooley's trait and heterozygous thalassemia.

In thalassemia minor, the life expectancy of the patient is *not* affected and symptoms of the disease are mild or even absent. Thus, the body adjusts or compensates for a slight degree of abnormality in the development and structure of the red cells. The bone marrow simply works harder and the red cell count is usually normal or may even be increased.

The results of other significant laboratory examinations in thalassemia minor are as follows.

The hemoglobin and hematocrit reading are decreased. The reticulocyte count may be slightly increased. The blood smear may show several target cells, basophilic stippling, and a few nucleated red cells. Abnormal hemoglobin examinations reveal that hemoglobin F is usually less than 10% and hemoglobin A_2 is usually increased. The red cell osmotic fragility test shows decreased values.

What laboratory examinations distinguish thalassemia minor from thalassemia major?

The more significant laboratory examinations which distinguish thalassemia minor from thalassemia major are summarized in Table 49.

Table 49

Laboratory Examinations Distinguishing Thalassemia Minor from Thalassemia Major

Examination	Thalassemia Minor	Thalassemia Major
Reticulocyte count	2% to 5%	5% to 30%
Abnormal hemoglobin examination	hemoglobin F 5% to 10%	hemoglobin F 40% to 90%
Erythrocyte survival time	normal	decreased
Serum iron	normal	increased

Thalassemia minor may team up with other traits and thus produce many combinations of intermediate diseases. For example, if a man with thalassemia minor marries a woman with sickle cell trait, their children might have various forms of intermediate diseases.

The student should carefully study the following Table 50 and the accompanying Plate 16.

Table 50—Results of Laboratory Examinations in Thalassemia Major

Laboratory Examinations	Results	Values in this Disease	Values in Health
White cell count	Increased	13,000 to 30,000 per cu. mm.	5,000 to 10,000 per cu. mm.
Red cell count	Decreased	1 to 4 million per cu. mm.	4 to 6 million per cu. mm.
Hemoglobin determination	Decreased	2 to 10 grams per 100 cc.	12 to 18 grams per 100 cc.
Differential white cell count	Myelocytes	1% to 3%	0%
	Metamyelocytes	4% to 8%	0%
Stained red cell examination	Target cells	present	absent
	Ovalocytes	present	absent
	Hypochromia	present	absent
	Anisocytosis	present	absent
	Poikilocytosis	present	absent
	Polychromatophilia	present	absent
	Basophilic stippling	present	absent
	Cabot rings	present	absent
	Howell-Jolly bodies	present	absent
	Nucleated red cells	10 to 50 per 100 white cells	0 per 100 white cells
Hematocrit reading	Decreased	8% to 30%	37% to 54%
Reticulocyte count	Increased	5% to 30%	1% to 2%
Red cell osmotic fragility test	Decreased	hemol. begins .40% hemol. ends .20%	hemol. begins .44% hemol. ends .34%
Icteric index	Increased	8 to 30 units	4 to 7 units
Serum bilirubin	Increased	1.5 to 3.0 mg. per 100 ml.	0.2 to 0.8 mg. per 100 ml.
Fetal hemoglobin determination	Hemoglobin F	40% to 90%	0% to 2%
Abnormal hemoglobin examination	Hemoglobin F	40% to 90%	0% to 2%
	Hemoglobin A_2	3% to 10%	0% to 3%
Mean corpuscular volume (MCV)	Decreased	60 to 80 cubic microns	80 to 90 cubic microns
Mean corpuscular hemoglobin (MCH)	Decreased	20 to 27 micromicrograms	27 to 32 micromicrograms
Mean corpuscular hemoglobin concentration (MCHC)	Decreased	26% to 30%	33% to 38%
Red cell mechanical fragility test	Increased	5% to 8% hemolysis	2% to 5% hemolysis
Erythrocyte survival time	Decreased	12 to 19 days (Ashby method)	55 to 65 days half-life (Ashby method)
Plasma hemoglobin determination	Increased	10 to 30 mg. per 100 ml.	2 to 3 mg. per 100 ml.
Urine urobilinogen	Increased	4 to 36 mg. in 24 hrs.	0 to 4 mg. in 24 hrs.
Fecal urobilinogen	Increased	280 to 2,000 mg. in 24 hrs.	40 to 280 mg. in 24 hrs.
Bone marrow examination	Increase in nucleated red cells	30% to 60%	8% to 30%
Siderocyte count	Increased	1% to 5%	0% to 1%
Serum iron	Increased	180 to 300 micrograms per 100 ml.	70 to 180 micrograms per 100 ml.

Plate 16—Blood Smears in Health and in Thalassemia Major
(Stain: Wright's; Mag.: 1000 ✕)

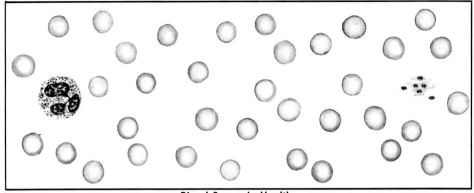

Blood Smear in Health

Note that the red cells are practically uniform in size, shape, and hemoglobin content. The white cell on the left side of the field is a neutrophilic segmented cell. The 6 small bluish-pink objects on the extreme right side of the field are platelets (thrombocytes).

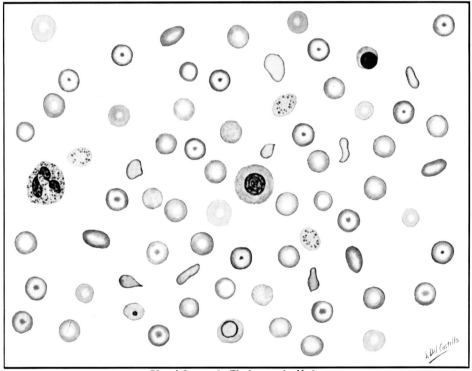

Blood Smear in Thalassemia Major

Note:

(1) target cells
   (red cells with bull's-eye in center)
(2) ovalocytes
   (oval shaped red cells)
(3) hypochromia
   (red cells with decreased color)
(4) anisocytosis
   (variation in size of red cells)
(5) poikilocytosis
   (variation in shape of red cells)

(6) polychromatophilia
   (gray appearance of some red cells)
(7) basophilic stippling
   (coarse granulation in some cells)
(8) Cabot ring
   (in red cell at 6 o'clock)
(9) Howell-Jolly body
   (red dot in red cell at 7 o'clock)
(10) nucleated red cells
   (in center and at 1 o'clock)

PAROXYSMAL NOCTURNAL HEMOGLOBINURIA

Paroxysmal nocturnal hemoglobinuria is also referred to by the letters P. N. H. and the Marchiafava-Micheli syndrome.

The word paroxysmal means a sudden intensification. Nocturnal means night. And hemoglobinuria means hemoglobin in the urine.

Thus, paroxysmal nocturnal hemoglobinuria is a sudden release of hemoglobin into the urine which occurs at night or during sleep.

The disease is thought to be caused by a defect in the structure of the red cells. This defect in structure apparently causes the red cells to rupture if they are subjected to an increase in the acidity of the blood.

Increased acidity of the blood, probably related to accumulated carbon dioxide, occurs during sleep. Thus, as the patient sleeps; increased acidity occurs, the red cells rupture, and hemoglobin is released into the urine.

Paroxysmal nocturnal hemoglobinuria is a rare disease. It is usually confined to adults, either male or female. And it usually runs a chronic prolonged course.

The results of the significant laboratory examinations are as follows.

The rupture of the patient's red cells is evidenced by the presence of hemosiderin, an iron compound, in the urine.

Thus, the following tests for urinary hemosiderin are positive: iron sulfide test and Prussian blue reaction.

The susceptibility of the patient's red cells to hemolysis is shown by the acid-serum test of Ham and the thrombin test of Crosby. Both of these tests are positive.

The following are below normal: red cell count, hemoglobin, hematocrit reading, white cell count, platelet count, and erythrocyte survival time.

The following tests are above normal: reticulocyte count, serum bilirubin, plasma hemoglobin, and urinary urobilinogen.

PAROXYSMAL COLD HEMOGLOBINURIA

Paroxysmal cold hemoglobinuria is also referred to by the initials P. C. H.

Paroxysmal cold hemoglobinuria is a condition which is precipitated by exposure to cold and characterized by the hemolysis of red cells in the blood and the passage of hemoglobin in the urine.

The rupture of the red cells is caused by an antibody in the patient's own plasma. The antibody apparently becomes fixed on the red cells at a temperature below normal body temperature (which may occur when the patient becomes chilled by sudden exposure to cold). Then, when the temperature rises to normal body temperature, the antibody causes the red cells to rupture.

The presence of these hemolytic antibodies or hemolysins may be revealed by several relatively simple laboratory tests. The usual tests, all of which show positive reactions, are as follows: Donath-Landsteiner test, Rosenbach's test, and Ehrlich's finger test.

This condition or disorder is rare and it is usually associated with syphilis. It is marked by sudden attacks and subsequent remissions. The attacks are characterized by weakness, headache, cramps, vomiting, and diarrhea. These are followed by chills and fever.

After an attack, the laboratory tests are affected as follows.

The various forms of hemoglobin, among them oxyhemoglobin and methemoglobin, discolor the urine.

Thus, the first voided urine may be red, brown, or black in color.

The breakdown of the red cells causes the red cell count, hemoglobin determination, and hematocrit reading to drop below normal and the serum bilirubin and plasma hemoglobin to rise above normal.

ACQUIRED AUTOIMMUNE HEMOLYTIC ANEMIA

The cause of this disease is unknown; thus, it is sometimes referred to as idiopathic acquired autoimmune hemolytic anemia.

In this anemia, the patient develops antibodies which hemolyze his own red cells. The results of the laboratory examinations are as follows.

The blood smear reveals anisocytosis, macrocytes and spherocytes, and sometimes a few nucleated red cells.

Because the spherocytes have a greater osmotic fragility than normal erythrocytes, increased values are frequently found in the red cell osmotic fragility test.

The direct Coombs' test on the patient's red cells is positive.

Additional laboratory tests showing values above or below normal are:

Below Normal	Above Normal	
red cell count	white cell count	urinary urobilinogen
hemoglobin determination	reticulocyte count	fecal urobilinogen
hematocrit reading	serum bilirubin	mechanical fragility test
erythrocyte survival time	plasma hemoglobin	

The mean corpuscular volume and mean corpuscular hemoglobin are normal. This anemia is considered a normocytic normochromic anemia.

ERYTHROBLASTOSIS FETALIS

The word, erythroblast, comes from two Greek words. The *erythro* portion means red; the *blast* portion means young cell. Thus, erythroblast means a young red cell.

The suffix, -*osis*, means an increase in. It follows that erythroblastosis means an increase in young red cells.

The name, erythroblastosis fetalis, therefore means an increase in the young red cells of the fetus.

Erythroblastosis fetalis is often referred to by the following terms: hemolytic disease of the newborn, icterus gravis neonatorum, erythroblastosis neonatorum, hydrops fetalis, and congenital anemia of the newborn.

The discussion of erythroblastosis fetalis will cover basic clinical information, factors affecting laboratory examinations, and results of laboratory examinations.

Basic Clinical Information

Erythroblastosis fetalis is a hemolytic anemia of the newborn caused by a reaction between fetal blood and maternal blood and characterized by a blood smear showing an increased number of nucleated red cells.

Erythroblastosis fetalis is caused by an antigen which is in or on the red cells of the fetus.

The red cells of the fetus, carrying the antigen, seep into the circulation of the mother. Here the antigens cause the production of antibodies. These antibodies accumulate in the circulation of the mother.

Then the antibodies leave the circulation of the mother, enter the fetus, and hemolyze his red cells.

The antigen may be any one of the following blood factors: Rh_0, A, B, C, E, AB, d, c, e, K, Lewis, Duffy, Kell, or Lutheran.

The blood factors Rh_0, A, and B are the most frequent offenders. These three blood factors account for about 96% of all the cases of erythroblastosis fetalis.

When blood factor Rh_0 is involved, the anemia is usually severe. But when blood factor A or blood factor B are involved, the anemia is usually mild.

Since blood factor Rh_0 causes the more severe anemia, we will consider this factor as the causative agent in our immediate discussions. We will briefly discuss blood factor A and blood factor B as the causative agents under the discussion of laboratory examinations.

The blood factor Rh_0 is also referred to as D or the Rh factor.

If your red cells have the Rh factor, you are Rh positive. If your red cells do not have the Rh factor, you are Rh negative.

About 85% of the population is Rh positive; the remaining 15% is Rh negative.

If a woman is Rh positive, she can usually rule out the possibility of having a child born with a severe case of erythroblastosis fetalis.

If a woman happens to be Rh negative, there is a slight possibility she may have an erythroblastotic baby.

It has been estimated, however, that only about 6% of all Rh negative women ever become affected by this condition. In addition, the condition usually does not develop until the third pregnancy. If it should develop, the woman herself is rarely, if ever, affected and the infant recovers in the vast majority of cases.

The background or medical history of the pregnant women is extremely significant.

For example, has she had any past pregnancies which produced Rh antibodies in her blood? Has she had any blood transfusions which produced Rh antibodies in her blood?

The presence of these Rh antibodies in her blood often foreshadows the possibility of an erythroblastotic baby.

If the physician suspects the possibility of an erythroblastotic baby, he orders a series of tests on the expectant mother and also on her husband. These tests usually include an Rh test on the husband and an Rh test and Rh titer on the expectant mother. Such tests aid in indicating the likelihood of an erythroblastotic baby.

If a baby is born with erythroblastosis fetalis, he usually recovers, with no serious aftereffects, in about 90% of the cases.

The damage to an erythroblastotic baby, caused by the breakdown of red cells, can usually be repaired; and the physician, nurse, and technologist, working smoothly as a team, can often save the life of this newborn infant.

The treatment is aimed at (1) removing the red cells so that they will not rupture inside the baby, (2) removing the antibodies in the plasma so they can not destroy additional red cells, and (3) removing the bilirubin produced by the ruptured red cells so it will not cause brain damage.

The above three objectives are accomplished by an exchange transfusion, that is, simultaneously removing the infant's blood and replacing it with compatible blood.

A new vaccine to combat erythroblastosis fetalis has recently been developed. It is called RhoGAM. When RhoGAM is injected into an Rh negative woman, it prevents the production of Rh antibodies.

This giant step forward in medical research appears to be stamping out the havoc caused by erythroblastosis fetalis.

Now let us consider the manner in which this disease affects the laboratory examinations.

Factors Affecting Laboratory Examinations

In this disease, the red cells of the fetus or newborn infant, attacked and besieged by antibodies, rupture; and their dying effects and remains cause a dreaded rise in the bilirubin of the blood. This pigment, bilirubin, in sufficiently high quantities, could cause brain damage or even death to the fetus or newborn infant.

The technologist may be present at birth and ordered to make the following tests on the newborn infant: white cell count, red cell count, hemoglobin determination, differential white cell count, stained red cell examination, reticulocyte count, serum bilirubin, urine bilirubin, Rh test, and direct Coombs' test.

In addition to the above tests on the infant, an indirect Coombs' test may be ordered on the mother.

The rupture of the red cells may start before birth, at birth, or after birth. Because of this, the results of the laboratory examinations vary considerably. A few examples follow.

The serum bilirubin may be normal at birth but rise rapidly in 4, 8, 12, or 24 hours.

The reticulocyte count may be normal at birth but rise rapidly the next day.

The blood smear may be normal at birth but reveal a shower of nucleated red cells a day or two later.

For the above reasons, laboratory tests may be repeated frequently during the first few days of life.

The test for bilirubin, in particular, is repeated frequently, for this test acts as a barometer of red cell destruction.

When the disease has gained a foothold, the laboratory tests are affected as follows.

Since the increased breakdown of red cells causes an increase in the bilirubin of the blood, the test for serum bilirubin shows increased values.

The increased breakdown of red cells causes the red cell count and hemoglobin determination to drop below normal.

The bone marrow, endeavoring to compensate for the hemolysis of red cells, becomes overactive and floods the circulation with immature red cells. The reticulocyte count therefore rises and a shower of nucleated red cells is seen in the blood smear.

A blood smear illustrating the shower of nucleated red cells in erythroblastosis fetalis will be shown in Plate 17, page 620.

Thus, the stained red cell examination shows anisocytosis, polychromatophilia, macrocytosis, and nucleated red cells.

The overactivity of the bone marrow also causes the white cell count to rise and the differential white cell count to show immature white cells.

As previously indicated, erythroblastosis fetalis is usually caused by the blood factors Rh_O, A, and B. Roughly speaking, about 50% of the cases of erythroblastosis are caused by Rh_O. The other 50% of the cases are caused by A and B.

If the disease is caused by Rh_O, the anemia is usually severe; if the disease is caused by A or B, the anemia is usually mild.

Thus, the abnormalities in the above discussed laboratory tests—red cell count, hemoglobin, etc.—are usually more pronounced in Rh_O incompatibility and usually less pronounced in A or B incompatibility.

(discussion continued on page 621)

Table 51

Results of Laboratory Examinations in
Erythroblastosis Fetalis Due to the Rh Factor

Laboratory Examinations	Results	Values in this Disease	Values in Health for Newborn Infant
White cell count	Increased	15,000 to 50,000 per cu. mm.	10,000 to 25,000 per cu. mm.
Red cell count	Decreased	1.0 to 5.0 million per cu. mm.	5.0 to 6.5 million per cu. mm.
Hemoglobin determination	Decreased	3 to 14 grams per 100 cc.	14 to 20 grams per 100 cc.
Differential white cell count	Myeloblasts	0% to 1%	0%
	Progranulocytes	0% to 3%	0%
	Neutrophilic myelocytes	3% to 13%	0% to 3%
	Neutrophilic metamyelocytes	6% to 12%	3% to 8%
Stained red cell examination	Anisocytosis	present	present
	Polychromatophilia	present	present
	Macrocytosis	present	present
	Nucleated red cells	10 to 500 per 100 white cells	0 to 5 per 100 white cells
Reticulocyte count	Increased	10% to 50%	2% to 6%
Serum bilirubin	Increased	3 to 35 mg. per 100 ml.	1 to 3 mg. per 100 ml.
Rh test	positive	positive	positive or negative
Direct Coombs' test	positive	positive	negative
Indirect Coombs' test (on mother)	positive	positive	
Rh test (on mother)	negative	negative	

PLATE 17

Blood Smear in Erythroblastosis Fetalis
(Stain: Wright's; Magnification: 950×)

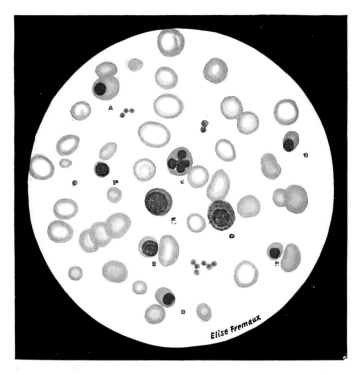

All the labelled cells (*A*, *B*, etc.) are nucleated red cells except cell *E* which is a lymphocyte. (Wintrobe, Tice, *Practice of Medicine*, courtesy of W. F. Prior Company.)

Now we must discuss additional tests, that is, those tests which point to Rh_0 as the offender and those tests which indicate A or B as the offender.

If the disease was caused by Rh_0, the following additional tests have the following results.

An Rh test on the baby is positive. An Rh test on the mother is negative. This sets up the possibility that a reaction could have occurred between the Rh positive fetus and the Rh negative mother.

A direct Coombs' test on the baby is positive, thus indicating that the infant's red cells were exposed to antibodies from the mother.

An indirect Coombs' test on the mother is positive, thus indicating that the blood of the mother contains antibodies.

If the disease was caused by A or B, the condition is usually referred to as ABO incompatibility. In these cases, the mechanism is similar to the mechanism of the Rh factor. It is an antigen-antibody reaction. The antigen, however, is not the Rh factor of the fetus but the group A or group B blood of the fetus.

If the disease was caused by A or B, the following additional tests have the following results.

Blood groupings reveal that the mother's blood is usually group O whereas the infant's blood is usually group A or group B.

A blood smear of the infant's blood shows spherocytes.

Since the spherocytes have a greater osmotic fragility than normal erythrocytes, increased values are found in the red cell osmotic fragility test.

The results of laboratory examinations in erythroblastosis fetalis due to the Rh factor are summarized in Table 51, page 620.

In studying the table, the student should bear in mind that the normal values for a newborn infant may differ greatly from the normal values for an adult.

For example, a white cell count of 20,000 per cu. mm. may be normal for a newborn infant but, of course, above normal for an adult.

When he performs the white cell count, the student should be alert to the following technical abnormality.

The nucleated red cells are not hemolyzed by the WBC diluting fluid. Under the low power objective of the microscope, the nucleated red cells appear as white cells. Consequently, the nucleated red cells are unknowingly included in the white cell count.

This inclusion of the nucleated red cells in the white cell count makes the white cell count erroneously high. A correction should therefore be made. The method of making the correction has been described in the procedure for the white cell count (page 138).

When he studies the blood smear, the student should also bear in mind that the blood smear of a *healthy* newborn infant usually shows a few nucleated red cells and a few immature white cells.

A final word about the classification of erythroblastosis fetalis. Since erythroblastosis fetalis is characterized by the hemolysis of red cells, it is classified as a hemolytic anemia. Because the red cells are usually larger than normal red cells, the anemia is usually macrocytic.

POSTHEMORRHAGIC ANEMIAS

This section considers the anemias resulting from a loss of red cells. The anemias which will be discussed are acute posthemorrhagic anemia and chronic posthemorrhagic anemia.

ACUTE POSTHEMORRHAGIC ANEMIA

Acute posthemorrhagic anemia is caused by the sudden loss of a large quantity of blood. For example, a man having 5 quarts of blood might lose 1 quart from a bleeding ulcer or 2 quarts from an injury in an automobile accident.

In acute posthemorrhagic anemia, the laboratory examinations are quite variable, changing with such factors as (1) the amount of blood lost, (2) the time interval between the loss of blood and the withdrawal of blood for the test, and (3) the recuperating mechanism of the body. A brief discussion follows.

The red cell count, hemoglobin determination, and hematocrit reading may often furnish misleading information.

If the red cell count, hemoglobin determination, and hematocrit reading are made *immediately* after the loss of blood, they are usually *above* normal. This is due to a sudden constriction of the blood vessels and the subsequent concentration of red cells.

If the red cell count, hemoglobin determination, and hematocrit reading are made *several hours* after the loss of blood, they are usually *below* normal. This is due to fluids leaving the tissues and "diluting" the blood.

Thus, the results of the red cell count, hemoglobin determination, and hematocrit reading should be interpreted with caution.

The loss of blood soon stimulates the bone marrow to produce more blood cells and the laboratory tests are affected as follows.

The white cell count begins to rise several hours after the loss of blood. It may range between 10,000 and 35,000 per cubic millimeter for about 2 days. But it returns to a normal of 5,000 to 10,000 per cubic millimeter about 4 days after the loss of blood.

The differential white cell count may show immature white cells, the condition known as a "shift to the left."

The platelet count also begins to rise several hours after the loss of blood. It may rise from a normal range of 150,000–400,000 per cubic millimeter to as high as 1,000,000 per cubic millimeter.

The increase in the number of platelets causes a decrease in the coagulation time.

The reticulocyte count begins to rise about 2 days after the loss of blood and reaches the peak of its rise about 6 days after the loss of blood. It usually rises from a normal range of 1%–2% to 5%–15%.

The stained red cell examination may show some abnormalities about 1 week after the loss of blood. The abnormalities may include macrocytosis, polychromatophilia, and a few nucleated red cells. These abnormalities disappear about 2 weeks after the loss of blood.

What happens to the red cell count and hemoglobin as the patient recuperates?

As the bone marrow slowly progresses in the production of red cells, the red cell count and hemoglobin gradually return to normal.

In a severe case of acute posthemorrhagic anemia, the red cell count may take 5 weeks to return to normal and the hemoglobin determination may take 7 weeks to return to normal.

Since iron is used in the manufacture of red cells, the iron in the plasma may take a temporary drop below normal.

In acute posthemorrhagic anemia, the volume occupied by the average red cell is within the normal limits. Thus, the mean corpuscular volume is normal. Since the mean corpuscular volume is normal, the anemia is considered a normocytic anemia.

CHRONIC POSTHEMORRHAGIC ANEMIA

Chronic posthemorrhagic anemia is caused by mild but prolonged periods of bleeding. This may occur in such conditions as menstrual disturbances, bleeding peptic ulcers, and bleeding hemorrhoids.

The loss of blood causes a decrease in the red cell count, hemoglobin determination, and hematocrit reading.

The blood smear reveals red cells which are slightly smaller than normal and slightly deficient in hemoglobin.

Since the volume occupied by the average red cell is below normal, the mean corpuscular volume is below normal.

Because the red cells are deficient in hemoglobin, the following are below normal: color index, mean corpuscular hemoglobin, and mean corpuscular hemoglobin concentration.

Since the red cells are small and lack the normal quota of hemoglobin, chronic posthemorrhagic anemia is a microcytic hypochromic anemia.

In the absence of treatment, chronic posthemorrhagic anemia may develop into an iron deficiency anemia. This has already been discussed on page 580.

Chapter 35

The Leukemias

LEUKEMIA is pronounced lu-ke′me-ah. The word comes from the Greek words for *white* and *blood*. Consequently, leukemia means white blood. The leukemias will be discussed under the following headings:

> Introduction to the Leukemias
> Granulocytic Leukemia
> Lymphocytic Leukemia
> Monocytic Leukemia and Plasmacytic Leukemia
> Aleukemic Leukemia and Leukemoid Reactions
> A Note to the Student

The student review questions for the leukemias are numbered 431–449 and begin on page 770 of the Appendix.

INTRODUCTION TO THE LEUKEMIAS

Leukemia is a disease of the blood forming tissues. It has two outstanding characteristics. One, the white cell count often rises 10 to 20 times above the normal values. Two, the differential white cell count shows many immature white cells.

For example, instead of the white cell count being a normal count of 5,000 to 10,000 per cubic millimeter, it may be 200,000 per cubic millimeter. And instead of the differential white cell count showing 0% neutrophilic myelocytes, it may show 35% neutrophilic myelocytes.

Although the cause of leukemia is unknown, many patients with the disease have had a lengthy exposure to x-rays, benzene, or aniline dyes.

Leukemia is fatal: death usually comes within a few months or a few years.

The disease strikes 1 in every 10,000 persons each year and the rate is rising.

No successful treatment is available but the life of the patient may be prolonged by chemotherapy, x-ray treatments, and blood transfusions.

Leukemia is classified according to (1) the white cell series which predominates and (2) the intensity and duration of the disease.

The predominating white cell series may be the granulocytic, lymphocytic, monocytic, or plasmacytic. Thus, we may have granulocytic leukemia, lymphocytic leukemia, monocytic leukemia, and plasmacytic leukemia.

Roughly speaking, if 100 patients have leukemia, 65% have granulocytic leukemia, 30% have lymphocytic leukemia, 4% have monocytic leukemia, and 1% have plasmacytic leukemia.

The intensity and duration of a disease give rise to the terms acute and chronic. For example, if a disease is severe and short, it is acute; if a disease is mild and prolonged, it is chronic.

The leukemias may be acute or chronic. Thus, we may have acute granulocytic leukemia and chronic granulocytic leukemia. It follows that we may have acute lymphocytic leukemia and chronic lymphocytic leukemia, acute monocytic leukemia and chronic monocytic leukemia, and acute plasmacytic leukemia and chronic plasmacytic leukemia.

If a patient has any of the acute leukemias, death usually comes within 4 months; if a patient has any of the chronic leukemias, death usually comes within 4 years.

Roughly speaking, if 100 patients have leukemia, 50% have an acute form of leukemia and 50% have a chronic form of leukemia.

The classification of the leukemias which has just been discussed is summarized in Table 52.

Table 52

Classification of the Leukemias

Granulocytic Leukemia
acute granulocytic leukemia
chronic granulocytic leukemia

Lymphocytic Leukemia
acute lymphocytic leukemia
chronic lymphocytic leukemia

Monocytic Leukemia
acute monocytic leukemia
chronic monocytic leukemia

Plasmacytic Leukemia
acute plasmacytic leukemia
chronic plasmacytic leukemia

Now let us discuss the four major leukemias: granulocytic, lymphocytic, monocytic, and plasmacytic. We will briefly consider several rare forms of leukemia under the section entitled Diseases and Anomalies Rarely Encountered.

GRANULOCYTIC LEUKEMIA

Granulocytic leukemia is divided into acute granulocytic leukemia and chronic granulocytic leukemia.

Acute granulocytic leukemia and chronic granulocytic leukemia have many similar aspects. But each disease will first be considered separately. Then the two diseases will be compared with respect to the results of laboratory examinations and color illustrations of blood smears.

ACUTE GRANULOCYTIC LEUKEMIA

Acute granulocytic leukemia is also referred to as acute myelogenous leukemia, acute myeloid leukemia, acute myelosis, and acute myeloblastic leukemia.

The discussion will cover basic clinical information, factors affecting laboratory examinations, and results of laboratory examinations.

Basic Clinical Information

Acute granulocytic leukemia may affect anyone: man, woman, or child.

The typical patient complains about being tired and weak and having pains in the bones and joints.

The doctor observes that the patient is pale, has a fetid odor, and a fever; he notices bleeding into the skin and finds tenderness in the bones and joints; sometimes he may also find an enlarged spleen, liver, and lymph nodes.

The diagnosis will be made from the results of the physical examination and laboratory examinations.

The routine laboratory examinations usually include a white cell count, red cell count, hemoglobin determination, color index, differential white cell count, stained red cell examination, and platelet count.

Additional laboratory examinations may include a bone marrow examination, alkaline phosphatase stain, and peroxidase stain.

Factors Affecting Laboratory Examinations

A cancer-like growth of the granulocytes in the bone marrow causes an outpouring of granulocytes into the blood stream.

The white cell count therefore rises from the normal range of 5,000–10,000 per cubic millimeter to values between 20,000 and 100,000 per cubic millimeter.

The white cell count, however, may be normal or drop below normal during the following: (1) remissions of the disease, (2) treatment with x-rays or chemicals, and (3) terminal stages of the disease.

The granulocytes pouring into the blood stream are seen in the blood smear.

The differential white cell count shows a shower of myeloblasts, a few progranulocytes, a few neutrophilic myelocytes, and a few neutrophilic metamyelocytes.

Some myeloblasts may show red rods called Auer bodies in their cytoplasm.

In performing the differential white cell count, it is sometimes difficult to identify blast cells, that is, the myeloblast of acute granulocytic leukemia and the lymphoblast of acute lymphocytic leukemia.

A means of identifying a questionable blast cell is a method which is known as "the company they keep method."

"The company they keep method" is somewhat similar to (1) seeing 100 Indians on a reservation, (2) being able to definitely identify 8 or 10 of the *adult* Indians as Pima Indians, and (3) therefore assuming that any *baby* Indians on the reservation are also Pima Indians.

Let us take an example with blood cells.

If a blood smear contains 3% to 9% neutrophilic segmented cells (adult cells), the chances are good that any questionable blast cell (baby cell) belongs to the same "tribe" or series.

The neutrophilic segmented cells (adult cells) belong to the granulocytic series. Hence, any questionable blast cell (baby cell) would probably belong to the granulocytic series.

The blast cell in the granulocytic series is called a myeloblast. Consequently, any questionable blast cell would probably be a myeloblast.

Since the white cells in acute granulocytic leukemia belong to the granulocytic series, many of the white cells contain granules. Hence, the peroxidase stain reveals that 5% to 25% of the white cells are peroxidase positive, that is, contain granules.

The cancer-like growth of the granulocytes in the bone marrow crowds out the areas which are normally reserved for the development of red cells and platelets. This decreases the production of red cells and platelets. Consequently, the red cell count and platelet count drop below normal.

The fall in the red cell count causes a drop in the hemoglobin values.

The fall in the platelet count, that is, the decrease in the number of platelets, causes an increase in the bleeding time and coagulation time; it also results in a positive capillary resistance test.

The stained red cell examination shows anisocytosis and a few nucleated red cells.

The bone marrow examination reveals an increase in myeloblasts.

In acute granulocytic leukemia, the granulocytes contain a decreased amount of alkaline phosphatase. Thus, decreased values are found in the alkaline phosphatase stain.

During treatment with x-rays or chemicals, the white cells are destroyed and this causes a rise in the uric acid of the blood and urine.

The results of the laboratory examinations will be summarized in Table 53 and the cells of the blood smear will be illustrated in the accompanying Plate 18 (page 630).

In diluting the blood for the white cell count, the student may wish to use the following technique.

Since the white cells are so numerous, it may be advisable to dilute the blood 1 in 100 rather than 1 in 20. This is accomplished by using a red cell pipet, drawing blood to the 1.0 mark and WBC diluting fluid to the 101 mark, and making the proper correction in the calculation. This method has been illustrated in the procedure for the white cell count on page 137.

CHRONIC GRANULOCYTIC LEUKEMIA

Chronic granulocytic leukemia is also referred to as chronic myelogenous leukemia, chronic myeloid leukemia, chronic myelosis, and splenomedullary leukemia.

The discussion will cover basic clinical information, factors affecting laboratory examinations, and results of laboratory examinations.

Basic Clinical Information

Although chronic granulocytic leukemia may affect anyone, it is most often found in the 20 to 50 year old patient.

The typical patient complains about being tired and weak and having a slight pain or feeling of discomfort on the left side just above the stomach. Thus, the symptoms are vague and meager.

The doctor observes that the patient has an enlarged spleen.

This single observation of the enlarged spleen may seem slight but it is significant, for the spleen is being flooded with white cells, and it increases in size as the disease increases in intensity.

The diagnosis will be made from the results of the physical examination and laboratory examinations.

The routine laboratory examinations usually include a white cell count, red cell count, hemoglobin determination, color index, differential white cell count, stained red cell examination, and platelet count.

Additional laboratory examinations may include a bone marrow examination and an alkaline phosphatase stain.

Factors Affecting Laboratory Examinations

In many respects, the factors affecting laboratory examinations are the same in both chronic granulocytic leukemia and acute granulocytic leukemia.

The cancer-like growth of the granulocytes in the bone marrow produces a great outpouring of granulocytes into the blood stream.

The white cell count therefore rises from the normal range of 5,000–10,000 per cubic millimeter to values between 100,000 and 800,000 per cubic millimeter. Thus, a marked leukocytosis is seen.

But the white cell count may also be normal or drop below normal during the following: (1) remissions of the disease, (2) treatment with x-rays or chemicals, and (3) terminal stages of the disease.

In chronic granulocytic leukemia, the differential white cell count shows a predominance of neutrophilic myelocytes.

The neutrophilic myelocytes usually rise from a normal value of 0% to values between 20% and 50%.

Sometimes the technologist may see the whole spectrum of the granulocytic series. Thus, you may find neutrophilic segmented cells, neutrophilic band cells, neutrophilic metamyelocytes, neutrophilic myelocytes, progranulocytes, and even a myeloblast.

The differential white cell count may also show an increase in basophils. These cells usually rise from a normal range of 0%–1% to 1%–12%.

The overgrowth of white cells in the bone marrow crowds out the areas which are normally reserved for the development of red cells. This decreases the production of red cells. The decrease in the production of red cells causes the red cell count and hemoglobin to drop below normal.

The stained red cell examination shows anisocytosis and a few nucleated red cells.

In the early stages of the disease, the platelet count may be increased; in the more severe or terminal stages of the disease, however, the platelet count may be normal or decreased.

Thus, the platelet count may range between 100,000 and 600,000 per cubic millimeter whereas the normal range is between 150,000 and 400,000 per cubic millimeter.

The stepped-up production of white cells taking place in the bone marrow is revealed by a bone marrow examination. This examination shows an increase in myeloblasts.

Since the granulocytes contain a decreased amount of alkaline phosphatase, decreased values are found in the alkaline phosphatase stain.

The results of the laboratory examinations are summarized in Table 53 and the cells of the blood smear are illustrated in the accompanying Plate 18 (page 630).

What single laboratory examination can usually make the distinction between acute granulocytic leukemia and chronic granulocytic leukemia?

The differential white cell count can usually make the distinction between acute granulocytic leukemia and chronic granulocytic leukemia.

In acute granulocytic leukemia, the differential white cell count shows a predominance of myeloblasts; in chronic granulocytic leukemia, the differential white cell count shows a predominance of neutrophilic myelocytes (Plate 18).

Table 53

**Results of Laboratory Examinations in
Acute and Chronic Granulocytic Leukemia**

Laboratory Examinations	Acute Granulocytic Leukemia	Chronic Granulocytic Leukemia	Values in Health
White cell count	20,000 to 100,000 per cu. mm.	100,000 to 800,000 per cu. mm.	5,000 to 10,000 per cu. mm.
Red cell count	1 to 3 million per cu. mm.	2 to 3 million per cu. mm.	4 to 6 million per cu. mm.
Hemoglobin determination	2 to 8 grams per 100 cc.	4 to 8 grams per 100 cc.	12 to 18 grams per 100 cc.
Color index	0.9 to 1.1	0.9 to 1.1	0.9 to 1.1
Differential white cell count			
Myeloblasts	20% to 90%	2% to 10%	0%
Progranulocytes	5% to 10%	5% to 15%	0%
Neut. Myelocytes	3% to 8%	20% to 50%	0%
Neut. Metamyelocytes	1% to 3%	15% to 25%	0%
Eosinophils	1% to 5%	3% to 7%	1% to 3%
Basophils	0% to 1%	1% to 12%	0% to 1%
Stained red cell examination			
Anisocytosis	present	present	absent
Nucleated red cells	2 to 8 per 100 white cells	4 to 12 per 100 white cells	
Platelet count	50,000 to 150,000 per cu. mm.	100,000 to 600,000 per cu. mm.	150,000 to 400,000 per cu. mm.
Bone marrow examination			
Myeloblasts	15% to 50%	5% to 15%	0% to 5%
Alkaline phosphatase stain	0 to 5	0 to 13	13 to 100
Peroxidase stain	5% to 25% of white cells are peroxidase positive		

Plate 18—Acute and Chronic Granulocytic Leukemia
(Stain: Wright's; Mag.: 1000 ✕)

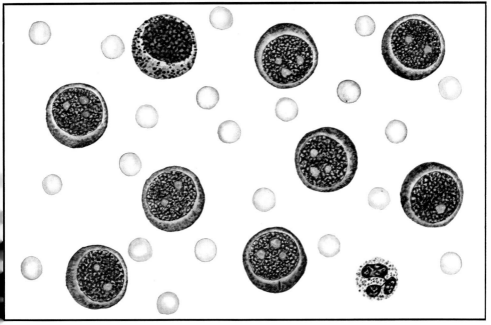

Acute Granulocytic Leukemia

All the white cells are myeloblasts except the neutrophilic segmented cell at 5 o'clock and the progranulocyte at 11 o'clock. Note the myeloblast at 6 o'clock; it has an Auer body (red rod) in the cytoplasm.

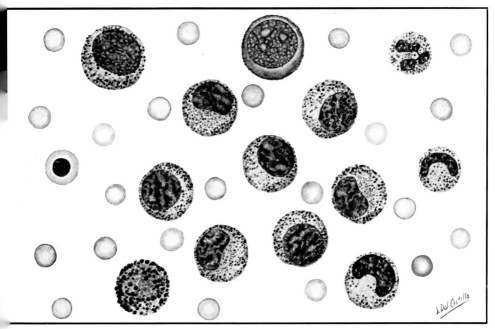

Chronic Granulocytic Leukemia

The 7 white cells in the central area are all neutrophilic myelocytes. The identity of the other cells is as follows: The cell at 1 o'clock is a neutrophilic segmented cell. At 3, a neutrophilic band cell. At 5, a neutrophilic metamyelocyte. At 7, a basophilic myelocyte. At 9, a nucleated red cell. At 11, a progranulocyte. And at 12, a myeloblast.

LYMPHOCYTIC LEUKEMIA

Lymphocytic leukemia is divided into acute lymphocytic leukemia and chronic lymphocytic leukemia.

Acute lymphocytic leukemia and chronic lymphocytic leukemia have many similar aspects. But each disease will first be considered separately. Then the two diseases will be compared with respect to the results of laboratory examinations and color illustrations of blood smears.

ACUTE LYMPHOCYTIC LEUKEMIA

Acute lymphocytic leukemia is also referred to as acute lymphatic leukemia, acute lymphoblastic leukemia, and acute lymphadenosis.

The discussion will cover basic clinical information, factors affecting laboratory examinations, and results of laboratory examinations.

Basic Clinical Information

Acute lymphocytic leukemia may affect anyone but it is most frequently encountered in a child.

The child usually complains about being very tired, having headaches, and having pains in the arms and legs.

The doctor observes that the child has bleeding into the skin, enlarged lymph glands, and an enlarged spleen.

The diagnosis will be made from the results of the physical examination and the laboratory examinations.

The routine laboratory examinations usually include a white cell count, red cell count, hemoglobin determination, differential white cell count, stained red cell examination, and platelet count.

Additional laboratory examinations may include a bone marrow examination and a peroxidase stain.

Factors Affecting Laboratory Examinations

In acute lymphocytic leukemia, a cancer-like growth of the lymphocytes in the lymph glands causes a great outpouring of immature lymphocytes into the blood stream.

The white cell count therefore rises from a normal range of 5,000–10,000 per cubic millimeter to values between 20,000 and 100,000 per cubic millimeter.

The white cell count, however, may be normal or drop below normal during the following: (1) remissions of the disease, (2) treatment with x-rays or chemicals, and (3) terminal stages of the disease.

42

The differential white cell count reveals that the lymphoblasts rise from a normal value of 0% to values between 15% and 75%.

The differential white cell count may also show many degenerating lymphocytes. These degenerating cells are called smudge cells and basket cells. Their presence indicates increased fragility or abnormal destruction of the cells.

A peroxidase stain usually shows that 95% to 100% of the white cells are peroxidase negative, that is, lack granules. Since the white cells lack granules, it indicates that the immature white cells are probably in the lymphocytic series rather than the granulocytic series.

The cancer-like growth of the lymphocytes produces hordes of lymphocytes which invade the organs of the body, including the bone marrow.

The lymphocytes take over the areas of the bone marrow which are normally used for the development of red cells and platelets. This decreases the production of red cells and platelets and results in a fall in the red cell count and platelet count.

The fall in the red cell count causes a drop in the hemoglobin values; the decrease in platelets causes an increase in the bleeding time.

The stained red cell examination may show anisocytosis and an occasional nucleated red cell.

A bone marrow examination reveals a greatly increased percentage of lymphoblasts.

The results of the laboratory examinations will be summarized in Table 54 and the cells of the blood smear will be illustrated in the accompanying Plate 19 (page 634).

CHRONIC LYMPHOCYTIC LEUKEMIA

Chronic lymphocytic leukemia is also referred to as chronic lymphatic leukemia and chronic lymphadenosis.

The discussion will cover basic clinical information, factors affecting laboratory examinations, and results of laboratory examinations.

Basic Clinical Information

Chronic lymphocytic leukemia may affect anyone but it is most frequently encountered in the male patient past the age of 50.

The typical patient complains about being tired and weak and having a swelling on the side of the neck.

The doctor observes that the lymph glands in the neck of the patient are enlarged and also that his spleen is enlarged.

The diagnosis will be made from the results of the physical examination and laboratory examinations.

The routine laboratory examinations usually include a white cell count, red cell count, hemoglobin determination, differential white cell count, stained red cell examination, and platelet count.

Additional laboratory examinations may include a bone marrow examination.

Factors Affecting Laboratory Examinations

The cancer-like growth of the lymphocytes in the lymph glands causes a great outpouring of lymphocytes into the blood stream.

The white cell count therefore rises from a normal range of 5,000–10,000 per cubic millimeter to values between 50,000 and 200,000 per cubic millimeter.

The white cell count, however, may be normal or drop below normal during the following: (1) remissions of the disease, (2) treatment with x-rays or chemicals, and (3) terminal stages of the disease.

The differential white cell count reveals that the lymphocytes rise from a normal range of 20%–35% to values between 75% and 95%.

At the beginning of the disease, the production of red cells and platelets may be normal.

When the disease gains a foothold, however, the lymphocytes invade the bone marrow. They crowd out the developing red cells and platelets. This decreases the production of red cells and platelets.

Consequently, the red cell count and platelet count fall below normal.

As the disease increases in intensity, the red cell count and platelet count gradually decline.

The stained red cell examination may show anisocytosis and a rare nucleated red cell.

A bone marrow examination reveals a greatly increased percentage of lymphocytes.

The results of the laboratory examinations are given in Table 54 and the cells of the blood smear are illustrated in the accompanying Plate 19 (page 634).

What single laboratory examination can usually make the distinction between acute lymphocytic leukemia and chronic lymphocytic leukemia?

The differential white cell count can usually make the distinction between acute lymphocytic leukemia and chronic lymphocytic leukemia.

In acute lymphocytic leukemia, the differential white cell count shows a predominance of lymphoblasts; in chronic lymphocytic leukemia, the differential white cell count shows a predominance of lymphocytes (Plate 19).

Table 54

Results of Laboratory Examinations in
Acute and Chronic Lymphocytic Leukemia

Laboratory Examinations	Acute Lympho- cytic Leukemia	Chronic Lympho- cytic Leukemia	Values in Health
White cell count	20,000 to 100,000 per cu. mm.	50,000 to 200,000 per cu. mm.	5,000 to 10,000 per cu. mm.
Red cell count	1 to 3 million per cu. mm.	3 to 5 million per cu. mm.	4 to 6 million per cu. mm.
Hemoglobin deter- mination	2 to 6 grams per 100 cc.	6 to 12 grams per 100 cc.	12 to 18 grams per 100 cc.
Differential white cell count			
Lymphoblasts	15% to 75%	0% to 3%	0%
Lymphocytes	10% to 25%	75% to 95%	20% to 35%
Platelet count	10,000 to 60,000 per cu. mm.	50,000 to 200,000 per cu. mm.	150,000 to 400,000 per cu. mm.
Bone marrow exam- ination			
Lymphoblasts	15% to 75%		0%
Lymphocytes		30% to 90%	5% to 15%
Peroxidase stain	95% to 100% of white cells are peroxidase neg- ative		

Plate 19—Acute and Chronic Lymphocytic Leukemia
(Stain: Wright's; Mag.: 1000 ✕)

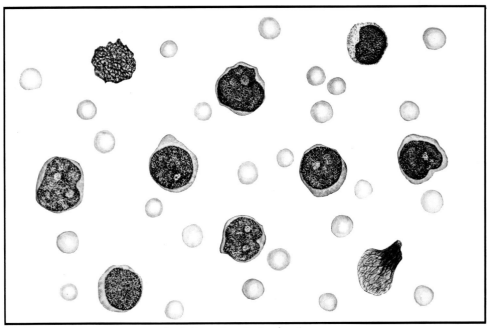

Acute Lymphocytic Leukemia

All the white cells are lymphoblasts except the lymphocyte at 1 o'clock, the basket cell at 5, the prolymphocyte at 7, and the smudge cell at 11.

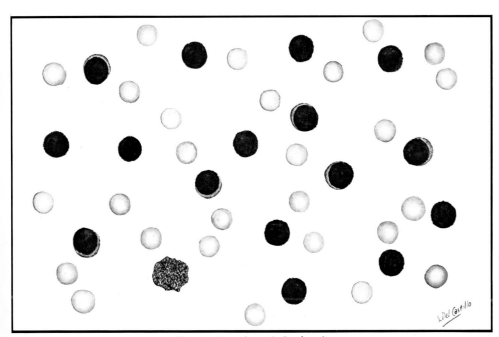

Chronic Lymphocytic Leukemia

All the white cells are lymphocytes except the smudge cell at 7 o'clock.

MONOCYTIC LEUKEMIA AND PLASMACYTIC LEUKEMIA

Monocytic leukemia and plasmacytic leukemia are rare, being found much less frequently than granulocytic and lymphocytic leukemia. A brief discussion of each disease is given below.

MONOCYTIC LEUKEMIA

Monocytic leukemia may be technically divided into acute monocytic leukemia and chronic monocytic leukemia. From the laboratory point of view, however, very little difference exists between the acute and chronic form of the disease. Consequently, the disease will be broadly discussed as simply monocytic leukemia.

The discussion of monocytic leukemia will cover basic clinical information, factors affecting laboratory examinations, and results of laboratory examinations.

Basic Clinical Information

Monocytic leukemia may affect anyone but it is most frequently found in the male patient past the age of 40.

The typical patient complains about being tired and weak and having occasional bleeding from the mouth.

The doctor observes that the gums of the patient are swollen and ulcerated; his lymph glands are enlarged; and his spleen and liver are slightly enlarged.

The diagnosis will be made from the results of the physical examination and laboratory examinations.

The routine laboratory examinations usually include a white cell count, red cell count, hemoglobin determination, differential white cell count, stained red cell examination, and platelet count.

Additional laboratory examinations may include a bone marrow examination.

Factors Affecting Laboratory Examinations

The origin of the monocytes is not clearly understood but they are found in the spleen, lymph nodes, and bone marrow.

Due to a cancer-like growth, the cells of the monocytic series flood the blood stream.

The white cell count rises from the normal range of 5,000–10,000 per cubic millimeter to values between 20,000 and 200,000 per cubic millimeter.

The differential white cell count reveals that the monocytes rise from the normal range of 2%–6% to values between 20% and 90%. In addition, several promonocytes and monoblasts may be seen.

The differential white cell count may also show many atypical forms of the monocytic series. Thus, many abnormal monocytes, promonocytes, and monoblasts may be seen.

The monocytes flooding the blood stream invade the bone marrow and hinder the development of red cells and platelets.

As a consequence, the red cell count and platelet count fall below normal.

The decrease in red cells causes a decrease in hemoglobin; the shortage of platelets causes an increase in the bleeding time.

A bone marrow examination reveals a great increase in monocytes.

In monocytic leukemia, the results of several laboratory examinations, especially the differential white cell count, may vary greatly from week to week.

And, in this connection, it should be stated that monocytic leukemia is often classified as either the Schilling type of monocytic leukemia or the Naegeli type of monocytic leukemia.

The Schilling type of monocytic leukemia is characterized by the presence of white cells which definitely belong to the monocytic series. Hence, the Schilling type of monocytic leukemia is referred to as true monocytic leukemia.

The Naegeli type of monocytic leukemia is characterized by the presence of (1) white cells which belong to the monocytic series and (2) white cells which appear to belong to the granulocytic series. Thus, the identity of some white cells is questionable.

The usual results of the laboratory examinations are given in Table 55, page 637, and the typical cells of the blood smear are illustrated in Plate 20.

PLASMACYTIC LEUKEMIA

Plasmacytic leukemia is also referred to as plasmocytic leukemia and plasma cell leukemia.

This disease is very rare and it has been stated that no hard and fast line exists between plasmacytic leukemia and multiple myeloma. In fact, many authorities consider plasmacytic leukemia as simply a phase of multiple myeloma.

The typical patient has an enlarged liver, spleen, and lymph nodes.

The significant laboratory findings are as follows.

The white cell count rises from a normal range of 5,000–10,000 per cubic millimeter to values between 20,000 and 60,000 per cubic millimeter.

PLATE 20

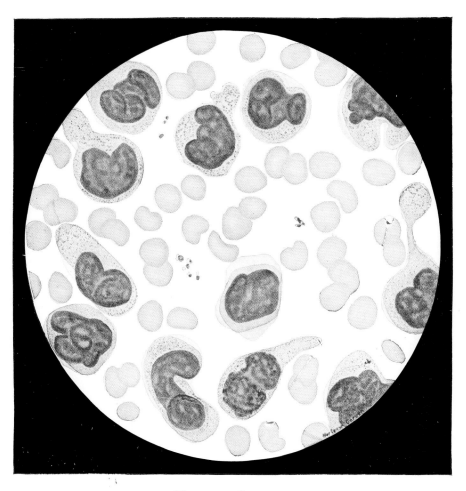

MONOCYTIC LEUKEMIA

The cell nearest the center, which lacks granules, is a promonocyte. All the other cells are monocytes. (Kracke, *Diseases of the Blood*, 2nd edition, Courtesy of J. B. Lippincott Company.)

The differential white cell count reveals that the plasmacytes rise from a normal value of 0% to values between 25% and 75%. The red cell count, hemoglobin, and platelet count drop below normal. A bone marrow examination reveals an increase in the percentage of plasmacytes.

The typical plasmacyte has a single small nucleus which is located near the edge of the cell and a deep blue cytoplasm. However, some plasmacytes may have two nuclei and some plasmacytes may have vacuoles in the cytoplasm. Typical plasmacytes have been illustrated in Plate 3, page 218, Plate 5, page 245, and Plate 15, page 526.

The results of the laboratory examinations in plasmacytic leukemia are summarized in Table 55.

Table 55

Results of Laboratory Examinations in Monocytic Leukemia and Plasmacytic Leukemia

Laboratory Examinations	Monocytic Leukemia	Plasmacytic Leukemia	Values in Health
White cell count	20,000 to 200,000 per cu. mm.	20,000 to 60,000 per cu. mm.	5,000 to 10,000 per cu. mm.
Red cell count	1 to 4 million per cu. mm.	2 to 4 million per cu. mm.	4 to 6 million per cu. mm.
Hemoglobin determination	2 to 12 grams per 100 cc.	4 to 12 grams per 100 cc.	12 to 18 grams per 100 cc.
Differential white cell count			
Monoblasts	2% to 10%		0%
Promonocytes	5% to 15%		0%
Monocytes	20% to 90%		2% to 6%
Plasmablasts		0% to 3%	0%
Proplasmacytes		0% to 6%	0%
Plasmacytes		25% to 75%	0%
Platelet count	40,000 to 150,000 per cu. mm.	40,000 to 150,000 per cu. mm.	150,000 to 400,000 per cu. mm.
Bone marrow examination			
Monocytes	20% to 60%		0% to 5%
Plasmacytes		15% to 75%	0% to 1%

ALEUKEMIC LEUKEMIA AND LEUKEMOID REACTIONS

In this section, we consider (1) leukemia which does not resemble leukemia and (2) some reactions which do resemble leukemia. The discussion will cover aleukemic leukemia and leukemoid reactions.

ALEUKEMIC LEUKEMIA

Aleukemic leukemia is also referred to as aleukemic lymphadenosis and aleukemic myelosis.

Aleukemic leukemia means white blood without white blood. It is a phase of leukemia in which the white cell count is normal or below normal and the differential white cell count may show only a few immature white cells.

Aleukemic leukemia occurs in 10% to 20% of all cases of leukemia. Its significance lies in the fact that, during the phase, the disease may easily be confused with other diseases such as aplastic anemia or agranulocytosis.

With the exception of the white cells, the laboratory findings and clinical picture are the same as those which have just been described for the various leukemias.

Because the white cell count is normal or below normal, the white cells in the differential white cell count are relatively few. These white cells may be concentrated, however, and the differential white cell count run on the concentrated specimen. The concentrated specimen of white cells is called a buffy coat preparation (for the procedure, see Buffy Coat Preparations, page 558).

As previously stated, in aleukemic leukemia, the differential white cell count may not show many immature white cells. A bone marrow examination then becomes the more significant laboratory examination. This examination usually reveals large numbers of immature white cells.

LEUKEMOID REACTIONS

Leukemoid reactions are reactions which resemble leukemia. Thus, the white cell count is high and the differential white cell count shows immature white cells. But the patient does not have leukemia.

The distinction between a leukemoid reaction and true leukemia is usually made by (1) careful clinical observations of the patient, (2) a continual check for changes in laboratory examinations, and (3) a bone marrow examination.

The more commonly encountered leukemoid reactions are neutrophilic leukemoid reactions and lymphocytic leukemoid reactions. These reactions are briefly discussed below.

Neutrophilic Leukemoid Reactions

A neutrophilic leukemoid reaction is accompanied by a white cell count of 20,000 to 100,000 per cubic millimeter and a differential white cell count showing immature neutrophils such as neutrophilic metamyelocytes and neutrophilic myelocytes.

Thus, from a laboratory viewpoint, a neutrophilic leukemoid reaction may resemble granulocytic leukemia.

A neutrophilic leukemoid reaction may be found in the following conditions: tuberculosis, meningitis, diphtheria, lobar pneumonia, malaria, syphilis, hemorrhage, hemolytic anemia, severe burns, tumors, Hodgkin's disease, myeloid metaplasia, mercury poisoning, and eclampsia

If it is difficult to distinguish between a neutrophilic leukemoid reaction and granulocytic leukemia, the alkaline phosphatase stain may be used.

The alkaline phosphatase stain reveals values above normal in a neutrophilic leukemoid reaction and values below normal in granulocytic leukemia.

Lymphocytic Leukemoid Reactions

A lymphocytic leukemoid reaction is accompanied by a white cell count of 20,000 to 150,000 per cubic millimeter and a differential white cell count showing 35% to 95% lymphocytes.

Thus, from a laboratory viewpoint, a lymphocytic leukemoid reaction may resemble lymphocytic leukemia.

A lymphocytic leukemoid reaction may be found in the following conditions: mumps, measles, chickenpox, whooping cough, infectious lymphocytosis, and infectious mononucleosis.

Of the above conditions, infectious mononucleosis probably gives the most trouble, for it is often difficult to differentiate between infectious mononucleosis and lymphocytic leukemia.

The distinction between infectious mononucleosis and lymphocytic leukemia can usually be made by the heterophil agglutination test.

The heterophil agglutination test is usually positive in infectious mononucleosis and negative in lymphocytic leukemia.

A NOTE TO THE STUDENT

What single laboratory examination can usually point a finger at granulocytic leukemia, lymphocytic leukemia, monocytic leukemia, or plasmacytic leukemia?

The differential white cell count can usually separate one leukemia from the other.

The differential white cell count shows cells of the granulocytic series in granulocytic leukemia, cells of the lymphocytic series in lymphocytic leukemia, cells of the monocytic series in monocytic leukemia, and cells of the plasmacytic series in plasmacytic leukemia.

If the cells are very immature, it usually points to the acute form of leukemia; if the cells are more mature, it usually points to the chronic form of leukemia.

Thus, the differential white cell count is an extremely significant examination in diagnosing the various leukemias and blood smears of the various leukemias are frequently given to students to study and identify.

In identifying blood smears of the various leukemias, (1) you first identify the predominating white cell series and (2) then note the age or maturity of the white cells.   A few examples are given below.

Example #1:

You are given a blood smear of leukemia.

You observe that most of the white cells belong to the granulocytic series.   Which leukemia are you dealing with?

You note that the white cells are mostly neutrophilic myelocytes.   Is the leukemia acute or chronic?

Example #2:

You are given a blood smear of leukemia.

You observe that most of the white cells belong to the lymphocytic series.   Which leukemia are you dealing with?

You note that most of the white cells are mature lymphocytes.   Is the leukemia acute or chronic?

Answers:

The leukemia in the first example would, of course, be chronic granulocytic leukemia and the leukemia in the second example would be chronic lymphocytic leukemia.

Chapter 36

Hemorrhagic Diseases

Hemorrhagic is pronounced hem″o-raj′ik. The word is derived from two Greek words: "blood" and "bursting forth." Hence, hemorrhagic means the bursting forth of blood.

The hemorrhagic diseases will be discussed under the following headings:

Introduction to the Hemorrhagic Diseases
Diseases of Vascular Defects
Diseases of Platelet Deficiencies
Plasma Coagulation Disorders

The student review questions for the hemorrhagic diseases are numbered 450–460 and begin on page 771 of the Appendix.

INTRODUCTION TO THE HEMORRHAGIC DISEASES

"When I think of abnormal bleeding, I think of
pipes, platelets, and plasma coagulation factors."
—Dr. Donald L. Duckworth

The hemorrhagic diseases deal with abnormal bleeding.

The abnormal bleeding may be produced by any one of the following 3 circumstances.

One, capillary walls that are weak and thus enable blood to seep into the tissues.

Two, platelets that are decreased in number or defective in structure and therefore fail in their function of blood coagulation.

Three, plasma coagulation factors which are deficient or abnormal and therefore fail in their function of blood coagulation.

Thus, the hemorrhagic diseases may be divided into 3 broad groups:

1. diseases of vascular defects
2. diseases of platelet deficiencies
3. plasma coagulation disorders

The diseases of vascular defects which we will consider are scurvy and hereditary hemorrhagic telangiectasia.

The diseases of platelet deficiencies which we will discuss are purpura hemorrhagica and symptomatic thrombocytopenic purpura.

The plasma coagulation disorders which we will consider are hemophilia and hemorrhagic disease of the newborn.

The classification of the hemorrhagic diseases is given in Table 56.

Table 56

Classification of the Hemorrhagic Diseases

Diseases of Vascular Defects
scurvy
hereditary hemorrhagic telangiectasia

Diseases of Platelet Deficiencies
purpura hemorrhagica
symptomatic thrombocytopenic purpura

Plasma Coagulation Disorders
hemophilia
hemorrhagic disease of the newborn

DISEASES OF VASCULAR DEFECTS

The diseases of vascular defects which we will discuss are scurvy and hereditary hemorrhagic telangiectasia.

SCURVY

Scurvy is also referred to as ascorbic acid deficiency, scorbutus, hypovitaminosis C, and Barlow's disease.

The discussion will cover basic clinical information, factors affecting laboratory examinations, and results of laboratory examinations.

Basic Clinical Information

Vitamin C is ascorbic acid and, in discussions, the terms are used interchangeably.

Scurvy is caused by a deficiency of vitamin C and the disease is characterized by abnormal bleeding.

The disease is relatively rare but it may sometimes be seen in elderly patients, food faddists, and infants.

The typical *adult* patient complains about being tired, listless, irritable, having no appetite, and having occasional bleeding from the mouth.

The typical *infant* patient resents being touched, even crying or screaming when moved.

The doctor observes that the patient has a foul odor, there is bleeding into the skin, and small hemorrhages around the hair follicles on the arms and legs; the doctor also notices that the patient's gums are spongy and swollen.

The diagnosis will be made from the results of the physical examination and laboratory examinations.

The laboratory examinations usually include a bleeding time, coagulation time, platelet count, clot retraction time, capillary resistance test, urine analysis, plasma ascorbic acid test, urinary ascorbic acid test, and vitamin C saturation test.

If the patient does have scurvy, treatment usually consists of bed rest and restoring vitamin C to the system by injection, oral medication, or the proper diet.

The outlook is favorable, most patients recover in a few weeks.

Factors Affecting Laboratory Examinations

In this disease, a deficiency of ascorbic acid causes the lining of the capillaries to weaken and blood seeps into the tissues.

The deficiency of ascorbic acid causes the plasma ascorbic acid test to drop from a normal range of 0.5–1.5 milligrams per 100 milliliters to less than 0.2 milligrams per 100 milliliters.

The urinary ascorbic test drops from a normal range of 6–18 milligrams per day to values approaching zero.

Table 57
Results of Laboratory Examinations in Scurvy

Laboratory Examinations	Values in Scurvy	Values in Health
Plasma ascorbic acid test	0 to 0.2 mg. per 100 ml.	0.5 to 1.5 mg. per 100 ml.
Urinary ascorbic acid test	0 to 3 mg. per day	6 to 18 mg. per day
Capillary resistance test	positive	less than 10 petechiae produced
Bleeding time	normal or increased	1 to 3 min. (Duke method)
Platelet count	normal	150,000 to 400,000 per cu. mm.
Coagulation time	normal	2 to 6 min. (capillary tube method)
Clot retraction time	normal	some retraction after 2 hrs. complete retraction after 24 hrs.
Urine analysis		
Albumin	positive	negative
Blood	positive	negative
Casts	present	absent
Vitamin C saturation test	unsaturated	saturated

Since the capillaries are weak, the capillary resistance test is positive.
The bleeding time may be normal or increased.
The platelet count, coagulation time, and clot retraction time are normal.
The urine shows albumin, blood, and casts.
The vitamin C saturation test reveals a depletion of vitamin C.
The results of the laboratory examinations in scurvy are summarized in Table 57.

HEREDITARY HEMORRHAGIC TELANGIECTASIA

Telangiectasia is pronounced tel-an"je-ek-ta'ze-ah. The word means a dilation of the capillaries resulting in the formation of small blood vessel tumors.

Hereditary hemorrhagic telangiectasia is also referred to as Osler's disease and the Rendu-Osler-Weber syndrome.

The discussion will cover basic clinical information, factors affecting laboratory examinations, and results of laboratory examinations.

Basic Clinical Information

Hereditary hemorrhagic telangiectasia is a disease of the blood which is characterized by the dilation, thinning, and spontaneous rupture of small capillaries resulting in abnormal bleeding.

The disease is inherited, it is relatively rare, and it may affect man, woman, or child.

The typical patient complains about bleeding from the nose and mouth.

The doctor observes that the skin of the patient, especially on the face and hands, is peppered with small lesions called telangiectases.

The diagnosis is usually made from the physical examination and history of the patient.

Laboratory examinations may include a red cell count, hemoglobin determination, bleeding time, coagulation time, and platelet count.

If the patient has hereditary hemorrhagic telangiectasia, treatment consists of medication and devices to control the bleeding.

The outlook varies from patient to patient. The patient may (1) live practically a normal life, (2) become an invalid because of the bleeding, or (3) suddenly die from severe hemorrhage.

Factors Affecting Laboratory Examinations

In this disease, the walls of the capillaries are thin and tend to rupture.

The resulting bleeding causes the red cell count and hemoglobin to drop below the normal values.

The bleeding time, coagulation time, and platelet count are usually normal.

The prolonged bleeding in the patient may eventually lead to a microcytic hypochromic anemia and the stained red cell examination will then show small pale red cells.

DISEASES OF PLATELET DEFICIENCIES

The word purpura is pronounced pur'pu-rah and it means purple.

Purpura is a condition caused by abnormal bleeding and characterized by the presence of small purplish red spots on the body. The purplish red spots are usually referred to as petechiae. An illustration of petechiae has been given in Figure 163, page 480.

The diseases of platelet deficiencies which we will discuss are purpura hemorrhagica and symptomatic thrombocytopenic purpura.

PURPURA HEMORRHAGICA

Purpura hemorrhagica is also referred to as hemorrhagica purpura, thrombocytopenic purpura, idiopathic thrombocytopenic purpura, primary thrombocytopenic purpura, splenic thrombocytopenic purpura, idiopathic thrombopenic purpura, essential thrombocytopenia, and Werlhof's disease.

The discussion will cover basic clinical information, factors affecting laboratory examinations, and results of laboratory examinations.

Basic Clinical Information

Purpura hemorrhagica is a disease of the blood characterized by a low platelet count, spontaneous bruising or bleeding, and the production of petechiae.

This disease is relatively rare, the cause is unknown, and it occurs most frequently in girls under 21.

The typical patient complains about nosebleeds, bleeding gums, and prolonged menstruations.

The doctor observes that the patient has a skin rash of pin-point petechiae, bruises on various areas of her body, and petechial spots in her mouth.

The diagnosis will be made from the results of the physical examination and laboratory examinations.

The laboratory examinations usually include a white cell count, red cell count, hemoglobin determination, differential white cell count, bleeding time, coagulation time, platelet count, clot retraction time, capillary resistance test, prothrombin time, prothrombin consumption test, and bone marrow examination.

If the patient does have purpura hemorrhagica, treatment usually consists of (1) medications, such as steroids, to control the bleeding, (2) iron or blood transfusions to relieve the anemia, and (3) possibly an operation to remove the spleen.

The spleen is thought to produce an anti-platelet factor which destroys platelets. Hence, it is believed that the spleen is repsonsible for the low platelet count. In any event, removal of the spleen is often beneficial.

The prognosis in this disease varies from patient to patient. The patient may (1) completely recover, (2) have rare occurrences of bleeding which may be mild or severe, or (3) have frequent occurrences of bleeding which may be mild or severe.

The duration of the bleeding periods is usually 2 to 14 days.

Factors Affecting Laboratory Examinations

In this disease, the number of platelets in the blood drops below normal; the cause may be either decreased production or increased destruction of platelets.

Table 58

Results of Laboratory Examinations in Purpura Hemorrhagica

Laboratory Examinations	Values in Purpura Hemorrhagica	Values in Health
White cell count	normal	5,000 to 10,000 per cu. mm.
Red cell count	normal or decreased	4 to 6 million per cu. mm.
Hemoglobin determination	normal or decreased	12 to 18 grams per 100 cc.
Differential white cell count	normal	normal
Platelet count	0 to 50,000 per cu. mm.	150,000 to 400,000 per cu. mm.
Bleeding time	increased	1 to 3 min.
Clot retraction time	increased	some retraction after 2 hrs.; complete retraction after 24 hrs.
Capillary resistance test	positive	less than 10 petechiae produced
Coagulation time	normal	varies with method
Prothrombin time	normal	11 to 16 seconds
Prothrombin consumption time	decreased	20 to 40 seconds
Bone marrow examination	number of megakaryocytes is normal or increased; platelet formation is decreased	normal

The laboratory examinations are affected as follows.

The platelet count is usually less than 50,000 per cubic millimeter against the normal range of 150,000 to 400,000 per cubic millimeter.

The shortage of platelets results in an increase in the bleeding time, increase in the clot retraction time, and a positive capillary resistance test. The coagulation time is normal.

During periods of bleeding, the red cell count and hemoglobin may drop below normal.

The following laboratory tests are useful in ruling out other diseases which may sometimes present a somewhat similar clinical picture.

The white cell count and differential white cell count are usually normal. These findings are useful in ruling out leukemia and many other diseases.

The prothrombin time is normal and the prothrombin consumption time is decreased, thus being useful in ruling out other hemorrhagic diseases.

A bone marrow examination reveals that the megakaryocytes are immature or abnormal. The number of megakaryocytes may be normal or even increased but their ability to produce platelets is greatly decreased. These findings thus differ from the reports in aplastic anemia and acute leukemia.

The results of the laboratory examinations are summarized in Table 58.

SYMPTOMATIC THROMBOCYTOPENIC PURPURA

Symptomatic thrombocytopenic purpura is also referred to as secondary thrombocytopenia.

Symptomatic thrombocytopenic purpura is a condition characterized by a decrease in the number of platelets which is due either to a toxic agent or some underlying disease.

Among the toxic agents that may be responsible for this condition are:

phenobarbital	ergot
sulfonamides	iodine
quinine	bismuth
phenylbutazone	benzol
ionizing radiation	streptomycin

Among the underlying diseases that may be responsible for this condition are:

anemia	lupus erythematosus
leukemia	septicemia
cancer	typhoid fever
Gaucher's disease	measles
tuberculosis	scarlet fever

The typical patient complains about nosebleeds, shows massive bruises and petehiae on various areas of the body, and reveals blood in the urine and feces.

43

If the physician suspects that the condition was caused by a toxic agent, he endeavors to elicit this information from the patient.

If the condition was caused by a toxic agent, the treatment consists of removal or avoidance of the toxic agent, blood transfusions, and medications.

If the condition was caused by an underlying disease, treatment consists of treating the underlying disease.

The laboratory examinations usually include a red cell count, hemoglobin determination, platelet count, bleeding time, and coagulation time.

The results of the laboratory examinations are as follows.

The red cell count and hemoglobin determination are below normal.

The platelet count is usually less than 100,000 per cubic millimeter against the normal range of 150,000 to 400,000 per cubic millimeter.

The bleeding time is increased but the coagulation time is normal.

To summarize: In symptomatic thrombocytopenic purpura, the platelet count is decreased, the bleeding time is increased, and the coagulation time is normal.

PLASMA COAGULATION DISORDERS

The discussion will cover classification of the plasma coagulation disorders, hemophilia, and hemorrhagic disease of the newborn.

CLASSIFICATION OF THE PLASMA COAGULATION DISORDERS

You will recall the 3 stages in the coagulation of blood:

Stage 1—formation of thromboplastin
Stage 2—formation of thrombin
Stage 3—formation of fibrin

These 3 stages have been discussed and illustrated under the theory of blood coagulation (page 392).

Each of these 3 stages are associated with various plasma coagulation disorders.

Stage 1 disorders include those conditions and diseases which have deficient blood thromboplastin formation.

Stage 2 disorders include those conditions and diseases which have deficient thrombin formation.

Stage 3 disorders include those conditions and diseases which have defective fibrin formation.

This basic grouping of the plasma coagulation disorders and a representative condition or disease is given in Table 59.

Table 59

Basic Grouping of the Plasma Coagulation Disorders

Group	Abnormality Involved	Representative Condition or Disease
Stage 1 disorders	deficient blood thromboplastin formation	hemophilia
Stage 2 disorders	deficient thrombin formation	hemorrhagic disease of the newborn
Stage 3 disorders	defective fibrin formation	afibrinogenemia

The plasma coagulation disorders are currently undergoing a great deal of investigation but the theoretical information involved has little practical significance for the student of medical technology.

In this discussion of the plasma coagulation disorders, we will consider hemophilia and hemorrhagic disease of the newborn.

HEMOPHILIA

Hemophilia is also referred to as classical hemophilia, hemophilia A, classic hemophilia A, factor VIII deficiency disease, antihemophilic globulin deficiency disease, and AHG deficiency disease.

The discussion will cover basic clinical information, factors affecting laboratory examinations, and results of laboratory examinations.

Basic Clinical Information

Hemophilia is a hemorrhagic disease which is characterized by a deficiency of Factor VIII.

Factor VIII is a plasma coagulation factor which is also referred to as antihemophilic globulin, AHG, and AHF.

Hemophilia is inherited, it is confined almost exclusively to males, and it is usually discovered in childhood.

The patient suffers from both internal and external bleeding.

The internal bleeding is frequently spontaneous and it is marked by the seepage of blood into the tissues and joints of the body.

The external bleeding may result from an injury to the body or the extraction of a tooth.

The usual treatment during periods of bleeding is complete bed rest and blood transfusions.

The prognosis is poor. The majority of patients die before reaching the age of 21. If a patient does survive to the age of 21, however, his chances of living a normal life span are good.

Medical research is currently seeking a simple effective method of furnishing the patient with Factor VIII.

Factors Affecting Laboratory Examinations

In hemophilia, a deficiency of Factor VIII results in a delay in the coagulation of blood.

The delay in the coagulation of blood causes an increase in the coagulation time.

The coagulation time may rise from a normal value of 2 to 6 minutes (by the capillary tube method) to values between 60 and 120 minutes.

The partial thromboplastin time is prolonged, the prothrombin consumption time is decreased, the thromboplastin generation test reveals a plasma defect, and the Factor VIII assay is decreased.

Normal values are found in the following laboratory tests: bleeding time, platelet count, clot retraction time, capillary resistance test, thrombin time, and prothrombin time.

During hemorrhages, the red cell count and hemoglobin drop below normal.

Thus, in hemophilia, the results of the laboratory examinations may be summarized as follows:

1. coagulation time greatly increased
2. partial thromboplastin time increased
3. prothrombin consumption time decreased
4. thromboplastin generation test reveals plasma defect
5. Factor VIII assay decreased
6. all other coagulation tests normal

HEMORRHAGIC DISEASE OF THE NEWBORN

Hemorrhagic disease of the newborn is also referred to as hemorrhagic diathesis newborn, neonatorum hemophilia, morbus hemorrhagicus neonatorum, vitamin K deficiency of the newborn, hemorrhagic diathesis in infancy, and melaena neonatorum.

The discussion will cover basic clinical information, factors affecting laboratory examinations, and results of laboratory examinations.

Basic Clinical Information

In hemorrhagic disease of the newborn, the infant is subject to slow bleeding into the intestinal tract, into the tissues, and beneath the skin.

The disease may occur during the first week of life, it is sometimes fatal, and the cause is considered to be a deficiency of vitamin K.

The administration of vitamin K tends to relieve the condition and the outlook is usually favorable.

Factors Affecting Laboratory Examinations

In this disease, the infant is affected by a delay in the synthesis of pro-thrombin.

The delay in the synthesis of prothrombin causes a shortage of pro-thrombin.

The shortage of prothrombin results in an increased prothrombin time.

The prothrombin time rises from a normal infant's range of about 40–45 seconds to 120–360 seconds.

The platelet count is normal and the coagulation time is usually increased.

Thus, in hemorrhagic disease of the newborn, the results of the laboratory examinations may be summarized as follows:

1. prothrombin time increased
2. platelet count normal
3. coagulation time usually increased

Chapter 37

Miscellaneous Blood Diseases

THE past three chapters discussed the three major classes of blood diseases: the anemias, leukemias, and hemorrhagic diseases.

This chapter considers miscellaneous blood diseases. It covers 6 blood diseases which are usually encountered and 17 blood diseases and anomalies which are rarely encountered. The material is presented as follows.

Polycythemia Vera and Agranulocytosis
Infectious Mononucleosis and Multiple Myeloma
Hodgkin's Disease and Gaucher's Disease
Diseases and Anomalies Rarely Encountered

The student review questions for the miscellaneous blood diseases are numbered 461–494 and begin on page 772 of the Appendix.

POLYCYTHEMIA VERA AND AGRANULOCYTOSIS

In the anemias, we saw a low red cell count and a low hemoglobin; but in polycythemia vera, we will see a high red cell count and a high hemoglobin.

In the leukemias, we saw a high white cell count; but in agranulocytosis, we will see a low white cell count.

We will first discuss polycythemia vera and then consider agranulocytosis.

POLYCYTHEMIA VERA

Polycythemia vera is also referred to by the following synonyms: erythremia, primary polycythemia, polycythemia rubra, polycythemia rubra vera, splenomegalic polycythemia, Vaquez's disease, and Osler's disease.

The discussion will cover definitions, basic clinical information, factors affecting laboratory examination, and results of laboratory examinations.

Definitions

First, let us briefly discuss and define the following terms:

1. polycythemia
2. polycythemia vera
3. secondary polycythemia
4. relative polycythemia
5. erythrocytosis

1. Polycythemia

Polycythemia is pronounced pol"e-si-the'me-ah. The prefix *poly* means many, the stem *cyt* means cells, and the suffix *hemia* means blood. Thus, polycythemia means many blood cells.

2. Polycythemia Vera

The word *vera* means true; thus, polycythemia vera means a true state of many blood cells.

Polycythemia vera is a disease of unknown cause characterized by an increased production of red cells resulting in the red cell count rising above the normal values.

3. Secondary Polycythemia

Secondary polycythemia is any condition or disease other than polycythemia vera in which the red cell count rises above the normal values. A few examples follow.

At high altitudes the oxygen content of the air is low. The lowered oxygen content of the air stimulates the bone marrow to manufacture more red cells. The increased manufacture of red cells causes the red cell count to rise above the normal values. The increase in the red cell count results in a secondary polycythemia.

In congenital heart disease, a sluggish heart fails to furnish the tissues with a normal supply of oxygen. The decrease in oxygen to the tissues stimulates the bone marrow to manufacture more red cells. The increased production of red cells causes the red cell count to rise above the normal values. The increase in the red cell count results in a secondary polycythemia.

Thus, a secondary polycythemia may be present in persons who live at high altitudes and in persons who have congenital heart disease.

4. Relative Polycythemia

A relative polycythemia is a form of secondary polycythemia which is due to a loss of fluid. An example follows.

In severe burns and in severe diarrhea, the body loses fluid. The loss of fluid makes the red cells more concentrated. The increased concentration of red cells causes the red cell count to rise above the normal values. The increase in the red cell count results in a relative polycythemia.

Thus, a relative polycythemia may be seen in a severe burn case and in severe diarrhea.

5. Erythrocytosis

Erythrocytosis means an increase in red cells. Obviously, an erythrocytosis occurs in both polycythemia vera and secondary polycythemia. The word erythrocytosis, however, is usually used in connection with secondary polycythemia.

Erythrocytosis is usually used in connection with secondary polycythemia because the "cause" of secondary polycythemia is known whereas the "cause" of polycythemia vera is, as yet, unknown.

When the cause of polycythemia vera becomes known, however, it should add to the confusion in terminology.

By Way of Summary

If the red cell count rises above the normal values, it may be due to:

1. polycythemia vera
2. secondary polycythemia
   a. decrease in oxygen
      (1) high altitudes
      (2) congenital heart disease
   b. loss of fluid
      (1) severe burn case
      (2) severe diarrhea

Basic Clinical Information

Polycythemia vera may affect anyone but it is found most frequently in the male patient past 40.

The typical patient complains about headaches, dizzy spells, stomach pains, intense itching, and difficulty in breathing; he may also complain about bed sweats, a ringing in his ears, and spots before his eyes.

The doctor observes that the face of the patient is red or ruddy, his lips and ears are purple, and his spleen is enlarged.

The diagnosis will be made from the results of the physical examination and laboratory examinations.

The routine laboratory examinations usually include a white cell count, red cell count, hemoglobin determination, differential white cell count, stained red cell examination, sedimentation rate, hematocrit reading, and platelet count.

Additional laboratory examinations may include a blood viscosity, blood specific gravity, total blood volume, total red cell volume, bone marrow examination, reticulocyte count, mean corpuscular volume, red cell osmotic fragility test, basal metabolic rate, blood uric acid, serum bilirubin, serum iron, alkaline phosphatase stain, and oxygen saturation of arterial blood.

If the patient does have polycythemia vera, treatment will be aimed at (1) removing the excess blood by blood-letting and (2) decreasing the production of blood by the action of radioactive phosphorus or busulfan.

The prognosis is variable. The patient may live 1 to 25 years. The average patient lives about 10 years.

Now let us consider the manner in which this disease affects the laboratory examinations.

Factors Affecting Laboratory Examinations

In polycythemia vera, the cell factories in the bone marrow are overactive. This overactivity causes an increase in the production of red cells, white cells, and platelets.

The increase in the production of red cells, white cells, and platelets results in the following examinations rising above their normal values:

red cell count
white cell count
platelet count

The increase in the number of red cells is responsible for an increase in the hemoglobin and hematocrit reading.

The overactivity of the cell factories causes the production and release of immature white cells and red cells.

Thus, the differential white cell count shows progranulocytes, neutrophilic myelocytes, and neutrophilic metamyelocytes.

The stained red cell examination may show a few nucleated red cells, anisocytosis, and polychromatophilia.

In polycythemia vera, what happens to the total blood volume?

The total blood volume rises above the normal values. To illustrate, a normal person has about 5 quarts of blood. But a patient with polycythemia vera may have about 8 quarts of blood.

What happens to the total red cell volume?

The total red cell volume also rises above the normal values. An example follows.

A normal person has about 5 quarts of blood, 40% being red cells. But a patient with polycythemia vera has about 8 quarts of blood, 60% being red cells. The normal person and the patient therefore have the following volume of red cells:

Normal = 5 qts. × 40% red cells = 2.0 qts. red cells
Patient = 8 qts. × 60% red cells = 4.8 qts. red cells

The normal person thus has 2.0 quarts of red cells and the patient with polycythemia vera has more than twice this amount, namely, 4.8 quarts of red cells.

Consequently, in polycythemia vera, the total red cell volume rises above the normal values.

What about the total plasma volume in the normal person and the patient with polycythemia vera?

The total plasma volume is found as follows:

Normal = 5 qts. × 60% plasma = 3.0 qts. plasma

Patient = 8 qts. × 40% plasma = 3.2 qts. plasma

Thus, the total plasma volume is about the same in the normal person and in the patient with polycythemia vera.

Therefore, in polycythemia vera, the increase in the total blood volume is due to the increase in the total red cell volume.

The blood volume in a normal person and in a patient with polycythemia vera is illustrated in Figure 181.

The increase in the total red cell volume causes the blood to be thicker or more viscous. For example, in health, the blood is about 5 times thicker

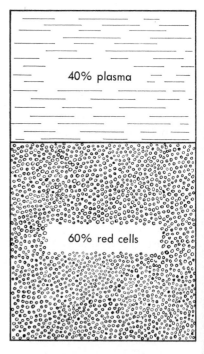

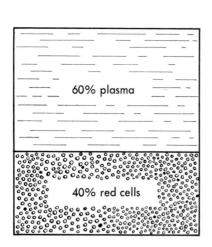

Blood Volume in a Normal Person   Blood Volume in a Patient
(about 5 quarts)   with Polycythemia Vera
                               (about 8 quarts)

FIG. 181.—Blood volume in a normal person and in a patient
with polycythemia vera.

Table 60
Results of Laboratory Examinations in Polycythemia Vera

Laboratory Examinations	Values in Polycythemia Vera	Values in Health
White cell count	10,000 to 50,000 per cu. mm.	5,000 to 10,000 per cu. mm.
Red cell count	6 to 12 million per cu. mm.	4 to 6 million per cu. mm.
Hemoglobin determination	18 to 24 grams per 100 cc.	12 to 18 grams per 100 cc.
Differential white cell count		
Progranulocytes	0% to 3%	0%
Neut. Myelocytes	3% to 8%	0%
Neut. Metamyelocytes	5% to 10%	0%
Neut. Band Cells	8% to 16%	2% to 6%
Neut. Seg. Cells	25% to 80%	55% to 75%
Stained red cell examination		
Anisocytosis	present	absent
Polychromatophilia	present	absent
Nucleated red cells	0 to 8 per 100 white cells	0 per 100 white cells
Sedimentation rate	decreased	varies with method
Hematocrit reading	54% to 74%	37% to 54%
Platelet count	200,000 to 3,000,000 per cu. mm.	150,000 to 400,000 per cu. mm.
Blood viscosity	12 to 33	5
Blood specific gravity	1.075 to 1.080	1.055 to 1.065
Total blood volume	84 to 130 ml. per kg. body weight	54 to 84 ml. per kg. body weight
Total red cell volume	36 to 110 ml. per kg. body weight	22 to 36 ml. per kg. body weight
Bone marrow exam	hyperplastic; normal percentage of cells	normal
Reticulocyte count	normal or increased	1% to 2%
Mean corpuscular volume (MCV)	normal or slightly decreased	80 to 90 cubic microns
Red cell osmotic fragility test	decreased values	hemol. begins .44% hemol. ends .34%
Basal metabolic rate	+15 to +35	−15 to +15
Blood uric acid	sometimes increased	2 to 4 mg. per 100 ml.
Serum bilirubin	normal	0.2 to 0.8 mg. per 100 ml.
Serum iron	normal	70 to 180 micrograms per 100 ml.
Alkaline phosphatase stain	values usually increased	13 to 100
Oxygen saturation of arterial blood	90% to 100%	90% to 100%

than water. But, in polycythemia vera, the blood is about 20 times thicker than water.

The increase in the thickness or viscosity of the blood causes the specific gravity of the blood to rise above the normal values.

When the medical technologist draws blood from a patient with poly-cythemia vera, he may notice that the blood is unusually dark and thick. He may also find that the thickness of the blood makes it difficult to prepare blood smears.

A bone marrow examination reveals that all the cell factories are over-active, but the respective percentage of red cells, white cells, and platelets is normal.

The reticulocyte count is normal or elevated.

The mean corpuscular volume (MCV) is normal or slightly decreased.

The red cells show an increased resistance to hypotonic saline solutions; therefore, decreased values are found in the red cell osmotic fragility test.

The basal metabolic rate is increased and the sedimentation rate is decreased.

The blood uric acid is sometimes increased.

The serum bilirubin and serum iron are normal.

What laboratory examination is useful in distinguishing polycythemia vera from chronic granulocytic leukemia?

The values for the alkaline phosphatase stain are usually increased in polycythemia vera but decreased in chronic granulocytic leukemia.

What laboratory examination is useful in distinguishing polycythemia vera from secondary polycythemia?

The oxygen saturation of arterial blood is normal in polycythemia vera but below normal in secondary polycythemia.

The results of the laboratory examinations in polycythemia vera are summarized in Table 60.

AGRANULOCYTOSIS

Agranulocytosis is pronounced ah-gran″u-lo-si-to′sis.

Agranulocytosis is also referred to by the following synonyms: malignant neutropenia, primary granulocytopenia, acute granulocytopenia, agranulo-cytic angina, and granulopenia.

The discussion will cover basic clinical information, factors affecting laboratory examinations, and results of laboratory examinations.

Basic Clinical Information

Agranulocytosis is a severe disease of the blood characterized by a low white cell count and a decrease in granulocytes.

Agranulocytosis is usually caused by a hypersensitivity to certain drugs and chemicals used in the treatment of disease.

Among the many drugs and chemicals that may be responsible for agranulocytosis are aminopyrine, sulfonamides, arsenicals, benzene, and barbiturates.

These drugs and chemicals either hinder the development of white cells in the bone marrow or cause the white cells to be removed from the blood stream.

This disease may affect anyone but it is most frequently found in the adult female patient.

The incidence of agranulocytosis is usually high among persons who work in doctor's offices, clinics, and hospitals. This is probably due to the fact that the personnel in the medical field are often prone to "self treatment."

The typical female patient complains about being extremely exhausted, having a sore throat, difficulty in swallowing, and sudden chills.

The doctor observes that the patient has a high fever, a rapid weak pulse, and ulcers in her mouth and throat. He may also find ulcers in her rectum and vagina.

The diagnosis will be made from the results of the physical examination and laboratory examinations.

The routine laboratory examinations usually include a white cell count, red cell count, hemoglobin determination, differential white cell count, stained red cell examination, hematocrit reading, and sedimentation rate.

Additional laboratory examinations may include a platelet count, bone marrow examination, and certain bacteriological examinations.

Why are bacteriological examinations necessary?

In this disease, the decrease in the number of white cells increases the susceptibility to infection; if infection is present or suspected, bacteriological examinations such as throat smears and blood cultures may be ordered.

If the patient does have agranulocytosis, treatment will be aimed at (1) discontinuing the use of the offending drug or chemical and (2) the administration of an antibiotic, such as penicillin, to combat any infection.

If the disease is caught in time and the treatment and bodily resistance are adequate, the outlook or prognosis is favorable. But, if the disease is not caught in time, and an overwhelming infection sets in, the outcome may be fatal.

Factors Affecting Laboratory Examinations

The toxic action of an offending drug or chemical greatly decreases the number of the disease fighting white cells, the granulocytes, in the blood stream.

Thus, the differential white cell count may show 0% to 10% neutrophilic segmented cells against a normal value of 55% to 75%.

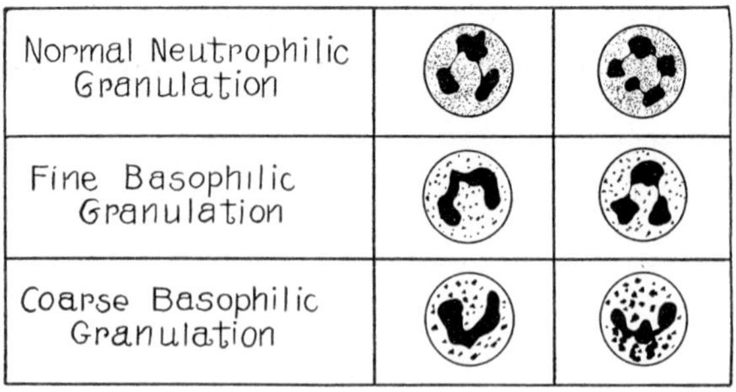

Normal Neutrophilic Granulation		
Fine Basophilic Granulation		
Coarse Basophilic Granulation		

FIG. 182.—Basophilic ("toxic") granulation of the neutrophilic leukocytes. The "toxic" granules vary in size depending on the seriousness of the damage to the cells in the marrow. (Haden, *Principles of Hematology.*)

In addition, the neutrophilic segmented cells usually show toxic granulation, that is, unusually large granules in the cytoplasm.

Toxic granulation of the white cells is illustrated in the accompanying Figure 182 and also in Plate 7, page 258.

The white cell count falls below the normal values of 5,000 to 10,000 per cubic millimeter, usually dropping to a count between 100 and 2,000 per cubic millimeter. This is referred to as a marked leukopenia.

Since the red cells are not affected, the following tests are normal:

red cell count
hemoglobin determination
stained red cell examination
hematocrit reading

The normal values obtained in the above tests are of great value to the physician in ruling out other diseases.

The sedimentation rate is increased.

The platelet count is usually normal but may sometimes be decreased.

The bone marrow examination is often useful in establishing the diagnosis.

If the patient has agranulocytosis, the bone marrow reveals that the development of the red cells and platelets is normal. This finding usually differs from the findings in aplastic anemia and granulocytic leukemia.

The development of the granulocytes in the bone marrow varies with the stage of the disease.

At the height of the disease, the development of the granulocytes is arrested. Thus, the cells of the granulocytic series are below their normal percentages.

Table 61

Results of Laboratory Examinations in Agranulocytosis

Laboratory Examinations	Values in Agranulocytosis	Values in Health
White cell count	100 to 2,000 per cu. mm.	5,000 to 10,000 per cu. mm.
Red cell count	normal	4 to 6 million per cu. mm.
Hemoglobin determination	normal	12 to 18 grams per 100 cc.
Differential white cell count		
Neutrophilic segmented cells	0% to 10%; cells usually show toxic granulation	55% to 75%
Stained red cell exam	red cells normal in size and color	red cells normal in size and color
Hematocrit reading	normal	37% to 54%
Sedimentation rate	increased	varies with method
Platelet count	usually normal	150,000 to 400,000 per cu. mm.
Bone marrow exam		
Granulocytes	decreased during disease; increased during recovery	30% to 70%
Nucleated red cells	normal	8% to 30%
Platelets (megakaryocytes)	normal	0% to 3%

During recovery from the disease, however, the development of the granulocytes is accelerated. Thus, the cells of the granulocytic series are above their normal percentages.

The results of the laboratory examinations in agranulocytosis are summarized in Table 61.

INFECTIOUS MONONUCLEOSIS AND MULTIPLE MYELOMA

In this section, we will meet two abnormal white cells: the abnormal lymphocyte seen in infectious mononucleosis and the abnormal plasmacyte found in multiple myeloma.

Let us first discuss infectious mononucleosis and then consider multiple myeloma.

INFECTIOUS MONONUCLEOSIS

Infectious mononucleosis is often referred to by the following terms: glandular fever, the letters I. M., benign lymphadenosis, and acute epidemic infectious adenitis.

The discussion will cover basic clinical information, factors affecting laboratory examinations, and results of laboratory examinations.

Basic Clinical Information

Infectious mononucleosis is an acute infectious disease which is characterized by the presence of atypical lymphocytes and a positive heterophil agglutination test.

Although the cause of infectious mononucleosis is unknown, it is generally considered to be a virus infection.

The disease is usually confined to children and young adults.

The typical patient complains about being tired and having a sore throat, headaches, and chills.

The doctor observes that the patient has a fever, enlarged lymph nodes in the neck, and an inflamed throat and palate. He may also find conjunctivitis, body rashes, and an enlarged liver.

Infectious mononucleosis is sometimes a difficult disease to diagnose and the physician often relies heavily on the laboratory reports of the medical technologist.

The routine laboratory examinations usually include a white cell count, red cell count, hemoglobin determination, differential white cell count, stained red cell examination, platelet count, slide test for infectious mononucleosis, and heterophil agglutination test.

Additional laboratory examinations may include a urine analysis, bleeding time, coagulation time, serum bilirubin, thymol turbidity, alkaline phosphatase stain, bone marrow examination, cerebrospinal fluid (CSF) examination, serum glutamic oxalic transaminase (SGO-T), and serum glutamic pyruvic transaminase (SGP-T).

If the patient does have infectious mononucleosis, treatment usually consists of simply confining the patient to bed.

The majority of patients recover in 2 or 3 weeks.

Now let us consider the manner in which this disease affects the laboratory examinations.

Factors Affecting Laboratory Examinations

An infection, probably virus in nature, causes atypical lymphocytes and a heterophil antibody to appear in the blood stream.

The atypical lymphocytes are seen in the blood smear and thus the differential white cell count becomes an extremely significant examination.

By finding and reporting the atypical lymphocytes, an alert medical technologist can often save the patient and physician a lot of trouble.

The search for the atypical lymphocytes should be made on the thin area of the blood smear. In this thin area, the cells are spread out. And it is much easier to notice any abnormalities.

The atypical lymphocytes are illustrated in Plate 21, page 666, and Plate 5, page 245.

In infectious mononucleosis, about 5% to 35% atypical lymphocytes will be seen in the differential white cell count.

The report of the differential white cell count should include the percentage of normal lymphocytes and the percentage of atypical lymphocytes. A sample report is given below:

Neutrophilic segmented cells	10%
Normal lymphocytes	60%
Atypical lymphocytes	30%

The above report informs the physician that 90% of the white cells are lymphocytes and that 1/3 of the lymphocytes are atypical lymphocytes.

Although the atypical lymphocytes discussed above are most frequently encountered in infectious mononucleosis, they may also be seen in several other diseases. Among these diseases are mumps, virus penumonia, and infectious hepatitis.

In infectious mononucleosis, the heterophil antibody which appears in the blood stream may be detected by the heterophil agglutination test.

The heterophil agglutination test is also referred to by the following names:

heterophile antibody test
Davidsohn test
Paul-Bunnell test

The heterophil agglutination test is a serological test for the heterophil antibody.

The word heterophil means love of another, and, in this case, the antibody in the patient's serum "loves" or reacts with the red cells of sheep.

The heterophil antibody is present in infectious mononucleosis and also in several other conditions such as serum sickness or as the result of a recent injection of horse serum.

Thus, to be effective, the heterophil agglutination test must be selective and capable of pointing an accusing finger directly at infectious mononucleosis.

The heterophil agglutination test is rather complicated. It consists of two separate tests. The first test is a *presumptive test* and the second test is a *differential test*.

Let us first discuss the *presumptive test* and then consider the *differential test*.

The presumptive test consists of making serial dilutions of the patient's serum, adding sheep cells, and inspecting the sheep cells for clumping.

In health, there may sometimes be clumping of the sheep cells in test tube #1 and #2 (see Table 62).

44

Table 62

Test Tube Numbers and the Corresponding Titers
in the Heterophil Agglutination Test

Test Tube Number	Titer (Dilution of Serum)
1	1:7
2	1:14
3	1:28
4	1:56
5	1:112
6	1:224
7	1:448
8	1:896
9	1:1,792
10	1:3,584
11	1:7,168

In infectious mononucleosis, however, there is clumping of the sheep cells in test tubes #1, #2, and #3 (or higher).

Thus, the presumptive test is positive through test tube #3 or higher. Test tube #3 is a dilution of 1:28 (see Table 62).

If the presumptive test was negative, that is, negative in test tube #3 and higher, the differential test does not have to be run. But, if the presumptive test was positive through test tube #3 or higher, the differential test should be performed.

The differential test consists of two parts. First, a guinea pig antigen test. Second, a beef cell antigen test.

Let us consider the first part of the differential test—the guinea pig antigen test.

The guinea pig antigen absorbs (or "neutralizes") the heterophil antibodies of (1) people who are normal, (2) people who have serum sickness, and (3) people who have recently received an injection of horse serum.

The guinea pig antigen, however, will not absorb (or "neutralize") the heterophil antibodies of people with infectious mononucleosis. These antibodies will then be able to clump the sheep cells.

The guinea pig antigen test is performed by adding the patient's inactivated serum to guinea pig antigen, removing the absorbed serum, making a serial dilution of this absorbed serum, adding sheep cells to the serial dilutions, and inspecting the preparation for clumping.

In infectious mononucleosis, the guinea pig antigen test is positive within 3 test tubes of the presumptive test. For example, if the presumptive test was positive through test tube #5, the guinea pig antigen test is positive through test tube #2, #3, or #4.

If the guinea pig antigen test is *not* positive within 3 test tubes of the presumptive test, it casts a shadow of doubt on either the physician's tentative diagnosis or the medical technologist's technique.

Now let us consider the second part of the differential test—the beef cell antigen test.

The beef cell antigen test is performed exactly like the guinea pig antigen test except that the guinea pig antigen is replaced by beef cell antigen.

The beef cell antigen absorbs (or "neutralizes") the heterophil antibodies of infectious mononucleosis; therefore, the patient's serum will fail to clump the sheep cells.

Thus, in infectious mononucleosis, the beef cell antigen test is negative.

A slide test for infectious mononucleosis has recently appeared on the market. The slide test has the advantage of simplicity. The trade names of several slide tests are Mono-Test, Hetrol Slide Test, and Monosticon Test.

Thus, a positive slide test for infectious mononucleosis is also of diagnostic significance.

Now let us discuss several tests which may be useful in ruling out other diseases being considered in a tentative diagnosis.

In infectious mononucleosis, the following tests are usually normal: red cell count, hemoglobin determination, and platelet count.

In leukemia, the above tests are usually *below* normal. Thus, the above tests are useful in distinguishing infectious mononucleosis from leukemia.

In the above connection, the bone marrow examination is also useful in ruling out leukemia and it is sometimes requested solely for this purpose.

In infectious mononucleosis, the bone marrow examination shows an increase in lymphocytes, many of them atypical lymphocytes.

The white cell count in infectious mononucleosis may be below normal, normal, or above normal. Thus, it is of little diagnostic significance.

The stained red cell examination shows that the red cells are normal in size and color.

In infectious mononucleosis, the urine may show albumin, bilirubin, and red cells.

The bleeding time may be above normal; the coagulation time is normal.

The following tests may rise above their normal values: serum bilirubin, thymol turbidity, serum glutamic oxalic transaminase (SGO-T), and serum glutamic pyruvic transaminase (SGP-T).

The values for the alkaline phosphatase stain drop below normal and a false positive test for syphilis may sometimes occur.

A cerebrospinal fluid examination may show an increase in lymphocytes, an increase in total protein, and a positive Pandy's test.

In infectious mononucleosis, some laboratory tests may be negative one day and positive several days later. Consequently, in doubtful cases, laboratory tests should be repeated.

The above repetition of laboratory tests applies especially to the differential white cell count, the slide test for infectious mononucleosis, and the heterophil agglutination test.

The results of the laboratory examination are summarized in Table 63 and the atypical lymphocytes are illustrated in the accompanying Plate 21.

Table 63—Results of Laboratory Examinations in Infectious Mononucleosis

Laboratory Examinations	Values in Infectious Mononucleosis	Values in Health
White cell count	2,000 to 40,000	5,000 to 10,000 per cu. mm.
Red cell count	usually normal	4 to 6 million per cu. mm.
Hemoglobin determ.	usually normal	12 to 18 grams per 100 cc.
Differential W.C.C.		
Normal lymphocytes	50% to 85%	20% to 35%
Atypical lymphocytes	5% to 35%	0%
Stained red cell exam	red cells are normal in size and color	red cells are normal in size and color
Platelet count	usually normal	150,000 to 400,000/cu. mm.
Slide test for I.M.	positive	negative
Heterophil agglutination		
I. Presumptive test	positive through: test tube #3 (or higher) titer 1:28 (or higher)	———
II. Differential test		
A. guinea pig antigen (Forssman antigen) test	must be positive within 3 test tubes of presumptive test; (see Table 62, page 664)	———
B. beef cell antigen test	0 (negative)	———
Urine analysis	may show albumin, bilirubin, and red cells	negative
Bleeding time	normal or increased	1 to 3 min. (Duke method)
Coagulation time	normal	varies with method
Serum bilirubin	normal or increased	0.2 to 0.8 mg. per 100 ml.
Thymol turbidity	normal or increased	0.4 to 4.0 units
Alkaline phosphatase stain	values decreased	13 to 100
Bone marrow examination	lymphocytes 15%–35%	lymphocytes 5%–15%
Cerebrospinal fluid (CSF)		
Lymphocytes	may be increased	0 to 10 per cu. mm.
Total proteins	may be increased	15 to 45 mg. per 100 ml.
Pandy's test	may be positive	negative
Serum glutamic oxalic transaminase (SGO-T)	normal or increased	8 to 50 units
Serum glutamic pyruvic transaminase (SGP-T)	normal or increased	5 to 45 units
Test for syphilis	may be positive	negative

PLATE 21

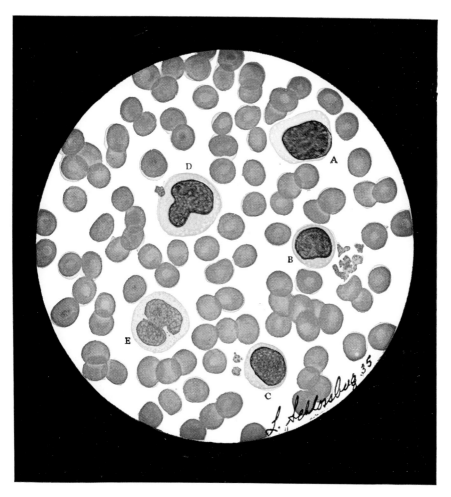

INFECTIOUS MONONUCLEOSIS. (WRIGHT'S STAIN, × 1200.)

A, Lymphocyte with moderately dense chromatin and vacuolated cytoplasm; *B,* small lymphocyte, normal except for a few vacuoles in the cytoplasm; *C,* lymphocyte with less dense chromatin in the nucleus and several azurophilic granules as well as a few vacuoles in the cytoplasm; *D,* lymphocyte which might be mistaken for a monocyte on account of its size and the shape of the nucleus. The coarse character of the chromatin and the blue, vacuolated cytoplasm contrast with the fine nuclear chromatin, fine granulation and gray-blue cytoplasm of a monocyte *(E).* *(Wintrobe, Tice, Practice of Medicine, courtesy of W. F. Prior Company.)*

MULTIPLE MYELOMA

Myeloma means marrow tumor; thus, multiple myeloma may be interpreted as simply meaning many tumors of the bone marrow.

Multiple myeloma is also referred to by the following terms: myeloma, plasmocytoma, plasma cell myeloma, myelomatosis, and Kahler's disease.

The discussion will cover basic clinical information, factors affecting laboratory examinations, and results of laboratory examinations.

Basic Clinical Information

Multiple myeloma is a malignant tumor of the bone marrow involving the plasmacytes and usually characterized by the production of excessive and abnormal proteins. The cause is unknown. This disease strikes 1 in every 100,000 persons each year and it is found most frequently in the male patient past the age of 50.

The typical patient complains about feeling weak and having pains in the back, chest, and extremities.

The doctor observes that the patient has small masses or swellings on the bones of the shoulders, ribs, and backbone.

The diagnosis will be made from the results of the physical examination, laboratory examinations, and x-ray examination of the bones.

The routine laboratory examinations usually include a white cell count, red cell count, hemoglobin determination, differential white cell count, stained red cell examination, sedimentation rate, urine analysis, test for Bence Jones protein, total serum proteins, and A/G ratio.

Additional laboratory examinations may include an electrophoresis of serum proteins, bone marrow examination, platelet count, bleeding time, test for serum cryoglobulins, serum calcium, uric acid, urea nitrogen, and nonprotein nitrogen.

If the patient does have multiple myeloma, treatment will be aimed at administering sedatives to relieve the pain and endeavoring to destroy the tumors with x-rays and chemicals.

The prognosis is poor, most patients die within 5 years.

Now let us consider the manner in which this disease affects the laboratory examinations.

Factors Affecting Laboratory Examinations

In multiple myeloma, a cancer-like growth of plasmacytes causes a slow destruction of bones and an excessive production of proteins.

The slow destruction of bones causes the calcium in the blood to rise above the normal values.

The excessive production of proteins causes the total serum proteins to rise above the normal values.

In health, the total serum proteins are about 6 grams per 100 milliliters of serum. These 6 grams consist of about 4 grams albumin and 2 grams globulin. This gives a normal albumin-globulin ratio of 4 to 2.

A ratio of 4 to 2 is usually expressed as 2:1 or 2/1.

In multiple myeloma, however, the total serum proteins may be increased to about 12 grams. These 12 grams are made up of about 4 grams albumin and 8 grams globulin. This gives an *abnormal* albumin-globulin ratio of 4 to 8.

A ratio of 4 to 8 is usually expressed as 1:2 or 1/2.

Thus, in multiple myeloma, the A/G ratio is said to be inversed, going from a normal of 2/1 to an abnormal of 1/2.

You will note that the albumin is about 4 grams in health and also about 4 grams in multiple myeloma.

Since the albumin remains practically constant, the inverse A/G ratio is due to the increase in globulin.

To summarize:

	Total Proteins	*Albumin*	*Globulin*	*A/G Ratio*
In health	6	4	2	2/1
In multiple myeloma	12	4	8	1/2

The excessive proteins soon clog the urinary tubules and the urine shows casts and also albumin.

As the excessive proteins continue to clog the urinary tubules and the waste materials accumulate in the blood, the following tests rise above their normal blood levels:

uric acid
urea nitrogen
nonprotein nitrogen

The excessive proteins in the blood may cause the red cells to assume a stacked formation called rouleau formation.

Thus, the stained red cell examination may show rouleau formation of the red cells; it may also show a few nucleated red cells.

The piling up or rouleau formation of red cells causes these red cells to fall faster in their plasma. Thus, increased values are found in the sedimentation rate.

An electrophoresis examination of the blood proteins reveals the presence of abnormal proteins.

One of these abnormal proteins—cryoglobulin—may sometimes be identified in the blood.

Another abnormal protein—the Bence Jones protein—may be found in the urine.

The finding of Bence Jones protein in the urine is significant, for this abnormal protein is rarely found in any other disease. It is present in multiple myeloma, however, in only about half the cases.

When the blood is diluted for the red cell count, the presence of excessive and abnormal proteins may produce a clumping of the red cells.

The clumping of the red cells is usually due to a reaction between the globulin in the blood and the mercury in Hayem's diluting fluid. The reaction results in the precipitation of the globulin and a bunching or clumping of the suspended red cells.

(The clumping of red cells, however, may also be caused by the presence of cold agglutinins in a patient's blood.)

If clumping of the red cells occurs, it will be noticed in the counting chamber during the red cell count and it will be impossible to make an accurate count unless the situation is remedied.

If clumping of the red cells occurs, the red cell count can be performed by proceeding as follows.

1. Obtain either physiological (0.85%) saline or Gower's solution.
2. Warm the solution until it is about body temperature (37° C.).
3. Using the solution as a diluting fluid, proceed to make another red cell count.
4. Make a notation of this abnormal clumping of red cells in your report.

As the disease advances, the cancer-like growth of plasmacytes in the bone marrow interferes with the normal production of red cells and platelets.

A decrease in the production of red cells and platelets causes a drop in the red cell count, hemoglobin, and platelet count.

A decrease in the number of platelets causes an increase in the bleeding time.

The white cell count is of little diagnostic significance because it may be below normal, normal, or above normal.

The differential white cell count may show a few plasmacytes, neutrophilic myelocytes, and neutrophilic metamyelocytes.

The bone marrow examination is significant. It reveals an increase in plasmacytes, proplasmacytes, and plasmablasts. Some of these cells may be normal, most are abnormal. These abnormal cells are referred to as "myeloma" cells.

The abnormalities in the myeloma cells may consist of the following:

1. The myeloma cells may vary greatly in size; the cells may be 2 to 6 times larger than a neutrophilic segmented cell.
2. The nucleus may be single, double, or triple; the nucleus may contain large nucleoli; the nucleus may be near the border of the cell.
3. The cytoplasm may contain large vacuoles.

The myeloma cells are illustrated in Figure 183.

The x-ray examination of the bones in multiple myeloma reveals characteristic punched-out lesions.

The results of the laboratory examinations in multiple myeloma are summarized in Table 64.

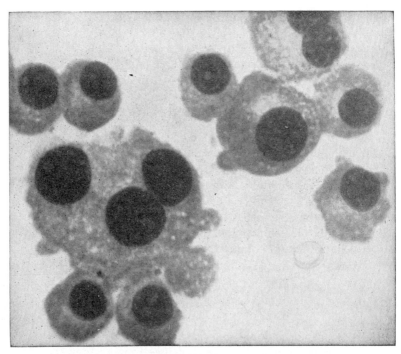

Fig. 183.—Myeloma cells. Bone marrow smear. (Reproduced from the 7th edition of "Clinical Laboratory Diagnosis" by Levinson and MacFate.)

Table 64

Results of Laboratory Examinations in Multiple Myeloma

Laboratory Examinations	Values in Multiple Myeloma	Values in Health
White cell count	4,000 to 16,000 per cu. mm.	5,000 to 10,000 per cu. mm.
Red cell count	3 to 5 million per cu. mm.	4 to 6 million per cu. mm.
Hemoglobin determin.	8 to 12 grams per 100 cc.	12 to 18 grams per 100 cc.
Differential W.C.C.		
Neutrophilic myelocytes	0% to 3%	0%
Neut. metamyelocytes	0% to 5%	0%
Plasmactyes	0% to 10%	0%
Stained red cell exam		
Nucleated red cells	0 to 6 per 100 white cells	0 per 100 white cells
Rouleau formation	present	absent
Sedimentation rate	increased	varies with method
Urine analysis		
Albumin	positive	negative
Casts	present	absent
Bence Jones protein	positive (in ½ of cases)	negative
Serum proteins		
Total proteins	usually increased	6.0 to 8.0 grams per 100 ml.
Albumin	usually normal	4.6 to 6.7 grams per 100 ml.
Globulin	usually increased	1.2 to 2.3 grams per 100 ml.
A/G ratio	usually 1/2	2/1
Electrophoresis exam		
Abnormal proteins	present	absent
Bone marrow exam		
Myeloma cells	10% to 90%	0%
Platelet count	100,000 to 400,000 per cu. mm.	150,000 to 400,000 per cu. mm.
Bleeding time	normal or increased	1 to 3 min. (Duke method)
Serum cryoglobulins	may be present	none
Serum calcium	usually increased	9.0 to 11.5 mg. per 100 ml.
Uric acid	usually increased	2 to 4 mg. per 100 ml.
Urea nitrogen (BUN)	usually increased	10 to 15 mg. per 100 ml.
Nonprotein nitrogen (NPN)	usually increased	25 to 35 mg. per 100 ml.

HODGKIN'S DISEASE AND GAUCHER'S DISEASE

In this section, we will meet two more abnormal cells: The Sternberg-Reed cell of Hodgkin's disease and Gaucher's cell of Gaucher's disease.

HODGKIN'S DISEASE

Hodgkin's disease is also referred to by the following terms: malignant lymphoma, lymphadenoma, lymphogranulomatosis, infectious granuloma, and malignant granuloma.

The discussion will cover basic clinical information, factors affecting laboratory examinations, and results of laboratory examinations.

Basic Clinical Information

Hodgkin's disease is an enlargement of the lymphatic tissue which usually begins in the neck and spreads throughout the body. The cause is unknown. This disease may affect man, woman, or child.

The typical patient complains about being tired and having chills, sweats, and intense itching sensations.

The patient may also complain about frequent fevers, loss of weight, and pains in the chest, back, or stomach.

The doctor observes that the patient has enlarged lymph nodes in the neck and that the spleen and liver are enlarged.

The diagnosis will be made from the results of the physical examination and laboratory examinations.

The routine laboratory examinations usually include a white cell count, red cell count, hemoglobin determination, differential white cell count, and stained red cell examination.

Additional laboratory examinations may include a bone marrow examination and a biopsy of the lymph nodes.

If the patient does have Hodgkin's disease, the treatment will be aimed at the regression and destruction of the tumors by means of chemicals and x-rays.

The prognosis is not favorable. Although death usually comes within 5 years, it may be delayed for as long as 25 years.

Factors Affecting Laboratory Examinations

In Hodgkin's disease, normal lymphatic tissue is being replaced by abnormal lymphatic tissue.

The abnormal lymphatic tissue contains a cell which is characteristic of the disease. This cell is known as the Sternberg-Reed cell.

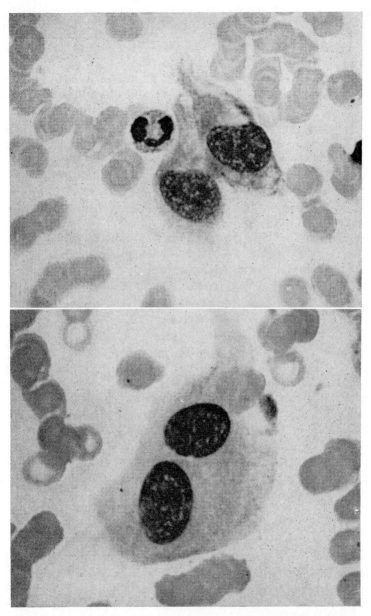

Fig. 184.—Sternberg-Reed cells. Two Sternberg-Reed cells lie near the neutrophilic segmented cell in the upper portion of the illustration. Note the difference
in size between the Sternberg-Reed cell and the neutrophilic segmented cell. Also
note the two nuclei in the Sternberg-Reed cell in the lower portion of the illustration.
The cytoplasm of the Sternberg-Reed cell stains a light blue. (Courtesy of Ludman
and Spear. Blood 12: 189, 1957.)

The Sternberg-Reed cell is also referred to by the following terms: Reed-Sternberg cell, Sternberg cell, and Dorothy Reed cell.

The Sternberg-Reed cell is about 5 times larger than a neutrophilic segmented cell.

The nucleus of the cell usually consists of 2 or 3 lobes. The nucleus also usually contains several light blue nucleoli which are as large as erythrocytes.

The cytoplasm of the cell stains light blue and may contain vacuoles.

The Sternberg-Reed cell is illustrated in Figure 184.

In Hodgkin's disease, the Sternberg-Reed cell is rarely found in the blood stream, occasionally found in a bone marrow examination, and often found in a biopsy of the lymph nodes.

Thus, a bone marrow examination and biopsy of the lymph nodes are of considerable diagnostic significance.

The biopsy of the lymph nodes is usually undertaken with caution, however, because the excision may activate a subclinical case.

The routine laboratory examinations are affected as follows.

Since the normal lymphatic tissue is being replaced by abnormal lymphatic tissue, the production of lymphocytes is decreased. As a result, the lymphocytes in the blood stream are decreased.

The differential white cell count reveals this decrease in lymphocytes and shows an increase in neutrophils, eosinophils, and monocytes.

The white cell count is usually slightly elevated, ranging between 10,000 and 20,000 per cubic millimeter.

The red cell count and hemoglobin are usually below normal.

The stained red cell examination reveals that the red cells are normal in size and color.

Thus, in Hodgkin's disease, the routine laboratory examinations are of little diagnostic significance; but the finding of the Sternberg-Reed cell in a bone marrow smear or biopsy of the lymph nodes is of paramount diagnostic significance.

GAUCHER'S DISEASE

The discussion will cover basic clinical information, factors affecting laboratory examinations, and results of laboratory examinations.

Basic Clinical Information

Gaucher's disease is inherited and confined mainly to Jews.

The disease is considered to be caused by a disturbance in the cellular metabolism of lipids.

Gaucher's disease may affect either male or female and it is most frequently discovered in childhood.

The typical patient complains about being tired and having a heavy dragging sensation in the stomach.

The patient may also complain about bleeding from the nose and mouth, having pains in the legs, and a swelling of the joints.

The doctor observes that the patient has a yellowish-brown pigmentation of the skin, the eyes have pale yellow deposits, and the spleen and liver are enlarged.

The diagnosis will be made from the results of the physical examination and laboratory examinations.

The routine laboratory examinations usually include a white cell count, red cell count, hemoglobin determination, differential white cell count, stained red cell examination, and platelet count.

Additional laboratory examinations may include a bone marrow examination or biopsy of the spleen.

If the patient does have Gaucher's disease, treatment will be aimed at relieving the discomfort of the patient. This may include medications, blood transfusions, and even removal of the spleen.

The prognosis varies from patient to patient. If the disease is mild, the patient may live practically a normal life. If the disease is severe, however, the patient may die an early death.

Factors Affecting Laboratory Examinations

A lipid substance, kerasin, accumulates in the reticulum cells. These cells are then referred to as Gaucher's cells. Gaucher's cells slowly "saturate" the spleen, liver, and bone marrow.

Gaucher's cell is usually about 5 times larger than a neutrophilic segmented cell but the diameter may range between 20 and 80 microns.

The nucleus of the cell is small, it is usually located near the border of the cell, and it may be single, double, or triple.

The cytoplasm of the cell is abundant and it is wrinkled or fiber-like in appearance.

Gaucher's cell is illustrated in Figure 185, page 676.

If special staining techniques are employed, Gaucher's cell will reveal the presence of kerasin.

In Gaucher's disease, Gaucher's cells are rarely found in the blood stream, occasionally found in a bone marrow examination, and often found in a biopsy of the spleen.

Thus, a bone marrow examination or biopsy of the spleen are of considerable diagnostic significance.

What changes occur in the routine laboratory examinations?

As Gaucher's cells slowly infiltrate the bone marrow, they crowd out the areas which are normally reserved for the production of white cells, red

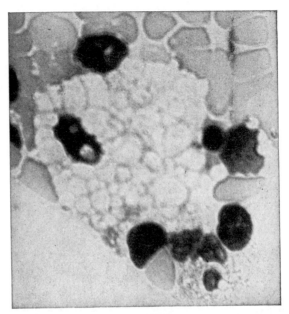

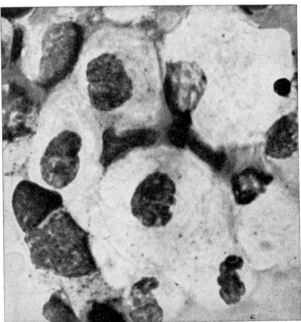

FIG. 185.—Pick's cell (upper illustration) and Gaucher's cell (lower illustration). Bone marrow smears. These cells are usually about 5 times larger than a neutrophilic segmented cell. Note that Pick's cell has a foamy cytoplasm whereas Gaucher's cell has a wrinkled or fiber-like cytoplasm. (Reproduced from the 7th edition of "Clinical Laboratory Diagnosis" by Levinson and MacFate.)

cells, and platelets. This decreases the production of white cells, red cells, and platelets. Consequently, the following examinations drop below normal:

> white cell count
> red cell count
> hemoglobin determination
> platelet count

The differential white cell count reveals a lymphocytosis and the stained red cell examination may show red cells which are normal in size but slightly deficient in hemoglobin.

The lipids of the blood are within the normal range of 400 to 900 milligrams per 100 milliliters.

The serum acid phosphatase is usually above the normal values of 0 to 1 Bodansky units.

If the lipid in the spleen is examined, it is found to be mostly cerebroside kerasin.

Thus, in Gaucher's disease, the routine laboratory examinations are of little diagnostic significance; but the finding of Gaucher's cells in a bone marrow examination or biopsy of the spleen is of considerable diagnostic significance.

DISEASES AND ANOMALIES RARELY ENCOUNTERED

In this section, we will briefly consider 17 diseases and anomalies rarely encountered.

The diseases and anomalies will be grouped and discussed under the following headings:

> Anemias Rarely Encountered
> Leukemias Rarely Encountered
> Hemorrhagic Diseases Rarely Encountered
> Additional Diseases Rarely Encountered
> Anomalies Rarely Encountered

ANEMIAS RARELY ENCOUNTERED

We will very briefly discuss the anemia of lead poisoning, chronic cold agglutinin disease, and primaquine sensitivity anemia.

Anemia of Lead Poisoning

Anemia of lead poisoning is caused by prolonged exposure to lead.

This anemia is sometimes seen in house painters who have used lead based paints for long periods of time.

The urine is positive for lead and coproporphyrin.

The stained red cell examination shows basophilic stippling.

The basophilic stippling seen in the anemia of lead poisoning has been illustrated in Plate 11, page 278.

Chronic Cold Agglutinin Disease

Chronic cold agglutinin disease is an acquired hemolytic anemia which is caused by cold autoantibodies.

In blood specimens of this disease, the red cells may agglutinate at room temperature and thereby cause difficulty in performing a red cell count.

The red cell count may be performed, however, by heating either Gower's solution or physiological (0.85%) saline solution to body temperature (37° C.) and using this solution as the RBC diluting fluid.

Primaquine Sensitivity Anemia

Primaquine sensitivity anemia is a hemolytic anemia caused by primaquine, an antimalarial drug.

LEUKEMIAS RARELY ENCOUNTERED

Many of the rare forms of leukemia are so rare that they appear to exist only by definition.

We will very briefly discuss basophilic leukemia, eosinophilic leukemia, neutrophilic granulocytic leukemia, thrombocytic leukemia, mast cell leukemia, histiocytic leukemia, and stem cell leukemia.

Basophilic Leukemia

Basophilic leukemia is a rare form of leukemia in which the predominating white cells are basophils.

Eosinophilic Leukemia

Eosinophilic leukemia is a rare form of leukemia in which the predominating white cells are eosinophils.

Neutrophilic Granulocytic Leukemia

Neutrophilic granulocytic leukemia is also referred to as myeloid granulocytic leukemia and neutrophilic leukemia.

Neutrophilic granulocytic leukemia is a rare (and doubtful) form of leukemia in which the predominating white cells are neutrophilic segmented cells.

Thrombocytic Leukemia

Thrombocytic leukemia is also referred to as megakaryocytic leukemia and hemorrhagic thrombocythemia.

Thrombocytic leukemia is a rare form of leukemia in which the predominating cells are thrombocytes (platelets).

Mast Cell Leukemia

A mast cell is a connective tissue cell which contains basophilic granules in the cytoplasm and closely resembles a basophil.

The mast cell is also referred to as a tissue basophil.

Mast cell leukemia is a rare form of leukemia which is characterized by the presence of large numbers of mast cells.

Histiocytic Leukemia

Histiocytic leukemia is also referred to as leukemic reticuloendotheliosis.

A histiocyte is a large phagocytic cell which is found in the reticuloendothelial system.

Histiocytic leukemia is a rare form of leukemia in which the predominating cells are histiocytes.

Stem Cell Leukemia

Stem cell leukemia is also referred to as undifferentiated cell leukemia, embryonal leukemia, hemoblastic leukemia, hemocytoblastic leukemia, lymphoidocytic leukemia, and blast cell leukemia.

A stem cell is also referred to as a hemohistioblast. This cell is the mother cell of red cells, white cells, and platelets. It may give rise to a rubriblast, myeloblast, lymphoblast, monoblast, plasmablast, or megakaryoblast.

Stem cell leukemia is a rare form of leukemia in which the predominating cell is so primitive and immature that its classification is difficult to determine.

HEMORRHAGIC DISEASES RARELY ENCOUNTERED

We will very briefly discuss purpura simplex and Glanzmann's disease.

Purpura Simplex

Purpura simplex is a condition which is characterized by a tendency to bruise easily.

This condition occurs most frequently in females and it is often associated with rheumatic fever and rheumatoid arthritis.

The capillary resistance test may be positive but other coagulation tests are negative.

45

Glanzmann's Disease

A functional defect in platelets is referred to as thrombasthenia (throm′-bas-the′ne-ah).

Glanzmann's disease is also known as hereditary hemorrhagic thrombasthenia.

This disease is characterized by a functional defect in the platelets (thrombasthenia), a normal platelet count, an increased bleeding time, and a prolonged clot retraction time.

ADDITIONAL DISEASES RARELY ENCOUNTERED

We will discuss acute infectious lymphocytosis, erythremic myelosis, and Niemann-Pick disease.

Acute Infectious Lymphocytosis

Acute infectious lymphocytosis is a disease of children.

The cause of this disease is unknown, the symptoms are variable, and it usually runs a benign course.

The white cell count is elevated, usually running between 20,000 and 50,000 cells per cubic millimeter.

The differential white cell count shows 60% to 95% small lymphocytes.

What distinguishes acute infectious lymphocytosis from infectious mononucleosis?

In acute infectious lymphocytosis, the lymphocytes are normal in appearance and the heterophil agglutination test is negative; in infectious mononucleosis, however, the lymphocytes are abnormal in appearance and the heterophil agglutination test is positive.

Erythremic Myelosis

Erythremic myelosis is also referred to as erythroleukemia and Di Guglielmo's disease.

Erythremic myelosis is characterized by an overgrowth of erythropoietic cells in the bone marrow.

Thus, erythremic myelosis may be looked upon as a cancer-like growth of the red cells, whereas leukemia may be looked upon as a cancer-like growth of the white cells.

The cause of erythremic myelosis is unknown and it usually runs a course similar to leukemia.

The blood smear shows a few immature white cells and many nucleated red cells.

Niemann-Pick Disease

Niemann-Pcik disease is also referred to as lipoid histiocytosis.

Niemann-Pick disease is closely related to Gaucher's disease.

Both Niemann-Pick disease and Gaucher's disease (1) are inherited, (2) occur most frequently in children of Jewish parentage, and (3) are associated with the abnormal metabolism of lipids.

Niemann-Pick disease, however, is more deadly than Gaucher's disease. In Niemann-Pick disease, the patient usually dies in infancy or childhood. The average patient seldom lives past the age of five.

The laboratory examinations are affected as follows.

The red cell count and hemoglobin are usually below normal.

The differential white cell count may show lymphocytes and monocytes which have large vacuoles of lipid material in their cytoplasm.

The serum cholesterol is usually above the normal range of 150 to 250 milligrams per 100 milliliters.

The serum acid phosphatase is usually above the normal range of 0 to 1 Bodansky units.

A bone marrow examination or biopsy of the spleen reveals a cell which is characteristic of this disease. This cell is a reticulum cell or histiocyte which is loaded with lipid. It is called Pick's cell.

Pick's cell is usually about 5 times larger than a neutrophilic segmented cell but the diameter may range between 30 and 50 microns.

The nucleus of the cell is small and generally located near the border of the cell.

The cytoplasm of the cell is abundant and foamy in appearance.

Pick's cell and Gaucher's cell have some similar characteristics but they differ on the following basis:

In structure, Pick's cell contains the lipid substance sphingomyelin; Gaucher's cell contains the lipid substance kerasin.

In appearance, Pick's cell has a foamy cytoplasm; Gaucher's cell has a wrinkled or fiber-like cytoplasm.

Pick's cell and Gaucher's cell are illustrated in Figure 185, page 676.

ANOMALIES RARELY ENCOUNTERED

An anomaly is a marked deviation from the normal standard.

Anomaly is the singular form of the word and anomalies is the plural form.

We will consider two anomalies: Alder's anomaly and Pelger-Huët's anomaly.

Alder's Anomaly

Alder's anomaly is also referred to as the Alder-Reilly anomaly.

Alder's anomaly is an inherited condition which is characterized by the presence of large coarse granules in the granulocytes. The large coarse granules appear in both the nucleus and cytoplasm. Sometimes the large coarse granules are also seen in the lymphocytes and monocytes.

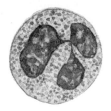 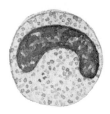 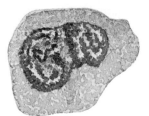

normal white cells

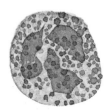 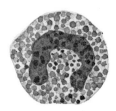 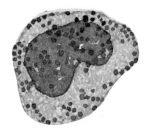

white cells in Alder's anomaly

FIG. 186—Normal white cells and white cells of Alder's anomaly. In the white cells of Alder's anomaly, note the large coarse granules in both the nucleus and cytoplasm. (Stain: Wright's; Magnification: 1500×.)

An illustration of the white cells in Alder's anomaly is given in Figure 186.

The abnormal granules of Alder's anomaly are similar to the toxic granules of agranulocytosis.

The abnormal granules of Alder's anomaly, however, are a permanent condition; but the toxic granules in agranulocytosis are only a temporary condition.

When Alder's anomaly is found in the blood, the patient is often afflicted with a deformity of the bones and joints.

Pelger-Huët's Anomaly

Pelger-Huët's anomaly is also referred to as Pelger's nuclear anomaly.

In this anomaly, the growth of the granulocytes appears stunted and the cells have difficulty in going through the final phases of development. Thus, very few band cells are able to blossom into segmented cells. The result is the formation of abnormal granulocytes which are referred to as Pelger's cells.

Pelger's cells are illustrated in Figure 187.

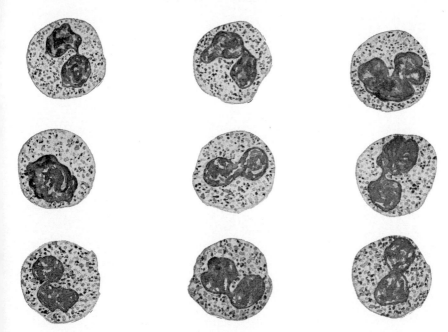

FIG. 187.—Pelger's cells. Note that the nucleus is abnormal in shape. The nucleus is also coarse and lumpy. (Stain: Wright's; Magnification: 1500×.)

Although Pelger's cells appear to be deformed granulocytes, they possess all the functional abilities of normal granulocytes.

Pelger-Huët's anomaly may be inherited or acquired; the acquired form may sometimes be seen in anemia and leukemia.

The significant laboratory examination is the differential white cell count which reveals a low percentage of neutrophilic segmented cells and a high percentage of Pelger's cells.

In some reports, Pelger's cells may be referred to as Pelger-Huët's cells.

STUDENT NOTES

Appendix

This appendix will cover the following:

Suggestions For a Short Introductory Course
Preparation of Solutions and Reagents
Dictionary of Miscellaneous Terms and Tests
Review Questions for National Registry and
State Board Examinations

The instructor in a clinic, hospital, private school, junior college, or university may find some useful material in the Suggestions For a Short Introductory Course. The student should make a superficial reading of the Preparation of Solutions and Reagents and a careful study of the Dictionary of Miscellaneous Terms and Tests and the Review Questions for National Registry and State Board Examinations.

SUGGESTIONS FOR A SHORT INTRODUCTORY COURSE

The instructor in a hospital laboratory finds that his students must "earn their keep" by performing routine laboratory tests.

The instructor in a private laboratory school finds that his students expect a practical economic approach to their study.

The instructor in biological sciences at a college or university finds that his students are hungry for some how-to knowledge of medical laboratory examinations.

These instructors may be interested in a practical and flexible introductory course in hematology.

The introductory course consists of 18 class meetings. A class meeting may last 2 or 3 hours, depending upon the size of the class. A small class may require 2 hours; a large class may require 3 hours.

The 18 class meetings may be completed in a few weeks or extended to several months. For example, the instructor in a hospital laboratory may have two class meetings a day. Whereas the instructor in a private school, college, or university may have one class meeting a week.

The 18 class meetings deal with the white cell count, red cell count, hemoglobin determination, and similar practical examinations.

The 18 class meetings may be increased to 19, 20, 21, etc. class meetings by simply performing additional tests.

The additional tests may include the reticulocyte count, eosinophil count, and tests of similar practical value.

The introductory course will be further discussed under the following headings:

SCHEDULE FOR THE INTRODUCTORY COURSE
OBTAINING BLOOD FOR THE VARIOUS TESTS
PREPARATION AND USE OF UNKNOWNS
PROCUREMENT AND USE OF ABNORMAL BLOOD SLIDES
NECESSARY EQUIPMENT AND REAGENTS

SCHEDULE FOR THE INTRODUCTORY COURSE

The schedule for the introductory course presents the home work and class work for the 18 class meetings.

The schedule includes numerous references to a complete blood count. The complete blood count is the backbone of the course. It consists of the following: white cell count, red cell count, hemoglobin determination, color index, differential white cell count, platelet estimation, and stained red cell examination.

The schedule for the introductory course is given below.

Class Meeting	Home Work	Class Work
1	Chap. 4	White cell count White cell count unknowns
2	Chap. 5	Red cell count Red cell count unknowns
3	Chap. 6	White cell count Red cell count Hemoglobin determination Color index
4	Chap. 7	Differential white cell count Platelet estimation
5	Chap. 8	Differential white cell count Platelet estimation Stained red cell examination
6	Review Chap. 4 through 8	Complete blood count
7	Chap. 1, 2	Finger puncture Complete blood count
8	Chap. 3	Finger puncture Complete blood count
9	Review Chap. 1 through 8	Finger puncture Complete blood count Written examination
10	Chap. 9, 10	Venipuncture Sedimentation rate Complete blood count Hematocrit reading
11	Chap. 17, 18	Bleeding time Coagulation time Complete blood count
12	Chap. 19	Platelet count Complete blood count White cell count unknowns
13	Chap. 34	Stained red cell examination on blood slide of iron deficiency anemia Stained red cell examination on blood slide of sickle cell anemia Complete blood count Red cell count unknowns Hemoglobin unknowns

Class Meeting	Home Work	Class Work
14	Chap. 35	Differential white cell count on blood slide of lymphocytic leukemia Differential white cell count on blood slide of granulocytic leukemia Complete blood count
15	Chap. 30	Stained red cell examination on blood slide of erythroblastosis fetalis Complete blood count Differential white cell count on blood slide of bone marrow
16	Chap. 37, Review Chap. 30, 34, 35	White cell count unknown Red cell count unknown Hemoglobin unknown Differential white cell count on blood slide of infectious mononucleosis Differential white cell count and stained red cell examination on blood slide of granulocytic leukemia
17	Review Chap. 30, 34, 35, 37	Complete blood count Differential white cell count and stained red cell examination on blood slide of bone marrow
18	Review	Practical examination Written examination

In the above schedule, the student performs 11 complete blood counts. This repetition may seem unnecessary but it is absolutely essential.

First, the repetition enables the student to discover and correct any mistakes in his procedure.

Second, the repetition enables the student to become familiar with the blood cells that are found in health. This background is necessary for the study of blood cells that are found in disease.

Third, the repetition enables the student to pick up his speed.

How fast should the student be?

When the student completes the course, he should be able to perform a complete blood count in 40 minutes. This is considered "slow." With practice, he should be able to run a complete blood count in 20 minutes.

OBTAINING BLOOD FOR THE VARIOUS TESTS

The introductory course calls for the use of blood containing an anticoagulant. Thus, oxalated blood, citrated blood, or Sequestrenized blood may be used.

The instructor in a hospital laboratory may obtain blood from a student or patient.

The instructor in a private school, college, or university may obtain blood from the following sources: students, hospitals, or blood banks. The average student, of course, is probably the best source of supply.

In class meetings 1 through 6, the instructor should issue about 1 cubic centimeter of anticoagulated blood to each student.

In class meetings 7, 8, 9, 11, and 12, the student is scheduled to obtain blood by performing a finger puncture. This finger puncture should be performed on a fellow student.

In class meeting 10, the student is scheduled to obtain blood by performing a venipuncture.

This venipuncture, of course, is optional.

The instructor in a private school, college, or university may wish to skip this venipuncture. For example, the class may be so large that the necessary supervision is impossible. In such cases, the instructor may simply issue oxalated blood to his students.

The instructor in a hospital laboratory may decide to have the students perform this venipuncture and several additional venipunctures. The additional venipunctures may be spliced into the latter portions of the course. They may be performed on fellow students or congenial patients.

PREPARATION AND USE OF UNKNOWNS

The introductory course calls for "unknowns." These unknowns are samples of blood. They are used to check the work of the student.

For example, the instructor prepares a test tube of blood having a high white cell count. He runs a count on this blood and finds the count to be 20,000. He issues this blood to a student and tells him to run a white cell count.

If the student obtains a white cell count between 18,000 and 22,000, his procedure is satisfactory. On the other hand, if the student obtains a white cell count above or below these values, he is making a mistake in his procedure. His mistake, of course, should be discovered and corrected.

The instructor will find that it saves time in the long run to discover and correct these mistakes during the first few class meetings.

The preparation of the white cell count, red cell count, and hemoglobin unknowns is given below.

Preparation of White Cell Count Unknowns

Obtain 10 cubic centimeters of oxalated blood. Put 5 cubic centimeters in one test tube and 5 cubic centimeters in another test tube. Centrifuge both test tubes at full speed for 30 minutes.

Using a medicine dropper, remove and discard most of the plasma from each test tube. Using the medicine dropper, remove and save about 0.5 cubic centimeter of the top layer of cells from each test tube. Transfer this top layer of cells to a small test tube.

The top layer of cells, of course, is the "white cream" containing the white cells.

This blood will have a high white cell count. The count may be anywhere from 20,000 to 200,000. Check the white cell count on this blood.

The above blood will serve as a white cell count unknown.

Prepare a second white cell count unknown as follows: Take a portion of the above blood and dilute it with either physiological saline or plasma which was removed from the original test tubes. Check the white cell count on this diluted blood.

Make a third white cell count unknown as follows: Obtain a sample of normal oxalated blood. Check the white cell count on this blood.

Thus, the white cell count unknowns may have values similar to those given below:

White cell count unknown #1 = 50,000
White cell count unknown #2 = 20,000
White cell count unknown #3 = 8,000

If you wish to make additional white cell count unknowns, proceed as follows: Make 10 samples of the #1 unknown and label them 1 through 10. Make 10 samples of the #2 unknown and label them 11 through 20. Make 10 samples of the #3 unknown and label them 21 through 30.

Thus, all bloods labelled 1 through 10 may have a white cell count of 50,000. All bloods labelled 11 through 20 may have a white cell count of 20,000. All bloods labelled 21 through 30 may have a white cell count of 8,000. These facts, of course, will only be known by the instructor.

When the white cell count unknowns are not being used, they should be stored in the refrigerator. They will keep for about 10 days.

What is an acceptable report on a white cell count unknown?

As a general rule, the report of the student and the count of the instructor should not differ by more than 2,000. If the count is extremely high, however, wider differences should be acceptable.

Preparation of Red Cell Count Unknowns

Obtain 8 cubic centimeters of oxalated blood. Put 4 cubic centimeters in one test tube and 4 cubic centimeters in another test tube. Centrifuge both test tubes at full speed for about 8 minutes.

Using a 2 milliliter volumetric pipet, remove about 2 cubic centimeters of plasma from one test tube and *transfer it to the other test tube*. The test tube containing the additional 2 cubic centimeters of plasma will now have a low red cell count. The test tube lacking the 2 cubic centimeters of plasma will now have a high red cell count.

Check the red cell count on each test tube.

After you have checked the count, each test tube will serve as a red cell count unknown.

Make a third red cell count unknown as follows: Obtain a sample of normal oxalated blood. Check the red cell count on this blood.

Thus, the red cell count unknowns may have values similar to those given below:

Red cell count unknown #1 = 2.5 million
Red cell count unknown #2 = 7.5 million
Red cell count unknown #3 = 5.0 million

If you wish to make additional red cell count unknowns, proceed as follows: Make 10 samples of the #1 unknown and label them 1 through 10. Make 10 samples of the #2 unknown and label them 11 through 20. Make 10 samples of the #3 unknown and label them 21 through 30.

When the red cell count unknowns are not being used, they should be stored in the refrigerator.

The red cell count unknowns are subject to a gradual but continual hemolysis of red cells. This causes a slight drop in the red cell count. It is therefore advisable to check the count before the unknowns are issued.

If the red cell count is checked every time the unknowns are issued, the unknowns may be used for at least 10 days.

What is an acceptable report on a red cell count unknown?

As a general rule, the report of the student and count of the instructor should not differ by more than 1 million. This wide leeway is due largely to the inherent error in the method of performing the red cell count.

Preparation of Hemoglobin Unknowns

The red cell count unknowns, of course, may also be used as the hemoglobin unknowns.

The hemoglobin unknowns will thus have values similar to the following:

Hemoglobin unknown #1 (RBC unknown #1) = 8 grams
Hemoglobin unknown #2 (RBC unknown #2) = 20 grams
Hemoglobin unknown #3 (RBC unknown #3) = 14 grams

PROCUREMENT AND USE OF ABNORMAL BLOOD SLIDES

As indicated in the schedule for the introductory course, the student will run differential white cell counts and stained red cell examinations on various abnormal blood slides.

A total of 7 blood slides is required. These slides may be put in a small slide box and issued to the student for class meetings 13 to 17. The safe return of the slides, of course, should be the responsibility of the student.

Blood slides of the following will be needed:

1. Iron deficiency anemia
2. Sickle cell anemia
3. Lymphocytic leukemia
4. Granulocytic leukemia
5. Erythroblastosis fetalis
6. Infectious mononucleosis
7. Bone marrow

The above blood slides may be obtained from hospital laboratories or medical supply houses.

If the instructor wishes, he may prepare his own blood slides. With a test tube of *fresh* oxalated blood, for example, he can make dozens of blood slides. The anticoagulated blood used to make the blood slides should be fresh, that is, it should not be over 2 hours old. If "old blood" is used, the white cells may be greatly distorted.

The blood slides should be stained and labelled with the name of the disease.

The instructor may also make "unknown" slides. For example, he can make a slide of sickle cell anemia and label the slide #10; he can make a slide of granulocytic leukemia and label the slide #20.

The instructor can use these "unknown" slides in various ways:

He may issue these "unknown" slides to his advanced students and have them run a differential white cell count and a stained red cell examination.

He may also use these "unknown" slides in the final practical examination. For example, he can issue an "unknown" slide to each student and have him run a differential white cell count and a stained red cell examination.

NECESSARY EQUIPMENT AND REAGENTS

In the introductory course, the following tests are performed: complete blood count, sedimentation rate, hematocrit reading, bleeding time, coagulation time, and platelet count.

These tests may be performed by various methods. For example, the sedimentation rate may be performed by the Westergren method, Cutler method, Landau micro method, or Wintrobe method.

In teaching the beginner, we have found the following methods satisfactory:

Test	*Method*
Complete blood count	
white cell count	microscopic method
red cell count	microscopic method
hemoglobin determination	Haden-Hausser method
color index	short method of calculation
differential white cell count	slide method (Wright's stain)
platelet estimation	
stained red cell examination	slide method (Wright's stain)
Sedimentation rate	Wintrobe method
Hematocrit reading	Wintrobe method
Bleeding time	Duke method
Coagulation time	capillary tube method
Platelet count	Rees and Ecker method

To perform the tests by the above methods, 50 items of equipment and reagents are required.

The complete blood count requires 35 items of equipment and reagents. These are listed below as items 1 to 35.

The remaining tests require 15 additional items of equipment and reagents. These are listed below as items 36 to 50.

If the instructor is not using the above methods, he may turn to his method of choice and find a list of the necessary equipment and reagents.

What is the price of the equipment and reagents?*

1. Microscope (must have oil immersion objective)
2. Microscope light
3. Counting chamber (for white cell counts and red cell counts)
4. Coverglass for counting chamber
5. Petri dish (to store counting chamber and coverglass)
6. White cell pipets
7. Red cell pipets
8. Rubber sucking tubes for pipets
9. 1% hydrochloric acid (diluting fluid for white cell count)
10. Hayem's solution (diluting fluid for red cell count)
11. Hemoglobinometer for hemoglobin estimation (Haden-Hausser preferred)
12. Suction device to attach to faucet (for cleaning pipets)
13. Stylets (for cleaning clogged pipets)
14. Medicine glasses (for holding test tubes of blood)

* A microscope costs $125 to $325. A counting chamber about $15. A hemoglobinometer about $20. A centrifuge about $90. The other items in the list will *average* about $1 per item. Thus, minus the microscope, the total cost will be about $175.

15. Glass slides (to make blood smears)
16. Round wooden applicator sticks (to place drop of blood on slide)
17. Staining rack and dish (to stain blood smears)
18. Wright's stain
19. Buffer solution for Wright's stain (pH 6.4 preferred)
20. Distilled water (to flush excess stain off slide)
21. Immersion oil
22. Lens paper
23. Xylene (to clean microscope lens)
24. Sterile blood lancets (for finger punctures)
25. 70% alcohol
26. Cotton balls
27. Test tubes of oxalated blood (for blood counts)
28. Small test tubes (no longer than 3 inches) to hold blood samples
29. Stoppers for the above test tubes
30. Several beakers (200 milliliter and 400 milliliter size)
31. Medicine droppers (to prepare unknowns)
32. Blood slides of iron deficiency anemia, sickle cell anemia, lymphocytic leukemia, granulocytic leukemia, erythroblastosis fetalis, infectious mononucleosis, and bone marrow
33. Small slide box to hold the above slides
34. Brush to clean slides
35. Bunsen burner (to "flame dry" clean slides)
36. Sterile 20 gauge needle
37. Sterile 10 cc. syringe
38. Tourniquet
39. Anticoagulant (Sequestrene preferred)
40. Serological test tubes and stoppers
41. Wax marking pencil
42. Wintrobe tubes
43. Wintrobe sedimentation rate rack
44. Wintrobe pipet (to fill Wintrobe tubes)
45. Centrifuge (to perform hematocrit reading and prepare unknowns)
46. Wintrobe tube cleaner (to clean Wintrobe tubes)
47. Filter paper (for bleeding time)
48. Capillary tubes (for coagulation time)
49. Rees and Ecker solution (for platelet count)
50. Funnel (to filter above solution)

PREPARATION OF SOLUTIONS AND REAGENTS

This section will consider *only* those solutions and reagents whose preparation has not been given in the text.

To obtain directions for preparing a particular solution, reagent, or stain which is not listed in this section, refer to the Index and then proceed to the page indicated.

First, let us consider the commonly used weights and measures and the balances employed in weighing.

The abbreviations, equivalents, and rough examples of the most commonly used weights and measures are summarized in Table 65.

Table 65.—Commonly Used Weights and Measures

Weights

Weight	Abbreviation	Equivalent	Rough Example
milligram	mg.	$\frac{1}{1000}$ of a gram	An eyelash weighs about 1 mg.
gram	G or Gm.	$\frac{1}{1000}$ of a kilogram	A large pea weighs about 1 gram
kilogram	kg. or kilo.	1000 grams	A kilogram is equal to 2.2 pounds

Measures

Measure	Abbreviation	Equivalent	Rough Example
cubic centimeter	cc.	$\frac{1}{1000}$ of a liter	There are about 15 drops of water in 1 cc.
milliliter	ml.	$\frac{1}{1000}$ of a liter	An ml. equals 1 cc. Thus, there are also about 15 drops of water in 1 ml.
liter	L.	1000 cc. or 1000 ml.	A liter is slightly larger than a quart
millimeter	mm.	$\frac{1}{10}$ of a centimeter	There are about 2.5 cm. or 25 mm. in 1 inch
cubic millimeter	cu. mm.	$\frac{1}{1000}$ of a cc.	In 1 drop of water, there are about 67 cu. mm.

For weighing, either a rough balance or an analytical balance may be used (Fig. 188).

The rough balance is easy to operate, requires very little time, and is sufficiently accurate for most weighings.

The analytical balance is rather difficult to operate, requires considerable time, but is extremely accurate.

The type of balance to be employed is specified with each weighing operation.

A Warning to the Beginner

Some solutions are very corrosive and could give you a severe burn.

Handle the solutions listed below with caution, being careful not to get any on your fingers, or especially, in your eyes or mouth.

glacial acetic acid
concentrated hydrochloric acid (HCl)
concentrated sulfuric acid (H_2SO_4)
concentrated nitric acid (HNO_3)
concentrated sodium hydroxide (NaOH)
concentrated potassium hydroxide (KOH)

If an accident occurs and you do get any of the above solutions on your body, *immediately flood the area with water*.

Potassium cyanide is a deadly poison. (It is used in the preparation of Drabkin's solution; Drabkin's solution is used in the cyanmethemoglobin method of performing the hemoglobin determination.) Avoid inhaling any cyanide fumes from any *concentrated* cyanide solutions. Dilute cyanide solutions are not dangerous unless, of course, they are swallowed in large quantities.

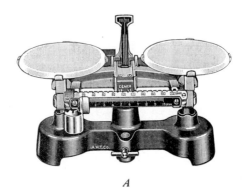

A

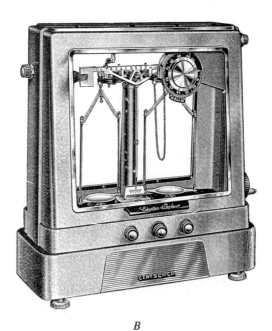

B

Fig. 188.—Analytical and rough balances.
A, rough balance; *B*, analytical balance.

Acetic Acid Solution

a. 2% acetic acid:
Place 98 cc. of distilled water in a container. Add 2 cc. of glacial acetic acid. Mix.

b. 10% acetic acid:
Place 90 cc. of distilled water in a container. Add 10 cc. of glacial acetic acid. Mix.

1% Ammonium Oxalate Solution

Using the rough balance, weigh out 1 gram of ammonium oxalate. Transfer to a container and add 99 cc. of distilled water. Mix. Store in the refrigerator. Filter before use.

Brilliant Cresyl Blue Solution

a. 1% methyl alcohol solution of brilliant cresyl blue:
Using the rough balance, weigh out 1 gram of brilliant cresyl blue. Place in a container and add 99 cc. of methyl alcohol. Mix and filter.

b. 1% physiological saline solution of brilliant cresyl blue:
Using the rough balance, weigh out 1 gram of brilliant cresyl blue. Place in a container and add 99 cc. of physiological (0.85%) saline. Mix and filter.

Calcium Chloride Solution

0.025 (fortieth) molar calcium chloride:
Using the analytical balance, weigh out 1.3875 grams of *anhydrous* calcium chloride. Place in a 500 cc. volumetric flask and add distilled water to the 500 cc. mark. Mix.

0.5% Copper Sulfate Solution

Using the analytical balance, weigh out 0.50 gram of *anhydrous* copper sulfate. Place in a 100 cc. volumetric flask and add distilled water to the 100 cc. mark. Mix.

Dacie's Solution

This is a diluting fluid which may be used for the red cell count.
Place 99 cc. of 3% trisodium citrate in a container. Add 1 cc. of concentrated formalin. Mix.

Discombe's Diluting Fluid

Discombe's modification of Dunger's fluid for the eosinophil count consists of the following: 0.1 gram of aqueous eosin, 10 cc. of acetone, and 90 cc. of distilled water.

Drabkin's Solution

Using the rough balance, weigh out 1.0 gram of sodium bicarbonate (C.P.). Place in a 1 liter volumetric flask. Obtain a bottle of potassium cyanide (C.P.). Cyanide compounds are poisonous! Handle with care! Using the analytical balance, weigh out 52 milligrams of the potassium cyanide. Add it to the volu-

46

metric flask. Using the analytical balance, weigh out 198 milligrams of potassium ferricyanide (C.P.). Add it to the volumetric flask. Now add distilled water to the 1 liter mark on the volumetric flask. Mix. Transfer the solution to a brown bottle. Store in the dark.

Dunger's Diluting Fluid

This diluting fluid for the eosinophil count consists of the following: 5 cc. of 2% aqueous eosin, 5 cc. of acetone, and 90 cc. of distilled water.

Eosin Solution

0.1% aqueous solution of eosin:
Using the rough balance, weigh out 0.2 gram of eosin. Transfer to a container and add 200 cc. of distilled water. Mix. Filter before use.

Gower's Solution

Using the rough balance, weigh out 62.5 grams of crystalline sodium sulfate. Place in a 1 liter volumetric flask. Add about 500 cc. of distilled water. Add 167 cc. of glacial acetic acid. Dilute to the 1 liter mark with distilled water. Mix.

Hayem's Solution

Using the rough balance, weigh out 2.5 gram of mercuric chloride, 5.0 gram of sodium chloride, and 25 grams of crystalline sodium sulfate. Place in a 1 liter volumetric flask and add distilled water to the 1 liter mark. Mix.

Hydrochloric Acid Solution

a. 1% (about 0.1 normal) hydrochloric acid:
Place 99 cc. of distilled water in a container. Add 1 cc. of concentrated hydrochloric acid. Mix.
b. 2% (about 0.2 normal) hydrochloric acid:
Place 98 cc. of distilled water in a container. Add 2 cc. of concentrated hydrochloric acid. Mix.
c. 0.1 N hydrochloric acid:
Using a 10 ml. volumetric pipet, place exactly 10 ml. of 1 N HCl in a 100 ml. volumetric flask. Add distilled water to the 100 ml. mark. Mix.

Lugol's Solution

Also referred to as Lugol's iodine solution, Lugol's stock solution, and liquor iodi fortis (U.S.P.).
Using the rough balance, weigh out 5 grams of iodine and 10 grams of potassium iodide. Transfer to a brown bottle. Add 100 cc. of distilled water. Mix.

14% Magnesium Sulfate Solution

Using the rough balance, weigh out 14 grams of magnesium sulfate (C.P.). Transfer to a 100 cc. volumetric flask. Add distilled water to the 100 cc. mark. Mix. Store in the refrigerator. Filter before use.

Manner's Diluting Fluid

This diluting fluid for the eosinophil count consists of the following: 50 grams of urea, 0.1 gram of phloxine, 0.6 gram of trisodium citrate, and 100 cc. of distilled water.

1% Methyl Alcohol Solution of Methylene Blue

Using the rough balance, weigh out 1 gram of methylene blue. Transfer to a bottle. Add 99 cc. of methyl alcohol. Mix. Store in the refrigerator. Filter before use.

New Methylene Blue N Solution

Using the rough balance, weigh out 0.5 gram of new methylene blue N, 1.4 grams of potassium oxalate, and 0.8 gram of sodium chloride. Place in a clean brown bottle. Add 100 cc. of distilled water. Mix well. Store in the refrigerator. Filter before use.

Normal Saline Solution

See physiological (0.85%) saline solution.

Physiological (0.85%) Saline Solution

Also referred to as normal saline solution and physiological (0.85%) sodium chloride. Using the analytical balance, weigh out 8.50 grams of sodium chloride. Transfer to a 1 liter volumetric flask. Add distilled water to the 1 liter mark. Mix. Store in the refrigerator.

Randolph's Diluting Fluid

This diluting fluid for the eosinophil count consists of the following: 0.1 gram of phloxine, 100 cc. of 1% calcium chloride, and an equal volume of propylene glycol which is added just before use.

Rees and Ecker Solution

Using the rough balance, weigh out 0.1 gram of brilliant cresyl blue and 3.8 grams of sodium citrate. Place them in a 100 cc. volumetric flask. Add 0.2 cc. of 40% formaldehyde. Dilute to the 100 cc. mark with distilled water. Mix. Transfer to a bottle. Store in the refrigerator. Filter before use.

Safranin Solution

a. 0.1% aqueous solution:
Using the rough balance, weigh out 0.2 gram of safranin. Transfer to a bottle. Add 200 cc. of distilled water. Mix. Filter before use.
b. 1% aqueous solution:
Using the rough balance, weigh out 1 gram of safranin. Transfer to a bottle. Add 99 cc. of distilled water. Mix. Filter before use.

0.1% Sodium Carbonate Solution

Using the rough balance, weigh out 1 gram of *anhydrous* sodium carbonate. Transfer to a large bottle. Add 1 liter of distilled water. Mix.

Sodium Chloride Solutions (for the osmotic fragility test)

Dry some chemically pure (C.P.) sodium chloride in an oven or desiccator and then prepare the solutions as follows.

a. 0.85% sodium chloride
Using the analytical balance, weigh out 8.50 grams of the sodium chloride. Transfer to a 1 liter volumetric flask. Add distilled water to the 1 liter mark. Mix. Store in the refrigerator.
b. 0.50% sodium chloride
Using the analytical balance, weigh out 0.50 gram of the sodium chloride. Transfer to a 100 cc. volumetric flask. Add distilled water to the 100 cc. mark. Mix. Store in the refrigerator.

Sodium Citrate Solution

a. 3.8% sodium citrate solution:
Using the rough balance, weigh out 3.80 grams of sodium citrate. Transfer to a 100 cc. volumetric flask. Add distilled water to the 100 cc. mark. Mix. *Note:* This 3.8% sodium citrate solution was the original anticoagulant used in the Westergren method of performing the sedimentation rate. However, experience has shown that double oxalate or Sequestrene are equally satisfactory as anticoagulants for this method.
b. sterile 3.8% sodium citrate solution:
First, prepare the 3.8% sodium citrate solution as directed above. Then, autoclave it for 20 minutes at 15 lbs. pressure. Store in the refrigerator.
c. 5% sodium citrate solution:
Using the rough balance, weigh out 5.0 grams of sodium citrate. Transfer to a 100 cc. volumetric flask. Add distilled water to the 100 cc. mark. Mix.

Sodium Oxalate Solution

a. 1.10% sodium oxalate solution:
Using the analytical balance, weigh out 1.10 grams of *anhydrous* sodium oxalate. Place in a 100 cc. volumetric flask and add distilled water to the 100 cc. mark. Mix.
b. 1.30% sodium oxalate solution:
Using the analytical balance, weigh out 1.30 grams of *anhydrous* sodium oxalate. Place in a 100 cc. volumetric flask and add distilled water to the 100 cc. mark. Mix.
c. 1.34% sodium oxalate solution:
Using the analytical balance, weigh out 1.340 grams of *anhydrous* sodium oxalate. Place in a 100 cc. volumetric flask and add distilled water to the 100 cc. mark. Mix.

Sterile Physiological (0.85%) Saline Solution

Prepare the physiological (0.85%) saline solution as directed above (page 697). Then autoclave it for 20 minutes at 15 lbs. pressure. Store in the refrigerator.

Tannen's Diluting Fluid

a. Prepare a 0.2% neutral red iodide solution as follows:
Using the rough balance, weigh out 0.5 gram of neutral red iodide. (This reagent may be obtained from your local medical supply house or Allied Chemical and Dye Corp., 40 Rector St., New York, N.Y.) Transfer the 0.5 gram of neutral red iodide to a large bottle. Add 250 cc. of distilled water. Shake for 5 minutes. Filter.

b. Pour the filtered neutral red iodide into a 100 milliliter volumetric flask until the 100 milliliter mark is reached. Add exactly 2.1 milliliters of 0.1 N NaOH. Mix well. Filter. Store at room temperature for 6 days and then filter again. This solution is stable.

Toison's Solution

This diluting fluid for the red cell count consists of the following: 1 gram of sodium chloride, 8 grams of sodium sulfate, 0.025 gram of methyl violet 5B, 30 cc. of glycerol, and 180 cc. of distilled water.

Türk's Solution

This diluting fluid for the white cell count consists of the following: 3 cc. of glacial acetic acid, 1 cc. of a 1% aqueous solution of gentian violet, and 100 cc. of distilled water. The function of the gentian violet is (1) to stain the nuclei of the white cells and thereby aid in identification and (2) to act as a preservative.

Wright's Stain and Buffer Solution

a. Wright's stain

Method One:
Using the rough balance, weigh out 3 grams of the powdered Wright's stain. Place in a container and add 1 liter of acetone-free methyl alcohol. Mix. Let stand for several days, mixing a few times each day. Filter before use.

Method Two:
Using the rough balance, weigh out 3 grams of powdered Wright's stain. Place in a container and add 30 cc. of glycerol. Mix thoroughly, grinding in a mortar if necessary. Place in a 37° C. incubator or water bath for a few days, stirring a few times each day. With constant stirring slowly add 1 liter of acetone-free methyl alcohol. Allow to "age" for a few days. Filter before use. This preparation of Wright's stain is recommended by many technologists.

b. Buffer solution
Wright's stain contains the acid stain eosin, which is red in color, and the basic stain methylene blue, which is blue in color. Consequently, the more acid (lower pH) the buffer solution, the more intense is the red coloration of the cells and the less pronounced is the blue coloration. On the other hand, the less acid (higher pH) the buffer solution, the less intense is the red coloration of the cells and the more pronounced is the blue coloration. Thus, it is apparent that the degree of acidity (pH) of the buffer solution is a very important factor in obtaining a good stain.

Experience has shown that a buffer solution which has a pH between 6.4 and 6.8 gives the best results. Some technologists prefer the color contrast which is obtained with a buffer solution of pH 6.4, whereas others like the buffer of pH 6.8. The best pH value is a matter of individual preference, and can be decided by experimentation.

Buffer solutions of various pH values are prepared by mixing two solutions of phosphate salts. The phosphate salt solutions should be kept in pyrex containers at refrigerator temperature. They are prepared as follows:

1. $\frac{M}{15}$Na$_2$HPO$_4$

Using the analytical balance, weigh out 9.470 grams of *anhydrous* secondary sodium phosphate, Na_2HPO_4, (or 11.870 grams of *hydrated* secondary sodium phosphate, $Na_2HPO_4.2H_2O$). Place in a 1 liter volumetric flask. Add distilled water to the 1 liter mark. Mix.

2. $\frac{M}{15}KH_2PO_4$

Using the analytical balance, weigh out 9.080 grams of primary potassium phosphate, KH_2PO_4. Place in a 1 liter volumetric flask. Add distilled water to the 1 liter mark. Mix.

To make a buffer solution of the desired pH, mix the quantities of phosphate solutions called for below.

pH	$\frac{M}{15}$ Na_2HPO_4	$\frac{M}{15}$ KH_2PO_4
6.4	26.7 cc.	73.3 cc.
6.5	31.8 cc.	68.2 cc.
6.6	37.5 cc.	62.5 cc.
6.7	43.5 cc.	56.5 cc.
6.8	49.6 cc.	50.4 cc.

DICTIONARY OF MISCELLANEOUS TERMS AND TESTS

Many terms and tests which the student will encounter have not been discussed in the body of the text.

For example, the term "Stat" is a common term meaning that a test should be performed immediately. This term will be frequently encountered. But it has not been mentioned in the body of the text.

Also, many tests useful in diagnosing blood diseases have not been discussed in the body of the text simply because they are not performed in the hematology department.

For instance, the Bence Jones protein examination may be useful in diagnosing multiple myeloma but this examination is performed in the urine analysis department.

These miscellaneous terms and tests will be covered in this section.

The student should first read the information dealing with the formation of words and then carefully study the terms and tests in the dictionary.

Formation of Words in Hematology

Words in hematology usually consist of one to three parts. These parts are called prefix, stem, and suffix. Consider a few examples.

The word erythrocyte is made up of two parts. The prefix *erythro* means red; the stem *cyte* means cell. Thus, erythrocyte means red cell.

The word hematology is also made up of two parts. The stem *hemat* means blood; the suffix *ology* means study. Thus, hematology is the study of blood.

An illustration of a word having all three parts is leukocytosis. This word means an increase in the number of white cells. It is broken down as follows:

prefix	stem	suffix
leuko	cyt	osis
white	cell	increase

These prefixes, stems, and suffixes were borrowed from the Latin and Greek during the early development of the English language; and even today, they serve as the building blocks of medical and scientific terminology.

The student can easily master hematologic words by keeping in mind the meaning of the prefixes, stems, and suffixes given in Table 66.

Table 66.—Prefixes, Stems, and Suffixes Used in the
Formation of Hematologic Words

Prefix, Stem, or Suffix	Meaning	Prefix, Stem, or Suffix	Meaning
a or an	without	mega	large
aniso	unequal	meniscus	crescent
anti	against	meta	after
auto	self	micro	small
baso	base	mono	one
bi	two	morpho	form
blast	germ	myelo	marrow
chrome	color	neo	new
crit	separate	nucleus	nut
cryo	cold	ology	study
cyte	cell	ortho	normal
emia	blood	osis	increase
eosin	dawn (red)	patho	disease
erythro	red	penia	poverty
globin	globe	phago	eat
granulo	granule	phile	love
hem or hemat	blood	plasia	formation
hyper	greater	poiesis	making
hypo	lesser	poikilo	variation
iso	same	poly	many
karyo	nut (nucleus)	post	after
leuk	white	pro	before
lympho	clear	pyro	fire
lysin	dissolve	reticulo	net
macro	large	thrombo	clot

absolute lymphocytosis

An increase in the total number of lymphocytes. It may be seen in mumps, whooping cough, German measles, infectious mononucleosis, lymphocytic leukemia, and acute infectious lymphocytosis. For further information, see Absolute Counts, pages 220, 222.

acetylcholinesterase

An enzyme found in erythrocytes.

acid hemolysin

A hemolysin is a substance which liberates hemoglobin from red cells. And an acid hemolysin is one which reacts best in an acid medium, that is, at a pH below 7.

activated clotting time

The activated clotting time is also referred to by the initials ACT and the activated coagulation time of whole blood. The activated clotting time is performed by drawing venous blood directly into a tube containing diatomite (Celite). Contact with the inert diatomite greatly shortens the clotting time, the normal values for this method being 1–2 minutes.

Adelson-Crosby method

This is a rather complicated method for determining the bleeding time. The normal values are 1–7 minutes and a blood loss less than 0.22 cubic centimeters.

agammaglobulinemia

The absence or deficiency of gamma globulin in the blood.

agglutinin

An antibody produced in the plasma in response to stimulation by a specific antigen.

agglutinogen

An antigen which stimulates the production of an agglutinin.

alkali (plural: alkalies)

A "strong" base. A group of compounds having marked basic properties such as the ability to neutralize acids, turn red litmus blue, etc. Examples are sodium carbonate and potassium carbonate.

anaphylaxis

A reaction to a foreign protein.

angina

A spasmodic choking pain.

anisochromia

Variation in the color of erythrocytes due to unequal hemoglobin content.

anoxia

Without oxygen. The reduction of oxygen in the tissues below physiological levels.

antibody

A substance which may be produced in the plasma in response to the presence of a specific antigen.

antibody titrations

A serial dilution of the serum is made, test cells are added, and the tubes are inspected for agglutination. Antibody titrations are usually performed in the blood bank department.

antigen

A substance which stimulates the production of an antibody.

antitrypsin test

A test based on the power of the serum to inhibit the action of trypsin. The antitryptic power of the serum is increased in cancer, nephritis, and many other diseases. The test is usually performed in the serology department.

aplasia
Lack of development of an organ.

aqueous
Watery. An aqueous solution is a solution prepared with water as the solvent.

Arneth classification
The Arneth classification is also known as the Arneth index, Arneth count, and Arneth formula. It is an old classification of the neutrophils which was based on the shape of the nucleus. The Arneth classification was rather complex and it was later simplified and modified by Schilling.

Arneth-Cooke count
Also called Cooke-Arneth count. A modification of the Arneth classification (see above).

artifact (or artefact)
Any artificial particle seen in cells, diluting fluids, urinary sediments, etc.

assay
1. The determination of the purity of a substance.
2. The amount of any particular constituent of a mixture.

autoantibodies
Antibodies which are capable of reacting on the patient's own red cells. For example, in paroxysmal cold hemoglobinuria, the patient develops antibodies which cause the hemolysis of his own red cells.

autoimmune hemolytic anemias
The autoimmune hemolytic anemias may be divided into 2 groups. One group is associated with warm antibodies. The other group is associated with cold antibodies.

azurophilic granules
Also referred to as azur granules and azurophil granules.
Granules that stain well with azure dyes. The granules are reddish in color. They may be large or small. Large azurophilic granules are often seen in the cytoplasm of lymphocytes. Small azurophilic granules are sometimes seen in the cytoplasm of monocytes. For illustration, see Plate 4, page 244.

Barr body
Sex chromatin.

basophilia
An abnormal increase in the number of basophilic (bluish staining) erythrocytes. If the erythrocytes contain coarse basophilic granules, it is called basophilic stippling. If the erythrocytes contain fine evenly distributed basophilic granules, it is called polychromatophilia. For illustration, see Plate 11, page 278.

Bence Jones protein examination
Bence Jones protein is a protein which was discovered by Bence Jones. It may be found in the urine in multiple myeloma and it has the following peculiar characteristics. It precipitates out at a temperature of about 50° C., partially or completely disappears when the temperature is raised to 100° C., and then reappears

upon cooling to room temperature (about 25° C.). The Bence Jones protein examination, which is performed in the urine analysis department, is also referred to as the heat precipitation test and the toluene sulfonic acid test.

beta thalassemia
A form of thalassemia in which beta chain synthesis is impaired.

Beutler's method
A method of performing the Heinz body stain.

Bl. & Coag. time
Bleeding and coagulation time.

blood dust
Blood dust is a term for the small "dancing" particles seen in blood. They are either round or dumbbell-shaped and they possess Brownian movement. Their origin is not definitely known. They are best observed using the dark-field condenser and the 95× (oil immersion) objective of the microscope. Blood dust is also referred to as hemoconia, hemokonia, and Müller's dust bodies.

blood dyscrasia
An abnormal or pathological condition of the blood.

blood urea nitrogen determination
Usually abbreviated BUN. A test for the waste product, urea nitrogen. The normal values are 10–15 milligrams per 100 milliliters of blood. Values above normal may be found in kidney disease and many other disorders. The determination is performed in the chemistry department.

blood volume determination
Also referred to as the total blood volume determination. The normal values are 54 to 84 milliliters per kilogram of body weight. Values above normal may be found in polycythemia vera. This determination is usually performed in the radioisotope department.

blood weight
About 8% of your weight is blood. Thus, if you weigh 100 pounds, you have about 8 pounds of blood.

Bl. & Ct.
Bleeding and clotting time.

buffer solution
A solution which will resist any change in acidity or alkalinity.

Bürker counting chamber
A counting chamber similar to the improved Neubauer ruling counting chamber (used in the white cell count and red cell count). The Bürker counting chamber has the same area (9 sq. mm.) and depth (0.1 mm.) as the improved Neubauer ruling counting chamber. The ruled lines, however, are slightly different.

capillary blood
Blood obtained from capillaries; for example, blood obtained from a finger puncture.

cascade or waterfall theory
A theory relating to the coagulation of blood.

CCV
Cell conductivity volume. The cell conductivity volume is directly related to the packed cell volume (hematocrit reading). Therefore, the cell conductivity volume is used as a measure of the packed cell volume (hematocrit reading) by some automatic cell counting instruments.

Charcot-Leyden crystals
Colorless, hexagonal, needle-like crystals. These crystals are derived from disintegrating eosinophils. They may be found in the sputum and bronchial secretions of patients with asthma and also in the feces of patients with parasitic infestations. Also called asthma crystals.

Chediak-Higashi anomaly
This is a rare inherited condition which is characterized by the presence of large granules and inclusion bodies in the cytoplasm of the white cells. It may occur in either sex and it is usually fatal. Also referred to as the Chediak-Higashi syndrome, anomalous panleukocytic granulation, and the Chediak-Steinbrinck-Higashi anomaly.

chloroma
A malignant tumor arising from myeloid tissue. It may occur anywhere in the body. And it is associated with granulocytic leukemia.

chromatin
The network of small fibers in the nucleus of a cell.

chromatin dust
Tiny red granules sometimes seen near the edge of erythrocytes in stained blood smears. These tiny granules are smaller than Howell-Jolly bodies. They are thought to be small particles of nuclear chromatin.

chromoprotein
A colored conjugated protein having respiratory functions. Example: hemoglobin.

chromosomal culture
An analysis of the chromosomes in white cells. In the future, this analysis may prove useful in our understanding of birth defects, some types of leukemia, and chromosomal abnormalities.

chromosome
A small rod-shaped body appearing in the nucleus of a cell during cell division. It contains the genes or hereditary factors of the species.

cold agglutinins
Agglutinins in the plasma which react best at temperatures between $0°$ C. and $20°$ C. These agglutinins are capable of reacting with red cells regardless of the blood group. They may even react on the patient's own red cells.

collagen disease
Collagen is a protein substance found in skin, tendon, bone, and cartilage. A collagen disease is a disease involving collagen tissue. For example, rheumatic

fever and systemic lupus erythematosus are collagen diseases. These diseases are usually accompanied by a high sedimentation rate.

collapsed vein

During a venipuncture, blood may cease to flow into a vein and the vein is said to be "collapsed." This may occur when a venipuncture is made on a small vein or a weak vein. It is caused by blood being withdrawn from the vein at a faster rate than it enters the vein.

complete antibody

An antibody which causes the agglutination of erythrocytes possessing the specific antigen when these erythrocytes are suspended in a saline solution.

Coombs' test

A test for the presence of Rh antibodies or blocking antibodies. The *direct* Coombs' test is performed on red cells and the *indirect* Coombs' test is performed on serum. These tests are usually performed in the blood bank department. Coombs' test is also referred to as Coombs' antiglobulin test, the antiglobulin test, and the antihuman globulin test.

coproporphyrin test

Coproporphyrin is a porphyrin formed in the intestine from bilirubin. Abnormal amounts of coproporphyrin may be present in the urine in some anemias. This test is performed in the chemistry department.

cord blood

Blood obtained from the umbilical vessels at birth.

counterstain

A stain used to make a previously applied stain more discernible.

C. P.

Chemically pure.

cu. μ

Cubic micron.

cryoglobulin test

Cryoglobulin is a serum globulin which precipitates, gels, or crystallizes spontaneously at low temperatures. The test is performed by placing serum in the refrigerator at 5° C. and then warming it to 37° C. If cryoglobulins are present a precipitate will form at the lower temperature and redissolve at the higher temperature. This test may be positive in multiple myeloma, collagen diseases, and many other disorders. The test is usually performed in the serology department.

cytogenetics

The branch of genetics concerned with the cellular elements involved in heredity, that is, the genes and chromosomes. Clinical cytogenetics deals with the relationship between chromosomal aberrations and pathological conditions.

cytology

The study of cells.

denaturation

The act of treating a protein with heat, acid, or alkali and thereby causing it to lose some of its original properties.

diathesis

A bodily condition or constitution predisposing to a disease.

dimorphism

The property of having or existing under two different forms.

Döhle bodies

Also referred to as Döhle's inclusion bodies and Amato bodies. These bodies are oval or spindle-shaped bodies which may be found in the cytoplasm of neutrophils. They stain light blue or blue-gray with Wright's stain. They are frequently seen in scarlet fever, measles, septicemia, burns, and pneumonia; they are sometimes seen in pernicious anemia, hemolytic anemia, and chronic granulocytic leukemia. These bodies are probably a by-product of the abnormal cellular metabolism which is found in toxic conditions.

Downey cells

An early grouping of the lymphocytes seen in infectious mononucleosis. Downey cell I was an atypical lymphocyte having many vacuoles in the cytoplasm. Downey cell II was an atypical lymphocyte with a nucleus like a plasma cell and having a few vacuoles in the cytoplasm. Downey cell III was an immature lymphocyte.

drumstick (drumstick appendage)

A nuclear lobule attached to the nucleus of a neutrophilic segmented cell. It is present in women but not in men. Hence, it may be useful in sex determination.

dyscrasia

A term generally used to indicate a morbid condition. An abnormal or pathological condition of the blood is referred to as a *blood dyscrasia*.

dyspnea

Difficulty in breathing.

dyspoiesis

An abnormality in the development of blood cells.

ecchymosis

Bleeding under the skin.

eclampsia

Convulsions.

emf

Erythrocyte maturation factor.

endothelioid cells

Large protoplasmic cells which are often seen in diseases of the blood-forming organs. They are believed by some investigators to be derived from the endothelial lining of blood and lymph vessels.

erythrocyte survival time

Also referred to as the red cell survival time and the red blood cell survival time. The normal values are a half-life of 55 to 65 days by the Ashby method and a half-life of 28 to 38 days by the radioactive chromium (Cr^{51}) method. The radioactive chromium (Cr^{51}) method is sometimes referred to as the radio-chromium (Cr^{51}) method. This determination is performed in the radioisotope department.

erythron

The tissue composed of the circulating red cells and their precursors.

etiology

A study of the cause of a disease.

fat cell

A connective tissue cell bloated with stored fat.

favism

An acute hemolytic anemia caused by eating fava beans. It is associated with an enzyme deficiency in the erythrocytes.

ferritin

An iron storing complex. One of the forms in which iron is stored in the body.

ferrokinetics

The turnover, or rate of exchange, of iron in the body.

Ferro-test

The trade-name of a test for serum iron and serum iron-binding capacity (sold by Hyland Laboratories).

folic acid

A widely distributed vitamin. It is an essential growth factor. A deficiency influences the development of the red cells in some cases of macrocytic anemia.

formiminoglutamic acid estimation

This acid accumulates in the urine during a deficiency of folic acid. Hence, its presence in increased amounts may indicate a deficiency of folic acid. The estimation, an electrophoretic analysis, is performed in the chemistry department.

Forssman antigen

An antigen made from the kidney of guinea pigs or horses. This antigen is capable of removing anti-sheep agglutinins from certain serums. It is used in the differential test for infectious mononucleosis. The test functions as follows: (1) The antigen removes the agglutinins if the patient does *not* have infectious mononucleosis. (2) But the antigen fails to remove the agglutinins if the patient does have infectious mononucleosis.

friable

Easily crumbled or pulverized.

g (or G)

1. An abbreviation for gram or grams.
2. Gravity or gravities. A unit of force. The symbol g is sometimes used in directions for centrifuging. It is similar (but not equivalent) to rpm (revolutions

per minute). 1 g is roughly 5 rpm; thus, 500 g is roughly 2,500 rpm. Also see
R. C. F. on page 720.

gamma
1. The third letter of the Greek alphabet, γ.
2. Microgram.
Thus, gamma = γ = microgram = μg = mcg.
And all the above may be used to represent one millionth (10^{-6}) part of a gram.
Rather confusing but true.

genotype
The fundamental hereditary constitution (or assortment of genes) of an individual.

granulocyte
Any cell containing granules. Usually used in reference to a white cell containing
neutrophilic, basophilic, or eosinophilic granules.

granulocytopenia
A poverty or decrease in granulocytes. The granulocytes may be neutrophilic,
eosinophilic, or basophilic.

grape cell
A plasma cell whose cytoplasm contains inclusion bodies which may be either
transparent bluish sacs or crystal-like in nature. This cell may be seen in disorders associated with hypergammaglobulinemia. A grape cell is also referred
to as a berry cell, a morular cell, and "Mott's cell."

Grawitz's degeneration
Basophilia. An abnormal increase in the blood of basophilic or bluish staining
erythrocytes. The staining may be either punctate, when it is called basophilic
stippling, or diffuse, when it is called polychromatophilia. For illustration, see
Plate 11, page 278.

Gumprecht shadow
A Gumprecht shadow is a smudge cell having a clear portion or "hole" in the
middle of the cell. It is often seen in chronic lymphocytic leukemia. For illustration of a smudge cell, see Plate 6, page 257.

halometer
An instrument for estimating the size of red cells by measuring the defraction
halos which they produce.

Hb A
Also referred to as A Hb, Hgb A, or A Hgb. The major normal adult hemoglobin.

Hb S
Also referred to as S Hb, Hgb S, or S Hgb. The hemoglobin responsible for
sickle cell trait and sickle cell anemia.

Hegglin's anomaly
A condition in which the blood smear shows white cells having spindle-shaped
or crescent-shaped bodies in their cytoplasm. These bodies resemble Döhle
bodies. The blood smear also shows giant platelets. The platelet count may be
below normal and the patient may have a mild bleeding tendency. This anomaly
is inherited and it remains with the individual throughout his or her lifetime.
Also referred to as the May-Hegglin anomaly.

hematin

An old outdated term for heme.

hematopoiesis

The formation and development of blood cells (which occurs mainly in the bone marrow). The formation and development of blood cells outside the bone marrow, that is, in the liver, spleen, and lymph nodes, is referred to as *extramedullary hematopoiesis.*

hematuria

Red cells in the urine.

heme

An iron-bearing compound which is the nonprotein pigment portion of hemoglobin.

hemochromatosis

A disorder of iron metabolism which is characterized by the deposition of excessive iron in the tissues.

hemoglobinemia

The presence of hemoglobin in the plasma of the blood.

hemoglobinuria

The presence of free hemoglobin in the urine.

hemolysin

A substance which liberates hemoglobin from red cells. For example, the bacterial hemolysin is a toxic substance produced by bacteria which has the ability to liberate hemoglobin from red cells (by simply dissolving the cells).

hemolysis

The liberation of hemoglobin from red cells. It may be caused by water, heat, cold, chemicals, or hemolysins.

hemolytic jaundice

A general term for either congenital hemolytic jaundice or acquired hemolytic jaundice.

hemorrhagic diathesis

A predisposition to abnormal hemostasis.

hemosiderin

An insoluble form of storage iron. It is visible microscopically with or without specific staining methods.

hemosiderinuria

The presence of hemosiderin in the urine.

hemostasis

1. The arrest of an escape of blood.
2. The checking of the flow of blood through any part or vessel.

heparin tolerance test

An outdated test of questionable value which was once used as "a test for hypercoagulability."

hof
The area of the cytoplasm of a cell encircled by the concavity of the nucleus.

homologous serum jaundice
Serum hepatitis. Also referred to as human serum jaundice.

hot-cold hemolysin
A hemolytic toxic substance of bacterial origin which lyses erythrocytes in the cold following warm incubation.

HPF
High power field. The field seen through the microscope when using the 45× (4 mm.) objective. The specimen is magnified 450 times (if the usual 10× eyepiece is used).

hyperchromemia
A high color index (of the red cells). A color index above the normal value of 0.9–1.1.

hyperchromic
Highly or excessively stained or colored.

hyperleukocytosis
An abnormal increase in the number of white cells.

hyperplasia
Abnormal increase in the number of cells.

hypofibrinogenemia
Abnormally low fibrinogen content of the blood.

IBC
Iron-binding capacity. A procedure measuring the ability of the plasma or serum to transport iron. See total iron-binding capacity, page 723.

icteric (icterus) index
A rough measure of the bilirubin in the blood. The normal values are 4 to 6 units. Values above normal may be found in hemolytic anemia. This test is run in the chemistry department.

idiopathic
A term describing any disease having a spontaneous origin and lacking an apparent cause.

immune antibodies
Antibodies which are not normally present but develop in response to some external stimulus. For example, in erythroblastosis fetalis, Rh antibodies develop in the mother in response to the stimulus of the Rh factor from the fetus.

incomplete antibodies
Antibodies which give no visible reaction with red cells suspended in saline. They may be detected by the antiglobulin (Coombs') test, by means of trypsinized red cells, and by titration in albumin.

47

infarct

An area of coagulation necrosis in a tissue due to local anemia resulting from obstruction of circulation to the area.

in vitro

Within a glass; observable in a test tube.

in vivo

Within the living body.

iron index

An index of iron in the blood calculated by dividing the value for the *whole* blood iron in milligrams per 100 milliliters by the red cell count in millions per cubic millimeter. For example,

$$\text{iron index} = \frac{\text{blood iron (in mg. per 100 ml.)}}{\text{RBC (in millions per cu. mm.)}} = \frac{40}{5} = 8$$

The normal values are 8 to 9.

iron sulfide test

Also referred to as the iron sulfide stain. A simple test for hemosiderin in urine. Positive in paroxysmal nocturnal hemoglobinuria. Usually performed in the chemistry department.

isoagglutinin

An agglutinin which will react with agglutinogens of the same species.

isotonic

A term describing a solution which has the same concentration or osmotic pressure as another solution or medium with which it is associated.

Example: If a salt solution of 0.85% is placed in contact with red cells, the salt solution and red cells have the same concentration. There is no transfer of water between the salt solution and the red cells. Hence, the salt solution has the "same tone" and is said to be isotonic.

isotopology

The study of isotopes.

I. U.

International units.

jaundice

A condition characterized by excessive bilirubin in the blood, the deposition of bile pigment in the tissues, and a tinge of yellow in the skin.

juvenile amaurotic idiocy

A fatal disease of infants and children characterized by paralysis and loss of vision. Also called amaurotic idiocy and amaurotic familial idiocy. The lymphocytes often contain vacuoles in the cytoplasm.

Kingsley's stain

A stain similar to Wright's stain. Used to stain blood smears for the differential white cell count.

Kupffer's cells

Cells present in the liver which have the power to engulf or phagocytize foreign material. These cells serve as part of the reticuloendothelial system. They are also referred to as stellate cells.

labile

Unstable.

lambda

1. The 14th letter of the Greek alphabet: Λ or λ.
2. In liquid measure, a lambda is one thousandth (10^{-3}) part of a milliliter or one millionth (10^{-6}) part of a liter. It is often referred to as a microliter which is usually abbreviated μl. Thus, lambda = Λ or λ = microliter = μl.

L:E ratio

Leuko-erythrogenetic ratio. A method of reporting the ratio of white cells to red cells found in a bone marrow smear. The L:E ratio *excludes* the mature granulocytes. Whereas the M:E (myeloid-erythroid) ratio *includes* the mature granulocytes.

leukemic hiatus

A blood smear showing a predominance of very mature and very immature cells of the granulocytic series. Hence, a gap or lack of cells between the neutrophilic segmented cell and the myeloblast of the granulocytic series. It is observed in many cases of acute granulocytic leukemia.

leukemic leukemia

Leukemia in which the white cell count is above the values found in health, that is, above the normal values of 5,000 to 10,000 per cubic millimeter.

leuko-agglutinin examination

A leuko-agglutinin is an agglutinin which acts upon a leukocyte or white cell. Leuko-agglutinins may be produced in the blood by transfusion reactions. The examination is usually performed in the blood bank department.

leukocytopenia

Another term for leukopenia. A white cell count below the normal values of 5,000 to 10,000 per cubic millimeter. See page 92.

leukopoiesis

The production of leukocytes or white cells.

lymphoma

A general term applying to any new and abnormal growth of lymphoid tissue.

lyse

To rupture or dissolve a cell.

lysin

An antibody which dissolves cells. For example, hemolysins are lysins which may dissolve red cells.

lysis

The dissolving of cells by a specific lysin.

m

Abbreviation for meter and also for the prefix *meta-*.

μ

Mu. The 12th letter of the Greek alphabet. It is equivalent to our small m. This μ is used as a symbol for the prefix *micro-* meaning one millionth. This μ is also used as a symbol for micron. Thus, the two symbols, μμ, stand for micromicron.

μ³

One micron cubed. A cubic micron.

macroglobulin

A globulin of high molecular weight.

macroglobulinemia

A condition characterized by an increase in the macroglobulins of the blood.

macrophage

A term for a large mononuclear wandering phagocytic cell which originates in the tissues.

macropolycyte

A large hypersegmented neutrophil.

Maragliano body

A round or elliptical body found as an artificial particle in degenerated or degenerating erythrocytes. The body resembles a vacuole. It is not to be considered a true erythrocyte inclusion body.

Maurer's dots

Red dots seen in stained erythrocytes infected with the malaria parasite *Plasmodium falciparum*.

megalocyte

An extremely large erythrocyte having a diameter of 12 to 25 microns. A megalocyte is larger than a macrocyte.

microcyte

A small erythrocyte. For illustration, see microcytosis, Plate 9, page 274.

microgram

One millionth (10^{-6}) part of a gram or one thousandth (10^{-3}) part of a milligram. Usually abbreviated μg. or mcg.

micromicro- (or pico-)

A prefix meaning one millionth of one millionth. Thus,

$$\frac{1}{1,000,000,000,000} \text{ or } 10^{-12}$$

For example, a micromicrogram is

$$\frac{1}{1,000,000,000,000} \text{ or } 10^{-12} \text{ of a gram.}$$

micromicrogram

Also referred to as a picogram. It is one millionth of one millionth (10^{-12}) gram. Usually abbreviated μμg or μγ.

micromicron

One millionth part of a micron. Abbreviated μμ.

micron (plural: microns or micra)

A unit of linear measure in the metric system.

It is $\dfrac{1}{1,000}$ of a millimeter. And it is often abbreviated μ.

millimicron

One thousandth $\left(\dfrac{1}{1000} \text{ or } 10^{-3}\right)$ part of a micron. It is abbreviated mμ or mmm.

mitochondria

Small granules or rod-shaped structures seen in the cytoplasm of myeloblasts and lymphoblasts (during a supravital stain). Mitochondria have been referred to as the "power plant of the cell."

mitosis

A type of cell division which functions as follows. The nucleus of the cell resolves into chromosomes. The cell then divides into two portions. The two portions separate. Each portion becomes a nucleus. And each nucleus starts a new cell.

moiety

A part or portion.

monocytopenia

A decrease in the normal percentage (2%–6%) of monocytes.

mononucleosis

An abnormally large *number* of monocytes (or lymphocytes) in the blood.

morphology

A study of the form or shape (of a cell). Usually used in reference to the red blood cell (RBC) morphology. This study is made in the stained red cell examination (page 267).

myeloblastoma

A tumor which may be present in a patient with granulocytic leukemia.

myelofibrosis

Replacement of bone marrow by fibrous tissue.

myelogram

A report of the percentage of each cell found in a bone marrow smear.

myeloid metaplasia
A condition characterized by the production of blood cells in areas other than the bone marrow, especially in the spleen, and having a blood smear showing immature white cells and immature red cells.

myeloproliferative disorders
Diseases accompanied by excessive cell production.
Examples: leukemia and polycythemia vera.

nano-
A prefix meaning one-billionth (10^{-9}).

neoplasm
Any new and abnormal growth; for example, a tumor is a neoplasm.

neutropenia
A decrease in the normal *number* of neutrophilic leukocytes in the blood. (Usually considered a drop below 2,000 per cu. mm.) It may be seen in agranulocytosis, aplastic anemia, irradiation (x-ray), many virus diseases such as measles and influenza, aleukemic leukemia, pernicious anemia, brucellosis, and Niemann-Pick disease. Also referred to as neutrocytopenia.

nonprotein nitrogen determination
Usually abbreviated NPN and also referred to as the total nonprotein nitrogen determination. This is a determination for the waste products in the blood, that is, the total amount of urea nitrogen, uric acid, and creatinine. The normal values are 25 to 35 milligrams per 100 milliliters of blood. Values above normal may be found in kidney disease, malignancy, and many other disorders. The NPN is performed in the chemistry department.

NRBC/100 WBC
The number of nucleated red blood cells per 100 white blood cells seen in a blood smear during the differential white cell count and stained red cell examination.

occult blood
Hidden blood, that is, blood which can not be detected except by chemical or microscopic means.

oligochromemia
Insufficiency of hemoglobin in the blood. May be seen in anemia.

orthochromia
Normal color or hemoglobin content of the erythrocytes.

osmotic pressure
Osmosis is the diffusion between two liquids or mediums of different densities which are separated by a semipermeable membrane. Example: When red cells are placed in an 0.5% salt solution, water passes through the cell membrane and enters the cell. The pressure exerted by this osmosis or passage of water is the osmotic pressure.

osteoblast
A cell which arises from a fibroblast and which, as it matures, is associated with the production of bone.

ovalocyte

An oval shaped erythrocyte. For illustration, see Plate 10, page 276.

oxidant drug

An oxidant is an oxidizing agent. Hence, an oxidant drug is a drug having the properties of an oxidizing agent. These drugs interfere with the respiratory functions of erythrocytes in some individuals.

panagglutinin

An agglutinin in serum which agglutinates the erythrocytes of all blood groups.

Papanicolaou smear

A smear for malignant cells. Often referred to as Pap's smear, Pap's vaginal smear, or Pap's stain for cancer cells.

Pappenheimer bodies

Basophilic iron-containing granules observed in various types of erythrocytes.

Paul-Bunnell test

Also called the Bunnell test. A serological test for infectious mononucleosis.

pencil cells

Elongated erythrocytes having the form or shape of a pencil. They may be seen in thalassemia and iron deficiency anemia.

peripheral blood

Blood obtained from the finger tip, vein, ear lobe, and toe or heel (in an infant).

pertussis

Whooping cough.

pessary cell

This cell is an abnormal erythrocyte with the following characteristics. The erythrocyte has a large central area of pallor due to a deficiency of hemoglobin. The small amount of hemoglobin in the erythrocyte is present as a narrow ring around the outer edge of the cell. The pessary cell is also referred to as an anulocyte or an erythrocyte showing "ring staining."

pH value

A value indicating the acid, neutral, or basic property of a dilute solution. A pH value between 0 and 7 is acid; the *lower* the number, the more acid the solution. A pH value of 7 is neutral. A pH value between 7 and 14 is basic; the *higher* the number, the more basic the solution. More technically speaking, the pH value deals with the hydrogen potential. It is the exponent (logarithm) of the hydrogen ion concentration with the minus sign dropped. For example,

hydrogen ion concentration	*pH value*	*solution*
10^{-1}	1	acid
10^{-7}	7	neutral
10^{-13}	13	basic

Note that the hydrogen ion is in *both* acid and basic solutions. But it is more concentrated in acid solutions and less concentrated in basic solutions.

phagocyte

Any cell that ingests microorganisms, other cells, or foreign particles. Examples: monocytes and neutrophilic segmented cells are phagocytes.

phagocytosis

The engulfing of microorganisms, other cells, and foreign particles by phagocytes.

phenotype

The outward visible expression of the hereditary constitution of an organism. Example: Hemoglobins A, S, etc.

pipette

An old spelling for pipet.

plasma volume test

Also referred to as the total plasma volume determination. This test is usually performed by a radioisotope procedure. It is run in the radioisotope department.

pleocytosis

An increase in the lymphocytes of the spinal fluid.

plethora

A condition marked by excess of blood, fullness of pulse, and vascular turgescence.

plumbism

A chronic form of poisoning produced by the absorption of lead or lead salts.

P. M. B.

Polymorphonuclear basophil. An old term for a basophilic segmented cell.

P. M. E.

Polymorphonuclear eosinophil. An old term for an eosinophilic segmented cell.

P. M. N.

Polymorphonuclear neutrophil. An old term for a neutrophilic segmented cell.

polycyte

A hypersegmented neutrophilic segmented cell which is normal in size.

porphobilinogen examination

Porphobilinogen is a chromogen which is used in the synthesis of heme. It may be found in the urine in porphyria, a metabolic disorder in which porphyrins are retained in the tissues. This examination is performed in the urine analysis or chemistry department.

porphyria erythropoietica

Also referred to as congenital porphyria. This is a form of porphyria in which the rubricytes and metarubricytes of the bone marrow contain excessive porphyrin.

porphyrin test
Porphyrins are complex organic compounds. They form the basis of the respiratory pigments in plants and animals. The porphyrin test is useful in detecting patients having porphyria (a metabolic disorder). The test is performed in the urine analysis or chemistry department.

posthemorrhagic
Occurring after hemorrhage.

precipitin test
Also referred to as a precipitation test. Any test in which a positive reaction consists of the formation and deposit of a precipitate. Example: An antigen-antibody reaction in which an antigen precipitates in the presence of a specific antibody.

proliferation
The reproduction or multiplication of cells.

protean
1. Assuming different shapes; changeable in form.
2. An insoluble derivative of protein, being the first product of the action of water, dilute acids, or enzymes.

prothrombinase
Thromboplastin. Extrinsic prothrombinase is extrinsic thromboplastin. Intrinsic prothrombinase is intrinsic thromboplastin.

pyknosis
A thickening or condensation. Usually refers to the condensation of the nucleus in a cell. The nucleus shrinks in size and the chromatin (network of small fibers) condenses to a solid mass or masses. Most generally used in reference to a degenerating cell.

pyogenic
Producing pus.

qns
Quantity Not Sufficient. Used when the amount of specimen is not sufficient to perform the test. Example: If only 2 cc. of urine is submitted for a urine analysis, the quantity is QNS for the specific gravity determination.

quality control
The term, quality control, is a term borrowed from industrial laboratories. In the medical laboratory, it may be considered as the use of commercially prepared agents to assist the medical technologist in performing laboratory examinations with accuracy, precision, and dependability. In days gone by, the conscientious medical technologist used the blood of a healthy student as a "quality control." The advent of the electronic era, however, made more precise controls not only more desirable but an absolute necessity. An excellent manual, "Quality Control in Hematology," may be obtained (free of charge) from Pfizer Diagnostics, 300 W. 43 St., New York City, N. Y. 10036.

quinidine purpura
Purpura produced by the drug quinidine. It is accompanied by a low platelet count.

radioactive

A property of those elements which have an atomic number above 83.

radioactive iodine uptake determination

This is a test for thyroid function; it is performed in the radioisotope department.

radioactivity

The disintegration of an atom's nucleus and the emission of electromagnetic particles.

Raynaud's phenomenon

A phenomenon in which cold or emotion produces intermittent periods of pallor and cyanosis (blue coloration) in the hands and feet.

R. C. F.

Relative centrifugal force. The formula or equation for the relative centrifugal force is: R. C. F. $= 0.000,011,18 \times r \times (rpm)^2$, where r is the rotating radius in centimeters of the centrifuge and rpm is revolutions per minute. The R. C. F. is sometimes referred to as gravity, gravities, g, or G. These terms are occasionally used in the directions for centrifuging a blood specimen. Also see g (or G) on page 708.

Reilly bodies

Bodies in the white cells of patients with gargoylism, a rare hereditary disorder. The bodies are said to be similar to (and may even be identical with) the large coarse granules that are seen in the white cells of Alder's anomaly.

relative lymphocytosis

An increase in the percentage of lymphocytes due to a decrease in the percentage of other white cells. May be seen in aplastic anemia and Gaucher's disease. For further information, see relative counts (pages 220, 222).

resolving power

The ability to reveal fine detail. It may be defined as the shortest distance that 2 lines can be placed side by side and still seen as 2 lines rather than as 1 blurred line. The term is generally used in reference to the lens of a microscope.

reticuloendothelial cell

A cell of the reticuloendothelial system. It has the power to engulf or phagocytize foreign material.

reticuloendothelial system

Also referred to as the R. E. S. system and the reticulo-endothelial system. This system is concerned with blood cell formation and destruction, the metabolism of iron and pigment, the storage of fatty materials, and defensive activities in immunity and inflammation. The system is located throughout the bone marrow, liver, spleen, and lymph nodes.

reticulum cell

Also referred to as a reticular cell. A fixed tissue cell and not a blood cell. It is found in the bone marrow, lymph glands, and spleen.

ribonuclease

An enzyme which catalyzes the depolymerization of ribonucleic acid.

Rieder cell
A white cell which may be seen in leukemia. It resembles a blast cell, that is, a myeloblast, lymphoblast, or monoblast. But the nucleus is deeply indented or lobulated (rather than round).

RISA method
RISA stands for radioiodinated serum albumin. It is a method of determining the blood volume. The test is performed in the radioisotope department.

"rolling" vein
A vein which "rolls" or moves during a venipuncture. Usually caused by having the needle approach the vein from the side rather than from above. May also be caused by failure to properly "fix" the vein and thus prevent its movement.

RPM
Also referred to as R. P. M., rpm, or r. p. m. Revolutions per minute. A term used in centrifuging.

rubella
1. Measles. 2. A virus disease similar to measles. Also referred to as German measles.

Russell bodies
Round glassy transparent bodies which may be seen in the cytoplasm (and sometimes the nucleus) of plasmacytes in plasmacytic leukemia and multiple myeloma.

saline
Salty. A saline solution is a solution containing salt.

Schilling hemogram
The Schilling method of reporting the differential white cell count. See Schilling classification, page 260.

Schilling test
Also referred to as the vitamin B_{12} absorption test and the Schilling test for P. A. This test is useful in the diagnosis of pernicious anemia. It is performed in the radioisotope department.

schistocyte
Also referred to as a schizocyte. Schistocytes are fragments of old erythrocytes. They may be wedge-shaped or any irregular shape. They are commonly seen in the hemolytic anemias.

Schüffner's dots
Red particles which may be seen in erythrocytes containing malaria parasites. Also referred to as Schüffner's granules and Schüffner's stippling.

segmentation index
An index which has been used in evaluating the shift to the right or hypersegmentation of granulocytes. The formula is:

$$\text{Segmentation index} = \frac{\text{granulocytes with 5 lobes or more}}{\text{granulocytes with 4 lobes}} \times 100$$

The normal values are 0–17.

serum hepatitis
A condition indistinguishable clinically from infectious hepatitis but caused by an immunologically distinct virus. This disease may be transmitted by inadequately sterilized needles or syringes.

serum iron determination
This determination may be useful in the diagnosis of anemia. The normal values are 70 to 180 micrograms per 100 milliliters of serum. The determination is usually performed in the chemistry department.

Sézary cell
A large lymphocyte about twice the size of a neutrophilic segmented cell. The outstanding feature of the cell is the nucleus. It occupies most of the cell and it may be round, convoluted, or bilobed. Two or three nuclei may sometimes be present in the same cell. The cytoplasm of the cell is pale and sparse and may contain vacuoles. This cell may occasionally be seen in proliferative disorders; it is frequently seen in the Sézary syndrome.

Sherman test
A test which may be useful in distinguishing between sickle cell trait and sickle cell anemia.

Sia water dilution test
A test for macroglobulinemia. This is a more refined method of performing the Sia test (page 556).

silicone
Any organic compound in which all or part of the carbon has been replaced by silicon.

sperm count
The sperm count may be useful in cases of infertility. The normal values are:
    number: 60–180 million per ml. (milliliter)
    motility: 75% of the sperm cells have the usual motility
    shape: 75% of the sperm cells have the usual shape (morphology)
The sperm count is usually performed in the bacteriology department and it is sometimes referred to as a semen analysis.

standard deviation
Also referred to as SD. A term expressing the accuracy of a determination. Used in quality control programs and often given with a report.

stasis
An arrest or stoppage in the flow of blood (or any other body fluid).

Stat
Immediately. A "Stat" request is a request to perform a test immediately. The test is usually an emergency procedure.

stercobilinogen
Fecal urobilinogen.

S. T. P.
Standard temperature and pressure. Standard temperature is $0°$ centigrade. Standard pressure is the pressure exerted by 760 millimeters of Hg (mercury) Thus, S. T. P. is $0°$ C. and 760 mm. pressure.

stroma

The structural portion of the erythrocyte. It is the portion which remains after the erythrocyte has been washed free of hemoglobin. When seen under the microscope, it appears as a "ghost" of a red cell or a shadow form.

supernatant fluid

The fluid "swimming" above a solid. Example: If a test tube of blood is centrifuged, the plasma which lies above the cells is supernatant fluid.

syndrome

A set or group of symptoms which occur together.

syneresis

A drawing together. Example: When blood clots, the clot shrinks or draws together and expresses a fluid, serum.

thick film

A thick blood smear. Usually made to concentrate the erythrocytes in a search for malaria parasites. Also called a thick smear, thick blood film, and thick blood smear.

Thoma hemocytometer

A counting chamber which may be used for the red cell count.

thrombocythemia

A fixed increase in the number of thrombocytes or platelets in the blood.

thrombopenia

A thrombocyte or platelet count below the normal values of 150,000–400,000 per cubic millimeter. Also referred to as thrombocytopenia.

thrombosis

The presence of a blood clot.

titer

The strength of a solution. Example: In the heterophile antibody test, the serum is diluted 1:7, 1:14, 1:28, etc. The greater the dilution, the weaker the serum. Also referred to as a titre.

titration

The act of finding the strength of a solution. Usually used in reference to a chemical analysis. For example, the strength of an acid solution may be found by performing a titration with a basic solution of known strength.

tortuous

Twisted.

total iron-binding capacity

Often referred to as the TIBC. The total iron-binding capacity (TIBC) consists of the serum iron *plus* the unsaturated iron-binding capacity (UIBC) of the serum. To make matters a bit confusing, the unsaturated iron-binding capacity (UIBC) is sometimes referred to as the serum iron-binding capacity (SIBC). Let us consider an example in the derivation of the total iron-binding capacity. If the serum iron is 100 micrograms per 100 ml. and the unsaturated iron-binding capacity is 200 micrograms per 100 ml., the total iron-binding capacity is 300 micrograms per 100 ml. The normal values for the total iron-binding capacity are 300–360 micrograms per 100 ml. of serum. Values above normal may be found in iron deficiency anemia. This determination is performed in the chemistry department.

total red cell volume determination

Also referred to as the erythrocyte volume test, red cell mass determination, and red blood cell mass determination. The normal values are 22 to 36 milliliters per kilogram of body weight. Values above normal may be found in polycythemia vera. This determination is performed in the radioisotope department.

transferrin

This substance is a protein, a beta globulin. Its function is to bind iron and enable it to be transferred for the manufacture of hemoglobin.

Trenner diluting pipets

Pipets which may be used to dilute the blood. A 1 in 20 dilution pipet is used for the white cell count. A 1 in 200 dilution pipet is used for the red cell count. These dilutions, of course, are the usual dilutions for the WBC and RBC.

μ

See μ (the Greek letter for m) under M (page 714).

uric acid determination

Uric acid is a waste product which is removed from the blood stream by the kidneys. The normal values are 2–4 milligrams per 100 milliliters of blood. Values above normal may be found in gout, leukemia, polycythemia vera, and many other disorders. The determination is performed in the chemistry department.

urobilinogen estimation

Urobilinogen is a colorless compound formed in the intestines by the reduction of bilirubin. A portion of the urobilinogen is excreted in the feces where by oxidation it becomes urobilin. Another portion of the urobilinogen is reabsorbed. The reabsorbed urobilinogen may be (1) re-excreted in the bile as bilirubin, or (2) it may sometimes be excreted in the urine. The urobilinogen in the urine may later be oxidized to urobilin. The urobilinogen estimation is performed in the chemistry department. The normal values for urinary urobilinogen are: 0.3–1.0 Ehrlich units/2 hr. or 0.05–2.5 mg./24 hr. Values above normal may be found in hemolytic anemia and liver disorders.

uroporphyrin test

Uroporphyrin is a porphyrin occurring in urine. The normal values are 10–30 micrograms per 24 hour specimen of urine. Values above normal may be found in patients with porphyria (a disturbance of porphyrin metabolism). This test is performed in the chemistry department.

venous blood

Blood obtained from a vein.

virocyte

An atypical lymphocyte said to be found in the blood during or following a virus infection. The virocyte is said to closely resemble the atypical lymphocyte seen in infectious mononucleosis.

vitro (vitrum)
Glass.

vivo (vivi-)
Living, alive, or life.

whole blood
Blood from which none of the elements have been removed.

REVIEW QUESTIONS FOR NATIONAL REGISTRY AND STATE BOARD EXAMINATIONS

This section contains 500 review questions for National Registry and State Board examinations.

Each review question is accompanied by a reference. The reference is the exact page in the text where the question was discussed and answered. Thus, an area of academic weakness may be quickly detected and readily reviewed.

A set of answers follows the 500 review questions; this set of answers may be used as a quick reference in oral quizzes.

These questions are not intended to "trick" the student. They are designed to assist the student in assimilating the material in the text. This, in turn, will increase the student's ability to recall the information during examinations.

The questions are of two types: (1) true or false questions and (2) multiple choice questions.

The student places a circle or bracket around the *best* answer to each question. Two examples are given below.

A monocyte is a white cell.   [T]   F

The word leukocytosis refers to:

a. a low white cell count
b. a low red cell count
c. a low platelet count
d. a high red cell count
[*e.*] a high white cell count

The student should always select the *best* answer to each question.

For example, the normal values which are given for the red cell count in women vary from textbook to textbook. Thus, the following authorities give the accompanying normal values:

Wintrobe	4.2 to 5.4 million per cu. mm.
Miale	3.6 to 5.0 million per cu. mm.
Goodale	4.6 to 4.8 million per cu. mm.

In view of the above, how should the student answer the question presented below?

The normal values for the red cell count in women are:

a. 5,000–10,000 per cu. mm.
b. 150,000–400,000 per cu. mm.
c. 3.0–4.0 million per cu. mm.
d. 4.0–5.5 million per cu. mm.
e. none of the above

Obviously, the *best* answer to the above question would be *d* and this is the answer the student should select.

After answering the questions, the student may wish to go over the questions and their answers just prior to his examination in hematology.

1. The average man has the following volume of blood:

 a. 10 quarts
 b. 2 quarts
 c. 1 liter
 d. 5 quarts
 e. 12 quarts   Ref. p.   2

2. For every 500 red cells there are approximately 30 platelets and only 1 white cell.   T   F   Ref. p.   2

3. Normal blood contains approximately the following per cent of plasma:

 a. 20%
 b. 30%
 c. 40%
 d. 50%
 e. 60%   Ref. p. 2, 3

4. The red cells, platelets, and most of the white cells are formed in the marrow of our bones; the most common sources of supply are the ribs, breastbone, and backbone.   T   F   Ref. p.   3

5. The monophyletic theory of blood formation states that a single mother cell produces all blood cells whereas the polyphyletic theory states that several mother cells are involved.   T   F   Ref. p. 3, 4

6. If a blood lancet is to be used again, it should be autoclaved or sterilized by heat, for this is the only type of sterilization that will kill the virus of infectious hepatitis.   T   F   Ref. p. 12

7. Needles and syringes may be sterilized by either dry heating in an oven at 170° C. for 2 hours or autoclaving at 15 pounds pressure for 20 minutes.
                                                     T   F   Ref. p. 32

8. The gauge number gives the diameter of a needle; the smaller the gauge number, the greater the diameter.   T   F   Ref. p. 32

9. In making a venipuncture of the forearm, which gauge needle would be most appropriate:

 a. 10
 b. 15
 c. 20
 d. 27
 e. 30   Ref. p. 32

10. In drawing blood for tests in hematology, which syringe is most frequently used:

    a. 1 cc.
    b. 2 cc.
    c. 5 cc.
    d. 10 cc.
    e. 20 cc.   Ref. p. 33

11. During a venipuncture, the tourniquet should be released *after* the needle is withdrawn from the arm.   T F   Ref. p. 57, 58

12. After making a venipuncture by the syringe method, the needle is removed from the syringe before the blood is transferred to a test tube.
                                              T F   Ref. p. 59

13. A hematoma may be caused by any of the following: (a) failure to have needle completely in vein, (b) failure to release tourniquet before withdrawing needle, (c) jerking needle out of vein, and (d) failure to apply pressure to wound after removal of needle.   T F   Ref. p. 68

14. The removal or inactivation of the calcium in the blood will prevent the blood from clotting.   T F   Ref. p. 77, 78

15. Which of the following anticoagulants does *not* react with calcium to prevent coagulation:

    a. double oxalate
    b. EDTA
    c. sodium citrate
    d. Sequestrene
    e. heparin   Ref. p. 78, 79

16. To obtain oxalated blood, the following anticoagulant is used:

    a. heparin
    b. Sequestrene
    c. sodium citrate
    d. Heller and Paul's mixture
    e. sodium fluoride   Ref. p. 78

17. The term, anticoagulated blood, is a general term applying to oxalated blood, Sequestrenized blood, heparinized blood, and citrated blood.
                                              T F   Ref. p. 77

18. If coagulation is prevented, centrifuging will separate the cells or formed elements from the:

    a. serum
    b. cell suspension
    c. packed cells
    d. diluted blood
    e. plasma   Ref. p. 82

48

19. When blood clots, the fluid that remains after separation of the clot is called:

    a. plasma
    b. whole blood
    c. cell suspension
    d. serum
    e. packed cells   Ref. p. 83

20. Serum differs from plasma in that it contains no fibrinogen—a substance used
    in the formation of the clot.   T   F   Ref. p. 83

21. If the red cells are placed in a hypotonic solution, water enters the red cells; if
    the red cells are placed in a hypertonic solution, water leaves the red cells.
                                                           T   F   Ref. p. 84, 85

22. Physiological saline, which is sometimes referred to as "normal" saline, is an
    isotonic solution.   T   F   Ref. p. 85

23. Physiological saline contains the following per cent of sodium chloride:

    a. 5.0
    b. 1.25
    c. 8.50
    d. 0.85
    e. 1.34   Ref. p. 86, 697

24. There is actually no difference between a normal physiological solution and a
    normal chemical solution.   T   F   Ref. p. 85, 86

25. The term leukopenia refers to a white cell count below:

    a. 10,000 cells per cu. mm.
    b. 20,000 cells per cu. mm.
    c. 5,000 cells per cu. mm.
    d. 15,000 cells per cu. mm.
    e. 25,000 cells per cu. mm.   Ref. p. 91, 92

26. A leukopenia may be found in:

    a. influenza
    b. agranulocytosis
    c. infectious hepatitis
    d. all of the above
    e. none of the above   Ref. p. 92

27. The normal range for the white cell count is:

    a. 1,000 to 3,000 per cu. mm.
    b. 10,000 to 15,000 per cu. mm.
    c. 5,000 to 10,000 per cu. mm.
    d. 8,000 to 12,000 per cu. mm.
    e. 4 to 6 million per cu. mm.   Ref. p. 91

28. A leukocytosis may be found in:

   a. appendicitis
   b. pneumonia
   c. leukemia
   d. all of the above
   e. none of the above   Ref. p. 92

29. The diluting fluid for the white cell count dissolves or hemolyzes the mature
    red cells—the erythrocytes.   T F   Ref. p. 96

30. In performing a white cell count, which of the following solutions may be
    employed as a diluting fluid:

   a. Gower's solution
   b. Drabkin's solution
   c. 2% acetic acid solution
   d. 10% nitric acid solution
   e. Hayem's solution   Ref. p. 96

31. When blood is drawn to the 0.5 mark and diluting fluid to the 11.0 mark in
    the white cell pipet, the dilution factor is:

   a. 10
   b. 20
   c. 200
   d. 22
   e. 16   Ref. p. 97

32. A hemocytometer is used in the microscopic or manual method for the white
    cell count.   T F   Ref. p. 105

33. In performing a white cell count with a counting chamber having an Improved
    Neubauer ruling, the white cells are counted in 4 "W" sections, each "W"
    section being composed of 16 small squares.   T F   Ref. p. 124, 126, 159

34. Each "W" section has an area of 1 square millimeter and a depth of 0.1
    millimeter.   T F   Ref. p. 132

35. If nucleated red cells are present in the blood, they are *not* dissolved by the
    white cell diluting fluid and are counted as white cells. T F   Ref. p. 138

36. In correcting a white cell count for the presence of nucleated red cells, the
    following formula is used:

$$\text{corrected WBC} = \text{uncorrected WBC} \times \frac{100}{100 + A}$$

where, 100 = white cells counted in the differential

   A = number of nucleated red cells seen while counting the differential
                                                  T F   Ref. p. 138, 139

37. When the red cell count rises above the normal values, it is referred to as an erythrocytosis.   T F   Ref. p. 143

38. The microscopic or manual method of performing a red cell count is subject to an error of about 10%.   T F   Ref. p. 144

39. Which of the following is a diluting fluid for the red cell count:

   a. distilled water
   b. 2% hydrochloric acid
   c. 1% acetic acid
   d. Gower's solution
   e. 0.1% sodium carbonate   Ref. p. 147

40. For the red cell count, the diluting fluid must be isotonic in order to prevent hemolysis of the red cells or crenation of the red cells. T F   Ref. pp. 84
                                                                            and 147

41. When blood is drawn to the 0.5 mark and diluting fluid to the 101 mark of the red cell pipet, the blood is diluted:

   a. 1 in 10
   b. 1 in 50
   c. 1 in 200
   d. 1 in 100
   e. 1 in 20   Ref. p. 147, 148

42. In performing a red cell count by the microscopic method, the first 4 or 5 drops are discarded from the pipet because this portion of the solution did not take part in the dilution of the blood.   T F   Ref. p. 153, 155

43. In the Improved Neubauer ruling, both the "W" sections and the "R" sections are subdivided into 16 squares.   T F   Ref. p. 159

44. In a counting chamber with the Improved Neubauer ruling, the central square millimeter is subdivided into:

   a. 100 small squares
   b. 16 small squares
   c. 400 small squares
   d. 80 small squares
   e. 200 small squares   Ref. p. 159

45. In performing a red cell count by the microscopic method, the red cells are counted in 5 "R" sections, each "R" section being subdivided into 16 small squares.   T F   Ref. p. 159, 160, 161

46. An "R" section has a depth of 0.1 mm. and an area of:

   a. 0.02 sq. mm.
   b. 1.00 sq. mm.
   c. 0.04 sq. mm.
   d. 0.08 sq. mm.
   e. 0.06 sq. mm.   Ref. p. 170

47. In making a red cell count by the microscopic or counting chamber method, the 5 "R" sections of the counting chamber have a total volume of:

  a. 0.1 cu. mm.
  b. 101 cu. mm.
  c. 200 cu. mm.
  d. 0.02 cu. mm.
  e. 0.85 cu. mm.   Ref. p. 170

48. In some diseases, such as multiple myeloma, the red cells may clump or agglutinate if Hayem's solution is used as a diluting fluid.   T   F   Ref. p. 173, 174

49. As the formation of hemoglobin increases within the red cell, the quantity of ribonucleic acid decreases.   T   F   Ref. p. 176

50. The function of hemoglobin is to carry oxygen from the lungs to the tissues and assist in the transport of carbon dioxide from the tissues to the lungs.
                                                           T   F   Ref. p. 176

51. When hemoglobin is carrying oxygen, it is known as oxyhemoglobin; when hemoglobin is conveying carbon dioxide, it is known as reduced hemoglobin.
                                                           T   F   Ref. p. 176

52. One gram of hemoglobin can hold approximately:

  a. 134 ml. oxygen
  b. 1.34 liters oxygen
  c. 13.4 ml. oxygen
  d. 0.134 ml. oxygen
  e. 1.34 ml. oxygen   Ref. p. 177

53. When the ferrous iron (Fe^{++}) in hemoglobin is oxidized to the ferric state (Fe^{+++}), a hemoglobin derivative, methemoglobin, is produced.
                                                           T   F   Ref. p. 177, 178

54. The normal number of grams of hemoglobin in an adult male is:

  a. 10 plus or minus 2 grams per 100 ml.
  b. 12 plus or minus 2 grams per 100 ml.
  c. 14 plus or minus 2 grams per 100 ml.
  d. 16 plus or minus 2 grams per 100 ml.
  e. 18 plus or minus 2 grams per 100 ml.   Ref. p. 178

55. The hemoglobin value of a newborn infant may be as high as 20 grams per 100 milliliters.   T   F   Ref. p. 178

56. The hemoglobin values may be affected by age, sex, altitude, pregnancy, and disease.   T   F   Ref. p. 178

57. The hemoglobin values decrease in high altitudes and increase at sea level.
                                                           T   F   Ref. p. 178

58. The hemoglobin values are below normal in anemia and leukemia and above normal in dehydration conditions and polycythemia vera.

                                                        T   F   Ref. p. 179

59. In determining the hemoglobin concentration with the Spencer hemoglobinometer, the blood is hemolyzed by stirring with an applicator containing:

    a. hydrochloric acid
    b. normal saline
    c. oxalic acid
    d. heparin
    e. saponin   Ref. p. 182

60. In the determination of hemoglobin, the Sahli-Hellige method and Haden-Hausser method convert hemoglobin to:

    a. methemoglobin
    b. oxyhemoglobin
    c. cyanmethemoglobin
    d. acid hematin
    e. sulfhemoglobin   Ref. p. 182

61. Dilute hydrochloric acid converts hemoglobin to:

    a. oxyhemoglobin
    b. alkaline hematin
    c. acid hematin
    d. cyanmethemoglobin
    e. sulfhemoglobin   Ref. p. 182

62. Drabkin's solution contains:

    a. calcium chloride
    b. magnesium sulfate
    c. sulfuric acid
    d. copper sulfate
    e. cyanide   Ref. p. 183

63. In the cyanmethemoglobin method for determining hemoglobin, the ferricyanide oxidizes the iron in hemoglobin to produce methemoglobin which reacts with cyanide to form cyanmethemoglobin.   T F   Ref. p. 183

64. The cyanmethemoglobin method for determining hemoglobin is the procedure used in the majority of hospital laboratories.   T F   Ref. p. 184

65. In the Sahli-Hellige method of determining hemoglobin, the diluent used to match the color of the *solution* with the standard is:

    a. distilled water
    b. normal saline
    c. oxalic acid
    d. physiological saline
    e. Drabkin's solution   Ref. p 192

66. In the cyanmethemoglobin method for determining hemoglobin, the diluent is:

    a. 1% hydrochloric acid
    b. normal saline
    c. ammonium hydroxide
    d. sodium carbonate
    e. Drabkin's solution   Ref. p. 200, 203

67. In the cyanmethemoglobin method for the determination of hemoglobin, the test tube is allowed to stand the following number of minutes to allow for the formation of cyanmethemoglobin:

    a. 15 min.
    b. 2 min.
    c. 5 min.
    d. 20 min.
    e. 10 min.   Ref. p. 200, 204

68. Hemoglobin is measured as cyanmethemoglobin in a spectrophotometer at a wavelength of:

    a. 540 millimicrons
    b. 620 millimicrons
    c. 360 millimicrons
    d. 450 millimicrons
    e. 720 millimicrons   Ref. p. 204

69. Which of the following cells is not present in normal blood:

    a. neutrophilic segmented cell
    b. monocyte
    c. lymphocyte
    d. plasmacyte
    e. neutrophilic band cell   Ref. p. 214

70. The youngest cell in the granulocytic series of white cells is the:

    a. progranulocyte
    b. neutrophilic segmented cell
    c neutrophilic band cell
    d. neutrophilic metamyelocyte
    e. myeloblast   Ref. Plate 2, p. 214

71. The immediate precursor of the neutrophilic band cell is the:

    a. neutrophilic segmented cell
    b. progranulocyte
    c. neutrophilic myelocyte
    d. myeloblast
    e. neutrophilic metamyelocyte   Ref. Plate 2, p. 214

72. The monoblast is the most immature cell in the monocytic series.
                                    T   F   Ref. Plate 2, p. 214

73. The immediate precursor of the progranulocyte is the:

   a. neutrophilic myelocyte
   b. neutrophilic band cell
   c. myeloblast
   d. neutrophilic segmented cell
   e. monoblast   Ref. Plate 2, p. 214

74. The neutrophilic segmented cell belongs to the following series:

   a. erythrocytic series
   b. plasmacytic series
   c. monocytic series
   d. granulocytic series
   e. none of the above   Ref. Plate 2, p. 214

75. The most *immature* cell in the lymphocytic series is the:

   a. lymphocyte
   b. prolymphocyte
   c. myeloblast
   d. lymphoblast
   e. plasmacyte   Ref. Plate 2, p. 214

76. Neutrophilic segmented cells are derived from:

   a. plasmablasts
   b. lymphoblasts
   c. erythroblasts
   d. monoblasts
   e. myeloblasts   Ref. Plate 2, p. 214

77. The immediate precursor of the myelocyte is the:

   a. metamyelocyte
   b. plasmablast
   c. lymphoblast
   d. progranulocyte
   e. monoblast   Ref. Plate 2, p. 214

78. The percentage distribution of the different types of white cells or leukocytes
   is called the differential white cell count.   T   F   Ref. p. 215

79. The normal percentages for neutrophilic segmented cells are:

   a. 2–6
   b. 1–3
   c. 0–1
   d. 55–75
   e. 20–35   Ref. p. 215

80. In a differential white cell count, the following cell would have the lowest normal range:

   a. neutrophilic segmented cell
   b. eosinophilic segmented cell
   c. basophilic segmented cell
   d. lymphocyte
   e. monocyte   Ref. p. 215

81. The normal percentages for monocytes are:

   a. 0–1
   b. 10–20
   c. 20–35
   d. 55–75
   e. 2–6   Ref. p. 215

82. Infants and children of pre-school age usually have more lymphocytes than neutrophilic segmented cells.   T   F   Ref. p. 215

83. An increased percentage of lymphocytes may be seen in whooping cough (pertussis).   T   F   Ref. p. 215

84. An increase in the percentage of basophils may be seen in all of the following, except:

   a. chronic granulocytic leukemia
   b. splenectomy (removal of spleen)
   c. hemolytic anemia
   d. chronic lymphocytic leukemia
   e. polycythemia vera   Ref. p. 215

85. An increase in the percentage of eosinophils may be seen in asthma, hay fever, and parasitic infestations.
                                             T   F   Ref. p. 215

86. In appendicitis, you would expect an increase in neutrophilic band cells and neutrophilic segmented cells.   T   F   Ref. p. 216

87. Neutrophilic segmented cells phagocytize or ingest bacteria.
                                             T   F   Ref. p. 216

88. Monocytes may also phagocytize or ingest bacteria.   T   F   Ref. p. 216

89. The function of all white cells is to phagocytize or ingest bacteria.
                                             T   F   Ref. p. 216

90. Lymphocytes may be produced in the bone marrow, lymphatic tissue, and spleen.   T   F   Ref. p. 216

91. With the exception of the lymphocyte, the life span of the average white cell in the blood stream is about:

    a. 120 days
    b. 1 month
    c. 5 weeks
    d. 10 days
    e. 200 days   Ref. p. 216

92. A neutrophilic leukocytosis is an increase in the percentage of neutrophilic cells and a monocytosis is an increase in the percentage of monocytes.
                                                          T F   Ref. p. 217

93. The largest cell found in normal blood is the:

    a. lymphocyte
    b. neutrophilic band cell
    c. neutrophilic segmented cell
    d. monocyte
    e. eosinophilic segmented cell   Ref. p. 218

94. Türk cell is an old name for a:

    a. lymphocyte
    b. monocyte
    c. neutrophilic myelocyte
    d. neutrophilic metamyelocyte
    e. proplasmacyte   Ref. p. 221

95. If a patient has a white cell count of 10,000 and a differential showing 30% monocytes and 70% lymphocytes, his absolute monocyte count would be:

    a. 7,000 per cu. mm.
    b. 10,000 per cu. mm.
    c. 3,000 per cu. mm.
    d. 3.5
    e. could not calculate from above data   Ref. p. 220

96. Wright's stain is a polychrome stain.   T F   Ref. p. 233

97. When using Wright's stain for blood smears, the buffer solution is usually added to the staining fluid after:

    a. 8–12 min.
    b. 6 min.
    c. 1 min.
    d. 10 min.
    e. 20–30 min.   Ref. p. 237

98. Neutrophilic segmented cells are 10 to 15 microns in diameter and monocytes are about 17 microns in diameter.   T F   Ref. p. 241

99. The lymphocyte has a:

   a. segmented nucleus
   b. kidney-shaped nucleus
   c. no nucleus
   d. spongy sprawling nucleus
   e. closely knit nucleus   Ref. p. 244

100. Azurophilic granules may be seen in the cytoplasm of:

   a. myeloblasts
   b. granulocytes
   c. erythrocytes
   d. lymphocytes
   e. rubriblasts   Ref. p. 244

101. Light gray or slate gray cytoplasm is characteristically seen in the:

   a. plasmacyte
   b. lymphocyte
   c. eosinophilic segmented cell
   d. monocyte
   e. basophilic segmented cell   Ref. p. 244

102. The nucleus of which cell appears buried under large purple or purplish-black granules:

   a. erythroblast
   b. lymphocyte
   c. monocyte
   d. eosinophilic segmented cell
   e. basophilic segmented cell   Ref. p. 244

103. The eosinophilic segmented cell has large red granules in the cytoplasm and a nucleus which is usually divided into 2 segments.   T   F   Ref. p. 244

104. Which cell has no granules in the cytoplasm and usually contains 1–3 nucleoli in the nucleus:

   a. neutrophilic metamyelocyte
   b. basophilic myelocyte
   c. eosinophilic myelocyte
   d. myeloblast
   e. monocyte   Ref. p. 245

105. In a neutrophilic metamyelocyte, the nucleus is indented or bean shaped and the cytoplasm contains small pink or brownish granules.
                                            T   F   Ref. p. 245

106. Which of the following is *not* characteristic of a neutrophilic myelocyte:

   a. has granules in the cytoplasm
   b. is absent in normal blood
   c. usually slightly larger than a neutrophilic segmented cell
   d. has nucleoli
   e. has a round or oval nucleus   Ref. p. 245

107. If progranulocytes are found in a blood smear, myelocytes should also be
present.   T F   Ref. p. 245

108. A "moth-eaten" or vacuolated cytoplasm may be seen in the abnormal lymphocyte of infectious mononucleosis.   T F   Ref. p. 245

109. In a plasmacyte, the nucleus is small and usually located near the edge of the
cell and the cytoplasm is deep blue.   T F   Ref. p. 245

110. Which cell is *not* an *immature* member of the granulocytic series:

   a. myeloblast
   b. neutrophilic metamyelocyte
   c. neutrophilic segmented cell
   d. progranulocyte
   e. neutrophilic myelocyte   Ref. p. 246

111. Differentiation of the granules in the white cell takes place as the cell goes from
a progranulocyte to a:

   a. metamyelocyte
   b. erythroblast
   c. myelocyte
   d. band cell
   e. myeloblast   Ref. p. 246

112. How would you distinguish a neutrophilic myelocyte from a neutrophilic
metamyelocyte:

   a. former has 1 nucleoli; latter has 3 nucleoli
   b. former has red granules; latter has purple granules
   c. former is small; latter is large
   d. former has granules; latter has no granules
   e. former has round or oval nucleus; latter has indented nucleus
                                                          Ref. p. 246

113. A smudge cell is the bare nucleus of a ruptured white cell and a basket cell is
the net-like nucleus from a ruptured white cell.   T F   Ref. p. 257, 258

114. A hypersegmented neutrophil has 5 to 10 segments in the nucleus and a vacuolated cell has vacuoles in the cytoplasm.   T F   Ref. p. 258

115. Toxic granulation of neutrophils may be caused by:

   a. overstaining of blood smear
   b. chemical poisoning in patient
   c. agranulocytosis in patient
   d. all of the above
   e. none of the above   Ref. p. 258

116. A decrease in platelets can be detected by a careful examination of the stained
blood smear.   T F   Ref. p. 259

117. "Shift to the left" is associated with the:

    a. erythrocytic development
    b. filament and non-filament classification
    c. Howell theory
    d. end taking out the tackle
    e. Schilling classification   Ref. p. 260

118. "Shift to the left" means:

    a. irreversible coagulation
    b. terminal leukemia
    c. increase in monocytes
    d. increase in immature cells
    e. decrease in erythrocytes   Ref. p. 260

119. A regenerative shift to the left is due to a depression of the cell factories in the bone marrow whereas a degenerative shift to the left is caused by a stimulus of the cell factories in the bone marrow.   T F   Ref. p. 260

120. The nucleated red cells are normally confined to the bone marrow; but, in some anemias and leukemias, they may be seen in the blood stream.
                                  T F   Ref. p. 268

121. As the red cell completes its development, the reticulocyte loses its reticulum and becomes an erythrocyte.   T F   Ref. p. 268

122. Red cells are produced mainly in the:

    a. liver
    b. gall bladder
    c. pancreas
    d. lymph nodes
    e. bone marrow   Ref. p. 268

123. The immediate precursor of the reticulocyte is the metarubricyte (orthochromic normoblast).
                              T F   Ref. pp. 269, 270

124. Both reticulocytes and erythrocytes have a nucleus.   T F   Ref. p. 270

125. The youngest cell in the erythrocytic series is the:

    a. rubriblast (pronormoblast)
    b. prorubricyte (basophilic normoblast)
    c. rubricyte (polychromatophilic normoblast)
    d. metarubricyte (orthochromic normoblast)
    e. reticulocyte   Ref. pp. 269, 270

126. Which cell has a nucleus which usually contains a few nucleoli:

    a. plasmacyte
    b. rubricyte
    c. metarubricyte
    d. rubriblast
    e. prorubricyte   Ref. p. 270

127. The oldest cell in the erythrocytic series is the:

   a. rubricyte
   b. prorubricyte
   c. erythrocyte
   d. metarubricyte
   e. reticulocyte   Ref. p. 268, 269, 270

128. The erythrocytic series is sometimes referred to as the normoblastic series.
                                              T   F   Ref. p. 269

129. The average normal erythrocyte has a diameter of:

   a.   3.0 microns
   b.   4.5 microns
   c.   7.5 microns
   d. 10.0 microns
   e.   9.5 microns   Ref. p. 274

130. Microcytosis is a decrease in the size of erythrocytes.   T   F   Ref. p. 274

131. *Abnormal* variation in the size of erythrocytes is called:

   a. hypochromia
   b. poikilocytosis
   c. ovalocytosis
   d. spherocytosis
   e. anisocytosis   Ref. p. 274

132. Macrocytosis is an increase in the size of erythrocytes. T   F   Ref. p. 274

133. Variation in the shape of erythrocytes is called:

   a. hypochromia
   b. anisocytosis
   c. poikilocytosis
   d. spherocytosis
   e. none of the above   Ref. p. 276

134. Target cells are also known as Mexican hat cells and leptocytes.
                                              T   F   Ref. p. 276

135. Target cells may be seen in thalassemia.   T   F   Ref. p. 276

136. Ovalocytosis, which is also called elliptocytosis, is an inherited abnormality.
                                              T   F   Ref. p. 276

137. Spherocytosis is the presence of sphere shaped erythrocytes which are thicker
     than normal disk shaped erythrocytes.   T   F   Ref. p. 276

138. Which of the following is *not* considered an erythrocyte inclusion:

    a. Howell-Jolly bodies
    b. basophilic stippling
    c. Cabot rings
    d. Heinz bodies
    e. Auer bodies   Ref. p. 278

139. When the hemoglobin in the erythrocytes is below normal, the condition is referred to as:

    a. microcytosis
    b. poikilocytosis
    c. anisocytosis
    d. hypocytopenia
    e. hypochromia   Ref. p. 278

140. Basophilic stippling is also referred to as punctate basophilia.
                                        T   F   Ref. p. 278

141. Basophilic stippling may be seen in erythrocytes in lead poisoning.
                                        T   F   Ref. p. 278

142. Cabot rings may be seen in:

    a. plasmacytes
    b. lymphocytes
    c. monocytes
    d. erythrocytes
    e. thrombocytes   Ref. p. 278

143. Howell-Jolly bodies may be seen in erythrocytes in severe anemias.
                                        T   F   Ref. p. 278

144. Polychromatophilia is also referred to as polychromasia and diffuse basophilia.
                                        T   F   Ref. p. 278

145. Rouleau formation, the arrangement of erythrocytes in rolls or stacks, may sometimes be seen in a normal blood smear.   T   F   Ref. p. 280

146. If the buffer solution used with Wright's stain is too acid, the erythrocytes will be colored a reddish color; if the buffer solution is too alkaline, the erythrocytes will be colored a dirty gray.   T   F   Ref. p. 280

147. A splitting of the nucleus in the red cell is known as:

    a. mononucleosis
    b. karyorrhexis
    c. anisocytosis
    d. polychromatophilia
    e. erythrocytosis   Ref. p. 284

148. Nucleated red cells may be distinguished from lymphocytes by the "company they keep" method of identification.   T   F   Ref. p. 284

149. The sedimentation rate is also referred to by the following terms: sed rate, erythrocyte sedimentation rate, ESR or E. S. R., sedimentation rate of erythrocytes, suspension stability of erythrocytes, and suspension stability of the blood.
                                                                     T   F   Ref. p. 300

150. The sedimentation rate is measured in mm. per hour and the normal values for the following methods are:

	men	*women*
Westergren	0–15	0–20
Wintrobe	0–10	0–20

                                                                     T   F   Ref. p. 300

151. You would expect an increase in the sedimentation rate in all of the following except:

    a. rheumatic fever
    b. rheumatoid arthritis
    c. cancer
    d. pregnancy
    e. polycythemia vera   Ref. p. 301

152. The sedimentation rate may be increased by changes in the normal ratio or percentage of the plasma proteins: albumin, globulin, and fibrinogen.
                                                                     T   F   Ref. p. 301

153. The sedimentation rate would be increased by such factors as rouleau formation of the red cells and tilting the sedimentation rate tube; whereas the sedimentation rate would be decreased by using blood which has stood for several hours and blood which has just been removed from the refrigerator.
                                                                     T   F   Ref. p. 301

154. Which of the following is not a method for performing the sedimentation rate:

    a. Westergren
    b. Wintrobe
    c. Cutler
    d. Landau
    e. Lee and White   Ref. p. 303

155. Which of the following could not be considered as a source of error in the sedimentation rate:

    a. excessive anticoagulant
    b. partially clotted blood
    c. use of cold unmixed blood
    d. air bubbles in blood column
    e. use of freshly drawn blood   Ref. p. 319

156. Blood which has been removed from the refrigerator should be allowed to return to room temperature and then thoroughly mixed before setting up a sedimentation rate.   T F   Ref. p. 319

157. The hematocrit reading may be referred to by all the following terms except:

   a. PCV
   b. Hct.
   c. cell pack
   d. MCV
   e. volume of erythrocytes   Ref. p. 320

158. When blood is centrifuged, the per cent occupied by the packed red cells is known as the hematocrit reading.   T F   Ref. p. 320

159. The normal values for the hematocrit reading in men are 40% to 54% whereas the normal values for women are 37% to 47%.   T F   Ref. p. 320

160. A high hematocrit reading is characteristically seen in:

   a. anemia
   b. leukemia
   c. infectious mononucleosis
   d. cancer
   e. polycythemia vera   Ref. p. 321

161. A low hematocrit reading may be seen in anemia whereas a high hematocrit reading may be found in dehydration conditions.   T F   Ref. p. 321

162. The hematocrit reading may be performed by the Wintrobe method, micro methods, and electronic methods.   T F   Ref. p. 322

163. The normal values for the reticulocyte count are:

   a. 5,000 to 10,000 per cu. mm.
   b. 40% to 54%
   c. 0 to 15 mm. per hr.
   d. 1% to 2%   .5 – 1.5 %
   e. 4 to 8 per cu. mm.   Ref. p. 331

164. A decrease in the production of red cells is indicated by:

   a. urobilinogen in urine
   b. leukocytosis
   c. thrombocytosis
   d. leukopenia
   e. reticulocyte count below normal   Ref. p. 332

165. The reticulocyte count drops below the normal values in aplastic anemia and rises above the normal values during a relapse in hereditary spherocytic anemia.   T F   Ref. p. 332

166. Reticulocytes are slightly larger than erythrocytes and contain a granular net-like substance. 　　　　　　　　　　　　　　　　T　F　　Ref. p. 333

167. A dye used for the staining of reticulocytes is:

    a. basic fuchsin
    b. sodium nitroprusside
    c. gentian violet
    d. brilliant cresyl blue
    e. potassium ferrocyanide 　　　　　　　　　　　　　　Ref. p. 334

168. The sickle cell examination is also referred to as a sickling examination, sickling of erythrocytes examination, RBC sickling test, and sickle cell phenomenon demonstration. 　　　　　　　　　　　　　T　F　　Ref. p. 340

169. The sickle cell examination is used to distinguish between sickle cell anemia and sickle cell trait. 　　　　　　　　　　　　T　F　　Ref. p. 341

170. Which of the following can *not* be used as an examination for the presence of Hb S:

    a. Scriver and Waugh method
    b. bisulfite method
    c. Sickledex method
    d. hemoglobin electrophoresis
    e. Duke method 　　　　　　　　　　　　　　　Ref. pp. 341, 519

171. The sickling of erythrocytes is due to the presence of an abnormal hemoglobin, Hb S, and its subsequent formation of tactoids or fluid crystals after the oxygen tension has been reduced. 　　　　　　　　T　F　　Ref. p. 341

172. Which reagent or equipment would not be used in any of the methods of performing the sickle cell examination:

    a. rubber bands
    b. 2% sodium metabisulfite
    c. petroleum jelly
    d. microscope
    e. 10% potassium permanganate 　　　　　　　　Ref. p. 342, 345

173. The osmotic fragility test is also referred to by the following terms: fragility test, F. T., RBC frag test, red cell fragility test, erythrocyte fragility test, red cell osmotic fragility test, and erythrocyte osmotic fragility test. 　　　　　　　　　　T　F　　Ref. p. 349

174. In the osmotic fragility test, the fragility of the red cells is said to be increased when the rate of hemolysis is increased. 　T　F　　Ref. p. 349

175. The fragility of the red cells is increased in:

    a. leukemia
    b. sickle cell anemia
    c. thalassemia major
    d. iron deficiency anemia
    e. hereditary spherocytic anemia 　　　　　　　　Ref. p. 350

176. The osmotic fragility test is increased in congenital hemolytic jaundice but decreased in obstructive jaundice.   T   F   Ref. p. 350

177. The Sanford method for the osmotic fragility test is performed by adding blood to a graded series of 12 hypotonic salt solutions and noting the extent of hemolysis after a period of 2 hours.   T   F   Ref. p. 350

178. The screening or presumptive test for the osmotic fragility of red cells is positive when hemolysis occurs in:

    a. 0.90% NaCl
    b. 0.85% NaCl
    c. 0.10 N NaCl
    d. 1.34% NaCl
    e. 0.50% NaCl   Ref. p. 353

179. In the Sanford method for the osmotic fragility test, the beginning of hemolysis for normal blood is 0.44% and the completion of hemolysis is 0.34%.   T   F   Ref. p. 356

180. The mean corpuscular volume (MCV) is the volume of the average erythrocyte.   T   F   Ref. p. 358

181. The normal range for the MCV is:

    a. 33%–38%
    b. 27 to 32 micromicrograms
    c. 14.5 grams
    d. 10–15 cc.
    e. 80 to 90 cubic microns   Ref. p. 358

182. The mean corpuscular hemoglobin (MCH) is the weight of hemoglobin in the average erythrocyte.   T   F   Ref. p. 358

183. The normal values for the MCH are:

    a. 14 to 18 grams per 100 ml.
    b. 33%–38%
    c. 80 to 90 cubic microns
    d. 27 to 32 micromicrograms
    e. 10 to 15 cc.   Ref. p. 358

184. The normal values for the MCHC are:

    a. 28–32 micromicrograms
    b. 33% to 38%
    c. 80 to 94 cu. microns
    d. 27% to 32%
    e. 80 to 90 micromicrograms   Ref. p. 358

185. To determine the MCV, you divide the:

    a. Hct × 10 by the Hb in grams
    b. Hb in grams by the RBC in millions
    c. RBC by the Hct
    d. RBC by the Hb in grams
    e. Hct × 10 by the RBC in millions   Ref. p. 364

186. To determine the MCH, you divide the:

    a. Hct by the RBC in millions
    b. Hct by the Hb in grams
    c. RBC by the Hct
    d. RBC by the Hb in grams
    e. Hb in grams × 10 by the RBC in millions   Ref. p. 366

187. The mean corpuscular hemoglobin concentration (MCHC) is determined by:

    a. multiplying the Hb in grams by 10 and dividing by the Hct
    b. multiplying the Hct by 100 and dividing by the Hb in grams
    c. dividing the Hb in grams by the Hct
    d. multiplying the Hb in grams by 100 and dividing by the Hct
    e. dividing the Hb in grams by the Hct times 10   Ref. p. 368

188. The color index is found by comparing the patient's hemoglobin and red cell count with a given set of standard values.   T   F   Ref. p. 371, 372

189. The normal range for the volume, color, and saturation indexes is:

    a. 0.0 to 1.0
    b. 0.5 to 1.0
    c. 1.0 to 1.5
    d. 1.0 to 2.0
    e. 0.9 to 1.1   Ref. p. 372

190. The mean corpuscular values present actual values whereas the red cell indexes present comparative values.   T   F   Ref. p. 373, 374

191. The color index may be found with the following formula:

$$\text{C. I.} = \frac{\text{Hb. in \%}}{\text{First 2 figures of RBC} \times 2}$$

T   F   Ref. p. 378

192. In the nomenclature for blood coagulation factors, Factor I is fibrinogen, Factor II is prothrombin, Factor III is thromboplastin, and Factor IV is calcium.   T   F   Ref. p. 386

193. Fibrinogen constitutes about 7% of the plasma proteins.
          T   F   Ref. p. 387

194. The synthesis of prothrombin takes place in the liver and requires the presence of vitamin K.   T   F   Ref. p. 387

195. Factor V (the labile factor) is consumed during the clotting of blood and is not found in the serum.   T F   Ref. p. 389

196. Parahemophilia is caused by a deficiency of factor:

   a. VIII
   b. VII
   c. V
   d. III
   e. I   Ref. p. 389

197. A deficiency of Factor IX (PTC) causes:

   a. hemorrhagic telangiectasia
   b. scurvy
   c. purpura hemorrhagica
   d. thrombocytopenic purpura
   e. Christmas disease   Ref. p. 391

198. Factor X is frequently referred to as the Stuart-Prower factor.
                                                   T F   Ref. p. 391

199. PTA (plasma thromboplastin antecedent) is an important factor which plays a role in the formation of plasma thromboplastin.   T F   Ref. p. 391

200. The end product of the first stage of coagulation is thromboplastin.
                                                   T F   Ref. p. 392, 393

201. The end product of the interaction between platelets and plasma factors other than fibrinogen is:

   a. prothrombin
   b. Factor I
   c. thrombin
   d. fibrin
   e. thrombocytes   Ref. Fig. 144, p. 393

202. The precursor of thrombin is:

   a. red cells
   b. fibrin
   c. NaCl
   d. fibrinogen
   e. prothrombin   Ref. p. 393, 394

203. The second stage of blood coagulation involves the conversion of prothrombin to thrombin.   T F   Ref. p. 394

204. In the third stage of coagulation, fibrinogen is converted into fibrin by:

   a. prothrombin
   b. calcium
   c. thromboplastin
   d. thrombin
   e. serum   Ref. p. 394

205. Platelets are necessary for normal clot retraction.   T   F   Ref. p. 394

206. The bleeding time is also referred to by the following terms: Bl. time, Bleeding t., skin bleeding time, capillary bleeding time, capillary contractility test,
capillary retractability test, and blood vessel retractability test.
                                                           T   F   Ref. p. 395

207. Which of the following is a method for testing capillary contractility:

   a. Westergren method
   b. Lee and White method
   c. Wintrobe method
   d. Ivy method
   e. Quick method   Ref. p. 395

208. The normal values for the bleeding time by the Duke method are:

   a. 11–16 seconds
   b. 2–12 minutes
   c. 0.9–1.1 min.
   d. 1–3 minutes
   e. 60–100 seconds   Ref. p. 395, 396

209. The method of performing the bleeding time by making a cut on the forearm
after application of a blood pressure cuff is called the:

   a. Macfarlane method
   b. Lee and White method
   c. Duke method
   d. Quick method
   e. Ivy method   Ref. p. 396

210. When doing a bleeding time by the method which employs a blood pressure
apparatus, the blood pressure cuff is inflated to:

   a. 10 mm. pressure
   b. 20 mm. pressure
   c. 30 mm. pressure
   d. 40 mm. pressure
   e. 50 mm. pressure   Ref. p. 396

211. The coagulation time is also referred to as the coag. time, clotting time, and
whole blood clotting time.   T   F   Ref. p. 402

212. Which of the following is *not* a method of performing the coagulation time:

   a. capillary tube method
   b. Dale and Laidlaw method
   c. silicone tube method
   d. Wintrobe method
   e. Howell method   Ref. p. 402

213. The normal values for the Lee and White method of performing the coagulation time are:

    a. 1–3 minutes
    b. 2–6 minutes
    c. 5–15 minutes
    d. 10–30 minutes
    e. 20–60 minutes   Ref. p. 402

214. Capillary blood methods have shorter clotting times than venous blood methods.   T   F   Ref. p. 402

215. The coagulation time using silicone coated glass tubes is longer than the coagulation time using ordinary glass tubes.   T   F   Ref. p. 402 and p. 404

216. If the method of performing the coagulation time calls for the temperature to be controlled, the correct temperature is:

    a. 56° C.
    b. 4° C.
    c. 76° C.
    d. 37° C.
    e. 98° C.   Ref. p. 404 and p. 411

217. Coagulation will be hastened by all of the following except:

    a. dirty test tubes
    b. tissue juices mixed with blood
    c. air bubbles in blood
    d. excessive agitation of blood
    e. temperature of 18° C.–20° C.   Ref. p. 413

218. The word platelet is another name for a thrombocyte.   T   F   Ref. p. 414

219. Platelets originate in the bone marrow from:

    a. myeloblasts
    b. lymphoblasts
    c. rubriblasts
    d. megakaryocytes
    e. none of the above   Ref. p. 414, 415

220. Platelets have a diameter of:

    a. 8–10 microns
    b. 6–8 microns
    c. 4–6 mm.
    d. 2–4 microns
    e. 10–12 mm.   Ref. p. 414

221. The life span of a platelet is about:

    a. 110 days
    b. 48 hours
    c. 9 days
    d. 4 weeks
    e. none of the above   Ref. p. 416

222. The normal values for the platelet count are:

   a. 50,000 to 100,000 per cu. mm.
   b. 5,000 to 10,000 per cu. mm.
   c. 500,000 to 750,000 per cc.
   d. 150,000 to 400,000 per cu. mm.
   e. none of the above   Ref. p. 416

223. When the platelet count drops below the normal values, it is referred to as a thrombocytopenia.   T F   Ref. p. 416

224. A thrombocytopenia may be found in purpura hemorrhagica (idiopathic thrombocytopenic purpura) and symptomatic thrombocytopenic purpura.
                                                          T F   Ref. p. 416

225. When the platelet count rises above the normal values, it is referred to as a thrombocytosis.   T F   Ref. p. 416

226. A thrombocytosis may be seen after splenectomy, in polycythemia vera, acute posthemorrhagic anemia, myeloproliferative disorders, metastatic carcinoma, and chronic granulocytic leukemia.   T F   Ref. p. 416

227. The platelet count may be below the normal values in newborn infants and before menstruation; the platelet count may be above the normal values at high altitudes and after severe exercise.   T F   Ref. p. 417

228. A platelet count below normal is usually associated with all of the following except:

   a. increased bleeding time
   b. increased clot retraction time
   c. decreased prothrombin consumption time
   d. positive capillary resistance test
   e. decreased coagulation time   Ref. p. 417

229. Which of the following methods is a *direct* method for the platelet count:

   a. Fonio
   b. Dameshek
   c. Olef
   d. Cramer and Bannerman
   e. Rees and Ecker   Ref. p. 417

230. The platelet count may be performed by all the following methods except:

   a. Fonio
   b. Dameshek
   c. Rees and Ecker
   d. Brecher-Cronkite
   e. Westergren   Ref. p. 417

231. In the Rees and Ecker method, the platelets are counted in a counting chamber or hemocytometer and the value obtained is multiplied by a dilution correction factor and a volume correction factor.   T F   Ref. p. 423, 428

232. If blood is drawn to the 0.5 mark of a red cell pipet and Rees and Ecker diluting fluid is drawn to the 101 mark, the dilution correction factor for the platelet count is 200.   T   F   Ref. p. 424, 428

233. In the Brecher-Cronkite method for the platelet count, a phase microscope is used which enables the platelets to be identified on the basis of their structure as well as their size and shape.   T   F   Ref. p. 429

234. In normal blood, there is partial retraction of the clot in 2 hours and complete retraction in 24 hours.   T   F   Ref. p. 433

235. The clot retraction time is usually increased if the platelet count is decreased.
                                                                      T   F   Ref. p. 434

236. The clot retraction time is usually increased in all of the following except:

   a. purpura hemorrhagica (idiopathic thrombocytopenic purpura)
   b. Glanzmann's disease (hereditary hemorrhagic thrombasthenia)
   c. aplastic anemia
   d. acute leukemia
   e. acute infectious lymphocytosis   Ref. p. 434

237. The clot retraction time may be performed by the single tube method, Macfarlane serum method, Tocantins method, Budtz-Olsen method, and Stefanini-Dameshek method.   T   F   Ref. p. 434

238. In the procedure for the clot retraction time, the blood is placed in a water bath at:

   a. 72° C.
   b. 98° C.
   c. 56° C.
   d. 37° C.
   e.   4° C.   Ref. p. 434

239. The fibrinogen deficiency test has the following normal values:

   a.   90 to 120 mg/100 ml plasma
   b.   10 to 15 mg/100 ml whole blood
   c. 200 to 400 mg/100 ml plasma
   d. 350 to 550 mg/100 ml plasma
   e. none of the above   Ref. p. 437

240. The fibrinogen deficiency test may be below the normal values in the following: congenital afibrinogenemia, congenital hypofibrinogenemia, severe liver damage, during or following surgery, severe hemorrhage, and complications during pregnancy.   T   F   Ref. p. 437

241. The fibrinogen deficiency test may be performed by all the following methods except:

    a. Fibrindex
    b. Warner-Lambert
    c. Fi-Test
    d. titration
    e. Wintrobe   Ref. p. 438

242. The prothrombin time is also referred to by the following terms: PT, pro time, prothrombin time test, P. T. test, and plasma prothrombin time.
                                                          T F   Ref. p. 443

243. The prothrombin time is a specific test for the quantitative measurement of prothrombin.   T F   Ref. p. 443

244. The normal values for the prothrombin time are:

    a. 1–3 minutes
    b. 28–40 seconds
    c. 2–6 minutes
    d. 60–82 seconds
    e. 11–16 seconds   Ref. p. 444

245. The prothrombin time is above the normal values in Dicumarol therapy, heparin therapy, fibrinogen deficiency, prothrombin deficiency, and vitamin K deficiency.   T F   Ref. p. 444

246. When the prothrombin time is used to control anticoagulant therapy, it is usually maintained:

    a. about 10 times the normal values
    b. slightly below the normal values
    c. within the normal values
    d. about 5 times the normal values
    e. about 2.5 times the normal values   Ref. p. 444

247. The prothrombin time may be performed by the following method:

    a. Wintrobe's method
    b. Westergren's method
    c. Rees and Ecker method
    d. Howell's method
    e. Quick's method   Ref. p. 445

248. In preparing the patient's plasma for the prothrombin time, which of the following anticoagulants is used:

    a. 0.1 ml. of Sequestrene
    b. 0.2 ml. of 10% ammonium oxalate
    c. 0.2 ml. of EDTA
    d. 0.5 ml. of 0.1 M (1.34%) sodium oxalate
    e. 0.1 ml. of 5% potassium oxalate   Ref. p. 455

249. In performing the prothrombin time, the correct temperature of the water bath is:

a. 4° C.
b. 56° C.
c. 76° C.
d. 48° C.
e. 37° C.   Ref. p. 460

250. The partial thromboplastin time is not capable of indicating a deficiency of factor VII or the functioning ability of platelets.   T F   Ref. p. 471

251. Which of the following is not used in performing the partial thromboplastin time:

a. 37° C. water bath
b. 0.02 M calcium chloride
c. partial thromboplastin reagent
d. normal control plasma
e. 0.5 ml. of patient's serum   Ref. p. 471

252. A partial thromboplastin time above 100 seconds would be considered abnormal.   T F   Ref. p. 472

253. Abnormal results of the prothrombin consumption time indicate a deficiency in the production of plasma thromboplastin.   T F   Ref. p. 475

254. In performing the prothrombin consumption time, you use the patient's serum rather than the patient's plasma.   T F   Ref. p. 475

255. A prothrombin consumption time below 18 seconds would be considered abnormal.   T F   Ref. p. 476

256. The plasma thrombin time may be affected by the concentration of fibrinogen in the patient's plasma.   T F   Ref. p. 476

257. Which of the following is not used in performing the plasma thrombin time:

a. normal control plasma
b. 37° C. water bath
c. thrombin solution
d. patient's plasma
e. thromboplastin reagent   Ref. p. 476

258. The normal range of the plasma thrombin time is:

a. 1–3 minutes
b. 2–6 minutes
c. 28–40 seconds
d. 12–15 seconds
e. none of the above   Ref. p. 477

259. The plasma recalcification time is also referred to as the plasma clotting time, recalcification time test, calcium clotting time, and calcium clotting time test.
                                                    T   F   Ref. p. 477

260. Plasma, if recalcified, will usually clot within 1–2 minutes.
                                                    T   F   Ref. p. 477

261. The plasma recalcification time is prolonged in all of the following except:

   a. classical hemophilia and Christmas disease
   b. deficiency of prothrombin or fibrinogen
   c. deficiency of factor V or factor X
   d. presence of a circulating anticoagulant
   e. polycythemia vera and pernicious anemia   Ref. p. 477

262. Which of the following is not used in performing the plasma recalcification time:

   a. patient's plasma
   b. 0.025 M calcium chloride
   c. 37° C. water bath
   d. stop watch or timer
   e. 0.85% sodium chloride   Ref. p. 478

263. Which of the following could be considered a normal range for the plasma recalcification time:

   a. 28–40 seconds
   b. 5–10 minutes
   c. 10–30 minutes
   d. 90–120 seconds
   e. 11–16 seconds   Ref. p. 478

264. The capillary resistance test is also referred to as the capillary fragility test, tourniquet test, cuff test, Rumpel-Leede test, R-L test, and the Rumpel-Leede phenomenon.   T   F   Ref. p. 479

265. A positive capillary resistance test is usually found in:

   a. polycythemia vera
   b. tuberculosis
   c. erythroblastosis fetalis
   d. agranulocytosis
   e. purpura hemorrhagica   Ref. p. 479

266. The capillary resistance test may be performed by either the tourniquet methods or the suction cup method.   T   F   Ref. p. 479

267. A positive capillary resistance is indicated by the appearance of petechiae:

   a. in the blood clot
   b. on the leg
   c. in the plasma
   d. on the arm
   e. in or on none of the above   Ref. p. 480

268. In the fibrinolysin test, a rapid lysis of the fibrin clot indicates the presence of an abnormal amount of fibrinolysin.   T F   Ref. p. 482

269. A euglobulin clot lysis time *below* the normal values indicates increased fibrinolytic activity.   T F   Ref. p. 484, 485

270. A circulating anticoagulant is an anticoagulant which circulates in the blood, hinders the normal clotting of blood, and causes a hemorrhagic syndrome.
                                              T F   Ref. p. 488

271. The Hicks-Pitney test is a modification of the thromboplastin generation test.
                                              T F   Ref. p. 489

272. Platelet adhesiveness is usually reduced in von Willebrand's disease.
                                              T F   Ref. p. 490

273. The prothrombin and proconvertin test (P and P test) is similar to the one-stage prothrombin time, the main difference being that the plasma is diluted in order to make the test more sensitive.   T F   Ref. p. 491

274. The Stypven time is a test performed exactly like Quick's one-stage prothrombin time except that Stypven (Russell's viper venom) is used in place of thromboplastin.   T F   Ref. p. 491

275. The thromboplastin generation test (TGT) is a long involved test which may be used to pinpoint deficiencies in the production of thromboplastin.
                                              T F   Ref. p. 491

276. Owren's thrombotest is used in the control of anticoagulant therapy, the normal range is 70%–130% activity, and the therapeutic range is generally considered to be 10%–20% activity.   T F   Ref. p. 491

277. The eosinophil count is also referred to as the direct eosinophil count, total eosinophil count, absolute eosinophil count, and circulating eosinophile count.
                                              T F   Ref. p. 494

278. The normal values for the direct eosinophil count are:

    a. 25%–35%
    b. 5,000–10,000 per cu. mm.
    c. 2%–6%
    d. 10–15 per cu. mm.
    e. 50–400 per cu. mm.   Ref. p. 494

279. When the eosinophil count drops below the normal values, the condition is known as an eosinopenia; when the eosinophil count rises above the normal values, the condition is known as an eosinophilia.   T F   Ref. p. 494

280. You would expect to find an eosinophilia in all of the following except:

    a. allergies
    b. skin diseases
    c. parasitic infestations
    d. chronic granulocytic leukemia
    e. hyperadrenalism (Cushing's disease)   Ref. p. 495

281. Which of the following is not a diluting fluid for the eosinophil count:

    a. phloxine diluting fluid
    b. Pilot's solution
    c. Tannen's diluting fluid
    d. Randolph's diluting fluid
    e. Rees and Ecker solution   Ref. p. 495

282. The eosinophil diluting fluid stains the eosinophils:

    a. blue
    b. yellow
    c. brown
    d. basophilic
    e. red   Ref. p. 495, 497

283. The Improved Neubauer ruling counting chamber has 2 sections. Each section
    has an area of 9 sq. mm. and a depth of 0.1 mm. Therefore, the *total* volume
    used in the eosinophil count is $2 \times 9 \times 0.1 = 1.8$ cu. mm.
                                        T   F   Ref. p. 496–498

284. The normal values for the spinal cell count are 0 to 10 white cells per cu. mm.
                                        T   F   Ref. p. 500

285. The spinal cell count rises above the normal values in meningitis, encephalitis,
    poliomyelitis, and latent syphilis.   T   F   Ref. p. 500

286. Spinal fluid often contains contagious material; therefore, particular precau-
    tions should be taken in handling the specimens.   T   F   Ref. p. 501, 502

287. The L. E. cell examination is also referred to as the LE cell test, Lupus Ery-
    thematosus test, L. E. preparation, and LE prep.   T   F   Ref. p. 506

288. The L. E. factor is a gamma globulin.   T   F   Ref. p. 506

289. The L. E. factor is frequently present in the plasma of patients with systemic
    lupus erythematosus; this L. E. factor acts upon a white cell and causes a
    chemical change in the nucleus.   T   F   Ref. p. 506

290. The L. E. cell is a neutrophilic leukocyte that has ingested a homogeneous
    globular mass of altered nuclear material.   T   F   Ref. p. 506

291. In an L. E. cell, the ingested material is round, smooth, and evenly stained; in
    a tart cell, the ingested material is irregular, coarse, and unevenly stained.
                                        T   F   Ref. p. 507

292. The Zimmer and Hargraves method of preparing the smear for the L. E. cell examination employs the use of:

    a. oxalated blood
    b. citrated blood
    c. capillary anticoagulated blood
    d. cell suspension
    e. clotted blood   Ref. p. 507

293. Which of the following is used in the Zinkham and Conley method of preparing the smear for the L. E. cell examination:

    a. clotted blood and blood plasma
    b. blood serum and citrated blood
    c. cell suspension and oxalated blood
    d. heparin and glass beads
    e. none of the above   Ref. p. 507, 508

294. Fetal hemoglobin is often referred to as F hemoglobin, hemoglobin F, Hb F, HbF, and Hb-F.   T F   Ref. p. 511

295. At birth, 50% to 90% of the hemoglobin is fetal hemoglobin.
                                                  T F   Ref. p. 511

296. After the age of 2 years, the blood contains the following per cent of Hb-F (fetal hemoglobin):

    a. 20%–30%
    b. 10%–20%
    c. 30%–40%
    d. 0%–2%
    e. none of the above values   Ref. p. 511

297. The fetal hemoglobin determination may be performed by the alkali denaturation method, blood slide methods, and electrophoretic methods.
                                                  T F   Ref. p. 512

298. Which hemoglobin is most resistant to alkali denaturation:

    a. Hb A
    b. Hb S
    c. Hb C
    d. Hb F
    e. Hb D   Ref. p. 512

299. In the alkali denaturation method for the fetal hemoglobin determination, which of the following is not used:

    a. hemoglobin solution (hemolysate)
    b. N/12 potassium hydroxide (alkali)
    c. stopwatch or timer
    d. acidified 50% saturated solution of ammonium sulfate
    e. patient's serum   Ref. p. 513

300. Hb A, Hb A₂, and Hb F are all normal hemoglobins.   T F   Ref. p. 518

301. Hemoglobin A has 2 alpha chains and 2 beta chains.   T F   Ref. p. 518

302. Hemoglobin A₂ has 2 alpha chains and 2 delta chains.   T F   Ref. p. 518

303. Hemoglobin F has 2 alpha chains and 2 gamma chains.   T F   Ref. p. 518

304. The hemoglobin diseases (hemoglobinopathies) are genetically transmitted.
                                                             T F   Ref. p. 519

305. If a person inherits a gene for normal hemoglobin A from one parent and a
     gene for abnormal hemoglobin S from the other parent, his hemoglobin pattern
     is said to be heterozygous.   T F   Ref. p. 519

306. If a person inherits a gene for abnormal hemoglobin S from both parents, his
     hemoglobin pattern is said to be homozygous.   T F   Ref. p. 519

307. In hemoglobin electrophoresis, which of the following migrate at the same
     speed:

     a. Hb A and Hb H
     b. Hb F and Hb C
     c. Hb G and Hb E
     d. Hb S and Hb D
     e. none of the above   Ref. p. 520, 521

308. Which hemoglobin moves the least during hemoglobin electrophoretic separa-
     tions on filter paper using 0.05 M barbital buffer solution at a pH of 8.6:

     a. S
     b. F
     c. A
     d. D
     e. C   Ref. p. 521

309. Hemoglobin electrophoretic separations may be carried out with the following
     media: filter paper, starch block, agar gel, acrylamide gel, and cellulose
     acetate.   T F   Ref. p. 521

310. In a normal bone marrow smear, you would expect to find the following
     number of myeloblasts:

     a. 7%–30%
     b. 5%–10%
     c. 15%–25%
     d. 0%–5%
     e. none of the above values   Ref. p. 523

311. In a normal bone marrow smear, you would expect to find the following
     number of neutrophilic band ("stab") cells:

     a. 1%–3%
     b. 2%–6%
     c. 5%–20%
     d. 10%–35%
     e. none of the above values   Ref. p. 523

312. In a normal bone marrow smear, you would expect to find the following number of lymphocytes:

a. 0%–5%
b. 20%–35%
c. 55%–75%
d. 5%–15%
e. none of the above values   Ref. p. 523

313. The M:E ratio (myeloid-erythroid ratio) is also referred to as the WBC: Nucleated RBC ratio and the average value is 4:1 with a normal range of 6:1 to 2:1.   T F   Ref. p. 522

314. An increased M:E ratio may be found in infections, granulocytic leukemia, leukemoid reactions, and a decrease in the number of nucleated red cells.
                                        T F   Ref. p. 522

315. A bone marrow examination is of particular interest to the physician in aplastic anemia, pernicious anemia, leukemia, purpura hemorrhagica, agranulocytosis, and multiple myeloma.   T F   Ref. p. 522

316. A megakaryocyte found in a bone marrow smear would be:

a. about the size of a myeloblast
b. about the size of 5 platelets
c. about the size of a monocyte
d. about the size of a prorubricyte
e. about 4 times the size of a myelocyte   Ref. Plate 15, p. 526

317. Bone marrow smears usually require a longer staining time than smears of peripheral blood.   T F   Ref. p. 525

318. A siderocyte is an erythrocyte containing free iron and a sideroblast is a nucleated red cell containing free iron.   T F   Ref. p. 529

319. The normal values for siderocytes are 0%–1%; increased values may be found in thalassemia major, lead poisoning, and following splenectomy (removal of the spleen).   T F   Ref. p. 529, 530

320. A Prussian blue reagent, which is freshly prepared by mixing a potassium ferrocyanide solution and dilute hydrochloric acid solution, is used for the siderocyte stain.   T F   Ref. p. 530

321. Heinz bodies may be present in erythrocytes in hemolytic anemia caused by drug poisoning and following splenectomy (removal of the spleen).
                                        T F   Ref. p. 532

322. If Heinz bodies are present in erythrocytes, they may be seen:

a. on wet unstained preparations of blood
b. after staining with a methyl violet solution
c. after staining with a brilliant cresyl blue solution
d. with all of the above methods
e. with none of the above methods   Ref. p. 532

50

323. Heinz bodies stain a deep purple with a methyl violet solution.
                                                        T   F   Ref. p. 532, 533

324. With the exception of the myeloblast, which is peroxidase negative, all cells of
the granulocytic series are peroxidase positive.   T   F   Ref. p. 535

325. All cells of the lymphocytic series and plasmacytic series are peroxidase
negative.   T   F   Ref. p. 535

326. The peroxidase stain may be useful in distinguishing between acute granulocytic leukemia and acute lymphocytic leukemia.   T   F   Ref. p. 536

327. In acute granulocytic leukemia, 5%–25% of the white cells are peroxidase
positive; in acute lymphocytic leukemia, 95%–100% of the white cells are
peroxidase negative.   T   F   Ref. p. 536

328. The peroxidase stain may be performed by all the following methods except:

    a. Sato and Sekiya method
    b. Goodpasture's method
    c. Kaplow's method
    d. Graham-Knoll method
    e. Sanford's method   Ref. p. 537

329. The alkaline phosphatase stain is also referred to as the alkaline phosphatase
score, alkaline phosphatase test, alkaline phosphatase activity of neutrophils,
leukocyte alkaline phosphatase test, LAP test, and alkaline phosphatase cytochemical test.   T   F   Ref. p. 539

330. An enzyme, alkaline phosphatase, is present in neutrophilic segmented cells,
neutrophilic band cells, and neutrophilic metamyelocytes.
                                                        T   F   Ref. p. 539

331. In the leukocyte alkaline phosphatase test, values below normal may be found
in chronic granulocytic leukemia whereas values above normal may be found
in neutrophilic leukemoid reactions.   T   F   Ref. p. 539

332. When the alkaline phosphatase stain is performed by the method of Kaplow,
the fixative is a mixture of formalin (36%–39% formaldehyde) and absolute
methanol (absolute methyl alcohol).   T   F   Ref. p. 541

333. The leukocyte alkaline phosphatase score is obtained by counting 100 neutrophils and grading the color and amount of granular precipitate, the following
grades being used: 0, 1+, 2+, 3+, and 4+.   T   F   Ref. p. 543, 544

334. Which stain is widely used for staining both blood smears and malaria smears:

    a. Feulgen stain
    b. peroxidase stain
    c. Pappenheim's stain
    d. alkaline phosphatase stain
    e. Giemsa stain   Ref. p. 545

335. The Feulgen reaction is specific for deoxyribonucleic acid (DNA).
T F   Ref. p. 546

336. The Ham test is also referred to as Ham's test for paroxysmal nocturnal hemoglobinuria, Ham's test for P. N. H., Ham's acidified serum test, acid-serum test, acid-serum hemolysis test, acid hemolysis test, and acid hemolysin test.   T F   Ref. p. 550

337. The Ham test involves mixing the patient's red cells with acidified serum and inspecting the mixture for hemolysis.   T F   Ref. p. 550

338. The Donath-Landsteiner test is also referred to as the Donath-Landsteiner reaction, Donath-Landsteiner hemolysin test, D-L hemolysin test, D-L antibody test, Donath-Landsteiner test for cold-warm hemolysins, and Donath-Landsteiner test for paroxysmal cold hemoglobinuria (P. C. H.).
T F   Ref. p. 552

339. The Donath-Landsteiner test is positive when a blood sample shows hemolysis:

  a. at 37 degrees F.
  b. at 4 degrees F.
  c. at 56 degrees C.
  d. after cooling at 4 degrees C. and rewarming to 56 degrees C.
  e. after cooling at 4 degrees C. and rewarming to 37 degrees C.
                                                  Ref. p. 553

340. The glucose-6-phosphate dehydrogenase deficiency test is also referred to as the G6PD deficiency test and the G-6-PD test.   T F   Ref. p. 554

341. The G6PD test is useful in diagnosing hemolytic anemia caused by oxidant drugs.   T F   Ref. p. 554

342. The Sia test is also referred to as the Sia test for macroglobulins, macroglobulinemia test, and euglobulin test.   T F   Ref. p. 556

343. The Sia test is performed by simply adding serum to distilled water and looking for the presence or absence of a heavy coarse precipitate.
T F   Ref. p. 556

344. The Thorn eosinophil test is also referred to as the Thorn ACTH test, ACTH stimulation test, and the eosinophil depression test.   T F   Ref. p. 556

345. The Thorn eosinophil test is a test for adrenal cortical function.
T F   Ref. p. 556

346. If the adrenal cortical function is normal, the eosinophil count is considerably *decreased* after an injection of ACTH.   T F   Ref. p. 557

347. A buffy coat is also referred to as the white cell cream or leukocytic cream.
T F   Ref. p. 558

348. A buffy coat preparation is a blood smear made from a concentrated specimen of white cells and it may be useful in searching for immature white cells seen in aleukemic leukemia, a phase of leukemia in which the immature white cells are few in number.   T   F   Ref. p. 559

349. The pigment carboxyhemoglobin, which is found in carbon monoxide poisoning, gives blood a brilliant cherry red color.   T   F   Ref. p. 562

350. Ehrlich's finger test is positive in paroxysmal cold hemoglobinuria (P. C. H.).
                                                                      T   F   Ref. p. 562

351. A method of determining the total plasma volume by injecting a suitable dye and measuring the resulting dilution is the:

    a. Feulgen stain
    b. Quick method
    c. LAP stain
    d. Sanford method
    e. Evans blue method   Ref. p. 562

352. Haptoglobin is a glycoprotein which binds free hemoglobin.
                                                                      T   F   Ref. p. 563

353. To calculate the hemolytic index, the following is required:

    a. Hb and hematocrit reading
    b. Hb and RBC
    c. Hb and urinary urobilinogen
    d. Hb and bilirubin
    e. Hb and fecal urobilinogen   Ref. p. 563, 564

354. Schumm's test is used to identify:

    a. plasma hemoglobin
    b. sulfhemoglobin
    c. methemoglobin
    d. oxyhemoglobin
    e. methemalbumin   Ref. p. 564

355. Normally, about 0.01% to 0.30% of the total hemoglobin is methemoglobin; increased amounts of methemoglobin may be found in toxic conditions caused by oxidizing drugs.   T   F   Ref. p. 565

356. The normal values for the plasma hemoglobin determination are 2 to 3 milligrams per 100 milliliters of serum; values above normal may occur in some cases of hemolytic anemia and in any condition associated with the sudden and extensive destruction of erythrocytes.   T   F   Ref. p. 565

357. If blood is shaken for 15 minutes and it turns a mauve-lavender color, the presence of sulfhemoglobin may be suspected.   T   F   Ref. p. 567

358. Teichmann's test for blood is performed by adding a crystal of sodium chloride and a drop of glacial acetic acid to 1 drop of the suspected specimen, mixing, gently heating the preparation, allowing it to cool, and then inspecting the preparation for rhombic shaped crystals of hemin.   T F   Ref. p. 568

359. A wet blood film examination may be used to study the red cells, white cells, platelets, and blood dust seen in a fresh specimen of blood.
                                                          T F   Ref. p. 568

360. A normal balance or equilibrium exists between red cell production and red cell destruction.   T F   Ref. p. 571

361. The normal daily output of red cells by the bone marrow is:

   a. 1 ml. of packed cells
   b. 5 ml. of packed cells
   c. 10 ml. of packed cells
   d. 20 ml. of packed cells
   e. 60 ml. of packed cells   Ref. p. 571

362. The life span of the erythrocyte in the blood stream is about:

   a. 2 months
   b. 30 days
   c. 10 days
   d. 5 weeks
   e. 120 days   Ref. p. 572

363. The morphological classification of the anemias deals with the size and hemoglobin content of the erythrocytes whereas the etiological classification is concerned with the cause of the anemia.   T F   Ref. p. 573

364. A MCV greater than 90 cubic microns indicates:

   a. spherocytosis
   b. macrocytic erythrocytes
   c. Howell-Jolly bodies
   d. hypochromia
   e. sickle cells   Ref. p. 573

365. Lack of development of an organ is referred to as:

   a. macrocytosis
   b. aplasia
   c. mononucleosis
   d. microcytosis
   e. polychromatophilia   Ref. p. 577, p. 703

366. Aplastic anemia is usually caused by the action of drugs, chemicals, or radiation on the bone marrow.   T F   Ref. p. 577

367. Aplastic anemia is characterized by a pancytopenia, that is, a poverty or decrease of all blood cells.   T F   Ref. p. 578

368. In aplastic anemia, you would expect the platelet count (thrombocyte count) to be:

    a. above normal
    b. 5,000 to 10,000 per cu. mm.
    c. 4.0 to 6.5 million per cu. mm.
    d. below normal
    e. normal   Ref. p. 578

369. In iron deficiency anemia, the blood smear shows hypochromia and micro-cytosis; in addition, it may also show anisocytosis and poikilocytosis.
                                                T F   Ref. p. 581

370. In iron deficiency anemia, the MCH is:

    a. normal
    b. increased
    c. 27 to 32 micromicrograms
    d. decreased
    e. 90 to 110 cubic microns   Ref. p. 581

371. In iron deficiency anemia, the mean corpuscular hemoglobin concentration (MCHC) is increased.   T F   Ref. p. 581

372. In iron deficiency anemia, there is an increase in:

    a. serum iron
    b. hemoglobin
    c. RBC
    d. total iron-binding capacity (TIBC)
    e. white cell count   Ref. p. 581

373. In iron deficiency anemia, the serum iron is:

    a. low and the TIBC is low
    b. low and the TIBC is normal
    c. low and the TIBC is high
    d. normal but the TIBC is low
    e. elevated and the TIBC is also elevated   Ref. p. 581

374. In iron deficiency anemia, the bone marrow is hyperplastic and shows an in-crease in nucleated red cells.   T F   Ref. p. 581

375. Pyridoxine deficiency most closely resembles:

    a. pernicious anemia
    b. erythroblastosis fetalis
    c. thalassemia major
    d. iron deficiency anemia
    e. hereditary spherocytic anemia   Ref. p. 582

376. Iron deficiency anemia is a microcytic hypochromic anemia.
                                                T F   Ref. p. 582

377. Pernicious anemia is caused by failure of the stomach to secrete an intrinsic factor.   T F   Ref. p. 584

378. The development of the macrocyte seen in pernicious anemia is associated with a deficiency of vitamin B_{12}.   T F   Ref. p. 585

379. A promegaloblast is a pernicious anemia type rubriblast.
                                                             T F   Ref. p. 587

380. In pernicious anemia, the color index shows increased values.
                                                        T F   Ref. p. 587, 589

381. The white cell abnormality most characteristic of pernicious anemia is the presence of:

    a. myeloblasts with Auer rods
    b. toxic granulation of neutrophils
    c. hypersegmented neutrophils
    d. atypical lymphocytes
    e. I. M. cells   Ref. p. 589

382. In pernicious anemia, the MCV is:

    a. decreased
    b. 33% to 38%
    c. 70 to 80 cubic microns
    d. increased
    e. normal   Ref. p. 590, 591

383. In pernicious anemia:

    a. the platelets and white cells are increased
    b. the platelets are increased but the white cells are decreased
    c. the platelets are decreased and the white cells are increased
    d. the platelets and white cells are decreased
    e. the platelets and white cells are normal   Ref. p. 590

384. In pernicious anemia, a gastric analysis reveals the absence of free hydrochloric acid, even after stimulation with histamine.   T F   Ref. p. 590

385. In pernicious anemia, the Schilling test is positive and thus becomes a useful diagnostic aid.   T F   Ref. p. 590

386. The serum vitamin B_{12} level, which can be determined chemically or by measuring the growth response of certain bacteria, is decreased in pernicious anemia.
                                                             T F   Ref. p. 590

387. Which test is *not* useful in the diagnosis of pernicious anemia:

    a. gastric analysis
    b. blood smear (differential and RBC morphology)
    c. Schilling test
    d. sedimentation rate
    e. bone marrow examination   Ref. p. 591

388. Pernicious anemia is classified as a macrocytic anemia and also as a megaloblastic anemia.   T   F   Ref. p. 592

389. Macrocytic anemia may be seen in all of the following, except:

    a. pernicious anemia
    b. tropical sprue
    c. idiopathic steatorrhea
    d. *Diphyllobothrium latum* infestation
    e. thalassemia major   Ref. p. 592

390. Macrocytic anemia may be seen following the administration of:

    a. 6-mercaptopurine
    b. 5-fluorouracil
    c. Dilantin
    d. mysoline
    e. all of the above   Ref. p. 592

391. When the erythrocyte breaks down in the hemolytic anemias, it liberates hemoglobin which decomposes into iron, globulin, and bilirubin.
                                                           T   F   Ref. p. 593

392. The one common finding in all hemolytic anemias is:

    a. presence of abnormal hemoglobin
    b. extracorpuscular abnormalities
    c. positive Coombs' test
    d. increased osmotic fragility
    e. increased hemolysis of red cells   Ref. p. 594

393. An increase in the breakdown of red cells causes the blood to show an increase
in bilirubin.   T   F   Ref. p. 594

394. An increase in the breakdown of red cells usually causes the urine and feces to
show an increase in urobilinogen.   T   F   Ref. p. 594

395. In the hemolytic anemias, increased destruction of red cells stimulates the bone
marrow to produce more red cells.   T   F   Ref. p. 594

396. An increase in plasma hemoglobin and the presence of methemalbumin in the
blood are signs of:

    a. posthemorrhagic anemia
    b. aplastic anemia
    c. increased red cell production
    d. chronic granulocytic leukemia
    e. increased red cell destruction   Ref. p. 594

397. In the hemolytic anemias, which of the following does *not* indicate increased RBC production:

   a. increase in reticulocyte count
   b. thrombocytopenia
   c. polychromatophilia in the blood smear
   d. increase in platelet count
   e. nucleated RBC's in the blood smear   Ref. p. 594

398. When erythrocytes from a patient with an intracorpuscular hemolytic anemia are transfused into a normal person, the transfused erythrocytes have a *decreased* life span.   T   F   Ref. p. 595

399. Hemolysis is caused by an intracorpuscular defect in all of the following, except:

   a. hereditary spherocytic anemia
   b. sickle cell anemia
   c. thalassemia major
   d. paroxysmal cold hemoglobinuria   Ref. p. 595, 596

400. When normal erythrocytes are transfused into a patient with an extracorpuscular hemolytic anemia, the normal erythrocytes have a *decreased* life span.
                                                     T   F   Ref. p. 595, 596

401. Hereditary spherocytic anemia is also referred to as congenital hemolytic anemia and hereditary spherocytosis.   T   F   Ref. p. 596

402. In hereditary spherocytic anemia, the spherocyte has a smaller diameter than a normal erythrocyte.   T   F   Ref. p. 598, 599

403. In hereditary spherocytic anemia, the red cell osmotic fragility test shows *increased* fragility.   T   F   Ref. p. 599

404. In hereditary spherocytic anemia, the erythrocyte survival time is decreased.
                                                     T   F   Ref. p. 599

405. In hereditary spherocytic anemia, polychromatophilic erythrocytes, which are slightly larger than normal erythrocytes, suggest the presence of reticulocytes.
                                                     T   F   Ref. p. 600

406. During a relapse in hereditary spherocytic anemia, the reticulocyte count may be 10% to 50%.
                                                     T   F   Ref. p. 602

407. Sickle cell anemia is an inherited disease which is usually confined to the Negro race.   T   F   Ref. p. 603

408. Sickled erythrocytes are also referred to as sickle cells, sickled red cells, sickle-shaped erythrocytes, drepanocytes, and menisocytes.   T   F   Ref. p. 604

409. In sickle cell anemia, the red cell osmotic fragility test shows *decreased* osmotic fragility.   T   F   Ref. p. 605

410. In sickle cell anemia, hemoglobin electrophoresis shows hemoglobins S and F; whereas in sickle cell trait, hemoglobin electrophoresis reveals hemoglobins S and A.   T   F   Ref. p. 605

411. Normal adult hemoglobin is called hemoglobin A and normal fetal hemoglobin is called hemoglobin F.   T   F   Ref. p. 608

412. In sickle cell anemia, the erythrocytes contain 75% or more of hemoglobin S; whereas in sickle cell trait, the erythrocytes contain 45% or less of hemoglobin S.   T   F   Ref. p. 608

413. In thalassemia major, fetal hemoglobin is produced in place of adult hemoglobin.   T   F   Ref. p. 609

414. There is a defect in cell structure and iron utilization in:

    a. hereditary spherocytic anemia
    b. sickle cell anemia
    c. erythroblastosis fetalis
    d. thalassemia major (Cooley's anemia)
    e. iron deficiency anemia   Ref. p. 609

415. Target cells, which are also referred to as Mexican hat cells and leptocytes, are longer and thinner than normal erythrocytes.   T   F   Ref. p. 610, 611

416. In thalassemia major, the plasma hemoglobin is above the normal range of:

    a. 2 to 3 milligrams per 100 ml.
    b. 2 to 3 micrograms per 100 ml.
    c. 20 to 30 milligrams per 100 ml.
    d. 2 to 3 grams per 100 ml.
    e. 10 to 15 grams per 100 ml.   Ref. p. 614

417. Which anemia is a microcytic hypochromic anemia:

    a. pernicious anemia
    b. aplastic anemia
    c. sickle cell anemia
    d. thalassemia major
    e. erythroblastosis fetalis   Ref. p. 612

418. In thalassemia major, the values for hemoglobin F are 40% to 90%; in thalassemia minor, the values for hemoglobin F are 5% to 10%.
                                                                          T   F   Ref. p. 613

419. Hemosiderin in the urine is highly suggestive of:

    a. pernicious anemia
    b. acute posthemorrhagic anemia
    c. paroxysmal nocturnal hemoglobinuria
    d. polycythemia vera
    e. infectious mononucleosis   Ref. p. 615

420. Paroxysmal cold hemoglobinuria is a rare disorder which is usually associated with syphilis.   T   F   Ref. p. 615, 616

421. In acquired autoimmune hemolytic anemia, the patient develops antibodies which hemolyze his own red cells; and thus a direct Coombs' test on the patient's red cells is positive.   T   F   Ref. p. 616

422. Erythroblastosis fetalis is a hemolytic disease of the newborn caused by a reaction between fetal blood and maternal blood and characterized by a blood smear showing an increased number of nucleated red cells.
    T   F   Ref. p. 617

423. In erythroblastosis fetalis caused by the Rh factor, a characteristic laboratory finding is a shower of nucleated red cells in the blood smear.
    T   F   Ref. p. 619

424. In erythroblastosis of the newborn, caused by ABO incompatibility, a blood smear may show spherocytes.   T   F   Ref. p. 621

425. Nucleated red cells in the blood smear of a newborn are found only in erythroblastosis fetalis.   T   F   Ref. p. 621

426. *Immediately* after the loss of blood in acute posthemorrhagic anemia, the red cell count and hemoglobin determination are *above* normal.
    T   F   Ref. p. 622

427. Sudden loss of a large quantity of blood may lead to:

   a. an increase in the white cell count
   b. an increase in the platelet count
   c. a "shift to the left" in the differential
   d. all of the above
   e. none of the above   Ref. p. 622

428. The reticulocyte count following acute hemorrhage is at its peak in:

   a. 1 hour
   b. 1 to 3 days
   c. 10 to 12 hours
   d. 5 to 7 days
   e. 12 to 14 days   Ref. p. 623

429. The anemia caused by acute blood loss is typically:

   a. microcytic
   b. macrocytic
   c. normocytic
   d. hypochromic
   e. megalocytic   Ref. p. 623

430. Chronic blood loss may lead to:

    a. pernicious anemia
    b. leukemia
    c. B$_{12}$ deficiency anemia
    d. iron deficiency anemia
    e. aplastic anemia   Ref. p. 623

431. The white cell count is always high in acute granulocytic leukemia.
                                      T   F   Ref. p. 626

432. In acute granulocytic leukemia, red rods called Auer bodies may be found in the cytoplasm of some myeloblasts.   T   F   Ref. p. 627, Plate 18 (630)

433. In acute granulocytic leukemia and acute lymphocytic leukemia, the platelet count is below normal.   T   F   Ref. p. 627 and p. 632

434. In acute granulocytic leukemia, a positive peroxidase reaction is of diagnostic value.   T   F   Ref. p. 627, 630

435. In chronic granulocytic leukemia, you would expect to find a:

    a. monocytosis
    b. lymphocytosis
    c. marked leukocytosis
    d. eosinopenia
    e. basopenia   Ref. p. 629

436. The presence of neutrophilic myelocytes in the blood in considerable numbers (20% to 50%) is suggestive of:

    a. acute lymphocytic leukemia
    b. chronic granulocytic leukemia
    c. iron deficiency anemia
    d. infectious mononucleosis
    e. agranulocytosis   Ref. p. 629

437. In chronic granulocytic leukemia, the basophils are usually increased.
                                      T   F   Ref. p. 629

438. In the early stages of chronic granulocytic leukemia, the platelet count may be increased; and in the more severe or terminal stages of the disease, the platelet count may be normal or decreased.   T   F   Ref. p. 629

439. In chronic granulocytic leukemia, the values for the alkaline phosphatase stain are above normal.   T   F   Ref. p. 629

440. In acute granulocytic leukemia, the predominating white cell is the myeloblast; whereas in chronic granulocytic leukemia, the predominating white cell is the neutrophilic myelocyte.   T   F   Ref. p. 629, 630

441. Chronic lymphocytic leukemia is most frequently seen:

   a. in a child between 3 and 10 years of age
   b. in infancy
   c. between the ages of 20 and 40
   d. in the male patient past the age of 50
   e. in the female patient   Ref. p. 632

442. Smudge cells may be seen in both acute and chronic lymphocytic leukemia.
                           T F   Ref. p. 632, Plate 19 (634)

443. In acute lymphocytic leukemia, the blood smear shows a predominance of lymphoblasts; whereas in chronic lymphocytic leukemia, the blood smear shows a predominance of lymphocytes.   T F   Ref. p. 633, 634

444. Monocytic leukemia is often classified as either the Schilling type or the Naegeli type.   T F   Ref. p. 636

445. Plasmacytic leukemia is often considered a phase of:

   a. lymphocytic leukemia
   b. chronic granulocytic leukemia
   c. multiple myeloma
   d. acute monocytic leukemia
   e. myelogenous leukemia   Ref. p. 636

446. The plasmacyte seen in plasmacytic leukemia may have all of the following, except:

   a. eccentrically placed nucleus
   b. deep blue cytoplasm
   c. vacuoles in the cytoplasm
   d. two nuclei
   e. nucleoli   Ref. p. 637

447. A neutrophilic leukemoid reaction may be found in many conditions; among these conditions are meningitis, tumors, and mercury poisoning.
                                            T F   Ref. p. 639

448. A lymphocytic leukemoid reaction may be seen in infectious mononucleosis.
                                            T F   Ref. p. 639

449. In identifying blood smears of the various leukemias, (1) you first identify the predominating white cell series and (2) then note the age or maturity of the white cells.   T F   Ref. p. 639, 640

450. Scurvy is caused by a deficiency of ascorbic acid which is commonly referred to as vitamin C.   T F   Ref. p. 642

451. Hereditary hemorrhagic telangiectasia (Rendu-Osler-Weber syndrome) is caused by:

    a. a stage 1 disorder
    b. a stage 2 disorder
    c. a stage 3 disorder
    d. a vascular defect
    e. a platelet deficiency   Ref. p. 642, 644

452. Purpura hemorrhagica is also known as idiopathic thrombocytopenic purpura and Werlhof's disease.   T   F   Ref. p. 645

453. Purpura hemorrhagica is a disease of the blood characterized by a low platelet count, spontaneous bruising or bleeding, and the production of petechiae.
                                           T   F   Ref. p. 645

454. In purpura hemorrhagica, there is:

    a. increased prothrombin consumption test
    b. markedly increased coagulation time
    c. decreased clot retraction time
    d. decreased platelet count
    e. increased prothrombin time   Ref. p. 646, 647

455. Symptomatic thrombocytopenic purpura is a condition characterized by a decrease in the number of platelets which is due either to a toxic agent or some underlying disease.   T   F   Ref. p. 647

456. The plasma coagulation disorders may be grouped under the 3 stages of blood coagulation.   T   F   Ref. p. 648, 649

457. Hemophilia is a hemorrhagic disease which is characterized by a deficiency of Factor VIII.   T   F   Ref. p. 649

458. Factor VIII is a plasma coagulation factor which is also referred to as anti-hemophilic globulin, AHG, and AHF.   T   F   Ref. p. 649

459. In hemophilia, the coagulation time is prolonged, but the bleeding time, platelet count, clot retraction time, and capillary resistance are normal.
                                           T   F   Ref. p. 650

460. In hemorrhagic disease of the newborn, the synthesis of prothrombin is delayed and the administration of vitamin K tends to relieve the condition.
                                         T   F   Ref. p. 650, 651

461. Polycythemia vera is also referred to as erythremia, primary polycythemia, and Osler's disease.   T   F   Ref. p. 652

462. In secondary polycythemia, there is:

    a. an increase in the platelet count
    b. a leukopenia
    c. anemia
    d. an increase in the red cell count
    e. hemolysis   Ref. p. 653

463. Secondary polycythemia may be due to loss of fluid or a decrease in oxygen (hypoxia).   T   F   Ref. p. 653, 654

464. In polycythemia vera, the total blood volume is increased; this is due to an increase in the total red cell volume.   T   F   Ref. p. 655, 656

465. In polycythemia vera, the vicosity of the blood is increased and this causes the specific gravity of the blood to rise above the normal values.
                                                                T   F   Ref. p. 656, 658

466. In polycythemia vera, which of the following is *not* increased:

   a. red cell count
   b. platelet count
   c. hematocrit reading
   d. total red cell volume
   e. sedimentation rate   Ref. p. 657, 658

467. Agranulocytosis is also referred to as malignant neutropenia, acute granulocytopenia, and granulopenia.   T   F   Ref. p. 658

468. Agranulocytosis is a severe disease of the blood characterized by a low white cell count and a decrease in granulocytes.   T   F   Ref. p. 658

469. Agranulocytosis may be caused by hypersensitivity to certain drugs and chemicals.   T   F   Ref. p. 658

470. In agranulocytosis, the granulocytes in the blood smear may have unusually large granules in the cytoplasm (toxic granulation).   T   F   Ref. p. 660

471. Infectious mononucleosis is an acute infectious disease which is characterized by the presence of atypical lymphocytes and a positive heterophil agglutination test.   T   F   Ref. p. 662

472. The search for the atypical lymphocytes of infectious mononucleosis should be made on the *thick area* of the blood smear.   T   F   Ref. p. 662

473. The heterophil agglutination test is also referred to as the heterophile antibody test, Davidsohn test, and Paul-Bunnell test.   T   F   Ref. p. 663

474. The heterophil agglutination test consists of a presumptive test and a differential test.   T   F   Ref. p. 663

475. The presumptive test for infectious mononucleosis uses:

   a. guinea pig antigen
   b. beef cells
   c. human red cells
   d. sheep cells
   e. none of the above   Ref. p. 663

476. In infectious mononucleosis, the presumptive test is positive, the guinea pig antigen (Forssman antigen) test is positive, and the beef cell antigen test is negative.   T   F   Ref. p. 663–666

477. In about half the cases of multiple myeloma, the urine reveals an abnormal protein, Bence Jones protein, which is rarely found in any other disease and is therefore of diagnostic significance.   T F   Ref. p. 669

478. In multiple myeloma, the blood smear may show a few plasmacytes and the bone marrow examination shows "myeloma" cells.   T F   Ref. p. 670

479. In a patient with multiple myeloma, you would *not* expect to find the following:

    a. rouleau formation
    b. increase in sedimentation rate
    c. increase in total serum proteins
    d. elevated alkaline phosphatase stain
    e. elevated serum calcium   Ref. p. 668–671

480. Which cell is characteristic of Hodgkin's disease:

    a. myeloma cell
    b. Gaucher's cell
    c. Pick's cell
    d. Sternberg-Reed cell
    e. Türk's cell   Ref. p. 672

481. In Hodgkin's disease, the differential white cell count shows a decrease in:

    a. neutrophilic band cells
    b. neutrophilic segmented cells
    c. eosinophils
    d. monocytes
    e. lymphocytes   Ref. p. 674

482. Which of the following is *not* characteristic of Gaucher's cell:

    a. cell is large (20 to 80 microns in diameter)
    b. nucleus is small
    c. nucleus is usually located near border of cell
    d. cytoplasm is abundant and looks wrinkled or fiber-like
    e. cytoplasm contains Auer bodies   Ref. p. 675

483. In chronic cold agglutinin disease, the red cells may agglutinate at room temperature.   T F   Ref. p. 678

484. Neutrophilic granulocytic leukemia, thrombocytic leukemia, mast cell leukemia, histiocytic leukemia, and stem cell leukemia are all rare forms of leukemia.   T F   Ref. p. 678

485. Mast cells closely resemble:

    a. eosinophils
    b. neutrophils
    c. basophils
    d. lymphocytes
    e. monocytes   Ref. p. 679

486. Purpura simplex is a condition which is characterized by a tendency to bruise easily; it occurs most frequently in females and it is often associated with rheumatic fever and rheumatoid arthritis.   T   F   Ref. p. 679

487. In Glanzmann's disease, you would expect to find a thrombasthenia, that is, a functional defect of the platelets.   T   F   Ref. p. 680

488. In acute infectious lymphocytosis, the lymphocytes are normal in appearance and the heterophil agglutination test is negative; in infectious mononucleosis, however, the lymphocytes are abnormal in appearance and the heterophil agglutination test is positive.   T   F   Ref. p. 680

489. Erythremic myelosis is also referred to as erythroleukemia and Di Guglielmo's disease.   T   F   Ref. p. 680

490. Erythremic myelosis is characterized by an overgrowth of erythropoietic cells in the bone marrow.   T   F   Ref. p. 680

491. Both Niemann-Pick disease and Gaucher's disease are (1) inherited, (2) found most frequently in children of Jewish parentage, and (3) associated with the abnormal metabolism of lipids.   T   F   Ref. p. 681

492. Pick's cell contains the lipid substance sphingomyelin and the cell has a foamy cytoplasm; Gaucher's cell contains the lipid substance kerasin and the cell has a wrinkled or fiber-like cytoplasm.   T   F   Ref. p. 681

493. Alder's anomaly is an inherited condition which is characterized by the presence of large coarse granules in the granulocytes.   T   F   Ref. p. 681

494. In Pelger-Huët's anomaly, the granulocytes:

 a. have nucleoli
 b. contain Auer rods
 c. have toxic granulation
 d. have large coarse basophilic granules
 e. fail to differentiate beyond the band stage   Ref. p. 682

495. Which of the following prefixes does not have the meaning indicated:

 a. aniso   unequal
 b. poly   many
 c. myelo   marrow
 d. hypo   lesser
 e. leuk   red   Ref. p. 701

496. About 8% of your body weight is blood; thus, if you weigh 100 pounds, you have about 8 pounds of blood.   T   F   Ref. p. 704

497. Cryoglobulin is a serum globulin which precipitates, gels, or crystallizes spontaneously at low temperatures.   T   F   Ref. p. 706

51

498. Döhle bodies are oval or spindle-shaped bodies which may be found in the cytoplasm of neutrophils in scarlet fever, measles, pernicious anemia, hemolytic anemia, and chronic granulocytic leukemia.   T F   Ref. p. 707

499. The erythrocyte survival time is also referred to as the red cell survival time and the red blood cell survival time; it may be performed by either the Ashby method or the radiochromium (Cr^{51}) method.   T F   Ref. p. 708

500. Myeloproliferative disorders are diseases accompanied by excessive cell production; for example, leukemia and polycythemia vera are myeloproliferative disorders.   T F   Ref. p. 716

ANSWERS TO REVIEW QUESTIONS

1.	d	26.	d	51.	T	76.	e	101.	d
2.	T	27.	c	52.	e	77.	d	102.	e
3.	e	28.	d	53.	T	78.	T	103.	T
4.	T	29.	T	54.	d	79.	d	104.	d
5.	T	30.	c	55.	T	80.	c	105.	T
6.	T	31.	b	56.	T	81.	e	106.	d
7.	T	32.	T	57.	F	82.	T	107.	T
8.	T	33.	T	58.	T	83.	T	108.	T
9.	c	34.	T	59.	e	84.	d	109.	T
10.	d	35.	T	60.	d	85.	T	110.	c
11.	F	36.	T	61.	c	86.	T	111.	c
12.	T	37.	T	62.	e	87.	T	112.	e
13.	T	38.	T	63.	T	88.	T	113.	T
14.	T	39.	d	64.	T	89.	F	114.	T
15.	e	40.	T	65.	a	90.	T	115.	d
16.	d	41.	c	66.	e	91.	d	116.	T
17.	T	42.	T	67.	e	92.	T	117.	e
18.	e	43.	T	68.	a	93.	d	118.	d
19.	d	44.	c	69.	d	94.	e	119.	F
20.	T	45.	T	70.	e	95.	c	120.	T
21.	T	46.	c	71.	e	96.	T	121.	T
22.	T	47.	d	72.	T	97.	c	122.	e
23.	d	48.	T	73.	c	98.	T	123.	T
24.	F	49.	T	74.	d	99.	e	124.	F
25.	c	50.	T	75.	d	100.	d	125.	a

ANSWERS TO REVIEW QUESTIONS (*continued*)

126.	d	151.	e	176.	T	201.	c	226.	T
127.	c	152.	T	177.	T	202.	e	227.	T
128.	T	153.	T	178.	e	203.	T	228.	e
129.	c	154.	e	179.	T	204.	d	229.	e
130.	T	155.	e	180.	T	205.	T	230.	e
131.	e	156.	T	181.	e	206.	T	231.	T
132.	T	157.	d	182.	T	207.	d	232.	T
133.	c	158.	T	183.	d	208.	d	233.	T
134.	T	159.	T	184.	b	209.	e	234.	T
135.	T	160.	e	185.	e	210.	d	235.	T
136.	T	161.	T	186.	e	211.	T	236.	e
137.	T	162.	T	187.	d	212.	d	237.	T
138.	e	163.	d	188.	T	213.	c	238.	d
139.	e	164.	e	189.	e	214.	T	239.	c
140.	T	165.	T	190.	T	215.	T	240.	T
141.	T	166.	T	191.	T	216.	d	241.	e
142.	d	167.	d	192.	T	217.	e	242.	T
143.	T	168.	T	193.	T	218.	T	243.	F
144.	T	169.	F	194.	T	219.	d	244.	e
145.	T	170.	e	195.	T	220.	d	245.	T
146.	T	171.	T	196.	c	221.	c	246.	e
147.	b	172.	e	197.	e	222.	d	247.	e
148.	T	173.	T	198.	T	223.	T	248.	d
149.	T	174.	T	199.	T	224.	T	249.	e
150.	T	175.	e	200.	T	225.	T	250.	T

ANSWERS TO REVIEW QUESTIONS (*continued*)

251.	e	276.	T	301.	T	326.	T	351.	e
252.	T	277.	T	302.	T	327.	T	352.	T
253.	T	278.	e	303.	T	328.	e	353.	e
254.	T	279.	T	304.	T	329.	T	354.	e
255.	T	280.	e	305.	T	330.	T	355.	T
256.	T	281.	e	306.	T	331.	T	356.	T
257.	e	282.	e	307.	d	332.	T	357.	T
258.	d	283.	T	308.	e	333.	T	358.	T
259.	T	284.	T	309.	T	334.	e	359.	T
260.	T	285.	T	310.	d	335.	T	360.	T
261.	e	286.	T	311.	d	336.	T	361.	d
262.	e	287.	T	312.	d	337.	T	362.	e
263.	d	288.	T	313.	T	338.	T	363.	T
264.	T	289.	T	314.	T	339.	e	364.	b
265.	e	290.	T	315.	T	340.	T	365.	b
266.	T	291.	T	316.	e	341.	T	366.	T
267.	d	292.	e	317.	T	342.	T	367.	T
268.	T	293.	d	318.	T	343.	T	368.	d
269.	T	294.	T	319.	T	344.	T	369.	T
270.	T	295.	T	320.	T	345.	T	370.	d
271.	T	296.	d	321.	T	346.	T	371.	F
272.	T	297.	T	322.	d	347.	T	372.	d
273.	T	298.	d	323.	T	348.	T	373.	c
274.	T	299.	e	324.	T	349.	T	374.	T
275.	T	300.	T	325.	T	350.	T	375.	d

ANSWERS TO REVIEW QUESTIONS (*continued*)

376.	T	401.	T	426.	T	451.	d	476.	T
377.	T	402.	T	427.	d	452.	T	477.	T
378.	T	403.	T	428.	d	453.	T	478.	T
379.	T	404.	T	429.	c	454.	d	479.	d
380.	T	405.	T	430.	d	455.	T	480.	d
381.	c	406.	T	431.	F	456.	T	481.	e
382.	d	407.	T	432.	T	457.	T	482.	e
383.	d	408.	T	433.	T	458.	T	483.	T
384.	T	409.	T	434.	T	459.	T	484.	T
385.	T	410.	T	435.	c	460.	T	485.	c
386.	T	411.	T	436.	b	461.	T	486.	T
387.	d	412.	T	437.	T	462.	d	487.	T
388.	T	413.	T	438.	T	463.	T	488.	T
389.	e	414.	d	439.	F	464.	T	489.	T
390.	e	415.	T	440.	T	465.	T	490.	T
391.	T	416.	a	441.	d	466.	e	491.	T
392.	e	417.	d	442.	T	467.	T	492.	T
393.	T	418.	T	443.	T	468.	T	493.	T
394.	T	419.	c	444.	T	469.	T	494.	e
395.	T	420.	T	445.	c	470.	T	495.	e
396.	e	421.	T	446.	e	471.	T	496.	T
397.	b	422.	T	447.	T	472.	F	497.	T
398.	T	423.	T	448.	T	473.	T	498.	T
399.	d	424.	T	449.	T	474.	T	499.	T
400.	T	425.	F	450.	T	475.	d	500.	T

BIBLIOGRAPHY

Abbott Laboratories, *The Use of Blood*, 1961.

Alba, Augusto: *Medical Technology, A Review for Licensure Examinations*, Berkeley, Berkeley Scientific Publications, 1964.

Alter, et al: *Medical Technology Examination Review Book*, Vol. 1 and 2, Flushing, Medical Examination Publishing Co., 1968.

Alumnae Association of Ursuline College, *Medical Technology Tests*, 1958.

Alvarez, et al: *Medical Writing*, New York, MD Publications, 1956.

Baker, F. J., Silverton, R. E., and Luckcock, Eveline D.: *An Introduction to Medical Laboratory Technology*, 4th Ed., Washington, Butterworths, 1966.

Baltimore Biological Laboratory Division, B-D Laboratories, Inc., *A Manual of Methods for the Coagulation Laboratory*, Baltimore, 1965.

Bauer, John D., Ackermann, Philip G., and Toro, Gelson: *Bray's Clinical Laboratory Methods*, 7th Ed., St. Louis, C. V. Mosby Co., 1968.

Berkeley Scientific Publications, *National and State Board Examination Questions and Answers for Medical Laboratory Technologists*, 1966 Ed.

Bessis, M.: *Life Cycle of the Erythrocyte*, Sandoz, 1966.

Best, Charles Herbert and Taylor, Norman Burke: *The Physiological Basis of Medical Practice*, 8th Ed., Baltimore, Williams & Wilkins Co., 1966.

BioQuest, Division of Becton, Dickinson and Company, *FibroSystem Manual of Methods for the Coagulation Laboratory*, 1968.

Boyd, William: *An Introduction to the Study of Disease*, 5th Ed., Philadelphia, Lea & Febiger, 1962.

Brown, H. Ivan: *Lectures for Medical Technologists*, Springfield, Charles C Thomas, 1964.

Cartwright, George E.: *Diagnostic Laboratory Hematology*, 4th Ed., New York, Grune & Stratton, 1968.

Catron, Dorothy A.: *American Medical Technologists Review Registry Questionnaire*, Virginia State Society of American Medical Technologists, 1969.

Collins, R. Douglas: *Illustrated Manual of Laboratory Diagnosis, Indications and Interpretations*, Philadelphia, J. B. Lippincott Co., 1968.

Dacie, J. V. and Lewis, S. M.: *Practical Haematology*, 3rd Ed., London, J. & A. Churchill Ltd., 1966.

Dade Reagents, Inc., *Coagulation Procedures Manual*, 1966.

Daland, Geneva A.: *A Color Atlas of Morphologic Hematology*, revised edition, Cambridge, Harvard University Press, 1959.

Darmady, E. M. and Davenport, S. G. T.: *Haematological Technique*, 3rd Ed., New York, Grune & Stratton, 1963.

Davidsohn, Israel and Carr, Mildred Tucker: *A Curriculum for Schools of Medical Technology*, 5th Ed., Registry of Medical Technologists of the American Society of Clinical Pathologists, 1964.

Davidsohn, Israel and Henry, John Bernard: *Todd-Sanford Clinical Diagnosis by Laboratory Methods*, 14th Ed., Philadelphia, W. B. Saunders Co., 1969.

Diggs, L. W., Sturm, Dorothy, and Bell, Ann: *The Morphology of Blood Cells*, North Chicago, Abbott Laboratories, 1954.

Diggs, L. W., Sturm, Dorothy, and Bell, Ann: *The Morphology of Human Blood Cells*, Philadelphia, W. B. Saunders Co., 1956.

Dolan, Francis E.: *Comprehensive Review for Medical Technologists*, St. Louis, C. V. Mosby Co., 1968.

Dorland's Illustrated Medical Dictionary, 24th Ed., Philadelphia, W. B. Saunders Co., 1965.

Eastham, R. D. and Pollard, B. R.: *A Laboratory Guide to Clinical Diagnosis*, Baltimore, Williams & Wilkins Co., 1964.

Eichelberger, James W., Jr.: *Laboratory Methods in Blood Coagulation*, New York, Hoeber Medical Division, Harper & Row, 1965.

Fishbein, Morris: *Medical Writing*, 2nd Ed., Philadelphia, The Blakiston Co., 1950.

French, Ruth M.: *Nurse's Guide to Diagnostic Procedures*, 2nd Ed., New York, The Blakiston Division, McGraw-Hill Book Co., 1967

Garb, Solomon: *Laboratory Tests in Common Use*, 4th Ed., New York, Springer Publishing Co., 1966.

General Diagnostics Division, Warner-Lambert Pharmaceutical Company, *Blood Coagulation*.

Goodale, Raymond H.: *Clinical Interpretation of Laboratory Tests*, 5th Ed., Philadelphia, F. A. Davis Co., 1964.

Gordon, Burgess L.: *Current Medical Terminology*, 3rd Ed., Chicago, American Medical Association, 1966.

Gradwohl, R. B. H.: *Clinical Laboratory Methods and Diagnosis*, Vol. 1 and 2, 5th Ed., St. Louis, C. V. Mosby Co., 1956.

Haden, Russell L.: *Principles of Hematology*, 3rd Ed., Philadelphia, Lea & Febiger, 1946.

Heilmeyer, Ludwig and Begemann, Herbert: *Atlas Der Klinischen Hämatologie Und Cytologie*, Bildband und Textband, Berlin, Springer-Verlag, 1955.

Hepler, Opal E.: *Manual of Clinical Laboratory Methods*, 4th Ed., Springfield, Charles C Thomas, 1949.

Hyland Laboratories, *Hyland Reference Manual of Coagulation Procedures*, 1964.

Israëls, M. C. G.: *Diagnosis and Treatment of Blood Diseases*, Springfield, Charles C Thomas, 1963.

Kahler, Carol: *Guide for Program Planning: Medical Laboratory Technician*, American Association of Junior Colleges, 1969.

Kolmer, John A.: *Clinical Diagnosis by Laboratory Examinations*, 3rd Ed., New York, Appleton-Century-Crofts, 1961.

Kracke, Roy R.: *Diseases of the Blood and Atlas of Hematology*, 2nd Ed., Philadelphia, J. B. Lippincott Co., 1941.

Lea & Febiger, *Manuscript Preparation and Book Publication*, 1965.

Leavell, Byrd S. and Thorup, Oscar A., Jr.: *Fundamentals of Clinical Hematology*, 2nd Ed., Philadelphia, W. B. Saunders Co., 1966.

Levinson, Samuel A. and MacFate, Robert P.: *Clinical Laboratory Diagnosis*, 7th Ed., Philadelphia, Lea & Febiger, 1969.

Maher, David J.: *Medical Technology, A Review for Board Examinations*, Berkeley, Berkeley Scientific Publications, 1968.

McDonald, George A., Dodds, T. C., and Cruickshank, Bruce: *Atlas of Haematology*, Baltimore, Williams & Wilkins Co., 1965.

Merck Sharp & Dohme Research Laboratories, *The Merck Manual of Diagnosis and Therapy*, 11th Ed., 1966.

Miale, John B.: *Laboratory Medicine Hematology*, 3rd Ed., St. Louis, C. V. Mosby Co., 1967.

Miller, Seward E.: *A Textbook of Clinical Pathology*, 7th Ed., Baltimore, Williams & Wilkins Co., 1966.

Morgan, Rose M.: *Guide Questions for Medical Technology Examinations*, Springfield, Charles C Thomas, 1966.

National Committee for Careers in Medical Technology, *Curriculum Guides for Re-Training in Medical Technology*, 1967.

National Committee for Careers in Medical Technology, *National Correlations in Medical Technology Education*, 1967.

National Council on Medical Technology Education, *Guide for Instructors: Medical Laboratory*, 1969.

Ortho Diagnostics, *Coagulation Procedures*, 1968.

Oser, Bernard L.: *Hawk's Physiological Chemistry*, 14th Ed., New York, The Blakiston Division, McGraw-Hill Book Co., 1965.

Page, Lot B. and Culver, Perry J.: *A Syllabus of Laboratory Examinations in Clinical Diagnosis*, Revised Edition, Cambridge, Harvard University Press, 1960.

Pfizer Diagnostics, *Quality Control in Hematology*, 1968.

Piney, A. and Wyard, Stanley: *Clinical Atlas of Blood Diseases*, 6th Ed., Philadelphia, The Blakiston Co., 1945.

Platt, William R.: *Color Atlas and Textbook of Hematology*, Philadelphia, J. B. Lippincott Co., 1969.

Quick, Armand J.: *Hemorrhagic Diseases and Thrombosis*, 2nd Ed., Philadelphia, Lea & Febiger, 1966.

Reich, Carl: *A Clinical Atlas of Blood and Bone Marrow*, Published by Abbott Laboratories.

Reich, Carl: *The Cellular Elements of the Blood*, Published by Ciba Corporation, 1962.

Ring, Alvin M.: *Laboratory Correlation Manual*, Springfield, Charles C Thomas Co., 1969

Schalm, Oscar W.: *Veterinary Hematology*, 2nd Ed., Philadelphia, Lea & Febiger, 1965.

Schudel, Lydia: *Manual of Blood Morphology*, 11th revised edition, Philadelphia, J. B. Lippincott Co., 1966.

Seiverd, Charles E.: *Chemistry for Medical Technologists*, St. Louis, C. V. Mosby Co., 1958.

Simmons, Arthur: *Technical Hematology*, Philadelphia, J. B. Lippincott Co., 1968.

Sirridge, Marjorie S.: *Laboratory Evaluation of Hemostasis*, Philadelphia, Lea & Febiger, 1967.

Sturgis, Cyrus C.: *Hematology*, 2nd Ed., Springfield, Charles C Thomas, 1955.

United States Government, Department of the Air Force, *Laboratory Procedures in Clinical Hematology*, 1962.

United States Government Printing Office, *Medical Laboratory Assistant, A Suggested Guide for a Training Program*, 1966.

United States Naval Medical School, *Hematology*, 1962.

Wells, Benjamin B. and Halsted, James A.: *Clinical Pathology, Interpretation and Application*, 4th Ed., Philadelphia, W. B. Saunders Co., 1967.

Whitby, Lionel E. H. and Britton, C. J. C.: *Disorders of the Blood*, 9th Ed., New York, Grune & Stratton, 1963.

White, Wilma L. and Frankel, Sam: *Seiverd's Chemistry for Medical Technologists*, 2nd Ed., St. Louis, C. V. Mosby Co., 1965.

Wintrobe, Maxwell M.: *Clinical Hematology*, 6th Ed., Philadelphia, Lea & Febiger, 1967.

Yale University School of Medicine, *Outline for Examination of Patients*, 1965.

Index

Bisulfite method
  for sickle cell examination, discussion
    of, 341
  for sickle cell examination, procedure
    for, 345
Bisulfite reagent
  for sickle cell examination, 345
Bl. & coag. time, 704
Bl. & Ct., 704
Bl. time
  see bleeding time, 395
Blast cell,
  method of identifying, 548, 627
Blast cell leukemia, 679
Bleeding t.
  see bleeding time, 395
Bleeding time, 395-401
  Adelson-Crosby method, as a method
    for bleeding time, 396
  conditions accompanied by abnormal
    values, 395
  definition, 395
  Duke method, discussion of, 396, pro-
    cedure for, 397
  error, causes of, 401
  frequency of performance, 396
  increased values, cause of, 395
  Ivy method, discussion of, 396, pro-
    cedure for, 399
  Macfarlane method, discussion of, 396
  normal values, 395, 396
  procedures, discussion of, 396
  sample report, 398, 400
  significance of, 395
  sources of error, 401
  student review questions, numbers for,
    395
  use of, 395, 396
Blocking antibodies
  see Coombs' test, 706
Blood
  anticoagulated, 77-81
  capillary, definition, 704
  cell, look under Cell
  characteristics of, 2
  citrated, 77-81
  clot, formation, illustration of, 393
  clot, retraction time, 433
  clotting time, 402
  coagulation, theory of, 384
  coagulation factors, list of, 386
  coagulation time, 402
  collection of, 5-74
  composition of, 2, 3
  cord, 706
  count, complete, 89
  diluted, 75
  disease, look under Disease

Blood (Continued)
  dust, 568, 704
  dyscrasia, definition, 704, 707
  examination, look under Test
  factor A, 617
  factor B, 617
  factor D, 617
  factor Rh, 617
  factors, 617
  film, 224, 568
  finger tip, on glass slide, 21
  formation of, 2
  function of, 4
  heparinized, 77-81
  infant, obtaining from, 72-74
  lancet, 12
  lancet, automatic, 397, 399
  occult, definition, 716
  oxalated, 77-81
  oxygen saturation, 658
  peripheral, definition, 717
  plasma, 81-83, 562, 653, 656
  platelet, 414, 415, 416
  preparations of, 75-88
  preparations, keeping time, 87
  presence of, test for, 561, 568
  sedimentation test, 300
  Sequestrenized, 77-81
  serum, 83
  slide, 21, 224, 297
  smear, look under Blood smear
  specific gravity of, 561, 562
  specimens, labelling of, 23, 28
  stains, 233
  suspension, cell, 84-87
  Teichmann's test for, 568
  test for, 561, 568
  thickness, in polycythemia vera, 656,
    657, 658
  tray, 7
  urea nitrogen determination, 704
  venous, definition, 724
  viscosity, 562, 656, 658
  volume, 2, 655, 656, 657, 704
  weight of, 704
  wet film, examination of, 568
  whole, definition, 725
Blood clot method
  for preparing smear, L. E. cell exami-
    nation, 507, 508
Blood smear
  abnormalities and irregularities in, 257,
    258
  area for identifying cells, 251, 255
  buffy coat, preparation of, 558
  from finger puncture, 21
  in L. E. examination, 507-510
  in leukemia, note for student, 639, 640

Lead
poisoning, anemia of, 677
Lee and White method
for coagulation time, discussion, 404,
procedure, 410
Leitz photrometer, 196, 197
Lempert
as method for platelet count, 417
Lens
achromatic, 118
on microscope, 118, 119
Leptocyte,
see target cells, 276, 610
Leukemia, 624-640
acute granulocytic leukemia, 626
acute lymphadenosis, 631
acute lymphatic leukemia, 631
acute lymphoblastic leukemia, 631
acute lymphocytic leukemia, 631
acute myeloblastic leukemia, 626
acute myelogenous leukemia, 626
acute myeloid leukemia, 626
acute myelosis, 626
aleukemic, buffy coat preparation for,
558, 559
aleukemic leukemia, 638
basophilic leukemia, 678
blast cell leukemia, see stem cell leukemia, 679
chronic granulocytic leukemia, 628
chronic lymphadenosis, 632
chronic lymphatic leukemia, 632
chronic lymphocytic leukemia, 632
chronic myelogenous leukemia, 628
chronic myeloid leukemia, 628
chronic myelosis, 628
classification, 624, 625
color plates, 630, 634, 636
definition, 624
discussion of, 624
embryonal leukemia, 679
eosinophilic leukemia, 678
granulocytic leukemia, 626
hemoblastic leukemia, 679
histiocytic leukemia, 679
introduction to, 624
leukemic hiatus, 713
leukemic leukemia, 713
leukemic reticuloendotheliosis, 679
leukemoid reactions, 638, 639
lymphocytic leukemia, 631
lymphocytic leukemoid reaction, 639
mast cell leukemia, 679
megakaryocytic leukemia, 679
monocytic leukemia, 635
myeloid granulocytic leukemia, 678
Naegeli type monocytic leukemia, 636
neutrophilic granulocytic leukemia, 678

Leukemia (*Continued*)
neutrophilic leukemia, 678
neutrophilic leukemoid reaction, **639**
note to student, for identification of
smears, 639
plasma cell leukemia, 636
plasmacytic leukemia, 636
plasmocytic leukemia, 636
prognosis, 625
Schilling type monocytic leukemia, 636
smears, system for identifying, **639**, 640
splenomedullary leukemia, 628
stem cell leukemia, 679
student review questions, numbers for,
624
tables, laboratory examinations, 630,
634, 637
thrombocytic leukemia, 679
true monocytic leukemia, 636
undifferentiated cell leukemia, 679
Leuko-agglutinin examination, 713
Leukocyte
as cell, look under *White cell*
count, look under *White cell count*
differential, look under *Differential
white cell count*
Leukocyte alkaline phosphatase test
see alkaline phosphatase stain, 539
Leukocytic cream, 558
Leukocytic series, 220, 221
Leukocytopenia
definition, 713
Leukocytosis
common types, cells in, 217
definition, 92
diseases accompanied by, 92
types of, in differential white cell
count, 216
various types, illustrations of, 218
Leuko-erythrogenetic ratio
see L:E ratio, 713
Leukopenia, 92
Leukopoiesis
definition, 713
site of, 216
Levy
see Speirs-Levy counting chamber, 496,
499
Lipid
in Gaucher's disease, 675, 677
in Niemann-Pick disease, 680, 681
in Pick's cell, 681
stain for, 548
Lipoid histiocytosis, 680
Lipshaw automatic stainer, 234
Liter, 693
LLF
see Laki-Lorand factor, 386

Ocular crossline disc, 336
O. D.
  optical density, in reading of spectro-
    photometer, 516
Oil immersion objective, 117, 118
Olef
  as method for platelet count, 417
Oligochromemia
  definition, 716
Oligocythemia, 143
-Ology, 1
One-stage method
  for prothrombin time, discussion of,
    445, procedure for, 453
Optical density, 205, 516
Ortho plasma coagulation control
  for PTT, 471
Orthochromatic megaloblast, 587
Orthochromia
  definition, 716
Orthochromic normoblast, 269
Osler's disease, 644, 652
Osmosis
  principle of, 84, 85
  see osmotic pressure, 716
Osmotic fragility test, 349-357
  basis of test, 349
  frequency of performance, 350
  in disease, 350
  normal and abnormal results, illustra-
    tion of, 356
  procedures, discussion of, 350
  sample report, 357
  Sanford method
    discussion of, 350
    procedure for, 354
  screening procedure
    discussion of, 350
    procedure for, 352
  significance of, 349
  solutions, preparation of, 697, 698
  student review questions, numbers for,
    349
Osmotic pressure, 716
Osteoblast
  definition, 176
Ovalocyte, 276, 717
Ovalocytosis, 276
Over-stained cells
  removal of stain, 240
Owren's thrombotest, 488, 491
Oxalate
  balanced, 78
  double, 78
  temperature of decomposition, 78
Oxalated blood, 77-81
  keeping time, 80, 81
Oxalated tube, 77, 78

Oxidant drug, 554, 717
  in formation of sulfhemoglobin, 567
Oxidizing agent
  and ferrous iron, 177
  in production of methemoglobin, 177,
    178
  see oxidant drug, 717
Oxydase reaction
  see peroxidase stain, 534
Oxydase stain
  see peroxidase stain, 534
Oxygen
  content of air, in hemoglobin values,
    178
  content of air, in red cell count, 142
  content of air, in sickle cell anemia,
    604
  content of blood, in sickle cell anemia,
    604
  pressure, in function of red cell, 571,
    572
  saturation, in polycythemia vera, 657,
    658
  supply, in red cell production, 571
  supply, in secondary polycythemia,
    653, 654
  tension, in sickle cell examination, 341
Oxygen method
  for hemoglobin determination, 180
Oxygenated
  hemoglobin, 177, 571
Oxyhemoglobin
  in function of hemoglobin, 176, 571
  in P.C.H., 616
  method, for hemoglobin determination,
    183, 198

P

P and P test, 491
"P.A. poly" cell, 258
Packed cell volume
  see hematocrit reading, 320
Panagglutinin
  definition, 717
Pancreas
  trypsin test, use of, 568
Pandy's test, 665
Panleukocytic granulation
  anomalous, see Chediak-Higashi
    anomaly, 705
Panmyelophthisis, 577
Panwarfin, 387
Papanicolaou smear, 717
Pappenheimer bodies, 717
Pappenheim's stain, 547
Pap's smear (or stain)
  see Papanicolaou smear, 717